BOUCHER'S
Prosthodontic Treatment for
Edentulous Patients

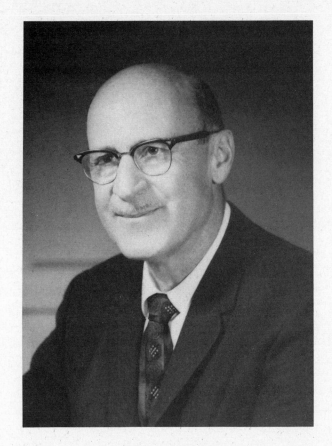

CARL O. BOUCHER

October 14, 1904–March 11, 1975

A respected teacher, a superb clinician,
a gifted editor and author, and a close personal friend.
He enriched the lives of his students,
his colleagues, and his patients.

JUDSON C. HICKEY
GEORGE A. ZARB
CHARLES L. BOLENDER

BOUCHER'S

Prosthodontic Treatment for Edentulous Patients NINTH EDITION

Judson C. Hickey, D.D.S., M.Sc.

Dean and Professor of Prosthodontics, Medical College of Georgia School of Dentistry; Member, Graduate Faculty of the Medical College of Georgia, Augusta, Georgia; formerly Chairman, Department of Prosthodontics, University of Kentucky College of Dentistry, Lexington, Kentucky; Editor, The Journal of Prosthetic Dentistry; Diplomate, American Board of Prosthodontics

George A. Zarb, B.Ch.D. (Malta), D.D.S., M.S. (Michigan), M.S. (Ohio State)

Professor and Chairman, Department of Prosthodontics, Faculty of Dentistry, University of Toronto; Section Editor, The Journal of Prosthetic Dentistry; Member of the School of Graduate Studies, University of Toronto, Toronto, Ontario; Fellow of the Royal College of Dentists of Canada

Charles L. Bolender, D.D.S., M.S.

Professor and Chairman, Department of Prosthodontics, University of Washington, School of Dentistry, Seattle, Washington

with 1123 illustrations, including 16 in color

THE C. V. MOSBY COMPANY

ST. LOUIS • TORONTO • PRINCETON   1985

MOSBY

A TRADITION OF PUBLISHING EXCELLENCE

Editor: Darlene Warfel
Assistant editor: Melba Steube
Manuscript editor: Carl Masthay
Book design: Jeanne Genz
Cover design: Tilford Smith
Production: Mary Stueck, Barbara Merritt, Graphic Works

NINTH EDITION

Printed in the United States of America

The C.V. Mosby Company
11830 Westline Industrial Drive, St. Louis, Missouri 63146

Library of Congress Cataloging in Publication Data

Boucher, Carl O.
   Boucher's Prosthodontic treatment for edentulous
patients.

   Bibliography: p.
   Includes index.
   1. Complete dentures. 2. Edentulous mouth.
I. Hickey, Judson C.   II. Zarb, George A. (George Albert), 1938-
III. Bolender, Charles L.   IV. Title.   V. Title: Prosthodontic
treatment for edentulous patients.   [DNLM: 1. Denture,
Complete.   2. Mouth, Edentulous.   WU 530 B753p]
RK656.B68   1985   617.6'92   84-19016
ISBN 0-8016-0815-5

TS/VH/VH   9   8   7   6   5   4   3   2   1   03/C/371

To our wives

Jean, Janet, and Mamie

and all students of prosthodontics

Preface

Proper prosthodontic treatment of edentulous patients requires that they be prepared orally, physically, and psychologically before treatment and that these aspects of their health be evaluated during and after clinical treatment. The provision of complete dentures is one important part of the total treatment plan. Every aspect of prosthodontic treatment of edentulous patients, except for certain laboratory procedures, requires clinical skills based on a knowledge and application of basic and behavioral sciences. The purpose of our book is to provide learning experiences that will correlate the basic, behavioral, and clinical skills of the dentist for the most effective comprehensive prosthodontic treatment of edentulous patients.

To accomplish our objectives, our book is organized so that technical considerations are described along with the basic fundamentals that control them. This type of organization allows students to prepare for each step in the treatment procedure and gives them the opportunity to acquire the necessary scientific and mechanical background to make the proper clinical judgments required for the successful treatment of their patients.

The clinical phases of denture construction are based on our own experiences in treating edentulous patients. This knowledge has been acquired from many sources over the years. It represents the actual procedures that we follow rather than a series of references or chapters selected from a number of authors writing in this discipline. For this reason, the bibliography for treatment procedures is compiled by topic and, for the most part, is presented alphabetically at the end of the text.

We recognize that more than one technique can produce good prosthodontic results. For that reason, we have included descriptions of different techniques for certain steps, such as impression making and the development of the occlusion with different occlusal forms. The choice of method for any patient will be made by the dentist on the basis of the individual conditions and the fundamentals involved.

Edentulous patients require competent, compassionate, and professional dental treatment, even though providing such treatment is difficult and time-consuming. An understanding of people, their problems, and their attitudes is necessary for the successful practice of prosthodontics. The challenge of overcoming the deficiencies of neglect or improper oral health care (for whatever reason) can be the most satisfying aspect of dental practice.

Many people have been of great assistance to us in the preparation of this book, and we wish to acknowledge and thank them for their contributions. Milton Burroughs, medical illustrator, Medical College of Georgia, School of Dentistry; and Margaret Hearn, medical illustrator, and Steve Burany, photographer, Faculty of Dentistry, University of Toronto, receive our special praise for the art work and photographs they provided. Our thanks to Horst Kroll for laboratory technical services and to Dr. Torsten Jemt for providing valuable suggestions for improvement.

Nancy Smith and Kathy Murray have our thanks for typing and proofing manuscripts and performing other duties related to this undertaking. We greatly appreciate the encouragement and patience of our wives, Jean Hickey, Janet Zarb, and Mamie Bolender. All others who have helped have our sincere thanks and appreciation.

Judson C. Hickey
George A. Zarb
Charles L. Bolender

Contents

SECTION ONE

The edentulous patient

1

Biomechanics of the edentulous state

Most patients regard tooth loss as mutilating, and a strong incentive to seek dental care for the preservation of a healthy dentition and socially acceptable appearance. Most dentists regard the loss of several teeth as posing the hazard of a greater mutilation—the destruction of part of the facial skeleton and the distortion of the morphology and function of soft tissues (Fig. 1-1).

The edentulous state represents a compromise in the integrity of the masticatory system. It is frequently accompanied by adverse functional and cosmetic consequences, which are varyingly perceived by the affected patient. The treatment of edentulous patients presents a range of biomechanical problems that involve individual tolerances and perceptions.

It is the objective of this text to provide an understanding of the effects of the edentulous condition, and to describe its clinical management. In this chapter, the clinical implications of an edentulous masticatory system are considered under these headings: modifications in areas of support, functional and parafunctional considerations, changes in morphologic face height, and cosmetic changes and adaptive responses.

MODIFICATIONS IN AREAS OF SUPPORT

The whole masticatory apparatus is involved in the process of trituration of food. Direct responsibility for these tasks falls on the teeth and their supporting tissues when natural teeth are present. The attachment of teeth in sockets is but one of many important modifications that took place during the period when the earliest mammals were evolving from their reptilian predecessors. The success of this modification is indicated by the fact that it appears to have been rapidly adopted throughout the many different groups of emerging Mammalia. Teeth function properly only if adequately supported. This support is provided by an organ composed of soft and hard connective tissues, the periodontium.

The periodontium attaches the teeth to the bone of the jaws, providing a resilient suspensory apparatus resistant to functional forces. It allows the teeth to adjust their position when under stress. The periodontium comprises hard connective tissues (cementum and bone) and soft connective tissues (the periodontal ligament and the lamina propria of the gingiva), which are covered by epithelium. The periodontium is regarded as a functional unit and is attached to the dentin by cementum and to the jawbone by the alveolar process. Continuity between these two hard-tissue components is maintained by the periodontal ligament and the lamina propria.

The periodontal ligament provides the means by which force exerted on the tooth is transmitted to the bone that supports it. The two principal functions of the periodontium are support and positional adjustment of the tooth, together with the secondary and dependent function of sensory perception. The patient needing com-

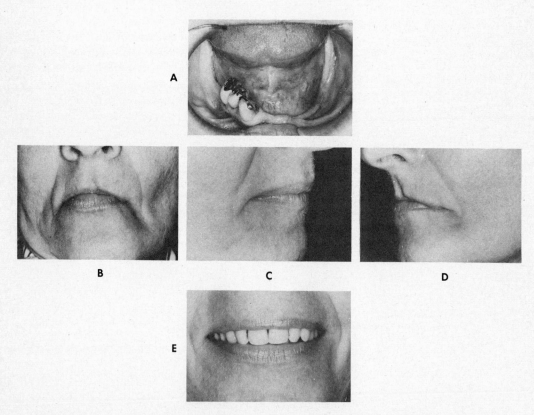

Fig. 1-1. Partial loss of mandibular dentition, **A,** and complete loss of maxillary dentition have seriously affected this middle-aged patient's cosmetic appearance, **B,** as well as functional status. Compare depleted soft-tissue support in **C** and **D** to support obtained by prostheses in **E.**

plete denture therapy is deprived of periodontal support, and the entire mechanism of functional load transmission to the supporting tissues is altered. Fig. 1-2 is an approximate diagrammatic representation of the masticatory system. Inevitably the biomechanical interactions of the components of this system are affected by the changes in the mechanism of tooth support when a patient becomes edentulous and undergoes complete denture treatment.

For appreciation of the many subtleties associated with the edentulous state and of the effects of the transition from the dentulous to the edentulous state, a brief comparison of the mechanisms of tooth support and denture support is essential. Such a review underscores the nature of the altered environment brought about by the loss of teeth.

MECHANISMS OF TOOTH SUPPORT

The mechanisms of tooth support have received a considerable amount of investigation during the past 20 years, and a number of conclusions have been drawn from observations in human and animal studies. As soon as teeth erupt into the oral cavity and occlusal contact is established, the nonfunctional orientation of the periodontal fibers changes into a functional arrangement. This fiber arrangement gives maximal stabilization to the tooth in the alveolar socket and at the same time allows a physiologic range of tooth mobility in all directions.

The occlusal forces exerted on the teeth are controlled by the neuromuscular mechanisms of the masticatory system. Reflex mechanisms with receptors in the muscles, tendons, joints, and the periodontal structures regulate mandibular movements. Through normal function the periodontal structures in a healthy dentition undergo characteristic mechanical stress. The most prominent feature of physiologic occlusal forces is their intermittent, rhythmic, and dynamic nature.

Gradual changes in force patterns occur during growth and eruption of the teeth. Abrupt alterations are produced as a result of loss or removal of an opposing or an adjacent tooth or the placement of a fixed or a removable prosthesis. The position normally occupied by a tooth in the dental arch depends on the balance of all the

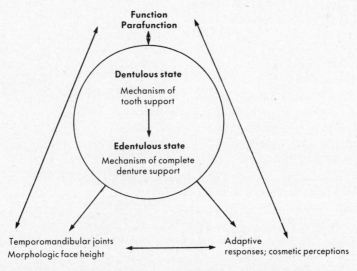

Fig. 1-2. Diagram of the masticatory system, relating the possible interaction between its various components in the context of a change in the mechanism of occlusal support.

forces acting on that tooth over an extended period of time. Sustained alterations in the magnitude or duration of the forces may cause the position of the tooth to change. This change is produced in the structural elements of the periodontium as a result of the position gradually assumed by the tooth in the alveolus.

The precise sequence of events that occur when force is applied to a tooth and then released is not clear, and likewise the relative importance of the constituent structural elements of the periodontium is not known. It appears, however, that in the healthy state the following factors are involved: (1) the magnitude, rate, and duration of the force; (2) the biologic status of the periodontal ligament, which is related to the previous loading history during the day; and (3) the long-term factors such as the patient's age and general systemic health. It appears that changes in force patterns acting on the teeth over extended periods of time elicit adjustments in the supporting tissues. Consequently the application of consistently greater loads during mastication tends to cause an increase in the width of the periodontal ligament and in both the number and density of principal fibers. Very little change of tooth position occurs, however. More sustained, but smaller, forces cause a change in tooth position, so that an equilibrium position is reestablished. The specific thresholds of force and time that are required for these changes to occur are unknown, and they vary in different people.

The greatest forces acting on the teeth are normally produced during mastication and deglutition, and they are essentially vertical in direction. Each thrust is of short duration, and for most people, at least, chewing is restricted to short periods of time during the day. Deglutition, on the other hand, occurs about 500 times a day (Powell, 1963), and tooth contacts during swallowing are usually of longer duration than those occurring during chewing (Glickman and associates, 1969). Loads of a lower order, but of a longer duration, are produced throughout the day by the tongue and perioral-circumoral musculature. These forces are predominantly in the horizontal direction. Estimates of peak forces from the tongue, cheeks, and lips have been made, and tongue force appears to exceed labiolingual force during activity. During rest or inactive periods, the total forces may be similar in magnitude.

During mastication, biting forces are transmitted through the bolus to the opposing teeth whether the teeth make contact or not. These forces increase steadily (depending on the nature of the food fragment), reach a peak, and abruptly return to zero. The magnitude, rise time, and interval between thrusts differ among persons and depend on the consistency of the food and the point in time in a specific chewing sequence. The direction of the forces is princi-

Table 1

Calculation of total time during 24 hours associated with direct functional occlusal force application to periodontal tissues

CHEWING	
Actual chewing time per meal	450 sec
4 meals a day	1800 sec
Each second 1 chewing stroke	1800 strokes
Duration of each stroke	0.3 sec
Total chewing forces per day	540 sec = 9 min

SWALLOWING	
Meals	
Duration of 1 deglutition movement	1 sec
During chewing 3 × per minute ⅓ of movements with occlusal force only	30 sec 0.5 min
Between meals	
Daytime: 25 per hour (16 hours)	400 sec 6.6 min
Sleep: 10 per hour (8 hours)	80 sec 1.3 min
	TOTAL 1050 sec = ca. 17.5 min

From Graf, H.: Dent. Clin. North Am. **13:**659-665, 1969.

pally perpendicular to the occlusal plane in normal function, but the forward angulation of most natural teeth leads to the introduction of a horizontal component that tends to tilt the teeth mesially as well as buccally or lingually. Upper incisors may be displaced labially with each biting thrust, and these tooth movements quite probably cause proximal wear facets to develop.

In healthy dentitions, teeth are not in occlusion except during the functional movements of chewing and deglutition and during the movements of parafunction. These various mandibular movements and their significance are described later. Graf (1969) calculated that the total time during which the teeth are subjected to functional forces of mastication and deglutition during an entire day amounts to approximately 17.5 minutes (Table 1). More than half of this time is attributable to jaw-closing forces applied during deglutition. Graf concluded that this total time and the range of forces seem to be well within the tolerance level of healthy periodontal tissues.

MECHANISMS OF COMPLETE DENTURE SUPPORT

The basic problem in the treatment of edentulous patients lies in the nature of the difference between the ways natural teeth and their artificial replacements are attached to the supporting bone.

The unsuitability of the tissues supporting complete dentures for load-bearing function must be immediately recognized. In normal function in the dentulous state, light loads are placed on the mucous membrane. With complete dentures, the mucous membrane is forced to serve the same purpose as the periodontal ligaments that provide support for natural teeth.

Masticatory loads

Masticatory loads are much smaller than those that can be produced by conscious effort and are in the region of 44 lb (20 kg) for the natural teeth (Picton, 1969). Maximum forces of 13 to 16 lb (6 to 8 kg) during chewing have been recorded

with complete dentures, but the average loads are probably much less than these. The forces required for chewing vary with the type of food being chewed. Prosthetic patients frequently limit the loading of supporting tissues by selecting food that does not require masticatory effect exceeding their tissue tolerance.

Area of support

The area of mucosa available to receive the load from complete dentures is limited when compared to the corresponding areas of support available for natural dentitions. Watt (1961) has computed the mean denture-bearing area to be 22.96 cm^2 in the edentulous maxillae and 12.25 cm^2 in an edentulous mandible. His estimate of the areas of periodontal membrane of natural teeth is approximately 45 cm^2 in each jaw—more than three and one-half times the average area of the basal seat of a mandibular complete denture. It must be remembered that the denture-bearing area (basal seat) becomes progressively smaller as residual ridges resorb. Furthermore, the mucosa demonstrates little tolerance or adaptability to denture wearing. This minimal tolerance can be reduced still further by the presence of systemic disease such as anemia, nutritional deficiencies, hypertension, or diabetes. In fact, any disturbance of the normal metabolic processes may lower the upper limit of mucosal tolerance and initiate inflammation.

Residual ridge

The residual ridge consists of denture-bearing mucosa, the submucosa and periosteum, and the underlying residual alveolar bone. Residual bone is that bone of the alveolar process that remains after teeth are lost. When the alveolar process is made edentulous by loss of teeth, the alveoli that contained the roots of the teeth fill in with new bone. This alveolar process becomes the residual ridge, which is the foundation for dentures.

Little is known about the changes that occur in the residual bone after tooth extraction and wearing of complete dentures. It is known that

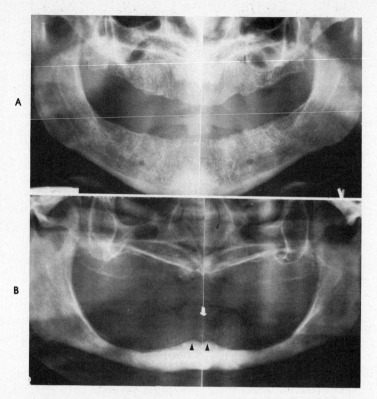

Fig. 1-3. A, Panoramic radiographs showing jaws of edentulous patients. **A,** Residual ridge reduction has occurred to a limited extent. **B,** Patient in this radiograph has worn complete dentures for 16 years, and advanced residual ridge reduction is evident. Notice the prominent superior genial tubercles.

(1) function can modify the internal structure of human bone, (2) pressure can cause its resorption, and (3) tension may bring about bone deposition in some situations. Alveolar bone supporting natural teeth receives tensile loads through a large area of periodontal ligament. The edentulous residual ridge receives vertical, diagonal, and horizontal loads applied by a denture with a surface area much smaller than the total area of the periodontal ligaments of all the natural teeth that had been present. Clinical experience underscores the frequently remarkable adaptive range of the masticatory system. On the other hand, edentulous patients demonstrate very little adaptation of the supporting tissues to functional requirements. One of the few solid facts in relation to edentulous patients is that denture

wearing is almost invariably accompanied by an undesirable bone loss (Fig. 1-3). The magnitude of this loss is extremely variable, and two concepts have been advanced concerning the question of the inevitability of loss of residual bone. One contends that as a direct consequence of loss of the periodontal structures, variable progressive bone reduction results. The other concept contends that residual bone loss is not a necessary consequence of tooth removal but is dependent on a series of poorly understood factors.

Clinical experience strongly suggests a definite relationship between healthy periodontal ligaments and maintained integrity of alveolar bone. Hence the dentist's commitment to preservation and protection of any remaining teeth (see Chapters 3 and 25) so as to minimize or avoid advanced residual-ridge reduction (Fig. 1-3).

It is apparent that the support for the complete denture is conspicuously limited in its adaptive ability and its inherent capability of simulating the role of the periodontium. The mechanism of support is further complicated by the fact that complete dentures move in relation to the underlying bone during function (Årstad, 1959; Woelfel and associates, 1962; Sheppard, 1963; Smith and associates, 1963). This movement is related to the resiliency of the supporting mucosa and the inherent instability of the dentures during function. Almost all "principles" of complete denture construction have been formulated to minimize the forces transmitted to the supporting structures or to decrease the movement of the prostheses in relation to them (Section three). Conclusions regarding denture stability are usually based on clinical experience, but denture instability has the potential of being traumatic to the supporting tissue. Movement of denture bases in any direction on their basal seats can cause tissue damage. In fact it is tempting to construe the recurrent movements of removable prostheses as parafunctional movement and a major factor for residual ridge reduction.

Brill (1967) has described the factors affecting the retention of complete dentures. He considers these factors as either physical or muscular. He points out the following three physical factors involved in denture retention and suggests that these are under the control of the dentist:
1. Maximal extension of the denture base
2. Maximal area of contact between the mucous membrane and the denture base
3. Intimate contact of the denture base and its basal seat

The musculature of the oral cavity can be used to increase the retention (and stability) of dentures. The buccinator, the orbicularis oris, and the intrinsic and extrinsic muscles of the tongue are the key muscles of this activity. Impression techniques, the design of the labial, buccal, and lingual polished surfaces of the denture, and the form of the dental arch should all be considered in the balancing of the forces generated by the tongue and perioral musculature and of the occlusal forces as well.

As the form and size of the denture-supporting tissues (the basal seat) change, the physiologic muscular forces become more important in denture retention. The newly inserted dentures will promote changes in the underlying mucosa (Östlund, 1958) and bone (Carlsson and Ericson, 1965).

Psychologic effect on retention

The dentures may have an adverse psychologic effect on the patient, and the nervous influences that result may affect the salivary secretions and thus affect retention. Eventually patients acquire an ability to retain their dentures by means of their oral musculature. This muscular fixation of dentures is probably accompanied by a reduction in the physical forces used in retaining their dentures. Quite clearly, the physical forces of retention can be improved and reestablished, up to a point, by careful and frequent attention to the denture status. This is done by periodic inspection and by relining and rebasing procedures (Section five).

FUNCTIONAL AND PARAFUNCTIONAL CONSIDERATIONS

The masticatory system appears to function best in an environment of continuing functional equilibrium (Moyers, 1969). This equilibrium is dependent on the interactions of the many components represented in Fig. 1-2. The substitution of a complete denture for the teeth/periodontium mechanism alters this equilibrium. An analysis of this alteration is the basis for understanding the significance of the edentulous state.

Occlusion

The primary components of human dental occlusion are (1) the dentition, (2) the neuromuscular system, and (3) the craniofacial structures. The development and maturation of these components are interrelated, so that growth,

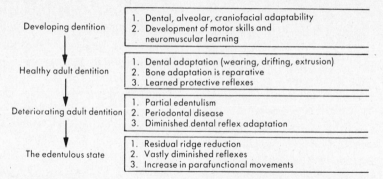

Fig. 1-4. Development and adaptation of occlusion. (After Moyers, R.E.: Dent. Clin. North Am. **13**:523-536, 1969.)

adaptation, and change actively participate in the development of an adult occlusion. The dentition develops in a milieu that is characterized by a period of dental alveolar and craniofacial adaptability (Fig. 1-4), which is also a time when motor skills and neuromuscular learning are developed. Clinical treatment at this period may take advantage of such responsive adaptive mechanisms; for example, teeth can be guided into their correct alignment by orthodontic treatment.

In a healthy adult dentition the dental adaptive mechanisms are restricted to wear, extrusion, and drifting of teeth. Bone adaptations are essentially of a reparative nature and are slow in their operation. Protective reflexes are learned so that one can avoid pain and inefficiency of the masticatory system. If and when an adult dentition begins to deteriorate, the dentist resorts to fixed or removable prosthodontic therapy in attempts to maintain a functional occlusal equilibrium. This period is characterized by greatly diminished dental and reflex adaptation and pathologic bone resorption. Obviously the presence of tooth loss and disease and the depletion of reparative processes pose a major prosthodontic problem. Finally, in the edentulous state there are few natural adaptive mechanisms left. The prosthesis rests on tissues that will change progressively and irreversibly. The artificial

occlusion serves in an environment characterized by constant change that is mainly regressive.

The design and fabrication of a prosthetic occlusion have led to fascinating controversies. Dental occlusion was studied first in the field of complete dentures, then in orthodontics, and then in periodontics. The pioneers encountered enormous mechanical difficulties in constructing reasonably fitting dentures that were both durable and esthetic. Inevitably these dentists had to be mechanically, rather than biologically, minded. Anatomy was the first of the biologic basic sciences to be related to prosthodontic services. Later histology and physiology were recognized as having an essential role in the treatment of edentulous patients. The emphasis on and application of these basic sciences lifted prosthodontics from the early mechanical art to the applied clinical science it is today.

Currently, complete denture service is characterized by an integration of biologic information with instrumentation, techniques, and use of materials. Narrow beliefs and dogmas are gradually being replaced by enlightened reasoning. Dentists are aware of the need for a better understanding of the physiology of the masticatory system and its application in complete denture service.

Complete dentures are designed so that their

occlusal surfaces permit both functional and parafunctional movements of the mandible. Orofacial and tongue muscles play an important role in retaining and stabilizing complete dentures. This is accomplished by arrangement of the artificial teeth to occupy a "neutral zone" in the edentulous mouth so that the teeth will occupy a space determined by the functional balance of the orofacial and tongue musculature. Thus the teeth in the dental arch need not necessarily be placed directly over the residual ridges.

Function: mastication and swallowing

Mastication consists of a rhythmic separation and apposition of the jaws and involves biophysical and biochemical processes including the use of the lips, teeth, cheeks, tongue, palate, and all the oral structures to prepare food for swallowing. During masticatory movements of the tongue and cheek muscles play an essential role in keeping the food bolus between the occlusal surfaces of the teeth. The control of mastication within the narrow limits of tolerance of the mouth requires considerable sensory information, since deviations from the normal path of mandibular movement can injure the tongue, buccal mucosa, and even the teeth and their supporting tissues. Here, again, the reader's attention must be drawn to the importance of the placement of the arch of artificial teeth in the making of complete dentures. The teeth must be placed within the confines of a functional balance of the musculature involved in controlling the food bolus between the occlusal surfaces of the teeth.

The comminution of twentieth century food does not demand a very vigorous masticatory performance. Mastication has other functions, however. It is necessary for full appreciation of flavor of foods and is therefore indirectly involved in the excitation of salivary and gastric secretions. Since mastication results in the mixing of food with saliva, it facilitates not only swallowing but the digestion of carbohydrates by amylase as well. Amylase activity, although of minor importance while the food is in the mouth, is nevertheless responsible for the continuation of carbohydrate digestion in the stomach, and this phase can account for as much as 60% of the total carbohydrate digestion. No reports of quantitative tests on the importance of chewing on the various stages of digestion were found, but Farrell (1956) investigated its effects on digestion as a whole. He concluded that masticatory efficiency as low as 25% is adequate for complete digestion of the foods tested. Other investigators (Manly and Braley, 1950) have noted that loss of teeth can lead to diminished masticatory efficiency. Patients did not compensate for the small number of teeth by more prolonged or larger number of chewing strokes— they merely swallowed larger food particles. Although it appears that the importance of a good dentition or denture in promoting digestion and utilization of food has not been adequately demonstrated, clinical experience indicates that the quality of the prosthetic service may have a direct bearing on the denture wearer's masticatory performance.

A study by Haraldsson and associates (1979) confirmed earlier findings that the maximal bite force in dentulous subjects is five to six times greater than in denture wearers. Edentulous patients are clearly handicapped in masticatory function and even clinically satisfactory complete dentures are poor substitutes for natural teeth.

Speed of masticatory movements. Ahlgren (1966) has comprehensively reviewed the speed of masticatory movements. In this study of children, he found greater inter- and intraindividual variations in the speed of masticatory movements than in patterns of movement. "Forms and speed of movements," he stated, "seem to be controlled by different neuromuscular mechanisms. Form of the masticatory movements is determined by an early conditioned reflex superimposed on a basic movement pattern and does not easily change. Speed of the masticatory movements on the other side is determined by the need of the occasion and, thus, easily influ-

enced by physical and psychological variables."*
According to Ahlgren, the more rapid opening
phase appeared to be a ballistic type of movement with relaxed antagonists, whereas the closing phase appeared to be a rapid tension movement with antagonistic control.

The results of studies of mandibular movement patterns of complete denture patients
indicate that these movements are similar in
denture-wearing patients and those with natural
teeth (Sheppard and associates, 1967 and 1968;
Sheppard and Sheppard, 1971). Recent reports
by Jemt (1983) have confirmed these observations. He stated that treatment of partially edentulous and edentulous patients improves both
their chewing efficiency and muscle activity.
This is also accompanied by a decreased duration of the occlusion phase, which contributes to
a decreased duration of elevator muscle activity.
Jent's observations are also supported by other
investigators (Hannam and others, 1977; Möller
and others, 1983).

Chewing occurs chiefly in the premolar and
molar regions, and both right and left sides are
used to about the same extent. The work of Hed-
egard and associates (1967) demonstrated that
the position of the food bolus during mastication
is dependent on the consistency of the food.
They observed that the tougher the consistency
of the food, the greater the patient preference
for using the premolar region. The latter observation was apparent even in patients who wore
bilateral, soft tissue–supported, mandibular
partial dentures opposing complete upper dentures. It is interesting to note in these studies
the obvious advantage accruing to a patient by
the replacement of missing premolar and molar
segments and by the fact that these patients did
not chew predominantly in the segments where
natural teeth were present.

Reference has been made to the importance
of making complete denture occlusion compatible with the forces developed during degluti-

*From Ahlgren, J.: Mechanism of mastication. Acta
Odontol. Scand. **24** (supp. 44):1-109, 1966.

tion. Tooth contacts made while swallowing are
fleeting in nature, and they occur many times
during a 24-hour day. Swoope and Kydd (1966)
suggested that the effects of the frequency and
duration of tooth contacts while swallowing may
be significant in denture base deformation. They
believe that swallowing may contribute to a
greater accumulated transfer of energy from the
denture base to the underlying mucosa in the
course of a day than mastication does.

Both the occurrence of tooth contacts and the
observations that the mandible braces itself
against the maxillae in denture patients during
swallowing, suggest that a complete denture
occlusion should be compatible with the forces
generated by mandibular movements of deglutition. It should be noted that electromyographic
swallowing patterns have been shown to be
influenced by changes of natural and complete
denture occlusion (Tellgren, 1961).

The pronounced differences between patients
with natural teeth and patients wearing complete dentures are conspicuous in this functional
context. These differences include (1) the mucosal mechanism of support as opposed to support
by the periodontium, (2) the movements of the
dentures during mastication, (3) the progressive
changes in maxillomandibular relations and the
eventual migration of dentures (described in the
discussion of morphologic face height), and (4)
the different physical stimuli to the sensori-
motor systems.

The denture-bearing tissues are constantly
exposed to the frictional contact of their overlying denture bases. Dentures move during mastication as a result of the dislodging forces of the
surrounding masculature (Woelfel and associates, 1962; Smith and associates, 1963). These
movements manifest themselves as displacing,
lifting, sliding, tilting, or rotation of the dentures. Furthermore, opposing-tooth contacts
occur with both natural and artificial teeth during function and parafunction both in the day
and during sleep.

Masticatory investigations up to now have

been limited to few subjects, and the occlusal contacts recorded were in selected experimental areas. Furthermore, the dentures used in the studies were designed so that the maximum intercuspation of the artificial teeth was in centric relation, or the terminal hinge position of the mandible at the selected vertical dimension. Other occlusal concepts that claim other condylar or muscular positions as preferable for complete denture construction have not been investigated for occlusal tooth-contact patterns. In all instances the frequency of tooth contact on the nonchewing side was greater than on the chewing side, irrespective of the side on which the patient chewed or the tooth form or arrangement used.

It appears that tissue displacement beneath the denture base probably results in tilting of the dentures and tooth contacts on the nonchewing side. Also, occlusal pressure on dentures displaces soft tissues of the basal seat and allows the dentures to move closer to the supporting bone. This change of position under pressure changes the relationship of the teeth to each other.

The presence of inanimate foreign objects (dentures) in an edentulous mouth are bound to elicit different stimuli to the sensori-motor system, which in turn influences the cyclic masticatory stroke pattern (Hardy, 1970). Both exteroceptors and proprioceptors are probably affected by the size, shape, position, pressure from, and mobility of the prostheses. The exact role and relative importance of mucosal stimuli in the control of jaw movements need clarification. Brill and associates (1959) have shown that the control of dentures by muscle activity is reduced if surface anesthetic is applied to the oral mucous membrane. Although it is tempting to assume that there is a correlation between oral stereognosis and purposeful oral motor activity, the results of most investigations up to now indicate that successful denture wearing possibly involves factors other than oral perception and oral performance (Berry and Mahood, 1966).

Table 2

Direction, duration, and magnitude of the forces generated during function and parafunction

	FORCE GENERATED	
	DIRECTION	DURATION AND MAGNITUDE
Mastication	Mainly vertical	Intermittent and light
		Diurnal only
Parafunction	Frequently horizontal as well as vertical	Prolonged, possibly excessive
		Both diurnal and nocturnal

Parafunction

Nonfunctional or parafunctional habits involving repeated or sustained occlusion of the teeth can be harmful to the teeth or other components of the masticatory system (Ramfjord and Ash, 1971). There are no epidemiologic studies about the incidence of parafunctional occlusal stress in normal or denture-wearing populations. However, clinical experience indicates that bruxism is common and is a frequent cause of the complaint of soreness of the denture-bearing mucous membrane (Thomson, 1968). In the denture wearer, parafunctional habits can cause additional loading on the denture-bearing tissues (Table 2). The unsuitability of the mechanism of denture support has already been recognized and described.

The neurophysiologic basis underlying bruxism has been studied experimentally both in animals and in man. The neuromuscular mechanism can be explained by an increase in the tonic activity in the jaw muscles. Emotional or nervous tension, pain or discomfort, the stresses of everyday life, and occlusal interferences are some of the factors that can increase muscle tonus and lead to nonfunctional gnashing and clenching.

The initial discomfort associated with wearing new dentures is known to evoke unusual patterns of behavior in the surrounding musculature. Frequently the complaint of a sore tongue is related to the habit of thrusting the tongue against the denture. The patient is usually unaware of the causal relationship between the painful tongue and its contact with the teeth. Similarly patients tend to occlude the teeth of new dentures frequently at first—perhaps to strengthen confidence in retention until the surrounding muscles become accommodated or because some accommodation in the chewing pattern is usually required and experimental closure of the teeth is part of the process of adaptation (Thomson, 1971). A strong response of the lower lip and mentalis muscle has been observed electromyographically in long-term complete denture wearers with impaired retention and stability of the lower denture (Tallgren, 1963). It is feasible and probable that the tentative occlusal contacts resulting may trigger a greater possibility for the development of habitual nonfunctional occlusion.

Yemm (1972) suggests that stress can induce increases in activity of the masseter and temporal muscles in denture wearers, which in turn can cause tooth contact and eventually soreness of underlying mucosal tissues. He infers that such widespread pressure is similar to the generalized soreness that develops with an excessive vertical dimension of occlusion in complete dentures. The mechanism whereby pressure causes soreness of the mucous membrane is probably related to an interruption or a diminution of the blood flow in the small blood vessels in the tissues. These vascular changes could very well upset the metabolism of the involved tissues. *The relationship between parafunction and residual ridge reduction has not been investigated. It is tempting, however, to include parafunction as a possible significant prosthetic variable that contributes to the magnitude of ridge reduction.*

Distribution of stress to denture-supporting tissues

The need for fulfilling the fundamental objectives of good prosthodontic treatment is under-scored by the preceding information. All possible methods should be undertaken to ensure continued tissue health by minimizing the potential traumatic effects of complete denture wear. The capability of the supporting tissues should be improved whenever possible by adequate preparation of both hard and soft tissues. Mucosal health may be promoted by hygienic and therapeutic measures, and tissue-conditioning techniques may be applied when appropriate. Complete denture base extension within morphologic and functional limits can reduce considerably the occlusal load on the unit area of mucosa. Resilient denture base lining materials may be used, and the masticatory loading may be decreased by reduction of the area of the occlusal table.

Currently, for practical purposes, denture bases are made of rigid materials. These may be one of various types of resins, metals, or combinations of them. The dentist must recognize that the prolonged contact of these bases with their underlying tissues is bound to elicit changes in the tissues. Furthermore, the tissues are susceptible to changes caused by the increased longevity of patients with the effects of aging on tissues, as well as by the functional and parafunctional demands that patients make on their denture-supporting tissues. Many dentists have been tempted to equate the prevalent residual ridge reduction in the edentulous population with excessive stresses that are imposed on these ridges. Up to now there is no specific evidence to indict any one factor as causing advanced ridge reduction. However, strong theoretical evidence exists to justify the development of permanently resilient lining materials in complete dentures. These materials could permit a wider dispersion of forces and result in a lower force per unit area being transmitted to the supporting tissues. Such a soft denture-lining material could effectively increase the thickness of the oral tissue by serving as an analog of the mucoperiosteum with its relatively low elastic modulus (Kydd and Mandley, 1967).

The distance increment between the hard

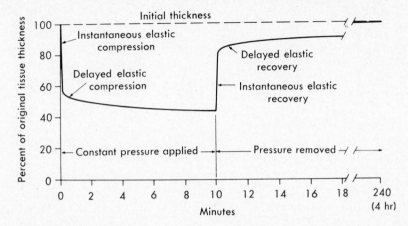

Fig. 1-5. Typical behavior of tissue under constant pressure loading up to 10 minutes. Typical behavior of pressure removal showing 90% recovery in 8 minutes. Total recovery requires 4 hours. (From Kydd, W.L., Daly, C.H., and Wheeler, J.B.: Int. Dent. J. **21:**430-441, 1971.)

denture base and the nonresilient bony support would be increased with hypothetical salutary long-term results. The Academy of Denture Prosthetics listed ideas for future research in denture base materials. The list enumerates the desirable qualities for the improvement of denture base materials and cites the following desirable properties:

1. Possessing variable consistency under varying mouth conditions
2. Selectively resilient—compatible with resiliency of the tissues
3. Resilient with quick recovery—able to recover shape quickly after deforming forces are removed
4. Compressible on tissue side but rigid on occlusal side
5. Shock absorbing
6. Controlling or reducing forces transmitted through the base to the underlying tissue
7. Possessing flexibility that can be controlled and varied in processing as desired

The work of Kydd and associates (1971) on pressures in the oral cavity has posed an excellent argument favoring the employment of soft lining materials. They argue that during function and parafunction, pressures are applied by the dentures, which will displace the soft tissues. These pressures deform the mucoperiosteum and interfere with circulation of blood, nutrients, and metabolites. Several studies have demonstrated changes in soft-tissue contour as a result of mechanical stress (Pfeiffer, 1929; Lytle, 1962; Årstad, 1959). Kydd and associates described the viscoelastic character of denture-supporting tissue (Fig. 1-5). There is an initial elastic compression of soft tissues that takes place instantly on application of load. After the elastic phase there is a delayed elastic deformation of the tissue that takes place slowly and continues to diminish in rate of change as duration of load is extended. An instantaneous elastic decompression occurs when the pressure is removed. This is followed by a continuing delayed elastic recovery. Histologically, the stressed oral mucosa has an altered morphologic pattern. The loaded epithelium demonstrates a decrease in the depth of the epithelial ridges, and the connective tissue papillae are obliterated. The extent of these alterations varies with the force and duration of the applied force. Human soft tissues take as long as 4 hours to recover after moderate loading for 10 minutes (Kydd and associates, 1971). They ask, "What

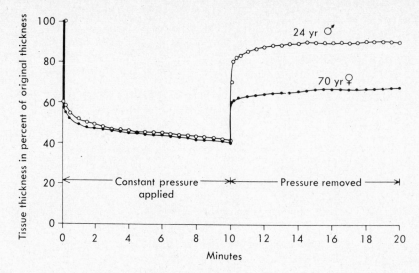

Fig. 1-6. Comparison of response to tissue loading and removal of load in an elderly and young adult. The compression curve is essentially the same. The removal of load shows definite differences in rate of recovery. Load was 11 g/mm². (From Kydd, W.L., Daly, C.H., and Wheeler, J.B.: Int. Dent. J. **21**:430-441, 1971.)

would be the effect of a defective removable partial denture stressing the supporting mucoperiosteum for hours?"

A change in tissue displaceability can also be demonstrated as being a function of age. A longer period of time is needed for the recovery of displaced mucosa in elderly people (68 to 70 years) when compared with young adults (21 to 27 years) (Fig. 1-6). It appears that any intraoral prosthesis can be intruded into the denture-supporting oral mucosa by up to 20% of its resting thickness with relatively small occluding forces (0.2 g/mm²). Lindan (1961) has shown that pressures as small as 0.13 g/mm² will displace human soft tissues to 95% of their resting thickness. This indicates that impression materials, for example, must flow readily and with minimal pressure when an impression is made.

Cutright and associates (1976) recorded pressures under complete maxillary dentures. They used a closed fluid system connected to a pressure transducer and recorder to register positive and negative pressures in four subjects at four locations. Each subject performed a number of controlled masticatory and nonmasticatory activities. Their findings indicate that a number of nonmasticatory activities (smoking, swallowing, speaking) created as much, or more, positive and negative pressures on the supporting tissues as the masticatory activities.

It has been observed that some patients swallow approximately one and a half times per minute while reading, which would total approximately 1500 swallows per day unrelated to eating or drinking. When converted to pounds of pressure, this amounts to about 3500 to 4200 pounds per day from swallowing alone.

The rapid fluctuation from positive to negative pressures indicates a pressure wave beneath the denture. This is attributable to rocking or movement or to a flow of fluid within the vascular channels that possibly creates trauma with each tooth contact. It is tempting to suggest that these pressures could affect the soft tissue and the blood and lymph vessels, perhaps causing sclerosis, diminished blood supply, and the many morphologic variants we encounter in our

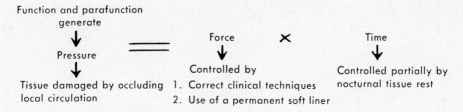

Function and parafunction
generate
↓
Pressure   ═══   Force   ×   Time
↓   ↓   ↓
Tissue damaged by occluding   Controlled by   Controlled partially by
local circulation   1. Correct clinical techniques   nocturnal tissue rest
                              2. Use of a permanent soft liner

Fig. 1-7. Increased denture base coverage and use of a soft liner diminish the force per unit area directed to basal seat. The pressure-time threshold may thus be raised.

edentulous patients. Cutright and associates concluded that the effect of these continually occurring, non–masticatory induced pressure changes and waves may well be of greater significance than that of mastication.

It appears that pressure may cause tissue damage by occluding the local circulation, subject to a force-time threshold. The harmful effect of pressure can be avoided by diminution or elimination of either factor. The amount of force generated by a patient's masticatory system is not controlled by the dentist. The dentist can seek to minimize force distribution by maximizing denture base coverage and developing an optimal denture occlusion. Occlusal surfaces of the artificial teeth can be made smaller, and the patient can be instructed to handle parafunctional habits through education and understanding. Forces can also be reduced or diluted by use of a permanently resilient liner if such materials are readily available (Fig. 1-7). The time factor can be controlled to a large extent by frequent rest periods for the denture-supporting tissues. Leaving the dentures out of the mouth during sleeping hours is recommended. Oral tissues were designed to be exposed to oral fluids and to be stimulated by the action of tongue, lips, and cheeks. Nocturnal rest can achieve this objective, along with a quantitative diminution in the duration of exposure of these tissues to stress.

The efficiency of temporary soft or treatment liners in routine prosthodontic practice has proved the value of such an approach in treating

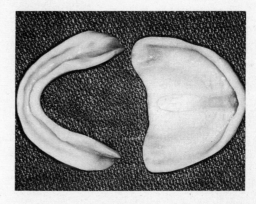

Fig. 1-8. Tissue-surface appearance of maxillary and mandibular complete dentures lined with a silicone rubber resilient liner.

soft-tissue problems. The contribution of permanent liners toward the maintenance of supporting-tissue integrity and morphology is still hypothetical, however.

A number of resilient liners with furtive claims to permanency have appeared on the market in recent years. Their major use, however, has been as a therapeutic measure for patients who cannot tolerate the stresses induced in denture use (Fig. 1-8). Clinical experience indicates almost universal tissue tolerance for these materials and acceptable patient reactions. At present, the materials have to be considered as temporary expedients, since none of the soft liners has a life expectancy comparable to that of the resin denture base.

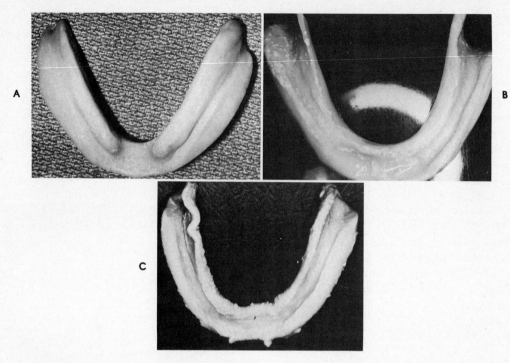

Fig. 1-9. A, Recently completed resilient liner on a mandibular denture. **B,** Six-month-old resilient liner with foci of yeast colonies already apparent. **C,** Neglected 12-month-old resilient liner, which has been almost totally replaced by yeast colonies.

The most frequently used liners are usually produced from silicone rubbers or acrylic resins. Recent reports also suggest the possible employment of hydrophilic polymers and fluoropolymers (Hayakawa, 1984) The research effort is in the direction of a material that is permanently resilient, does not absorb fluids, adheres to denture base materials, and is clemically stable. The silicone rubber resilient liners, when properly used, are the most appropriate of the various types available, but they too are only temporary expedients. These materials may support yeast growth (e.g., *Candida albicans*) (Fig. 1-9); they must be observed regularly by the dentist and replaced when unsatisfactory. The use of proper cleansers and home care habits have contributed to the employment of these materials with significantly beneficial results. It must be empha-sized that the use of these materials does not preclude adherence to the fundamental principles of complete denture construction. When used intelligently, resilient liners can be an excellent adjunct in prosthodontics.

CHANGES IN MORPHOLOGIC FACE HEIGHT AND TEMPOROMANDIBULAR JOINTS
Face height

Numerous descriptions of temporomandibular joint function have evolved as a result of several research methods. The basic physiologic relation between the condyles, the disks, and their glenoid fossae appears to be maintained during maximal occlusal contacts and during all movements guided by occlusal elements. It seems logical that in the treatment with complete dentures, the dentist should seek to maintain or restore this basic physiologic relation. Posselt (1952) showed that the border movements of the mandible were reproducible and that all other movements took place within the confines of his classic "envelopes of motion." His work was confirmed by several investigators, notably Ahlgren (1966) and Nyffenegger and associates (1971). These researchers concluded that the passive hinge movement had a constant and definite rotational and reproducible character. The reproducibility of the posterior border path is of tremendous practical significance in the treatment of prosthodontic patients and is described in Section three. However, this reproducibility has been established in healthy young persons only. It must be recalled that most edentulous patients have experienced a period with variations on the theme of a mutilated dentition. In the course of this period, pathologic or adaptive changes of the temporomandibular joints may have occurred (Posselt, 1952). Several authors suggest that structural alterations can take place in the temporomandibular joints (Blackwood, 1959, 1963, 1966a,b, 1968; Johnson, 1962; Moffett and associates, 1964; McNamara, 1972). These investigations are mainly based on autopsy studies; hence the results are only speculative (Carlsson and Oberg, 1979).

Although the terminal stage of skeletal growth is usually accepted as being at 20 to 25 years of age, it is recognized that growth and remodeling of the bony skeleton continue well into adult life. Such growth accounts for dimensional changes in the adult facial skeleton. Tallgren (1957) has shown that morphologic face height increases with age in persons possessing an intact or relatively intact dentition. However, a premature reduction in morphologic face height occurs with attrition or abrasion of teeth. This reduction is even more conspicuous in edentulous and complete denture–wearing patients.

Maxillomandibular morphologic changes take place slowly over a period of years and depend on the balance of osteoblastic and osteoclastic activity. The articular surfaces of the temporo-mandibular joints are also involved, and at these sites growth and remodeling are mediated through the proliferative activity of the articular cartilages. In the facial skeleton any dimensional changes in morphologic face height or the jawbones as a result of the loss of teeth are inevitably transmitted to the temporomandibular joints. It is not surprising, then, that these articular surfaces undergo a slow but continuous remodeling throughout life. Such remodeling is probably the means whereby the congruity of the opposing articular surfaces is maintained, even in the presence of dimensional or functional changes in other parts of the facial skeleton (Blackwood, 1968).

The reduction of the residual ridges (Figs. 1-10 and 1-11) tends to cause a resultant reduction in total face height and an increase in mandibular prognathism. Tallgren (1972) has shown that in complete denture wearers the mean reduction in height of the mandibular process, as measured in the anterior region, was 6.6 mm, approximately four times greater than the mean reduction occurring in the maxillary process. The cephalometric observations of Atwood (1957) and the longitudinal studies of Tallgren (1957, 1966, 1972) support the hypothesis that the vertical dimension of rest position of the jaws does not remain stable and can be altered over a period of time. Their statements usurp the previously popular concept of a stable vertical dimension of rest positions (Niswonger, 1934; Brodie, 1941; Thompson, 1943; Ballard, 1955).

It is obvious that complete dentures constructed to conform to clinical decisions regarding jaw relation records are placed in an environment that retains considerable potential for change. Thus concepts of reproducible and relatively unchangeable mandibular border movements may not identically apply to edentulous patients as they do to those with healthy dentitions. Practical methods that recognize these facts are described in subsequent chapters. It must be reemphasized, however, that the recognition that jaw relations are not immutable does

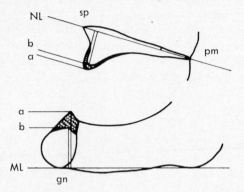

Fig. 1-10. Measurements of alveolar resorption. Anterior height of upper and lower alveolar ridges at two stages of observation (*a* and *b*). The difference, *a* − *b*, represents the reduction in height of alveolar ridges between stages of observation. *Shaded area,* Area of resorption. (From Tallgren, A.: J. Prosthet. Dent. **27**:120-132, 1972.)

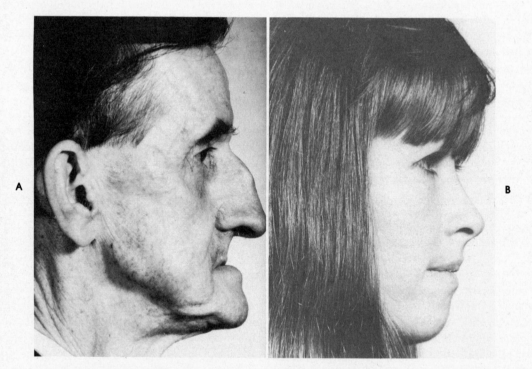

Fig. 1-11. A, A 67-year-old man who has worn unserviced dentures for almost 20 years, with a resultant reduction in total face height and an increase in mandibular prognathism. **B,** Contrast his appearance to that of a 24-year-old woman who recently acquired complete dentures but posed for this picture with her dentures out of her mouth.

not invalidate the clinical requirement of using a centric relation record as a starting point for developing a prosthetic occlusion.

Centric relation. Concepts of centric relation of the upper and lower jaws have been a dominant factor in prosthodontic thinking on occlusion. Centric relation is defined as the most posterior relation of the mandible to the maxillae at the established vertical relation. Centric relation coincides with a reproducible posterior hinge position of the mandible, and it may be recorded with a high degree of accuracy. It is considered to be an essential relationship in any prosthodontic treatment.

The use of centric relation has its physiologic justification as well. In the vast majority of patients, unconscious swallowing is carried out with the mandible at or near the centric relation position. The unconscious or reflex swallow is important in the developing dentition. The act and frequency of swallowing are important influences in the movement of teeth within the muscle matrix, and this movement determines the tooth position and occlusal relations (Moyers). The erupting teeth are guided into occlusion by the surrounding musculature (the muscle matrix), whereas the position of the mandible is determined by its location in space during the act of unconscious swallowing. The contacts of inclined planes of the teeth aid in the alignment of the erupting dentition. It must be remembered that in this developmental period most of the mandibular activities have not yet been learned, at least not in their adult form.

The occlusion of complete dentures is designed to harmonize with the primitive, unconditioned reflex of the patient's unconscious swallow. Tooth contacts and mandibular bracing against the maxillae occur during swallowing by complete denture patients. This suggests that complete denture occlusions must be compatible with the forces developed during deglutition to prevent disharmonious occlusal contacts that can cause trauma to the basal seat of dentures. During swallowing the mandible is in centric relation, or that position of maximum mandibular retrusion relative to the maxillae at the established vertical dimension of occlusion. It is conceded, however, that most functional natural tooth contacts occur in a mandibular position anterior to that of centric relation, a position referred to as centric occlusion.

In complete denture prosthodontics the position of maximum planned intercuspation of teeth, or centric occlusion, is established to coincide with the patient's centric relation. The centric occlusion position occupied by the mandible in the dentate patient cannot be registered with sufficient accuracy when the patient becomes edentulous. In other words, the muscle memory pattern of the mandibular musculature would not be effective in edentulous patients. Clinical experience supports the conviction that the recording of centric relation is an *essential starting point* in the design of an artificial occlusion.

However, one must realize that an integral part of the definition of centric relation—at the established vertical relation—has potential for change. This change is brought about by alterations in denture-supporting tissues and facial height morphology and by morphologic changes in the temporomandibular joints. An appreciation for the dynamic nature of centric relation in denture-wearing patients recognizes the changing functional requirements of the masticatory system. It accounts for different concepts and techniques of design of occlusions, which is described in Section three.

Temporomandibular joint changes

Several authors claim that impaired dental efficiency resulting from partial tooth loss and absence of, or incorrect, prosthodontic treatment can bring about temporomandibular joint pain and dysfunction or even degenerative changes in the joints. Published clinical reports on patients with functional disorders of the masticatory system have also included patients who are denture wearers (Franks, 1965; Carlsson and Svärdström, 1971; Zarb and Thompson, 1970). It is possible that these denture wearers' difficulties started before the offending teeth were removed, though Bergman and Carlsson (1972) reported that half of the 54 complete denture patients they interviewed complained of general joint pain after only 1 year of prosthetic treatment.

Although the relationship between occlusion and degenerative joint disease is not completely clear, the dentist is tempted to believe that a depleted or inadequate dentition care obviously load the temporomandibular joints. The hypothesis that degenerative joint disease is a process rather than a disease entity has been advanced. The process involves joint changes that cause an imbalance in adaptation and a degeneration that results from alterations in functional demands on or in the functional capacity of the joints.

Research strongly suggests that purely dental factors may be important in the etiology of degenerative joint disease of the mandibular condyles (Kopp and associates, 1976). The involvement of the temporomandibular joints in degenerative diseases is well documented (Toller, 1973); however, it must be appreciated that the onset of a degenerative condition, though low in incidence, occurs more frequently in the adult years. Since the greater number of denture wearers is adult, the treatment of such patients suffering from degenerative joint conditions is very much the concern of the dentist. Clinical experience indicates that the application of sound prosthodontic principles, accompanied by appropriate supportive therapy, is usually adequate to provide the patients with comfort (Zarb, 1981).

One of the difficulties in the management of degenerative joint involvement is that of achieving rest of the joints. Because of the necessity for mastication and for the avoidance of tensional habits, voluntary or even enforced rest may be difficult to achieve.

COSMETIC CHANGES AND INDIVIDUAL ADAPTIVE RESPONSES
Cosmetic changes

There is little doubt that tooth loss can adversely affect a person's cosmetic appearance.

Table 3

Morphological changes associated with the edentulous state

1. Deepening of nasolabial groove
2. Loss of labiodental angle
3. Decrease in horizontal labial angle
4. Narrowing of lips
5. Increase in columella-philtral angle
6. Prognathic appearance

Such patients seek dental treatment for both functional and cosmetic reasons, and dentists have been successful in restoring or improving many a patient's appearance (Fig. 1-12).

Table 3 lists some of the conspicuous and clinically challenging cosmetic features that frequently accompany the edentulous state. It must be emphasized that one or more of the listed items can be encountered in persons with intact dentitions, since the compromised facial support of the edentulous state is *not* the exclusive cause of these morphologic changes. In clinical practice we frequently encounter situations where a patient's weight loss, age, heavy tooth attrition, and so on, can manifest orofacial changes usually suggestive of a compromised, or absent, dental support for the overlying tissues. Some patients fail to appreciate the fact that those aspects of their facial appearance for which they are seeking a solution are merely magnified or else are unrelated to their edentulous predicament.

These patients can cause the dentist considerable frustration. Experience suggests that *early communication about a patient's cosmetic expectations should be established so as to avoid later misunderstanding.* Patients should be asked to provide photographs of their preedentulous appearance, and relevant details from these photographs should be carefully analyzed and discussed with the patient. If this is not possible, photographs of siblings, or of children who resemble the patient, could be helpful.

Careful explanation of prosthodontic objectives and methods is the basis for good commu-

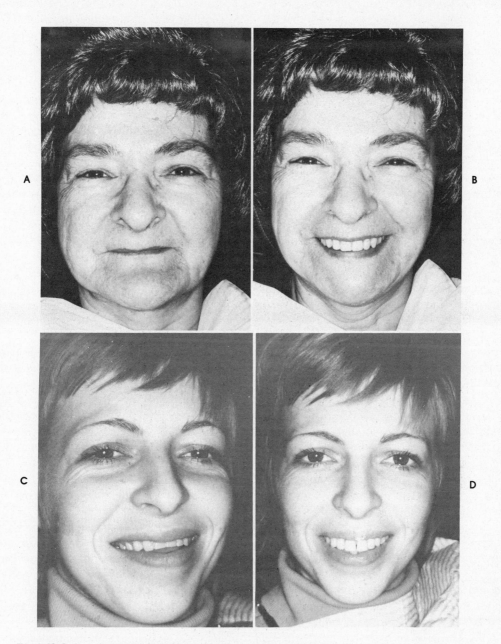

Fig. 1-12. Before, **A,** and after, **B,** clinical views of edentulous patient who has been treated by construction of complete upper and lower dentures. Before, **C,** and after, **D,** clinical views of a patient whose old cosmetically unsatisfactory dentures were replaced. The patient's youth and appealing smile are brought out by new tooth arrangement.

nication with all patients. This is particularly so when its become apparent to the dentist that the patient's cosmetic desires exceed morphologic or functional realities.

Adaptive response to complete dentures

The process whereby an edentulous patient can accept and use complete dentures is a complex one. It requires adaptation related to learning, muscular skill, and motivation. It is the patient's ability and willingness to accept and learn to use the dentures that ultimately determine the degree of success of the clinical treatment. Helping a patient adapt to complete dentures can be one of the most difficult but one of the most rewarding aspects of clinical dentistry (Zarb, 1982).

Learning means the acquisition of a new activity or change of an existing one. Muscular skill refers to the capacity to coordinate muscular activity so as to execute movement. The acceptance of complete dentures is accompanied by a process of habituation. Glaser (1966) defines habituation as a "gradual diminution of responses to continued or repeated stimuli." The tactile stimuli that arise from the contact of the prostheses with the richly innervated oral cavity are probably ignored after a short time. Since each stage of the decrease in response is related to the memory trace of the previous application of the stimulus, storage of information from the immediate past is an integral part of habituation. Difficulty in the storage of information of this type accompanies old age, and this accounts for the difficulties of older patients in getting used to dentures. Furthermore, stimuli must be specific and identical to achieve habituation (Greenwood and Lewis, 1959). This is what probably prevents the transfer of habituation evoked by an old familiar denture to a new denture that inevitably gives rise to a new range of stimuli. Fish describes several clinical applications of adaptation problems that may be encountered. The patient who has worn a complete upper denture opposing a few natural anterior mandibular teeth will usually find a complete lower

denture difficult to adapt to. Such a patient has to contend with an alteration in size and orientation of the tongue. The tongue frequently responds to the loss of posterior teeth and alveolar bone by altering its shape so as to bring its lateral borders into contact with the buccal mucosa. The insertion of a new denture imposes a new environment for the tongue, and the intrinsic tongue musculature reorganizes to change the tongue shape to conform to the altered space available. A degree of retraining of tongue activity also takes place. Furthermore, the posterior residual ridges are now exposed to new sensations from the overlying prosthesis. Tactile stimuli from the tongue and frictional contact with food are replaced by pressures transferred via the denture base. Also, control of the upper denture frequently has to be unlearned, since the posterior part of the tongue will no longer be required to counter the dislodging effect on the denture produced by the remaining mandibular dentition.

It must be realized that edentulous patients expect and are expected to adapt to the dentures more or less instantaneously and that the adaptation must take place in the context of the patient's oral, systemic, emotional, and psychologic states.

Facility for learning and coordination appears to diminish with age. Advancing age tends to be accompanied by progressive atrophy of elements of the cerebral cortex, and a consequent loss in the facility of coordination occurs. Certainly patient motivation frequently dictates the speed with which adaptation to dentures occurs. It is imperative that the dentist determine the patient's motivation in seeking treatment, cultivate this motivation, and seek to foster it if it is lacking or absent.

A distinct need exists for dentists to be able to understand a patient's motivation in seeking prosthodontic care and to identify problems before starting treatment. Emotional factors are known to play a significant role in the etiology of several dental problems. Moulton (1955) related complete denture problems to the emotional state of the wearer. The interview and clinical examination are obvious ways to observe patients and form the best treatment relationship. Successful management begins with identification of anticipated difficulties before treatment starts and with careful planning to meet specific needs and problems. Dentists must train themselves to reassure patients, to perceive their wishes, and to know how and when to limit patient expectations. An essential accompaniment to a denture design that is physically compatible with the oral complex is a good interpersonal relationship between dentist and patient. It is up to the dentist to explore the patient's symptoms and tensions. The way in which patients handle other illnesses and dental situations will aid in the prediction of future problems. Moulton pointed out that the secure patient will adjust readily, cope with discomfort, and be cooperative.

The whole area of prosthodontist-patient interpersonal relationship has not been adequately studied or emphasized by the dental profession. Although the taking of a health history can be effective, a great deal of experience and training is necessary to conduct a patient interview effectively and profitably. Unfortunately the rigors of dental practice prevent the majority of dentists from taking the time to carry out a thorough patient interview. Bolender and associates (1969) showed a connection between emotional problems and denture problems. They used one of the health questionnaires (The Cornell Medical Index), which had already been shown to be efficient and accurate (Brodman and associates, 1952). This questionnaire can be used as a guide for a structured personal interview with the patient. It is a useful adjunct to establishing a prognosis for the proposed treatment.

Adaptive potential of patients

The absence of a yardstick to gauge a patient's adaptive potential is one of the most challenging facets of treating edentulous patients. *The success of prosthetic treatment is predicated not only on manual dexterity, but also on the ability of the dentist to relate to patients and to understand their needs.* One cannot overemphasize the importance of empathy on the part of the dentist. The ability to understand and recognize the problems of edentulous patients and to reassure them has proved to be of great clinical value.

REFERENCES

Ahlgren, J.: Mechanism of mastication, Acta Odontol. Scand. 24(supp. 44:)1-109, 1966.

Årstad, T.: The resiliency of the edentulous alveolar ridges, Oslo, 1959, Oslo University Press.

Atwood, D.A.: A cephalometric study of the clinical rest position. II. The variability in the rate of bone loss following the removal of occlusal contacts, J. Prosthet. Dent. 7:544-552, 1957.

Ballard, C.F.: Consideration of the physiological background of mandibular posture and movement, Dent. Pract. 6:80-89, 1955.

Bergman, B., and Carlsson, G.E.: Review of 54 complete denture wearers; patients' opinions 1 year after treatment, Acta Odontol. Scand. 30:399-414, 1972.

Berry, D.C., and Mahood, M.: Oral stereognosis and oral ability in relation to prosthetic treatment, Br. Dent. J. 120:179-185, 1966.

Blackwood, H.J.J.: Development, growth and pathology of the mandibular condyle, Thesis presented to the Queen's University of Belfast, 1959.

Blackwood, H.J.J.: Arthritis of the mandibular joint, Br. Dent. J. 115:317-326, 1963.

Blackwood, H.J.J.: Cellular remodeling in articular tissue, Proceedings of the Third International Conference on Oral Biology, International Association for Dental Research, 1966a.

Blackwood, H.J.J.: Growth of the mandibular condyle of the rat studied with tritiated thymidine, Arch. Oral Biol. 11:493-500, 1966b.

Blackwood, H.J.J.: In Schwartz, L., and Chayes, C.M.: Facial pain and mandibular dysfunction, Philadelphia, 1968, W.B. Saunders Co., pp. 102-109.

Bolender, C.L., Swoope, C.C., and Smith, D.E.: The Cornell Medical Index as a prognostic aid for complete denture patients, J. Prosthet. Dent. 22:20-29, 1969.

Brill, N.: Factors in the mechanism of full denture retention, Dent. Pract. 18:9-19, 1967.

Brill, N., Lammie, G.A., Osborne, J., and Perry, H.: Mandibular positions and mandibular movements, Br. Dent. J. 106:391-400, 1959.

Brodie, A.G.: Growth pattern of human head from third month to eighth year of life, Am. J. Anat. 68:209-262, 1941.

Brodman, K., Erdman, A.J., Jr., Lorge, I., and Wolff, H.G.: Cornell Medical Index–Health Questionnaire. II. As a diagnostic instrument, J.A.M.A. 145:152-157, 1951. III. Evaluation of emotional disturbances, J. Clin. Psychol. 8:119-124, 1952. IV. Recognition of emotional disturbances in a general hospital, J. Clin. Psychol. **8:**289-293, 1952.

Carlsson, G.E., and Oberg, T.: Remodelling of the TMJ. In Zarb, G.A., and Carlsson, G.E.: Temporomandibular joint function and dysfunction, St. Louis, 1979, The C.V. Mosby Co.

Carlsson, G.E., and Svärdström, G.: Ett bettfysiologiskt patientmaterial, Sven. Tandlak. Tidskr. **64:**889-899, 1971.

Cutright, D.E., Brudvik, J.S., Gay, W.D., and Selting, W.J.: Tissue pressure under complete maxillary dentures, J. Prosthet. Dent. **35:**160-170, 1976.

Farrell, J.H.: The effect of mastication on the digestion of food. Br. Dent. J. **100:**149-155. 1956.

Franks, A.S.: Masticatory muscle hyperactivity and temporomandibular joint dysfunction, J. Prosthet. Dent. **15:**1122-1131, 1965.

Glaser, E.M.: The physiological basis of habituation, London, 1966, Oxford University Press.

Glickman, I., Pameijer, J.H., Roeber F., and Brion, M.: Functional occlusion as revealed by miniaturized radio transmitters, Dent. Clin. North Am. **13:**667-679, 1969.

Graf, H.: Bruxism, Dent. Clin. North Am. **13:**659-665, 1969.

Greenwood, R.M., and Lewis, P.D.: Factors affecting habituation to localized heating and cooling, J. Physiol. **146:**10P-11P, 1959.

Hannam, A.G., De Con, R.E., Scott, T.D., and Wood, W.W.: The relationship between dental occlusion, muscle activity and associated jaw movements in man, Arch. Oral Biol. **22:**25, 1977.

Hardy, J.C.: Development of neuromuscular systems underlying speech production. In Wertz, R.T., editor: Proceedings of the Workshop [on] Speech and the Dentofacial Complex: The State of the Art, ASHA Rep. No. 5, Washington, D.C., 1970, American Speech-Hearing Association, pp. 49-68.

Haraldsson, T., Karlsson, U., and Carlsson, G.E.: Bite force and oral function in complete denture wearers, J. Oral Rehabil. **6:**41-48, 1979.

Hedegård, B., Lundberg, M., and Wictorin, L.: Masticatory function: a cineradiographic investigation, Acta Odontol. Scand. **25:**331-353, 1967.

Hayakawa, I., Kawae, M., Tsuji, Y., and Masuhara, E.: Soft denture liner of fluoroethylene copolymer and its clinical evaluation, J. Prosthet. Dent. **51:**310-313, 1984.

Jemt, T., Lundquist, S., and Hedegård, B.: Group function or canine protection, J. Prosthet. Dent. **48:**719-724, 1982.

Jemt, T., Hedegård, B., and Wickberg, K.: Chewing patterns before and after treatment with complete maxillary and bilateral distal-extension mandibular removable partial dentures, J. Prosthet. Dent. **50:**566-570, 1983.

Johnson, L.C.: Joint remodelling as the basis for osteoarthritis, J. Am. Vet. Med. Assoc. **141:**1237-1241, 1962.

Kopp, S., Carlsson, G.E., Hansson, T., and Öberg, T.: Degenerative disease in temporomandibular joint osteoarthrosis, Scand. Dent. J. Res. **85:**434-441, 1976.

Kydd, W.L., Daly, C.H., and Wheeler, J.B.: The thickness measurement of masticatory mucosa *in vivo*, Int. Dent. J. **21:**430-441, 1971.

Kydd, W.L., and Mandley, J.: The stiffness of palatal mucoperiosteum, J. Prosthet. Dent. **18:**116-121, 1967.

Laney, W.R.: Processed resilient denture liners, Dent. Clin. North Am. **14:**531-551, 1970.

Lindan, P.: Etiology of decubitus ulcers: an experimental study, Arch. Phys. Med. **42:**774-783, 1961.

Lönberg, P.: Changes in the size of the lower jaw on account of age and loss of teeth (Acta Genetica et Statistica Medica, supp.), Stockholm, 1951, S. Karger.

Lundberg, M., Wictorin, L., and Hedegård, B.: Masticatory function; a cineradiographic investigation, Acta Odontol. Scand. **25:**383-395, 1967.

Lytle, R.B.: Soft tissue displacement beneath removable partial and complete dentures, J. Prosthet. Dent. **12:**34-43, 1962.

Manly, R.S., and Braley, L.C.: Masticatory performance and efficiency, J. Dent. Res. **29:**448-462, 1950.

McNamara, J.: Neuromuscular and skeletal adaptation to altered orofacial function. Monograph No. 1, Craniofacial growth series, Ann Arbor, Mich., 1972, University of Michigan.

Moffett, J.C., Johnson, L.C., McGabe, J.B., and Askew, H.C.: Articulator remodelling in the adult human temporomandibular joint, Am. J. Anat. **115:**119, 1964.

Möller, E., Sheikholeslam, A., and Lous, I.: Response of elevator activity during mastication to treatment of functional disorders, Scand. J. Oral Dent. Res. **92**(1):64-83, 1984.

Moulton, R.: Oral and dental manifestations of anxiety, Psychiatry **18:**261-273, 1955.

Moyers, R.E.: Development of occlusion, Dent. Clin. North Am. **13:**523-536, 1969.

Niswonger, M.E.: The rest position of the mandible and the centric relation, J. Am. Dent. Assoc. **21:**1572-1582, 1934.

Pfeiffer, K.: Untersuchung über die Resilienz der durch die Prothesen beanspruchten Gewebe und ihre Bedeutung für die Okklusion der Prothesen, Schweiz. Monatsschr. Zahnheilkd. **39:**401-461, 1929.

Picton, D.C.A.: In Melcher, A.H., and Bowen, W.H., editors: Biology of the periodontium, New York, 1969, Academic Press, Inc., pp. 363-419.

Posselt, U.: Studies in the mobility of the human mandible, Acta Odontol. Scand. **10**(supp. 10):3-160, 1952.

Powell, R.N.: Tooth contact during sleep, master's thesis, University of Rochester, 1963 (I.A.D.R. **41:**72, 1963, abstract).

Ramfjord, S.P., and Ash, M.M.: Occlusion, ed. 2, Philadelphia, 1971, W.B. Saunders Co.

Sheppard, I.M., Rakoff, S., and Sheppard, S.M.: Bolus placement during mastication, J. Prosthet. Dent. **20:**506-510, 1968.

Sheppard, I.M., and Sheppard, S.M.: Denture occlusion, J. Prosthet. Dent. **26:**468-476, 1971.

Sheppard, I.M., Sheppard, S.M., and Rakoff, S.: Mandibular sideshift and lateral excursions, J. Oral Med. **22:**115-118, 1967.

Smith, D.E., Kydd, W.L., Wykhuis, W.A., and Phillips, L.A.: The mobility of artificial dentures during comminution, J. Prosthet. Dent. **13:**839-856, 1963.

Swoope, C.C., Jr., and Kydd, W.L.: The effect of cusp form and occlusal surface area on denture base deformation, J. Prosthet. Dent. 16:34-43, 1966.

Tallgren, A.: Changes in adult face height due to ageing, wear and loss of teeth and prosthetic treatment; a roentgen cephalometric study mainly on Finnish women, Acta Odontol. Scand. 15(supp. 24):1-122, 1957.

Tallgren, A.: An electromyographic study of the response of certain facial and jaw muscles to loss of teeth and subsequent complete denture treatment, Odontol. Tidskr. 69:384-430, 1961.

Tallgren, A.: Electromyographic study of the behaviour of certain facial and jaw muscles in long-term complete denture wearers, Odontol. Tidskr. 71:425-444, 1963.

Tallgren, A.: The reduction in face height of edentulous and partially edentulous subjects during long-term denture wear; a longitudinal roentgenographic cephalometric study, Acta Odontol. Scand. 24:195-239, 1966.

Tallgren, A.: The continuing reduction of the residual alveolar ridges in complete denture wearers: a mixed-longitudinal study covering 25 years, J. Prosthet. Dent. 27:120-132, 1972.

Thompson, J.R.: The constancy of the position of the mandible and its influence on prosthetic restorations, Illinois Dent. J. 12:242-247, 1943.

Thomson, J.C.: Diagnosis in full denture intolerance, Br. Dent. J. 125:388-391, 1968.

Thomson, J.C.: The load factor in complete denture intolerance, J. Prosthet. Dent. 25:4-11, 1971.

Toller, P.A.: Osteoarthrosis of the mandibular condyle, Br. Dent. J. 134:223-231, 1973.

Watt, D.M.: Morphological changes in the denture-bearing area following the extraction of maxillary teeth, doctoral dissertation, University of Edinburgh, 1961.

Woelfel, J.B., Hickey, J.C., and Allison, M.L.: Effect of posterior tooth form on jaw and denture movement, J. Prosthet. Dent. 12:922-939, 1962.

Yemm, R.: Stress-induced muscle activity: a possible etiologic factor in denture sorness, J. Prosthet. Dent. 28:133-140, 1972.

Zarb, G.A., and Thompson, G.W.: Assessment of clinical treatment of patients with temporomandibular joint dysfunction, J. Prosthet. Dent. 24:542-554, 1970.

Zarb, G.A.: Degenerative arthritis of the temporomandibular joint, Proceedings from Symposium at Northwestern University, Chicago, 1981.

Zarb, G.A.: Oral motor patterns and their relation to oral prostheses, J. Prosthet. Dent. 47:472, 1982.

2

Tissue response to complete dentures: the aging edentulous patient

A significant percentage of patients seeking complete denture treatment have already worn one or more sets of complete dentures. Their experiences should of course be analyzed by the dentist, and the resultant analysis used to design dentures that will significantly increase the possibilities of success with the new treatment. This approach will be reviewed in subsequent chapters. However it must be emphasized that long-term wear of dentures can lead to changes in the oral tissues. Furthermore these changes, or varying signs in wear and tear of denture-supporting tissues, must be reconciled with the possibility of similar or other tissue changes relating to aging. The purpose of this chapter is twofold: a review of the most frequently encountered sequelae of long-term denture wearing and a summary of the relevant oral changes associated with the aging edentulous masticatory system.

SOFT-TISSUE CHANGES

The response of human skin to everyday wear and tear is to become keratinized and tough. The oral mucosa does not behave in the same manner. Even in the dentulous state, the mucosa demonstrates a low tolerance to injury or irritation. This tolerance is further depleted if systemic disease is present. The mucosa does not appear to be suited to a complete denture load–

bearing role and demonstrates little or no ability to respond to this altered function. Östlund described denture-bearing mucosal changes as bordering on the pathologic but without frank clinical inflammation. He demonstrated a decrease in the keratinization of denture-bearing mucosa and a decrease in mucosal thickness. In his study, women wearing dentures appeared to have a thinner mucosa than men wearing dentures do and to demonstrate a greater predisposition to mucosal injury. He also showed that approximately one third of denture wearers with a clinically normal-appearing mucosa showed histologic evidence of severe injury. The extent of the injury was also related to the duration of the denture-wearing experience.

Cytologic examination of the denture-bearing mucosa has also demonstrated a depletion in keratinized cell counts (Zarb and associates, 1969). This depletion was related to both habits and duration of wear and to the clinical status of the dentures. The response of the oral epithelium to the placement of prostheses is controversial however, and some investigators (Kapur and Shklar, 1963; McMillan, 1972) maintain that the tissue response to denture wearing is an individual one. The pathologic significance of the noted changes has not been adequately explained. It is reasonable to suggest, however, that mucosal inflammation results from denture wear, and wherever inflammation is present, the process of bone resorption may be accelerated.

It appears that if the tolerance of the mucosal tissues is exceeded (as by an overextended denture border) injury and inflammation will result, and the denture cannot be worn. If, on the other hand, initial tolerance is high and the trauma tolerable, a fibrous response is elicited, and so the residual ridge is replaced with flabby hyperplastic tissue. Dentures are frequently worn over such tissue without discomfort. In between these two extremes lie the majority of patients, in whom chronic mucosal irritation proceeds quietly and painlessly. Mucosal and underlying bone changes are brought about, often irreversibly. It may be that the character

of the underlying bone determines the tolerance and the response of the denture-bearing mucosa.

Changes in both hard and soft tissues under complete dentures are common. They start soon after patients have been treated with such prostheses. Bergman and his associates (1964, 1972) showed a high incidence of mucosal inflammation within 1 year of denture construction and concluded that a new complete denture with a clinically good fit is no guarantee that mucosal inflammation will not develop in time. They also showed that there was a causal relationship between trauma and denture stomatitis and that the stomatitis was greater in those patients in whom the residual ridge was displaceable. They corroborated the results of Nyquist (1952), and underscored the importance of excising hyperplastic ridge tissue before prosthodontic therapy is started. Habits of denture wearers did not influence the incidence of mucosal irritation, but their observation period was of short duration. Round-the-clock denture wearing over a lifetime is conducive to an overloaded mucosal environment. This is especially valid when the incidence of nocturnal parafunction is remembered.

Clinical observation of many patients who have worn dentures continually reveals that they are more likely to have pseudoepitheliomatous hyperplasia and papillary hyperplasia.

Two examples of soft-tissue response to long-term denture wearing are frequently encountered: soft-tissue hyperplasia and denture stomatitis. Although these conditions are discussed separately, they can occur concurrently.

Soft-tissue hyperplasia

Hyperplasia of the soft tissues under or around a complete denture is the result of a fibroepithelial response to complete denture wearing. It is often asymptomatic and may be limited to the tissues around the borders of the dentures in the vestibular, lingual, or palatal regions, or it may occur on all or part of the residual ridge area (Fig. 2-1). Its etiology is mul-

A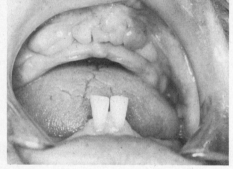

B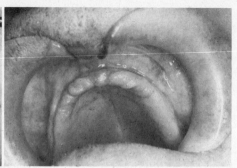

C

Fig. 2-1. A, Anterior maxillary residual ridge hyperplasia extends from one canine area to another. This patient wore a maxillary denture opposing four natural mandibular teeth. B, Entire maxillary alveolar ridge has been replaced by flabby hyperplastic tissue. C, Hyperplastic response involves both ridge and labial vestibule. Here again, two natural mandibular teeth opposed maxillary complete denture for several years.

tifactorial, and the following can be listed as probable causes:

1. Changes in the alveolar sockets after extractions
2. Trauma from denture wearing
3. Gradual residual ridge reduction
4. Changes in soft-tissue profile and temporomandibular joint function
5. Changes in the relative proportions of both jaws
6. Habits and duration of wear
7. Various aberrant forces to which the supporting tissues are subjected (e.g., natural lower anterior teeth opposing a complete upper denture), including parafunctional mandibular movement habits (Fig. 2-1, A and C)
8. Excessive forces on limited segments of the dental arches because of a lack of balancing contacts in eccentric jaw positions

The hyperplasia occurring around the border of a denture may be a fibrous growth referred to as *epulis fissuratum* (Fig. 2-2). It occurs in the free mucosa lining the sulcus or at the junction of the attached and free mucosa. It apparently develops as a result of chronic irritation from ill-fitting or overextended dentures. However, since residual ridges resorb, even the best fitting dentures gradually develop overextensions as a result of the dentures' settling into different positions on the basal seat. Clinical examination reveals that these tissues are usually hyperemic and swollen. Surgical excision of epulis fissuratum is indicated, but only after a period of prescribed tissue rest to reduce the edema. Clinical experience supports the value of advising patients to rest the irritated/overloaded tissues (keeping the dentures out with dentist's reduction of offending flanges) and to institute a program of regular and vigorous massage of the damaged site. Fig. 2-3 demonstrates the efficacy of such an approach. The "home treatment" program for this patient brought about the desired result in 6 weeks and obviated the need for a

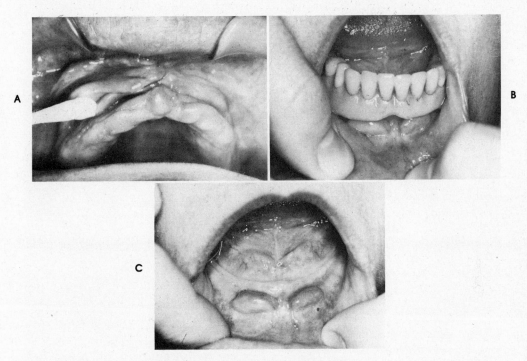

Fig. 2-2. Epulis fissuratum occurring around border of a maxillary denture, **A,** and around labial border of a mandibular denture, **B** and **C.**

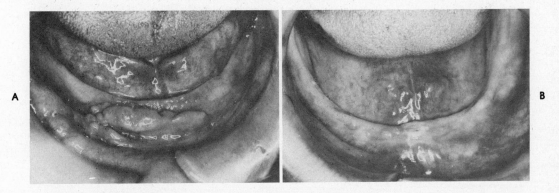

Fig. 2-3. A, Mucosal response to chronic irritation from a labial flange was treated by reduction of flange, tissue rest, use of a conditioner, and program of vigorous and regular finger massage. **B,** Impressive resolution of the soft tissue enlargement 6 weeks later.

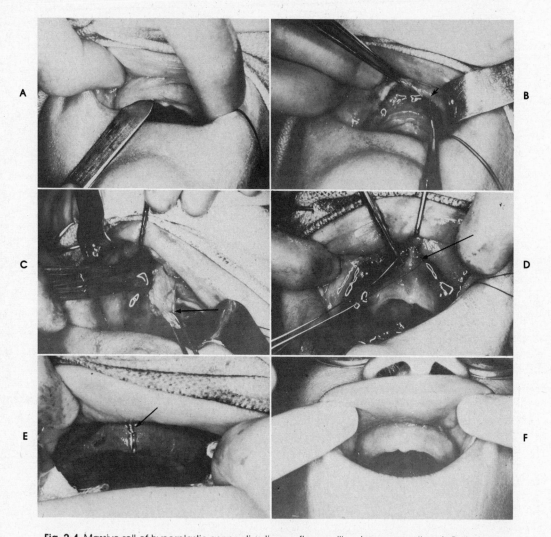

Fig. 2-4. Massive roll of hyperplastic connective tissue after maxillary bone resorption. **A,** Roll of movable connective tissue between upper lip and ridge. **B,** Incision is made so that as much oral mucosa as possible will be saved. **C,** Hyperplastic tissue is being removed. **D,** Ligature wire is passed around anterior nasal spine to support a splint. **E,** Acrylic resin splint is wired into position *(arrow)*. It should be pointed out that wiring of a splint is not always essential other than when a mucosal or skin graft is used to extend the depth of a vestibule. **F,** Residual ridge 6 months after surgery.

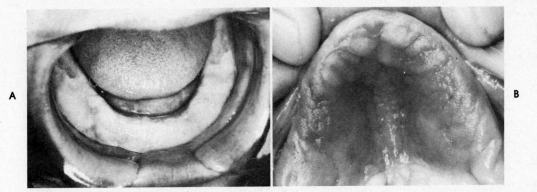

Fig. 2-5. A, Enlarged labial and buccal vestibule as a result of sulcus-deepening procedure with skin graft placement. **B,** Denture stomatitis of maxillary denture–bearing mucosa. A generalized hyperemic response is present.

surgical intervention. Although such a positive result is not always possible, it is clear that the inflammatory reduction makes a conservative surgical intervention possible.

During the surgical procedure all healthy mucous membrane is retained, and great care must be taken to avoid excising any attached mucosa, since otherwise the depth of the sulcus will be reduced (Fig. 2-4). If attached mucosa is absent over the residual ridge, a graft is usually placed and a splint is then placed to maintain the patency of the sulcus. Infrequently, the patient's old mandibular denture is modified to serve as a splint that is circumferentially wired into place for the first postoperative week. The modified old denture or the newly fabricated splint is usually lined with a plasticized resin treatment liner. This is worn postoperatively until adequate epithelization has taken place, which usually takes about 6 to 8 weeks. At that time the old dentures can be relined, or new ones can be made (see Chapter 6).

Hyperplastic tissue, which may replace the bone of the residual ridge, is incompatible with the demand for healthy denture-supporting tissues and should be excised. Many efforts have been made either to build dentures over these flabby ridges (Kelly, 1972) or to seek to convert them into firm ridges by the injection of sclero-

sing solutions into them (Laskin, 1970). Clinical experience supports the value of surgical excision of the hyperplastic tissue in most patients where it exists. Here, again, principles of tissue rest and surgical principles of extreme conservation are indispensable. The risks of sulcus obliteration are often high, and the need for a vestibuloplasty must always be kept in mind. Obwegeser (1959) reported a high incidence of success for oral sulcus–deepening procedures accompanied by a skin graft placement (Fig. 2-5, *A*). The use of the modified old denture or the fabrication of splints for use after sulcus deepening is similar to that described earlier.

Wallenius and Heyden (1972) carried out a histochemical study of flabby ridges and demonstrated extensive inflammatory reactions of the fibrotic tissues. There was a positive correlation between the degree of inflammation and vascular reactions and bone resorption. The flabby hyperplastic ridges found in denture wearers should be excised to minimize the progressive resorption of residual ridges. Nordenram and Landt (1969) found lesions of denture hyperplasia to have a higher incidence in the older patients (50 to 80 years), a higher incidence in women (81.2%) than in men, an incidence of 44.5% in patients with a long-term denture-wearing experience (15 years), an absence of symptoms or discomfort in 37.2% of patients, and an almost equal incidence in the upper and lower jaws, with the anterior part of either jaw being the most common site.

Denture stomatitis

Denture stomatitis is a chronic inflammation of the denture-bearing mucosa (the basal seat), and it may be localized or generalized in nature (Fig. 2-5, *B*). Some investigators (Nyquist, 1952; Bergman and associates, 1964) believe that trauma from ill-fitting dentures or a parafunctional habit is the predominant etiologic factor. Bergendal (1982) observed that nocturnal denture wear was related to denture stomatitis. A few authors have suggested a hypersensitivity to some component of the denture material with consequent allergic response or infection with *Candida albicans* and poor oral denture hygiene, (Bergendal, 1982; Budtz-Jørgensen and Bertram, 1970).

The possibility that denture stomatitis is of an allergic nature was investigated by Turrell (1966), and he concluded that the concentration of residual monomer in properly cured acrylic resin is unlikely to elicit a clinical response. It is possible for denture base materials to acquire antigenic properties as a result of a continuous absorption of such fluids as cleansing agents, foods, or drugs. Also, as dentures become increasingly ill-fitting, tissue trauma is produced that could make tissues more susceptible to any allergen imbibed by the dentures over the years. Infection from poor oral and denture hygiene can aggravate the condition.

Definite conclusions have not been reached concerning the allergic potentiality of nonmetallic denture base materials. It is recognized, however, that a denture that has been worn for some time may absorb fluids that may be capable of promoting an allergic response. Clinic experience indicates that this is a tenable perspective and that the majority of stomatitis conditions are caused by trauma and a superimposed fungal infection (Budtz-Jørgensen and Bertram, 1970).

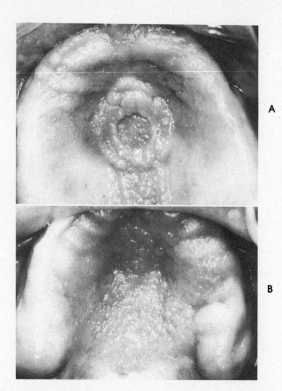

Fig. 2-6. Palatal papillomatosis. **A,** Condition is localized to midpalatal region as result of patient's wearing a maxillary denture with a suction cup. **B,** Papillomatosis covers entire palatal surface and extends distally past the location where posterior palatal seal of the denture would contact palatal mucosa.

Most patients with denture stomatitis are unaware of their lesion, since it is frequently asymptomatic. A small number of the patients complain of a burning or itching sensation that is usually related to both the palatal and glossal mucosa. The inflammation varies in intensity; it may be localized in isolated areas or may involve the entire basal seat. It tends to occur more frequently in the maxillary arch than in the mandibular arch. Occasionally a granular type of palatal inflammation—papillary hyperplasia, or papillomatosis—is seen (Fig. 2-6). Papillary hyperplasia should not be considered to be an entirely innocuous lesion. Some authors (Shaffer and associates, 1974) suggest that the best treatment is surgical excision.

The incidence of papillary hyperplasia is related to the presence of relief chambers in dentures (Fig. 2-7) and to the relief-chamber effect that can develop as a result of uneven settling of a maxillary denture. Some believe that the chronic irritation resulting from a make-and-break alternating vacuum created under the denture elicits the papillary inflammatory response. The appearance of papillary projections covering variable amounts of the hard palate is characteristic. It must be emphasized that this lesion is frequently camouflaged by a thick mucus-saliva film, and the palatal mucosa should be carefully dried before it is examined. The frequency of papillomatosis appears to be higher in patients who wear their denture throughout the 24-hour day (Love and associates, 1967), and patients should be urged to rest the tissues of the mouth by removing their dentures at night or other comparable periods.

Recent research by Bergendal (1982) concluded that the presence of microbial plaque and yeasts on the fitting surface of the denture base appeared to be of critical importance for development and maintenance of denture stomatitis.

Treatment of denture stomatitis. The best treatment for denture stomatitis is to prevent it. Good oral and dental hygiene and rest for the tissues of the basal seat are essential. Other treatment of denture stomatitis includes the construction of new well-fitting dentures after achievement of a healthy condition of the mucosa, the use of tissue conditioners in existing or treatment dentures, indirect relining of existing dentures with autopolymerizing resins (Olsson and Bergman, 1971), use of antifungal drugs (Cawson, 1963a, b; Budtz-Jørgensen and Bertram, 1970), the use of a 2% solution of chlorhexidine gluconate (Budtz-Jørgensen and Löe, 1972), or gingival massage with a toothbrush or fingers.

The following clinical procedures are recommended and are employed singly or in combination, depending on the severity of the condition.

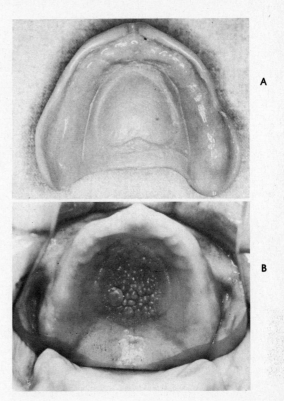

Fig. 2-7. Arbitrary relief chamber in a maxillary denture, **A,** has caused a papillomatosis response, **B.** Note conformity of lesion to outline of relief areas.

1. Oral and denture hygiene accompanied by tissue rest. Tissue rest is achieved by removal of the dentures or by use of a tissue conditioner, occlusal adjustment, and technical improvement of the existing dentures.

2. Antifungal therapy. One can be instituted antifungal therapy after an elective verification of *Candida* infection using a palatal smear. A therapeutic dose of one nystatin tablet taken three times a day for 10 to 14 days is usually sufficient to control the infection. Antifungal therapy may be required for up to 4 weeks for some patients. If the dentures are not relined with a tissue conditioner, they must be kept impeccably clean, and a chelating agent with a mixture of enzymes (MacCallum and associates,

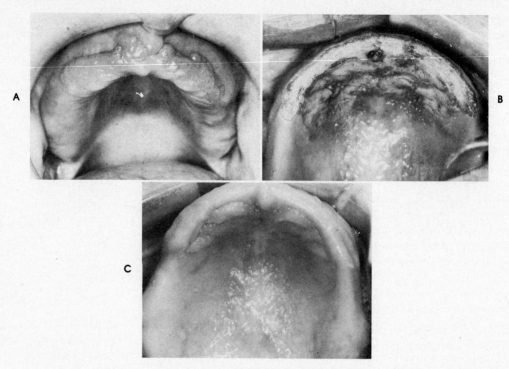

Fig. 2-8. A, Papillomatosis and anterior maxillary ridge hyperplasia have been treated surgically. **B,** Immediate postoperative appearance of the surgically treated palate. **C,** Six weeks later, epithelization is complete.

1968) or chlorhexidine (Budtz-Jørgensen and Löe, 1972) may be used. This form of therapy is usually applied when there is generalized stomatitis, especially of a symptomatic nature.

Recent research (Bergendal, 1982) demonstrated that nystatin treatment was promptly followed by recolonization of yeasts. It is therefore suggested that antimycotic drugs should not be used in the routine treatment of denture stomatites. Furthermore patients whose microbial plaque and yeast scores from the denture base decreased when the denture stomatites healed also showed an accompanying disappearance of their angular cheilitis and glossitis.

3. Surgical excision of papillomatosis (Fig. 2-8). Excision is only undertaken after other methods of treatment have been used. The surgery is easier and more conservative after pretreatment

because of the diminished inflammation. Electrosurgery is frequently used to excise maxillary papillary hyperplasia. Recently cryosurgery has been used with good results. A treatment liner should be placed inside the denture postoperatively and changed weekly until epithelization is completed. It must be emphasized that papillomatosis is an irreversible lesion, which by virtue of its morphology can act as an excellent nidus for the accumulation of plaque and fungal growth. Its surgical elimination is frequently necessary as a prerequisite for optimal hygiene. When it occasionally extends to or past the junction of the hard and soft palate, great care must be paid to its excision, since scar band formation in this area can seriously interfere with the development of a future posterior palatal seal. The maxillary denture may be rebased or a new

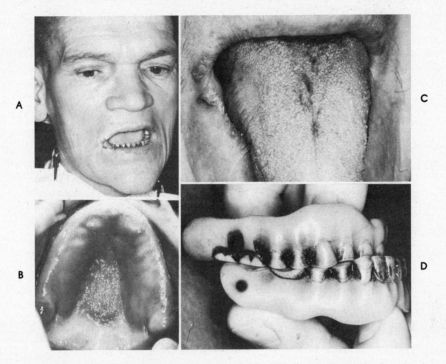

Fig. 2-9. Angular cheilitis, **A,** accompanying a case of denture stomatitis, **B.** The tongue also demonstrates presence of a glossitis, **C.** Gross loss of vertical dimension of occlusion and patient neglect are self-evident, **D.**

denture constructed when healing is completed after an interval of 6 to 8 weeks.

Denture stomatitis is occasionally accompanied by an angular stomatitis (a painful inflammation of the corners of the mouth), which is also known as *angular cheilitis,* or *perlèche* (Fig. 2-9). For several years this clinical condition was attributed to a reduction of the vertical dimension of occlusion or to riboflavin and thiamine deficiency. Although either of these situations can predispose to an angular stomatitis, Cawson (1963a, b), Mäkilä (1969), and Bergendal (1982) have shown that this condition is usually secondary to a denture stomatitis and usually the result of *Candida* infection from contaminated saliva. Angular stomatitis can respond to antifungal therapy and supplementary antifungal ointment application at the lesion's site (Fig. 2-10). How-

ever its recurrence is frequently related to denture stomatitis, and a combined treatment approach is mandatory. Mäkilä indicated its higher incidence in women and in denture wearers. Age does not seem to affect its incidence nor does the duration of the edentulous period. It can occur unilaterally or bilaterally and is infrequently accompanied by an atrophic glossitis.

Denture sore mouth

Rarely, one encounters mucosal complaints that do not fit into the general description of denture stomatitis. These complaints are conveniently grouped as a "denture sore mouth" syndrome, and the condition is usually determined when the treatment methods just outlined have been unsuccessful. Clinical experience suggests

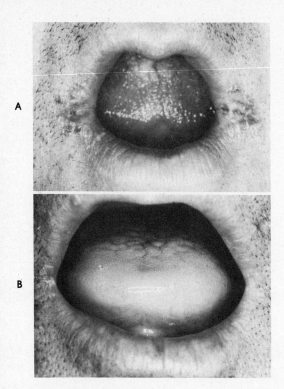

Fig. 2-10. Angular stomatitis lesion that responded to antifungal therapy. **A,** Before. **B,** After.

that denture sore mouth is probably the result of an underlying abnormal metabolic or hormonal function or a nutritional deficiency, for example, alcoholism.

Patients with psychologic problems may occasionally fall into this picture. The symptoms are a bizarre spectrum of itching, painful, irritated, and tender denture-bearing mucosa. Clinical findings are frequently negative, and it appears that in such patients mucosal tolerance is extremely low, without any visible clinical or laboratory signs. It should be pointed out that these symptoms can also be produced by tranquilizers used in the management of psychiatric disorders, and so these drugs can further complicate the diagnosis.

Iron deficiency, insufficient protein, and incomplete intestinal absorption have been cit-ed as contributory factors. Patients presenting with this syndrome should be referred to a physician for a thorough systemic analysis, which may identify the underlying cause of causes of the sore mouth. Medical treatment may consist of a high-protein diet, avoidance of local irritants, slow-release hydrogen chloride supplement in the achlorhydric patient, ascorbic acid tablets dissolved sublingually, and occasionally psychiatric help. Perhaps because of the rather vague nature of denture sore mouth, there is no real consensus about its treatment.

EFFECTS OF AGING

Time leaves its imprint on every living thing, and this principle applies to all the successive levels of organization—molecule, cell, tissue, organ, and organism. A diagrammatic representation (Fig. 2-11, *A*) of the human life-span reveals a period of gradual development of increasing body efficiency in childhood and adolescence until what we call maturity is reached. After a long period of little change, a gradual decline in powers, especially physical ones, occurs. This is commonly referred to as the period of senescence. The time at which age changes become evident is quite variable, and many of the changes can actually occur early. Almost as soon as human beings have passed adolescence, deteriorative changes begin in some tissues. Therefore the curve begins to slope downward slightly from the point of maturation. Degenerative changes in joints have been detected as early as 25 to 30 years of age (De Palma, 1957; Davies, 1961). The vascular changes characteristic of old age can be detected almost as early (McMillan, 1969). Other changes such as reduction in muscle strength begin later.

Much evidence has accumulated to indicate that this state of ultimate decline is an intrinsic part of the nature of all multicellular organisms. The aging process is insidious and is characterized by individual variation in onset and rate of decline. It includes biologic changes in cardiac output, secretion of digestive juices, decrease in muscular coordination, and decline in endocrine

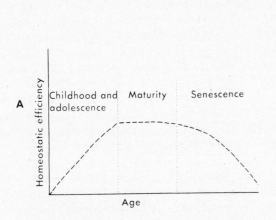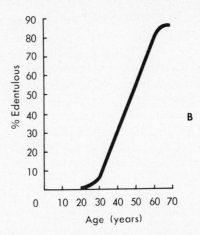

Fig. 2-11. A, Simple diagram of human life-span. **B,** Composite picture of correlation between age (years) and incidence of the edentulous state in several Western countries. (**A,** Modified from Miles, A.E.W.: Proc. R. Soc. Med. **65:**801-806, 1972.)

activity. On the psychologic level, the aging process is characterized by an increase in reaction time, a slowing of the learning process, and a decline in memory and intellectual efficiency. These changes are reflected in a gradual diminution of the individual's adaptability. Homeostasis of the *milieu intérieur* is maintained with greater difficulty. Many aspects of aging have been studied in a representative population, and the inadequacy of any single criterion of biologic age was demonstrated. An assessment of the biologic age in relation to the chronologic age is an important aid to correct treatment planning. A chronologically old person in whom these changes have been delayed is said to be biologically young. If, however, the changes occur comparatively early in life, a patient is described as being biologically old even though he or she may be young in years. The clinician has no alternative but to make subjective judgments, which are imprecise but nonetheless valuable.

Although most living tissues retain a capacity to repair or renew themselves, the dentition is a notable exception. Surveys in various parts of the world confirm the high percentage of edentulous patients among elderly people (Fig. 2-11, *B*). Hence the popular conviction that geriatric

dentistry consists largely in the oral rehabilitation of edentulous patients. The outlook for future decades also appears to be one of prosthodontic treatment for the elderly patient.

Regardless of what happens in preventive and restorative dentistry, a number of 40-year-old persons of today will be the geriatric edentulous patients of tomorrow, and many of this group have already lost their teeth. Furthermore, life expectancy is longer today, and there are more people. Patients who started wearing complete dentures in their thirties or forties will pose staggering prosthodontic problems, and time and long-term denture wearing will continue to exact a biologic price from their oral supporting tissues.

ORAL ASPECTS OF AGING

The oral aspects of aging have received increasing attention (Shepherd, 1967; Krogman, 1962; Taylor and Doku, 1963; Winkler, 1977). The effects of aging on the edentulous geriatric patient include (1) oral mucosa and skin changes, (2) residual bone and maxillomandibular relation changes, (3), tongue and taste changes, (4) salivary flow changes and nutritional impairment, and (5) psychologic changes.

Oral mucosa and skin changes

The clinical picture is one of atrophy. The epithelial layers are less in number, and the mucosa and submucosa show a decrease in thickness. This actual thinning of the tissues, coupled with its depleted repair potential, renders the denture-bearing mucosa of the basal seat friable and easily traumatized (Fig. 2-12). Massler (1971) attributes the vulnerability of mucosa to a shift in the water balance from the intracellular to the extracellular compartment of the tissues. Diminished kidney function may also result in dehydration of the tissues. The tissue cells may become nutritionally deficient. Younger edentulous patients tend to have denture-bearing mucosa and submucosa of considerable thickness. On the other hand, edentulous mucosa of the elderly is frequently thin and tightly stretched, and it blanches easily. Lammie (1960) believed that a mucosa of reduced thickness is associated with reduced residual ridge height. He postulated that epithelial atrophy, which results in a reduction in the number of epithelial cell layers and the thickness of the underlying connective tissues, also manifests itself in a reduction of the surface area of the oral mucosa. This in turn applies pressure to the underlying ridge. The externally applied molding force meets more or less resistance from the bone itself, and this is the action involved in the resorption process. Newton (1964) studied age changes in the collagen fibers of the oral mucosa. He showed that these shorten to a degree compatible with the concept of a contracting mucosa acting as a molding force on alveolar bone.

An atrophying denture-bearing mucosa is frequently encountered during menopause. The reduction in estrogen output is known to have an atrophic effect on epithelial surfaces. The number of cell layers is reduced as is the potentially for keratinization. In addition, there is a reduction in surface area that affects the genital epithelium, oral mucosa, and skin. Clinical experience indicates that hormonal replacement therapy can be beneficial in such patients to create a more favorable oral environment of the dentures.

It must be clear to the reader that the points made in Chapter 1, in the discussion of stress

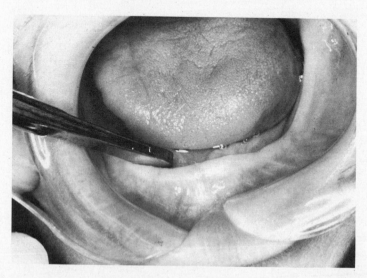

Fig. 2-12. Thin, nonresilient, mandibular denture–bearing mucosa, which blanches easily and is easily traumatized.

distribution to denture-supporting tissues, become particularly relevant when one is dealing with patients with compromised mucosal support. These patients' mucosal tissues need extra care, that is, frequent application of soft liners (tissue conditioners), as well as counseling in tissue handling and cleansing.

Similar changes take place in the skin, which may appear loose and wrinkled, or tight, smooth, and thin. A person's skin is changing throughout life. Lee (1962) described young skin as smooth and having a dull sheen because of the almost microscopic pattern of tiny grooves that divide the surface into rhomboidal areas. This network of fine grooves is the outward view of the pattern of the junction between the epithelium and its supporting lamina propria. As the skin ages, its surface loses its fine pattern, and the skin loses its elasticity. The concomitant atrophy occurring in the structures beneath the skin leads to even more noticeable changes in the face. The muscles, fat, and connective tissue all diminish in bulk. There is more skin than is needed to cover them, and so it droops into folds and exaggerates the creases, which become

more obvious (Figs. 2-13 to 2-15). Although the position of these creases is not constant for all persons, there is a certain uniformity in their distribution. As the elastic property of the skin is decreased, the lines in the base of the creases become more permanent.

These skin changes cannot be compensated for by prosthodontics, and they can severely compromise the esthetic opportunities of the denture service. The skin changes should be brought to the patient's attention before the denture treatment is started, as mentioned in the previous chapter.

Residual bone and maxillomandibular relation changes

The gross reduction of the height of maxillary and mandibular residual ridges is often a result of long-term wear of complete dentures (Chapter 1). It has been assumed that ridge resorption is an inevitable accompaniment of denture wearing, but there is a lack of longitudinal analyses of residual ridge height in edentulous people who have not worn dentures (Campbell, 1960).

Disuse atrophy. Flat residual ridges, distal to

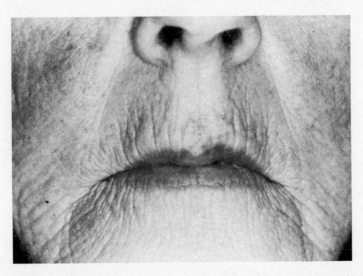

Fig. 2-13. Age changes in skin around mouth. Loss of elasticity results in network of wrinkles, which are conspicuous and impossible to camouflage by prosthetic therapy.

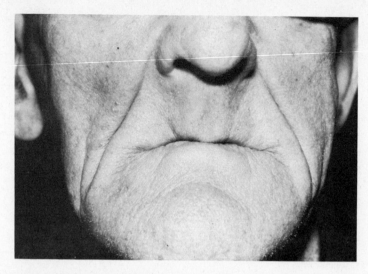

Fig. 2-14. Age changes in skin of face. Natural folds and creases are exaggerated, and with time the lines in the base of the creases become permanent.

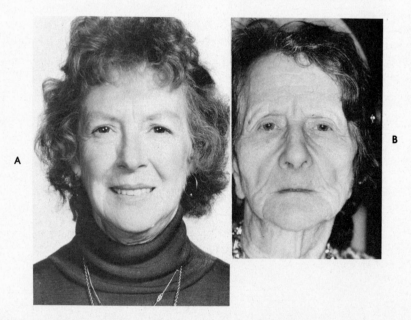

Fig. 2-15. Both patients **A** and **B** are in their sixties. Patient **A** demonstrates facial skin changes that do not parallel her chronologic age, or the resultant effects of long-term denture wear. The cosmetic aspects of her prosthodontic treatment are not likely to be very demanding at a morphologic level. On the other hand, patient **B** combines the cosmetic sequelae illustrated in Figs. 2-13 and 2-14. Optimal prosthodontic treatment will compensate only minimally for the biologic and chronologic effects of aging.

natural teeth, are frequently seen, and several dentists have attributed ridge reduction in these regions to disuse atrophy. Carlsson and associates (1967) carried out a clinical and radiographic study of the changes in ridge height in partially edentulous patients. Bilateral distal extension mandibular edentulous spans were restored by removable partial dentures in some persons and not restored in others. No disuse atrophy was observed over the 2-year follow-up period. The fact that atrophy of residual ridges has not yet been demonstrated in controlled research reinforces the notion that denture wearing is potentially stressful and damaging to the underlying bone.

Changes in the size of the basal seat. Aging is frequently accompanied by osteoporotic changes in the human skeleton, but the relationship between this condition and the jaws has not been adequately studied.

By observing the axial inclination of the natural teeth in a human skull, one can envision the direction of residual ridge reduction subsequent to tooth loss (Figs. 2-16 to 2-18). Maxillary teeth generally flare downward and outward so that

bone reduction is generally upward and inward. Since the outer cortical plate is thinner than the inner cortical plate, resorption from the outer cortex would be greater and more rapid. As the maxillary residual ridges are reduced, the maxillae become smaller in all dimensions and the denture-bearing (basal seat) surface decreases.

The anterior mandibular teeth generally incline upward and forward to the occlusal plane, whereas the posterior teeth either are vertical or incline slightly lingually. The outer cortex is generally thicker than the lingual cortex, except in the molar region. Also, the width of the mandible is greatest at its inferior border. As a result, the mandibular residual ridge appears to migrate lingually and inferiorly in the anterior region and to migrate buccally in the posterior region. Consequently, the mandibular arch appears either to remain static or to become wider posteriorly as resorption progresses. This discrepancy in relative jaw sizes can pose several technical problems for the dentist because failure to place the artificial teeth in the positions of the natural teeth can jeopardize denture support and stability. Obviously, the

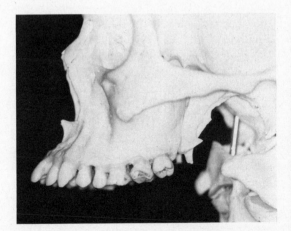

Fig. 2-16. Direction of roots and alveolar process of anterior maxillary teeth is clearly suggested. This is the direction of residual ridge reduction that usually takes place.

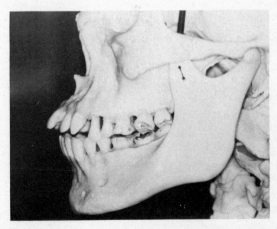

Fig. 2-17. In the mandible, the pattern of residual ridge reduction tends to be downward and backward. Relate to Fig. 1-10 to compare the morphologic pattern of resorption as deduced from longitudinal studies.

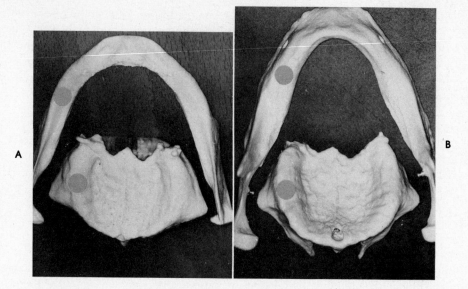

Fig. 2-18. Maxillae and mandibles in different stages of resorption and compared to illustrate the clinical observation that the maxilla becomes narrower and the mandible wider, as progressive resorption modifies jaw morphology. The centers of the ridges are almost aligned in **A,** but not in **B** after resorption has taken place.

attempt to restore the original arch contour occupied by the natural teeth can be limited by the effects of aging on the adjacent and surrounding tissues.

There are changes also in the vertical maxillomandibular relations with the passage of time (see Chapter 1). Muscle changes occur, and these changes, coupled with residual ridge reduction, bring about a spatial alteration in the position of the mandible relative to that of the maxillae. These changes must be recognized and assessed in the context of the patient's desired or anticipated facial support from new dentures. An accurate assessment must be made of the proposed interarch and interocclusal distances in the elderly person receiving complete dentures.

Such an assessment must take into account the possibility that a certain amount of the reduction of vertical dimension of occlusion (or increased freeway space) is permanent, and an attempt to restore a so-called normal vertical may cause the patient discomfort.

Tongue and taste changes

A common nodular varicose enlargement of the superficial veins on the undersurface of the tongue is frequently seen (Fig. 2-19). Bean (1956) noted an association between these sublingual varicosities and the minute spidery nevi that tend to appear on the skin in advanced age. Kleinman (1967) confirmed that these varicosities do not have any significant association with cardiac or pulmonary dysfunction. Occasionally these varicosities may lead to cancerphobia, and the patient should be reassured about their insignificance.

The tongue frequently becomes smooth and glossy or red and inflamed in appearance. A variety of symptoms can center on the lingual mucosa with complaints of soreness, burning, or abnormal taste sensations. These sensations are common in both elderly people and postmenopausal women. It is not uncommon for these symptoms to be related to the posterior region of the tongue margin, that is, the region of the foliate papillae (Miles, 1972). These papillae can

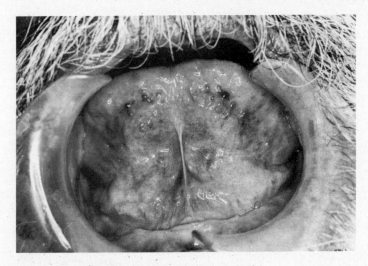

Fig. 2-19. Varicose enlargement of superficial veins on undersurface of tongue. These varicosities appear to be innocuous.

appear red and projecting and may be a cause for alarm for some patients who must be reassured that this is not a proliferating neoplasm. On the other hand, persistent soreness in this region can occur and is usually eliminated by excision of the sore papillae. Vitamin B therapy has been frequently administered to patients complaining of a sore or burning tongue. The clinical results have often been successful. It must be remembered that the tongue can undergo various changes with age, and there appears to be a tendency for the number of taste buds to diminish. Focal collections of chronic inflammatory cells are also common, and this may be because of ingress of microorganisms or their toxins through the thin epithelium of this region.

Tongue thrusting associated with nervous tension or with attempts to control a lower denture can also lead to a sore tongue. The size of the tongue probably does not vary with age. However, tooth loss can lead to a wider tongue by virtue of an overdevelopment of some parts of the tongue's intrinsic musculature. Constant and habitual attempts to keep a loose maxillary denture in place can cause these changes. The effect of this on subsequent denture wearing must not be overlooked.

Lingual tissue changes may be accompanied by alterations in the sense of taste. Taste bud atrophy may lead to loss of appetite, which in turn can adversely affect tongue comfort as a manifestation of nutritional deficiency. Older patients frequently blame their dentures for a changed sense of taste and a burning sensation of their tongue. Reassurance and diet counseling are necessary to overcome these symptoms.

Salivary flow changes and nutritional impairment

A dryness of the mouth may be evident in some patients. This xerostomia may be related to medication the patient is taking, usually for gastric complaints or for depression and insomnia. It also may reflect a diminution in salivary flow resulting from atrophy of the salivary glands. Regardless of the cause, it may lead to a diminished facility for mastication, digestive upsets, and sometimes poor retention of the dentures. The dryness of the mucosa renders it more susceptible to frictional irritation from denture movement and may interfere with patients' ability to wear their dentures.

Some older patients, on the other hand, may produce excessive saliva on insertion of new dentures. This effect is a transient one and can be controlled by explanation of the cause to the patient, reassurance, and antisialagogue administration, if necessary.

Degenerative changes. The cumulative degenerative changes that develop are often accompanied by a reduced neuromuscular coordination. This manifests itself as impaired adaptability and a consequent reduction of masticatory ability. It is possible that several or all of the biologic changes accompanying aging can be present in any one patient. Collectively, they can be the cause of nutritional impairment by altering dietary and nutritional habits (Jamieson, 1958).

Dietary problems. Most dietary problems in the elderly may be said to be caused by the following*:

1. Low income and the lack of knowledge of how to spend the money available for food to the best advantage
2. Physical handicaps, debility, and a lack of mobility, which make shopping and food preparation difficult
3. Poor facilities for food preparation
4. Poor dentitions, especially dentures, which may cause the wearer to reject some essential foods that are difficult to chew, without the inclusion of a suitable substitute
5. Existing food habits which may result in the choice of a poor diet
6. Depression, boredom, anxiety, and loneliness, which give little or no incentive for the preparation of nourishing meals

Studies of the elderly have shown that they are susceptible to subclinical, if not frank clinical, malnutrition. The relationship between the integrity of the masticatory system throughout the life-span and the nutritional status of a person has not been thoroughly or conclusively elucidated. However, clinical experience indicates that mucosal tissue intolerance in edentulous

*From Ettinger, R. L.: Diet, nutrition, and masticatory ability in a group of elderly edentulous patients, Aust. Dent. J. **18:**12-19, 1973.

patients frequently responds to nutritional supplements and dietary counseling. Patient instruction in the use and the shortcomings of their complete dentures and diet counseling are integral parts of prosthodontic therapy.

Current research suggests that systemic processes are operant in alveolar ridge resorption. Although such resorption can occur in any age group, it tends to be more conspicuous in the elderly edentulous patient. Among the many recognized systemic influences that affect bone resorption and resistance, calcium deficiencies and calcium-phosphorus imbalances have been specifically implicated (Wical and Swoope, 1974). Wical and Brusse (1979) investigated the effects of calcium and vitamin D dietary supplements on postextraction alveolar bone resorption. Their 1-year results demonstrate a retardation in bone resorption, and they make a good case for consideration of such ridge reduction as a manifestation of osteoporosis. This is an exciting hypothesis and one that expands the complexity and research scope of residual ridge resorption. Hopefully, longitudinal observation of a large number of patients treated with such supplements will be undertaken, especially since the efficacy, safety, economy, and convenience of such a dietary supplement method make it a rational prosthetic procedure.

Psychologic changes

It is important to have some understanding of the psychology of human aging to be able to appreciate the difference between behavioral disorders that are associated with organic brain disease and those that are not. Organic brain damage creates an almost impossible predicament for prosthetic treatment. In senile dementia, for example, an irreversible deterioration of intellectual faculties develops, and the patient is frequently hostile, withdrawn, and virtually incapable of adjusting to any prosthesis. Such patients are probably best treated by the eradication of oral disease and dietary changes to accommodate to their modified dentition or their nonexistent prostheses.

Geriatric patients can demonstrate a high incidence of depression and feelings of insecurity and experience vague and often bizarre pains and fears. Nervous habits like tooth clenching may develop, and this places extra stress on tissues that already have a diminished capacity to deal with the loadings. Older patients are also more likely to be using drugs, and care must be taken to understand the clinical dental implications of such drug use.

Tissue distortion can result from medication taken for edema caused by kidney or cardiac dysfunction, from fatigue, or from changes in fluid intake. Tissue distortion can seriously affect impression making, and it is recommended that morning appointments be organized to ensure minimal tissue distortion from edema.

Reassurance, tolerance, and a versatile clinical approach can usually help the elderly obtain satisfactory prosthodontic results.

REFERENCES

Bean, W.B.: Changing incidence of certain vascular lesions of the skin with aging, Geriatrics 11:97-102, 1956.

Bergendal, T.: Treatment of denture stomatitis, doctoral thesis, Stockholm, 1982.

Bergman, B., and Carlsson, G.E.: Review of 54 complete denture wearers; patients' opinions 1 year after treatment, Acta Odontol. Scand. 30:399-414, 1972.

Bergman, B., Carlsson, G.E., and Hedegård, B.: A longitudinal two-year study of a number of full denture cases, Acta Odontol. Scand. 22:3-26, 1964.

Budtz-Jørgensen, E., and Bertram, U.: Denture stomatitis I and II, Acta Odontol. Scand. 28:71-92, 283-304, 1970.

Budtz-Jørgensen, E., and Löe, H.: Chlorhexidine as a denture disinfectant in the treatment of denture stomatitis, Scand. J. Dent. Res. 80:457-464, 1972.

Campbell, R.L.: A comparative study of the resorption of the alveolar ridges in denture wearers and non-denture-wearers, J. Am. Dent. Assoc. 60:143-153, 1960.

Carlsson, G.E., Ragnarsson, N., and Åstrand, P.: Changes in height of the alveolar process in edentulous segments, Odontol. I. 75:193-208, 1967.

Cawson, R.A.: Denture sore mouth and angular cheilitis, Br. Dent. J. 115:441-449, 1963a.

Cawson, R.A.: Symposium on denture sore mouth. II. The role of Candida, Dent. Pract. 16:138-142, 1963b.

Davies, D.V.: In Bourne, G.H., and Wilson, E.M.H., editors: Structural aspects of ageing, London, 1961. Pitman Medical Publishing Co., Ltd., pp. 25-37.

De Palma, A.F.: Degenerative changes in the sternoclavicular and acromioclavicular joints in various decades, Springfield, Ill., 1957, Charles C Thomas, Publisher.

Ettinger, R.L.: Diet, nutrition, and masticatory ability in a group of elderly edentulous patients, Aust. Dent. J. 18:12-19, 1973.

Jamieson, C.H.: Geriatrics and the denture patient, J. Prosthet. Dent. 8:8-13, 1958.

Kapur, K., and Shklar, G.: The effect of complete dentures on alveolar mucosa, J. Prosthet. Dent. 13:1030-1037, 1963.

Kelly, E.: Changes caused by a mandibular removable partial denture opposing a maxillary complete denture, J. Prosthet. Dent. 27:140-150, 1972.

Kleinman, H.Z.: Lingual varicosities, Oral Surg. 23:546-548, 1967.

Krogman, W.M.: Geriatric research and prosthodontics, J. Prosthet. Dent. 12:493-515, 1962.

Lammie, G.A.: The reduction of the edentulous ridges, J. Prosthet. Dent. 10:605-611, 1960.

Laskin, D.M.: A sclerosing procedure for hypermobile edentulous ridges, J. Prosthet. Dent. 23:274-278, 1970.

Lee, J.H.: Dental aesthetics, Bristol, 1962, John Wright & Sons, Ltd.

Love, W.D., Goska, F.A., and Mixson, R.J.: The etiology of mucosal inflammation, J. Prosthet. Dent. 18:515-527, 1967.

MacCallum, M., et al.: Which cleanser? Dent. Pract. 19:83-89, 1968.

Mäkilä, E.: Prevalence of angular stomatitis; correlation with composition of food and metabolism of vitamins and iron, Acta Odontol. Scand. 27:655-680, 1969.

Massler, M.: Oral aspects of aging, Postgrad. Med. 49:179, 1971.

McMillan, D.R.: The cytological response of palatal mucosa to dentures, Dent. Pract. 22:302-304, 1972.

McMillan, G.C.: In Bittar, E.E., and Bittar, N., editors: The biologic basis of medicine, ed. 6, New York, 1969, Academic Press, Inc., pp. 235-255.

Miles, A.E.W.: Changes in oral tissues with advancing age, Proc. R. Soc. Med. 65:801-806, 1972.

Newton, A.V.: Factor affecting the resilience of connective tissues, Dent. Pract. 14:289-292, 1964.

Nordenram, A., and Landt, H.: Hyperplasia of the oral tissues in denture cases, Acta Odontol. Scand. 27:481-491, 1969.

Nyquist, G.: A study of denture sore mouth, Acta Odontol. Scand. 10(supp. 9):11-154, 1952.

Obwegeser, H.: Die submuköse Vestibulumplastik, Dtsch. Zahnaerztl. Z. 14:749, 1959.

Olsson, K.A., and Bergman, B.: A comparison of two prosthetic methods for the treatment of denture stomatitis, Acta Odontol. Scand. 29:745-753, 1971.

Shaffer, W.G., Hine, M.K., and Levy, B.M.: Oral pathology, ed. 2, Philadelphia, 1974, W.B. Saunders Co.

Shepherd, R.W.: Prosthetic treatment for the older patient, Aust. Dent. J. 12:339-342, 1967.

Taylor, R.G., and Doku, H.C.: Dental survey of healthy older persons, J. Am. Dent. Assoc. 67:63-70, 1963.

Turrell, A.S.W.: Aetiology of inflamed upper denture-bearing tissues, Br. Dent. J. 118:542-546, 1966.

Wallenius, K., and Heyden, G.: Histochemical studies of flabby ridges, Odontol. Revy 23:169-179, 1972.

Wical, K.E., and Brusse, P.: Effects of calcium and vitamin D supplement on alveolar ridge resorption in immediate denture patients, J. Prosthet. Dent. **41**:4-11, 1979.

Wical, K.E., and Swoope, C.C.: Studies of residual ridge resorption. II. The relationship of dietary calcium and phosphorus to residual ridge resorption, J. Prosthet. Dent. **32**:13-22, 1974.

Winkler, S.: The geriatric complete denture patient, Dent. Clin. North Am. **21**(2):403-425, 1977.

Zarb, G.A., Lewis, D., and Scrivener, W.: The effects of removable prostheses on the oral tissue—a cytologic assessment, I.A.D.R. Program and Abstracts, 47th General Meeting, No. 452, p. 153, Houston, Texas, 1969.

SECTION TWO

Preparing patients for complete dentures

3

Diagnosis and treatment planning for patients with some teeth remaining

Dentists have been very successful in treating edentulous patients with complete dentures. However, the profession's commitment to avoid the edentulous state continues, and this commitment has led to expanded knowledge and clinical skills. As a result, earlier and improved operative and prosthodontic treatment, combined with the effectiveness of modern endodontic and periodontal therapy, usurped the old myth that tooth loss inevitably accompanies old age. These same therapeutic modalities can also be applied to those persons who, as a result of earlier neglect, come for treatment with broken-down dentitions. These patients can frequently have their masticatory systems restored to near normal without having to consider prosthodontic intervention as an interim postponement of the edentulous state (Zarb and associates, 1978).

Patients with some teeth remaining, who request complete dentures, should be carefully diagnosed to ensure that treatment alternatives to complete dentures are thoroughly considered. The decision to retain or remove even one tooth is a serious one, and all alternatives must be explored before a final decision is made. The removal of teeth is an irreversible procedure, underscoring the significance and importance of a correct diagnosis.

Diagnosis consists of planned observations to determine and evaluate the existing conditions,

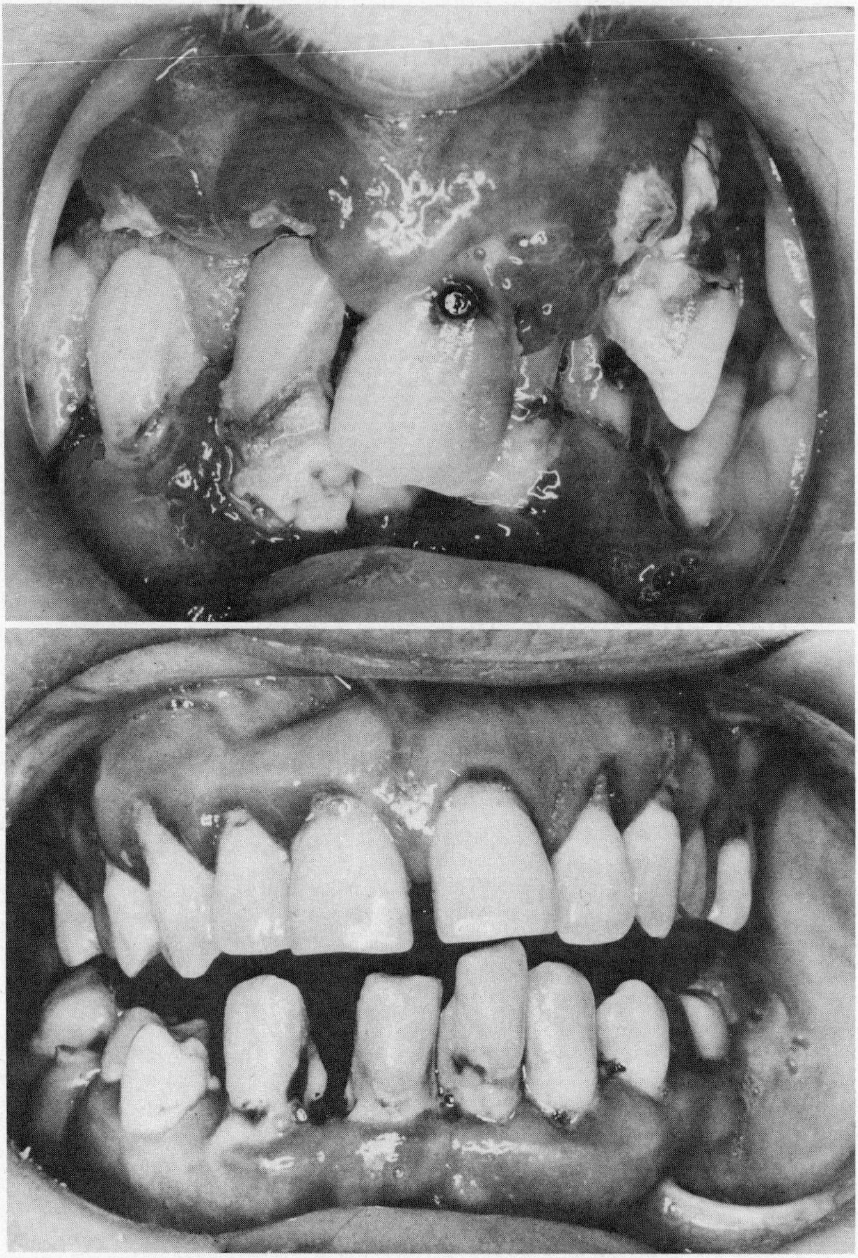

Fig. 3-1. Advanced neglect makes both patients, **A** and **B,** candidates for immediate denture therapy. The full-mouth radiographic survey, **C,** of the patient in **B,** combined with an assessment of poor patient motivation, confirm decision to place such a patient in total extraction treatment group.

which lead to decision making based on the conditions observed. All the facts must be known before they can be correlated in such a way that judgments and decisions can be made. Only then can treatment plans be developed to best serve the needs of each individual patient.

Those patients with some teeth remaining who may need complete denture service tend to fall into the following three groups, each of which poses special problems and decisions:

1. Patients with or without severely depleted dentitions characterized by extensive caries or advanced periodontal disease (Fig. 3-1). Immediate dentures are usually prescribed for such patients, and this topic is described in Chapter 26.

2. Patients with depleted dentitions (Fig. 3-2) or, infrequently, failed reconstructions with one or more teeth that can serve as overdenture abutments. These potential abutments may require minimal preparation or else entail several procedures (e.g., endodontic or periodontal therapy, gold coping) to enhance their longevity. The objective in retaining teeth under complete dentures is alveolar bone preservation (Fig. 3-3) and is discussed in Chapter 25. The overdenture, or tooth-supported complete denture, concept has led to a dramatic increase in the number of patients who have been spared the edentulous predicament.

3. Patients who are edentulous in only one arch, most frequently the maxillary one. A characteristic clinical picture emerges in such patients and includes one or more of the following: (1) few anterior mandibular teeth present, (2) variable hyperplastic replacement of the anterior maxillary ridge secondary to anterior upward settling of the maxillary denture, and (3) loss of vertical dimension of occlusion (Fig. 3-4). Infrequently, an intact or restored maxillary

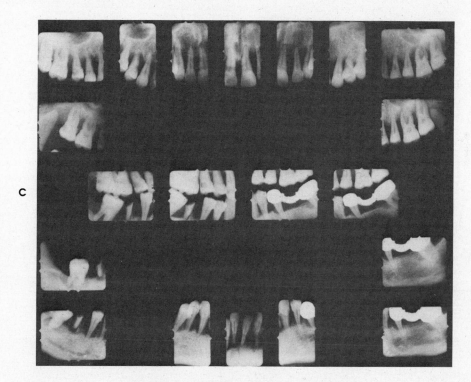

C

Fig. 3-1, cont'd. For legend see opposite page.

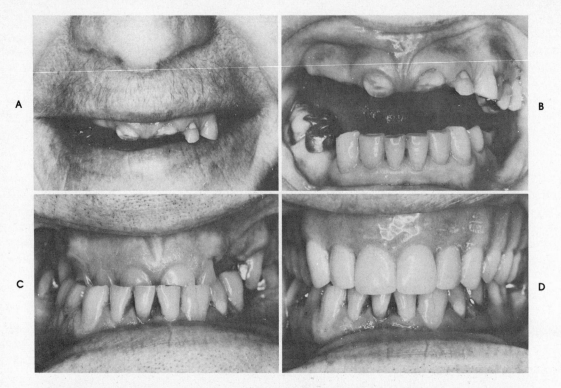

Fig. 3-2. A and **B,** This middle-aged patient had complaints of mandibular dysfunction and dissatisfaction with appearance. Recovery of loss of vertical dimension of occlusion and bilateral function could easily be accomplished by treatment with overdenture technique, which is illustrated in another patient in **C** and **D.**

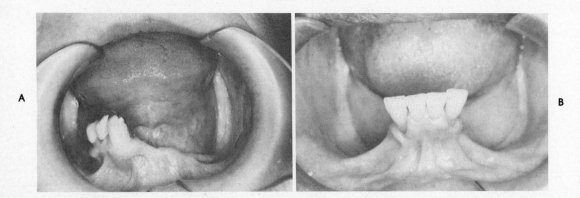

Fig. 3-3. Level of alveolar bone around retained teeth is in dramatic contrast to missing or resorbed alveolar bone where natural teeth once were.

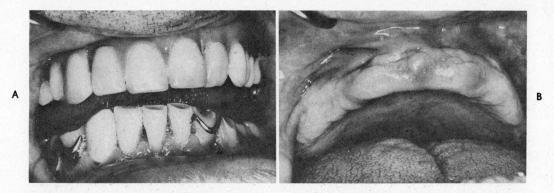

Fig. 3-4. A, Single maxillary denture opposing a partially edentulous mandible with an unserviced bilateral distal extension prosthesis. A collapse in vertical dimension of occlusion has occurred and anterior maxillary ridge has been replaced by hyperplastic tissue, **B.**

dentition is opposed by an edentulous mandible, and in these patients the mandible appears to be very susceptible to residual ridge resorption (Fig. 3-5). In previous editions of this text, we favored the sacrifice of the remaining teeth in such situations. However, clinical experience has demonstrated that such drastic action is only rarely needed, and modifications in technique and the materials used allow for a more conservative approach. The single denture opposing a natural dentition is discussed in Chapter 27.

DIAGNOSTIC PROCEDURES

To make the correct decisions, certain steps should be followed in an orderly sequence, and this is preferably done in two appointments. The first appointment should allow the dentist and the patient to become acquainted with each other and allow the dentist to obtain essential information from the patient. This information consists of a thorough history, a radiographic survey, and diagnostic casts. After thorough consideration of the diagnostic information, the dentist discusses the proposed treatment with the patient at the second appointment, along with the sequence in which this treatment will be carried out and the anticipated fee for service.

The first contact of the patient with the dental office is usually by telephone. The call may be received by an assistant, a secretary, a receptionist, or the dentist. At this time certain general, but important, information can be obtained, such as the following:

1. The patient's name, address, and telephone number are important for making future contacts as may be necessary. This information also can be an indication of the socioeconomic status of the patient and may provide a clue to the desires and expectations of the patient.

2. The means by which the patient selected you as the dentist is important. Was the patient referred by a dentist? Another patient? A physician? Or was your name obtained from the telephone book or other listing? The information about the way the patient found you will guide you in discussions regarding office policy, arrangement of appointments, and the type of service that will be expected. If the patient was referred by a dentist, radiographs and diagnostic casts may be available from that dentist. If not, the patient may wish to have that dentist make them so that they will be available to you at the first appointment. Otherwise, these records should be made at the first appointment with you.

3. The type of treatment the patient is seeking will make it possible to arrange adequate time for the first appointment. If it is treatment for a

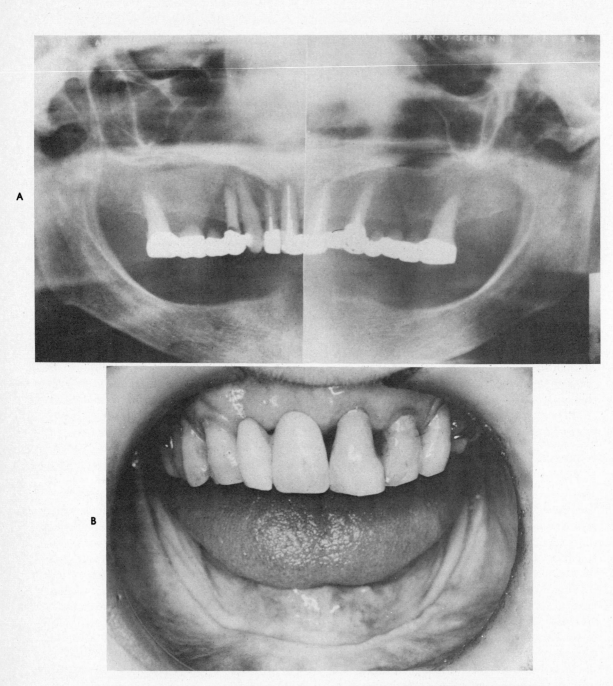

Fig. 3-5. A, This patient never wore a lower denture, and the edentulous mandibular ridge opposed a restored maxillary dentition for several years. Usually, mandibular ridge demonstrates advanced resorption in such patients, especially if a denture is worn, **B.** (See Chapter 27.)

toothache, an emergency visit can be arranged. If it is for new dentures, an appointment for making preliminary records can be made.

First appointment

The purpose of the first appointment is to allow the dentist to become acquainted with the patient so that evaluation of the problems involved in diagnosis and treatment can begin. It also provides an opportunity for the patient to become acquainted with and evaluate the dentist. Since the success or failure of prosthodontic treatment depends greatly on mutual confidence and rapport between the dentist and the patient, this appointment is extremely important. The things that are said and the questions that are asked and answered will determine to a great extent the way the dentist and patient will react to each other. Therefore the first contact should be pleasant but serious and dignified. The dentist's attitude should be one of kindness and concern for all patients and their problems. A planned office procedure will help to put patients at ease and develop the mutual respect that is essential.

The patient is met by the receptionist, assistant, or dentist at the reception room and conducted to the dental chair. After being comfortably seated, the patient is asked for the information that is necessary for the business records. This will verify or correct the information that had been received by telephone when the appointment was made. At this time the patient can supply information about age and general health by filling out a questionnaire that was devised for this purpose (Fig. 3-6).

When the dentist meets the patient for the first time, the receptionist or assistant makes the necessary introduction. Then the dentist carries on some conversation on general topics for a few moments and tries to avoid answering questions about the patient's dental problems at this time. Instead, this time is for making certain observations of the patient. These include the *apparent age* (i.e., physiologic age rather than chronologic age), facial appearance and expression (esthe-

tics), speech (phonetics), lip support, vertical jaw relations, and general health and attitude of the patient as determined from an analysis of the health questionnaire. Each of these observations will be taken into consideration as the diagnosis is made.

Mandibular dysfunction

Temporomandibular joint (TMJ) problems, or problems of mandibular dysfunction, are frequently encountered in patients with depleted dentitions. Although the cause of mandibular dysfunction appears to be multifactorial (Rugh, 1982), it seems that occlusion is the etiologic factor that can be best controlled and adjusted by the dentist. Current research of the epidemiologic and microscopic and macroscopic postmortem varieties suggests that the incidence of dysfunction is related to a decreased number of residual teeth. It is not surprising therefore that the temporomandibular joints of patients who are candidates for immediate or tooth-supported complete dentures may demonstrate arthritic or degenerative changes that will modify the treatment strategy and sequence in some ways. Hard research evidence is lacking to support the claim that occlusal therapy by itself is of value in the treatment of all types of mandibular dysfunction. However an understanding of the pathogenesis of degenerative arthritis gives strength to the belief that the arthritic process is influenced by adverse joint loading, which can result from depleted dentitions (Carlsson and others, 1979; Zarb, 1981).

A nonarthritic mandibular dysfunction is diagnosed on the basis of reported symptoms and clinical findings (Table 4). A degenerative arthritis is similarly recognized but usually is confirmed by means of temporomandibular joint radiographs. The dentist's treatment strategies for most types of mandibular dysfunction emphasize rest for the masticatory system plus elimination of occlusion discrepancies and restoration of support for the vertical dimension of occlusion. Quite frequently, recording jaw relations accurately will be a problem with these

Text continued on p. 62.

Instructions:

This history is designed to assist us in finding out more about you and your problems (if any). Please circle the correct answer YES or NO. We will check your answers with you.

Mr. Mrs. Miss Ms_____

Address_____

City_____Zone_____

Phone (HOME)_____(BUSINESS)_____

Occupation_____Age_____

Bus. Address_____Birth date_____

Referring doctor_____

Address & phone_____

Name of spouse_____

Occupation_____

Number of children_____

Ages_____

Family physician: (name, address, tel.)_____

_____

When did you last see him and why?_____

Do you take any medication? (how much and why)_____

Other doctors?_____

SECTION I MEDICAL

Has a doctor ever told you that you have a heart condition (heart murmur, heart leakage, heart attack . . . or angina pectoris, for example)?	NO	YES
Have you ever had rheumatic fever or rheumatic heart disease?.	NO	YES
Have you ever been told that your blood pressure is too high? Too low?	NO	YES
Have you ever been told that you have diabetes?.	NO	YES
Do you bleed abnormally following a cut, a tooth extraction, or other operation?	NO	YES
Do you have any allergies (hay fever, asthma, for example)?.	NO	YES
Are you allergic to any drug or medicine (aspirin, sulfas, penicillin, or Novocaine, for example)?	NO	YES
Have you ever had a lung, liver, or kidney disease?	NO	YES
Have you ever had syphilis?	NO	YES

Fig. 3-6. Sample of a health questionnaire.

SECTION II CARDIOVASCULAR

Do you get out of breath easily? . . . .   NO   YES

Do you have difficulty breathing when you are lying down? . . . .   NO   YES

Are your ankles often badly swollen? . . . .   NO   YES

Have you ever had a stroke? . . . .   NO   YES

Nervous system

Have you ever been treated for an emotional disturbance? . . . .   NO   YES

Have you ever been treated for epilepsy? . . . .   NO   YES

Have you fainted more than twice in your life? . . . .   NO   YES

Have you ever been treated for any other disease of the nerves? . . . .   NO   YES

Respiratory system

Have you ever had a sinusitis? . . . .   NO   YES

Have you ever coughed up blood? . . . .   NO   YES

Have you ever lived with anyone who had tuberculosis? . . . .   NO   YES

Gastrointestinal

Do you have frequent spells of diarrhea? . . . .   NO   YES

Have you ever vomited blood? . . . .   NO   YES

Have you suffered from any other stomach trouble? . . . .   NO   YES

Have you ever had jaundice? . . . .   NO   YES

Endocrine system

Does a blood relative of yours have diabetes? . . . .   NO   YES

Have you ever taken thyroid tablets? . . . .   NO   YES

Are you taking, or have you ever taken, ACTH or cortisone? . . . .   NO   YES

Blood

Have you ever had anemia? . . . .   NO   YES

Are you a hemophiliac? . . . .   NO   YES

Have you ever had any other blood diseases? . . . .   NO   YES

Bones and joints

Do you have arthritis? . . . .   NO   YES

Have you ever had more than one fractured bone? . . . .   NO   YES

Have you ever had more than one dislocation? . . . .   NO   YES

Have you ever had a bone infection? . . . .   NO   YES

Have you gained or lost much weight recently . . . .   NO   YES

Has your doctor given you a special diet? . . . .   NO   YES

Fig. 3-6, cont'd. Sample of a health questionnaire.

Bones and joints—cont'd

Have you ever had radiation treatments for any disease? . . . .   NO   YES

Have you ever had a tumor or cancer? . . . .   NO   YES

Have you ever had an operation? . . . .   NO   YES

Do you smoke? . . . .   NO   YES

Alcoholic beverages? . . . .   NO   YES

Physical activities? . . . .   NO   YES

(Women) Are you pregnant? . . . .   NO   YES

Do you feel you are in good health at the present time? If not, please specify:_____   NO   YES

Summary of medical history

Do you have dental insurance?
Carrier _____   Group Policy No. _____   Cert. or Soc. Ins. No._____

Dental history:
How often do you brush your teeth? . . . .   NO   YES

What kind of toothbrush and toothpaste do you use? . . . .   NO   YES

Do you use anything else? . . . .   NO   YES

Do you wear a prosthesis: (denture or bridge)? . . . .   NO   YES

Complete upper   Partial upper   Bridges   Upper   Right

Complete lower   Partial lower   Lower   Left

Have you received treatment by a dentist in the past year? . . . .   NO   YES

Have you ever experienced prolonged bleeding following a tooth extraction? . . . .   NO   YES

Have you ever experienced dizziness, or have you ever fainted, while undergoing dental treatment?

. . . .   NO   YES

Have you ever experienced any difficulty when dental anesthetics (such as Novocaine) were administered?

. . . .   NO   YES

Have you ever been treated for a gum disease (such as pyorrhea or trench mouth)? . . . .   NO   YES

Fig. 3-6, cont'd. Sample of a health questionnaire.

CC, HPC, PDH

_____
_____
_____
_____
_____
_____
_____
_____

ON EXAMINATION (Extra-oral, functional analysis, soft and hard tissues, prostheses)

_____
_____
_____
_____
_____
_____
_____
_____

IMPRESSION AND DIAGNOSIS   **PROPOSED TREATMENT AND PROGNOSIS**

_____   _____
_____   _____
_____   _____
_____   _____

Fig. 3-6, cont'd. Sample of a health questionnaire.

Table 4

Common symptoms in diseases related to the function of the masticatory system*

SYMPTOMS REPORTED BY PATIENTS	CLINICAL FINDINGS BY DENTIST
Joint noise(s)	Clicking, crepitation of TMJ
Pain in face, jaws, and ears and headache	Pain or tenderness with palpation of masticatory muscles and TMJ
Pain on opening mouth	Pain with mandibular movement
Difficulty in opening mouth wide and in chewing	Impaired, mandibular mobility, irregularity, deviation, locking of mandible

*Modified from Carlsson, G.E.: J. Dent. **4**:265-270, 1976.

patients, and this fact must be taken into consideration when the treatment plan is made and appointments are scheduled. Recommended treatment strategies are fairly routine, and tend to include (1) symptomatic treatment, (2) control or reduction of contributory factors, and (3) treatment of pathologic sequelae.

The making of maxillomandibular relation records is one of the most critical procedures in providing prosthodontic treatment for patients. The health of the temporomandibular joints is a key factor in the assessment the ability of patients to cooperate with the dentist when jaw relation records are made. The health of the temporomandibular joints can be estimated by a simple test. The patient is asked to open the mouth wide and relax, then to move the jaw to the left and relax, and finally to move the jaw forward and relax. If the patient has difficulty coordinating these movements or following the instructions correctly, problems in recording the jaw relations can be anticipated.

The next test consists in placing a fingertip on the face over each of the condyles and instructing the patient to open the mouth slightly and move the jaw rapidly from side to side and then to open wide and close rapidly. Any possible clicking or crepitus in the joints can be detected by the fingers. If these conditions exist, more difficulty in recording jaw relations can be anticipated. Naturally, this means that more time will be required for making jaw relation records and that changes in maxillomandibular relations may occur after the dentures have been in use for some time. Such changes are especially likely if the patient reports tenderness when fingertip pressure is applied by the dentist.

Patient's dental history

It is important that the dentist know about the patient's dental history, and this can be determined when the right kinds of questions are asked. Some of these are general, and some are specific. Some will reveal simple but important facts, and others will stimulate or encourage the patient to discuss dental problems, troubles, and complaints. Any significant comments should be noted on the patient's record card for further study and consideration at the next appointment. Up to this point, the questions are preliminary.

After the preliminary conversation, in which the patient is encouraged to talk and the dentist and assistant are good listeners, the discussion can be directed toward the patient's present dental problem by the question, What do you have in mind for us to do for you? The response will indicate considerations that are of major concern to the patient. It may be to obtain new dentures for one or more reasons such as to improve the patient's appearance or to eat better. These should be carefully noted because they could influence the diagnosis and the treatment procedures to be used. For example, if a patient's major concern is appearance, it will most likely require more time to solve the problem at the try-in stage than if the concern is only about eating.

As each of the patient's objectives or complaints are mentioned, they should be carefully noted on the patient's chart, but the dentist should refrain from making any comments about them in relation to the previous treatment received by the patient.

Intraoral examination

With this background information recorded, the dentist should carry out an intraoral examination. The remaining teeth are charted to show their location and condition. If the patient is wearing removable prostheses, the occlusion of these restorations should be observed before they are removed. Any disharmony in the occlusion or between centric relation and centric occlusion should be noted because it could explain some of the difficulties that the patient has been experiencing. These observations also provide information about the patient's coordination and ability to move the mandible to the centric position as well as to carry out multidirectional contact movements when instructed to do so.

Existing prostheses should be cleaned and laid aside while the teeth and oral cavity are observed. The mobility of the remaining teeth should be tested, and the depth of the gingival sulcus should be measured. The clinical crowns should be examined visually and by use of a sharp explorer. If teeth have restorations, the margins of the restorations, the occlusal surface contours, the general shape of each tooth and its restorations, and the materials of which the restorations are made should be observed and recorded. This information provides evidence of the quality of home care and professional care the teeth and mouth have received. If this care has been inadequate, the decision to retain or remove remaining teeth becomes easier to make. If the patient cannot be trained and motivated to give his teeth adequate care, their restoration by crowns, inlays, and other operative dentistry procedures will be futile. This problem should be thoroughly discussed with the patient so that a similar observation and evaluation can be made at the second appointment, at which time the final decision can be made.

Diagnostic casts and a radiographic survey are essential for the completion of the diagnosis.

Diagnostic casts

Diagnostic casts that may be used as part of the preextraction records are essential if the correct decisions are to be made. Therefore diagnostic casts must be available before the final decision is made regarding the removal of any teeth. The impressions for making diagnostic casts can be made in alginate (irreversible hydrocolloid) impression material in stock trays.

The making of the impressions for diagnostic casts is an important diagnostic procedure in itself. It will reveal unusual sensitivity of the mucous membranes, a tendency toward gagging, tolerance of the patient to procedures in the oral cavity, coordination of tongue activity, and other factors important to the diagnosis.

When teeth remain in both dental arches, the casts made in these impressions are preferably mounted on a simple hinge articulator. A wax interocclusal record can serve for relating the casts to each other on the instrument. If the impressions and interocclusal record are made at the first appointment, the casts can be mounted and studied before the second appointment (Fig. 3-7). When bilateral centric stops are absent, an articulatory mounting is impractical.

Perhaps the most important diagnostic information to be obtained from mounted diagnostic casts is related to the occlusion. This information is essential because it will determine for many patients whether teeth that might be saved should be saved. For example, periodontal therapy may be able to save some teeth that actually should be removed to develop a favorable occlusal plane or to avoid rotating or tipping forces on opposing, usually maxillary, dentures.

A third molar that is tipped forward can exert horizontal forces against its opposing tooth in eccentric occlusions, and this can dislodge a maxillary denture (Fig. 3-8). If the occlusal sur-

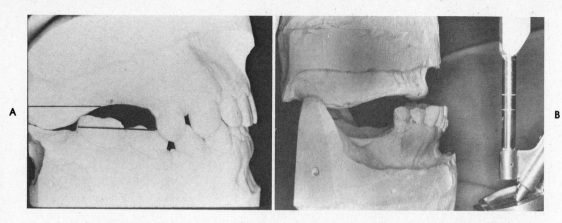

Fig. 3-7. Mounted diagnostic casts reveal existing conditions and potential problems. **A,** Mandibular occlusal plane is unfavorable and needs to be leveled; the tuberosity encroaches on interarch space. **B,** A Class III jaw relationship is evident. Note that this mounting on a semiadjustable articulator necessitated use of occlusion rims.

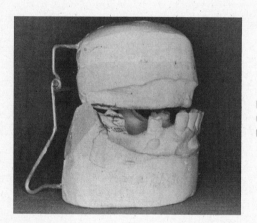

Fig. 3-8. Example of a third molar that could dislodge a maxillary denture if it is not extracted or its occlusal morphology is not altered.

face cannot be reshaped so that is is parallel to and on the occlusal plane, the tooth should be removed. One may do the reshaping by grinding on its occlusal surface or by making a full coverage crown. Endodontic therapy may be necessary if the tooth is to be saved.

Interarch space problems. Diagnostic casts, which are mounted or hand held, will reveal the amount of interarch space. This is important information because a lack of space in this part of the mouth has caused many dentures to fail. If a tooth is extruded so that its occlusal surface is above the occlusal plane, it should be removed unless it can be shortened sufficiently to be on the same plane with the other teeth in that dental arch.

Extremely large maxillary tuberosities make it necessary to locate the back end of the occlusal plane too low, to omit some posterior teeth, or more frequently to shorten the denture bases from their correct border extent and contour (Fig. 3-9). If there is insufficient space between

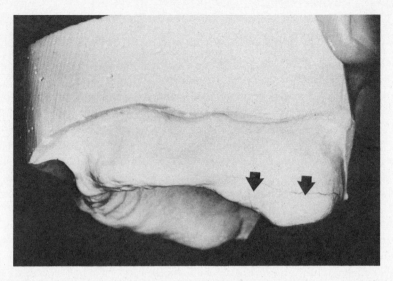

Fig. 3-9. Retention of this large tuberosity would compromise occlusal plane and distal extension of mandibular denture. If reduction is feasible, it should be done.

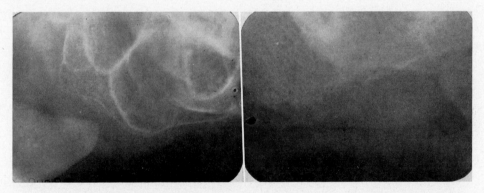

Fig. 3-10. Thick layer of fibrous connective tissue on tuberosity does not provide firm foundation for denture. The bulk of the tissue will cause interference between denture bases and prevent proper location of back end of occlusal plane.

the residual ridges, the denture bases will interfere with each other and cause the dentures to tip away from the basal seats in the anterior part of the mouth. In this situation, the lower denture base will wear away over the retromolar pads, and holes will be worn through the maxillary denture base, leading to reduced retention in both dentures. The fact that a patient may have been wearing dentures does not rule out this difficulty.

Although lack of adequate space between the ridges is easily recognized on the mounted casts, radiographs will show whether large tuberosities are bone or are simply an overgrowth of fibrous connective tissue in the tuberosity region (Fig. 3-10).

The large fibrous tuberosity can usually be moved from side to side when grasped by a thumb and forefinger. If it is movable in this test, it should be removed.

If the tuberosity is firm and hard and the radiographs show that it is composed of a thin layer of soft tissue over bone, it may have to be accommodated in the design of the denture. If it seems necessary to shorten a large bony tuberosity, care must be taken to avoid opening into the maxillary sinus. Such a surgical procedure may be contraindicated by a patient's systemic health.

The problem of insufficient interarch space in the posterior part of the mouth can be avoided for most people if the soft tissue distal to the last upper and lower molars is excised at the same time those teeth are removed.

Radiographs

Radiographs are essential for evaluating the conditions existing in every patient needing prosthodontic service. The dentist must know the conditions under the mucous membrane and the condition of the surfaces that can be seen.

The presence of abnormalities in edentulous jaws or in the edentulous segments of partially edentulous jaws is most often unsuspected because of the absence of clinical signs or symptoms. Abnormalities can and do occur, however, and have been demonstrated in a high percentage of patients on radiographic examination. These may be foreign bodies, retained tooth roots, unerupted teeth, or varied pathoses of developmental, inflammatory, or neoplastic origin (Fig. 3-11). Of these, the retained root is most commonly present. Various surveys have shown retained roots to be present in one out of every four edentulous patients, and an Australian study found evidence of tooth roots in 33% of 538 edentulous patients (Ettinger, 1971). A histologic survey of a series of retained tooth roots suggests that in the absence of clinical or roentgenographic abnormality, the retained tooth root can be regarded as having been accepted by the tissues (Herd, 1973). The decision to extract such roots preprosthetically tends to be an elective one. However, some situations are specific indications for their removal, e.g., the root's occupying a superficial submucosal position after progressive alveolar ridge resorption.

Radiographs also confirm the depth of periodontal pockets and provide information about pulpless teeth. They can show the amount of bone lost around the remaining teeth and in the

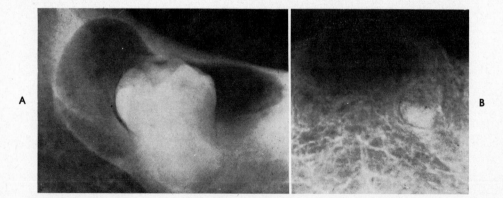

Fig. 3-11. A, Unerupted third molar with follicular cyst approaching crest of ridge; patient was wearing dentures without being aware of condition. **B,** Extremely thin process in mandibular anterior region that simulates a cyst or residual area; small fragment of root in residual area to patient's right; cementoma below and to patient's left.

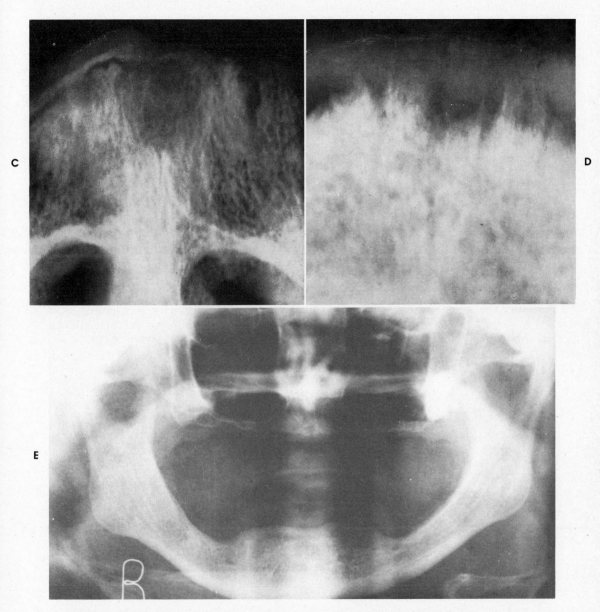

Fig. 3-11, cont'd. C, Maxillary anterior ridge thinned to point of separation; loose process causing pain in area. **D,** Thin anterior mandibular ridge with large nutrient canals is painful to pressure and ridge of flabby tissue. In **E,** a retained root is visible in left tuberosity region.

edentulous regions. They also can show the relative thickness of the submucosa covering the bone in edentulous regions, the location of the mandibular canal, and the mental foramen in relation to the basal seat for dentures. They can give an indication of the quality of the bone that supports the teeth and will support the dentures, though this is not as reliable as it should be because of variations in radiographic techniques, since variations in exposure time and developing procedures cause difficulty. In general, however, the more dense (radiopaque) the bone appears to be, the better the bony foundation and the less likelihood there is for rapid change in the basal seat when dentures are worn.

Sharp spicules of bone on ridge crests are also apparent on properly exposed dental radiographs, and these conditions may affect decisions about the location of the occlusal plane and about the types of impressions and the design of denture base that have to be used. An orthopantomogram should be taken routinely. It is also advisable to compensate for the unreliability of radiographic interpretation of the anterior regions where distortions frequently occur. This can be achieved by adjunctive use of periapical or standard occlusal films.

TREATMENT PLAN

Once all the intraoral and general physical and mental conditions have been noted on appropriate record cards or sheets, the treatment plan can be developed. This includes which teeth are to be saved and how, the sequence in which teeth should be removed, the amount and type of oral surgery that might be required, and the type of prosthesis that is indicated. Should it be an overdenture, an immediate overdenture (some teeth are extracted at the same time as the immediate denture is inserted), or an immediate denture? Or should all of the teeth be removed and a waiting time arranged so that the tissues can heal somewhat before impressions are made or the dentures are inserted? Only in the rare cases of seri-

ous systemic health problems is the latter treatment chosen (see Chapter 26).

Deciding whether to extract the remaining teeth

The loss of all remaining teeth can be a terrible psychologic shock to patients, even though some of them may not admit it. Consequently the dentist must have empathy for patients who must lose their teeth. The dentist should explore every possibility for saving them. It is when patients recognize that the dentist does not want them to lose their teeth that the necessary feeling of confidence can be developed.

Even patients who say that they want to get rid of their teeth so that they will not have to see dentists anymore really do not want to lose their teeth. They are only trying to prepare their defenses against future difficulties they do not understand. If the dentist removes the teeth without adequate reason, physical, mental, and even legal problems may arise.

The answer so far as the dentist is concerned is simple: to get all the facts and consider all possibilities before making the decision to remove the remaining teeth. Many diagnostic factors are involved. To ignore or fail to recognize any of them could lead to incorrect decisions.

The facts to be learned before the remaining teeth are to be removed include the following:

1. The general health of the patient will determine the extent and sequence of any surgical procedures that may be necessary. In most instances it may be more desirable for the patient to retain loose or broken teeth than to have them removed. In other patients it may be that their health can be improved if infected teeth are removed.

2. The age of the patient can be a determining factor in the decision to have the remaining teeth removed. If the patient is young and the bone is not fully calcified, the remaining teeth should probably be saved regardless of the cost of restoring them or the attitude of the patient toward the discomfort involved. The experience

of many edentulous young people is that they lose much too much alveolar bone in a short time after they lose their teeth.

If the patient is old and feeble, it may be better to save the few remaining teeth. If, however, elderly persons have loose, extruded teeth that are endangering their health, the teeth should be removed.

3. Highly mobile teeth that have been extruded from their sockets and teeth with radiographic evidence of infection either at their apices or along their sides should be removed.

It is fundamental that natural teeth should not be removed unless there is a valid reason for doing so. These reasons may include one or more of the following conditions:

1. Advanced periodontal disease with severe bone loss around the teeth
2. Severely broken-down clinical crowns (subgingival) that cannot be adequately restored; fractured roots
3. Periapical or lateral abscesses that cannot be successfully treated
4. Unfavorably tipped or inclined teeth that pose problems for their use as abutments for fixed or removable prostheses
5. Extruded or tipped teeth that interfere with the proper location of the occlusal plane

It must be emphasized that a number of techniques and skills are available to the dentist to cope with conditions 4 and 5, reducing the numbers of candidates for total extractions and immediate dentures. There has been a corresponding increase in the number of overdenture patients as a result, attesting to the profession's growing awareness that alveolar bone must be preserved at all costs.

Preextraction records

No patient should ever be made completely edentulous or treated with complete overdentures without first having preextraction records of the existing dental and facial conditions made. It requires only a few minutes to make diagnos-

tic impressions and casts if these have not been made before. The diagnostic casts may or may not be mounted on an articulator, but failure to make them is a serious breach of the trust placed in the dentist by the patient. In fact, it is probably valid to suggest that failure to make preextraction records may constitute professional negligence.

The color of the natural teeth should be recorded on the patient's record card. This will reassure the patient of the dentist's interest in the patient's well-being, but equally important, this record made before the teeth are removed will be valuable to the dentist. It will save time and help to avoid errors in tooth color selection when the dentures are made.

Photographs of the patient will be most helpful when the prosthetic work is completed, and they will be even more helpful as years go by and the patient needs modification to, or replacement of the dentures. The photographs are easily made in the dental office.

The pictures that are most useful are (1) full face with lips closed, (2) full face with a smile, (3) close-up of the teeth together and with the lips separated, (4) full face with the mouth open wide, and (5) profile of the face with the teeth in centric occlusion and the lips relaxed.

REFERENCES

Carlsson, G.E., Kopp, S., and Öberg, T.: Arthritis and allied diseases. In Zarb, G.A., and Carlsson, G.E., editors: Temporomandibular joint—function and dysfunction, Copenhagen, 1979, Munksgaard, International Booksellers & Publishers Ltd., Chapter 10.

Ettinger, R.W.: Roentgenographic evaluation of the edentulous patient, Aust. Dent. J. **16:**210-219, 1971.

Herd, J.R.: The retained tooth root, Aust. Dent. J. **18:**125-131, 1973.

Rugh, J.: Psychological factors in the etiology of masticatory pain and dysfunction, American Dental Association President's Conference on TMJ, Chicago, 1982.

Zarb, G.A.: Degenerative arthritis of the temporomandibular joint, Proceedings of the Northwestern Symposium on Temporomandibular Joint Dysfunction, Chicago, Nov. 1981.

Zarb, G.A., Bergman, B., Clayton, J.A., and MacKay, H.F., editors: Prosthodontic treatment for partially edentulous patients, St. Louis, 1978, The C.V. Mosby Co.

4

Diagnosis and treatment planning for patients with no teeth remaining

The procedures used in diagnosis and treatment planning for patients who have no teeth are similar to those used for patients who still have some teeth at the time treatment begins. These basic procedures have been discussed in Chapter 3. The same sequence of appointments should be followed, and the same diagnostic aids should be used. There are, however, some additional observations to be made. These are critical because the problems faced by dentists in treating edentulous patients are progressively more difficult to solve after the last teeth have been removed.

Treatment by fixed partial prosthodontics is somewhat simplified by the fact that restorations are cemented to retained teeth. Removable partial prostheses are retained by clasps or internal attachments. Complete dentures are maintained in position by the forces of adhesion, cohesion, interfacial surface tension, atmospheric pressure, and their adaptation to supporting and surrounding structures of the edentulous oral cavity.

For this adaptation to be effective, the procedures used in making the dentures must be coordinated with the basic anatomy of the patients, but equally important, the procedures used must be coordinated with the individual variations within the mouth of each patient.

Clinical experience proves the importance of developing refined mechanical skills, the *un-*

availability of a panacea for all edentulous patient problems, and above all the importance of *treating* the patient instead of just constructing dentures for the patient. We cannot overemphasize the importance of such an objective. It is probably far easier to acquire the skills of complete denture construction (challenging as these may be) than to acquire those necessary to treat a patient's aspirations and expectations. But both skills must be mastered if our patients are to be happier and if we are to receive greater satisfaction and pleasure from our work. Whereas in this text, we describe the diagnostic and clinical skills for treating the edentulous patient, we must reiterate our commitment to treating the whole patient and not just the mouth. Clinical skills alone, without compassion or awareness, distort the image of a true professional.

PATIENTS RECENTLY MADE EDENTULOUS

Patients who have had their teeth removed less than 6 months previously have problems different from those who have had some denture-wearing experience. Likewise, the problems faced by dentists in treating recently edentulous patients are different from the problems is treating patients who have been edentulous for a long time.

The first difference is in the patient's awareness of the difficulties involved and in their expectations regarding dentures, and the second is in the biologic aspects of the treatment.

New problems of the recently edentulous patient

Patients who are edentulous and have never attempted to wear dentures face problems that they do not know exist. At best, they are not aware of any difficulties and assume that the dentures will be placed in their mouth and that they will continue to use the same eating habits as with their natural teeth. In a few people—the delicate eaters—this may be true. Most people will find it necessary to reduce the size of the morsels of food taken at one time and to reduce the amount of force applied on the dentures dur-

ing mastication. Patients should be made aware of the fact that chewing should be *into* the food, rather than *through* the food being chewed. The education of patients as to these facts should begin with the second examination appointment and continue through the entire treatment sequence.

Patients' concepts of the permanence of dentures

Many recently edentulous patients expect their new teeth to last them the rest of their lives. Some even believe that by obtaining complete dentures they will no longer require the services of dentists. Of course, this is not true or possible. Changes occur in the basal seats for the dentures, and these will allow the positions of the dentures to change in relation to their foundation and to each other.

When teeth are removed, there remain the cavities in the bone (alveoli), which contained the roots of the teeth, and sharp ridges around each alveolus. Blood clots will form in the alveoli and form a matrix for the deposition of new bone in the tooth sockets. It would be nice if the new bone would entirely fill the alveolus, but this does not happen often.

At the same time that bone is forming in the tooth socket, the bony edge of the socket is resorbing in its attempt to become rounded. When these two processes proceed ideally, the resultant residual ridge is considered to be favorable, with a more or less flat crest and nearly vertical sides. When the residual ridge assumes this form, it provides good support for vertical forces applied through the dentures and resistance to horizontal forces that tend to cause the dentures to skid, slide, or rotate on their basal seats.

Unfortunately, in many people the tooth sockets do not completely fill with new bone, and the edges of the sockets do not always round off as desired (Fig. 4-1). These conditions can cause problems for both the dentist and the patient. The mucosa covers the edges of bone around the sockets, but this tissue will be pinched between

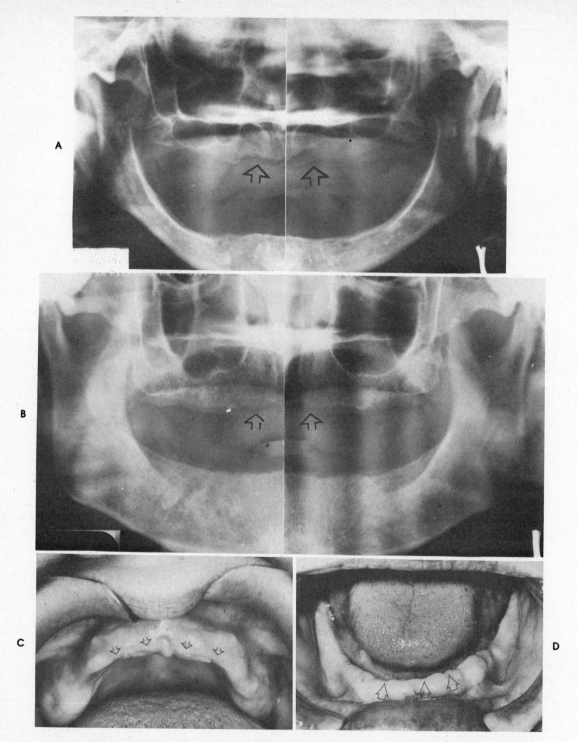

Fig. 4-1. A and **B,** Radiographic evidence of failure of maxillary sockets to round off. Contrast this to the well-healed mandibular ridges. Clinical evidence of gentle, **C,** to more conspicuous, **D,** residual ridge discrepancies. Both clinical situations can be treated conservatively, but alternate strategies (e.g., soft liners or preprosthetic surgery) may be initiated if healing of underlying bone is unfavorable and particularly if clinical symptoms persist.

the denture base and the bone during mastication or whenever tooth contacts are made. These tissues can be tender and even painful when closing pressure is applied on new dentures. In time, the bone will change enough to eliminate the sharp points and tender spots.

The residual ridges may have undercuts after tooth extraction, which make the insertion and removal of impressions and dentures painful and sometimes difficult. At the time of the second examination appointment, the dentist must determine whether surgical reduction of the undercuts is necessary. This can best be determined by palpation of the tissues *and* a survey of the diagnostic casts. The cast placed on a surveyor can be tipped to determine the most favorable angle of insertion for the denture. It is hardly ever necessary to have any bone removed from the labial side of the ridges. Some reduction of undercuts may be necessary in the tuberosity region, but only rarely is this necessary in the premolar region. No more bone should be removed than is absolutely necessary. The resiliency of the mucosa will compensate for most undercuts. Then time and normal bone changes will further ease the problem.

It is important that the patient be informed about inevitable changes *before* any impressions are made. To postpone giving the patient this information until later will almost certainly lead to misunderstanding between the dentist and the patient, who will look on this information as excuses. The patient must be warned in advance that the dentures will become progressively looser as the residual ridges change their form.

Changes in the bone supporting the basal seat continue as long as the patient lives. They vary greatly in amount from patient to patient, but they are unavoidable. Recent extraction patients should be warned of these changes, which are more rapid in the first year after teeth are removed than they will be later on.

The same basic observations and diagnostic aids are used for partially edentulous and recently edentulous patients. Radiographs are essential for making diagnoses for people who have lost their teeth, and diagnostic casts often reveal problems that would not otherwise be noticed before too late. The same as for other types of prosthodontic patients, the critical observations and decisions are made at the second examination appointment when all the diagnostic aids are available.

PATIENTS EDENTULOUS FOR A LONG TIME

When patients have been edentulous for a long time, the problems they present are progressively more difficult to treat, and these problems must be recognized before adequate treatment procedures can be planned.

Mental attitudes

Traditionally, prosthodontic therapy for edentulous patients could be depicted by the following equation: clinical skill + knowledge = successful care. Some dentists have even enlarged the equation to: clinical skill + knowledge + prompt payment of professional fees = successful care, a cynical and semifacetious formula for success. Although clinical experience does actually support such a formula for the majority of patients who require care for their natural dentitions, the prosthodontic experience demands a much more profound understanding of the patient as a whole. During the past few years there have been strong and exciting initiatives in dental education to place the patient's well-being alongside the dentist's clinical expertise as a major educational and treatment objective. The modern equation for prosthodontic treatment now includes both technical and patient management skills, with the latter being based on a keen understanding of a patient's mental attitude.

Attitude studies on satisfied denture patients are not available, but psychologic inventories have been used to assess the personality characteristics of the difficult denture patient. Such studies (Bolender and associates, 1969; Nairn and Brunello, 1971) have shown that a high proportion of such patients score highly on indices of neuroticism. Neurosis is regarded as a chronic anxiety state at the physiologic level and is known to affect the performance of tasks requiring neuromuscular coordination (Levitt, 1971). Both learning and skilled performance show optimal relationships with moderate levels of anxiety, whereas levels of anxiety that are too high or too low appear to be incapacitating. Although this suggests that only the most anxious patients should experience difficulty with their dentures, clinical experience suggests that such a conclusion may be a narrow and restrictive one. It should be pointed out, however, that cheerful extroverts are rarely found in the ranks of difficult denture patients who frequently complain unceasingly, although no causative factors can be found for their problems.

The House classification. Many years ago Dr. Milus House proposed a general classification of patients' mental attitudes. This classification is based on extensive clinical experience rather than on scientific yardsticks or psychologic inventories. It has stood up well to the test of time and deserves discussion at some length:

1. *Philosophic*. Patients in the philosophic class are willing to accept the judgment of their dentists without question. They accept their oral situation and know that their dentist will do the best that can be done. They have an ideal attitude for successful treatment, provided that the biomechanical factors are reasonably favorable.

2. *Indifferent*. Indifferent patients have little concern for their teeth or oral health. They have little appreciation for the efforts of their dentists and often seek treatment because of the insistence of their families. They will give up easily if problems are encountered with their new teeth. Indifferent patients will require more time for their instruction on the value and use of dentures. Their attitude can be very discouraging to dentists who treat them.

3. *Critical*. Patients in the critical group are those who find fault with everything that is done for them. They were never happy with their previous dentists, and this is usually because the previous dentists did not follow their instructions. They will bring with them a collection of

dentures made by a number of different dentists and will tell their new dentist exactly what is wrong with each one. Careful observation and listening will reveal that the big mistakes had been the result of dentists trying to follow the directions of the patient.

Critical patients will try the temper and patience of any dentist attempting to treat them. A failure to recognize critical patients during diagnosis is certain to cause each new dentist many problems. A firm control of these patients is essential. They must not be allowed to even think that they are directing the treatment. The dentist must be the doctor who directs all treatment and decisions. These patients can be traumatic in a dental practice if they are not properly controlled, but their successful treatment can be most rewarding. The first and most important phase of treatment is carried out at the first professional contact. These people can be helped, despite themselves, when one identifies them early and works for a revision of their attitude. Many of these patients are in poor health, which affects their personalities and makes them tend to look for trouble. Often consulation with their physicians will provide information that will explain their attitudes. Medical consultation is always advisable for critical patients before treatment is started.

4. *Skeptical*. Patients who may be classed as skeptical are those who have had bad results with previous treatment and are therefore doubtful that anyone can help them. They are often in poor health, with severely resorbed residual ridges and other unfavorable conditions. They have tried to be good patients, but their problems seem to them to be insurmountable. Often they will have had a recent series of personal tragedies such as a loss of a spouse, business problems, and other things not directly related to their denture problems. They think the world is against them and simply doubt the ability of anyone to help them with problems that are greater than anyone else has to bear. They need kind and sympathetic help as much as they need new dentures.

A careful and thorough examination can be

the start of successful treatment. The dentist should take more time than usual in making examinations of skeptical patients, since care and attention to detail at this time will help the patient begin to develop confidence in the new dentist. A hurried or cursory examination will destroy the confidence and trust that is essential for satisfactory treatment. These patients can be made into excellent patients if dentists recognize them and handle them properly, but it will take extra time before, during, and after treatment.

From the preceding discussion it is obvious that not the least important factor in the diagnosis of patients needing complete denture service is their mental attitude. This is not a mechanical problem or a biologic problem. It is one that requires an understanding of people and the ways in which they may react to the situations they face. Dentists, with their background education in psychology, can learn to detect patient attitudes and reactions during diagnostic appointments. They can then modify their own attitudes and reactions so that mutual confidence, which is so essential, can be established.

In this process, dentists must establish within themselves empathy for the patient. If they are unable to do this, the results of any treatment they prescribe are most likely to be less than successful. Dentists must have a sense of real concern for the health, comfort, and welfare of their patients to establish the necessary mutual confidence. Clinical experience has proved the merits of a "tender loving care" approach to dental patients. This should be done before treatment is started and continued throughout the treatment planning and the treatment itself.

Desires and expectations

To establish rapport and confidence, the dentist must find out just what the patient's desires and expectations are. The dentist must inquire into the history of the patient's denture experience and listen carefully to the comments and complaints made by the patient. Questions such as, What difficulties are you having with your present dentures? may stimulate the patient to

tell of looseness, soreness, or difficulty in eating or talking. An evaluation by the dentist of the existing dentures in relation to the patient's complaints can reveal much information about the patient's mental attitude toward dentures and dentists. This can guide the dentist in what things to say and what things not to say to gain the confidence of the patient without promising more than is possible.

The question by the dentist, Are you happy with the way you look with your present dentures? can prompt a flood of comments that will be helpful later on in the arrangement of teeth for esthetics. This question should be asked during the examination appointment rather than after treatment has been started.

DIAGNOSIS OF THE PATIENT WITH NO TEETH REMAINING

The examination of edentulous mouths should be visual, palpatory, and radiographic, and it should be made after some preliminary questioning by the dentist.

The questions should relate primarily to the patient's oral, dental, and general health. The answers will often reveal the causes for difficulties the patient may have had with previous dentures and will point to the use of procedures that might avoid these same problems. In addition, the answers will often reveal the mental attitudes of patients and thus bring out the real problems of some edentulous patients. This is discussed in more detail later in the chapter.

Examination charts and records

As information about each patient is accumulated, a record of this information must be made and kept for further study and later use. The information gained during the examination of the patient will be helpful in determining the method of treatment, but equally important from a practical viewpoint, it will determine the amount of the fee to be charged that would be fair to both the patient and the dentist. Since there are great variations in the difficulty of treating different patients, it is essential that the differences be recorded for future reference.

DIAGNOSTIC CHART

STUDENT_____   PATIENT'S NAME_____

Extraction history:

Maxillary   Periodontal disease _____   Caries _____   Both _____   Year _____

Mandibular Periodontal disease _____   Caries _____   Both _____   Year _____

Earlier denture experience: None _____   Previous set(s) _____

Good _____   Poor _____

Age of present denture: _____   Duration of edentulism _____

Type of denture: U & L _____   Upper _____   Other _____

Immediate denture(s):   Upper _____   Lower _____   Both _____

Denture worn: Constantly _____   Intermittently _____   Day only _____   Rarely or never _____

Tooth material: Resin _____   Porcelain _____

Tooth form: Cusped _____   Cuspless _____

Denture base material: Resin _____   Other _____

Further prosthetic treatment since last dentures were made: Yes _____   No _____

If yes, explain: _____

Patient evaluation: (subjective)

Comfort	Good _____	Fair _____	Poor _____
Chewing efficiency	Good _____	Fair _____	Poor _____
Esthetics	Good _____	Fair _____	Poor _____
Articulation	Good _____	Fair _____	Poor _____
Soreness	Good _____	Fair _____	Poor _____
Food trapping	Good _____	Fair _____	Poor _____

Clinical assessment of prostheses (if present)

Interocclusal distance   Adequate _____   (+) _____   (−) _____

Stability   Satisfactory _____   Defective _____

Occlusion   Correct _____   Incorrect _____

Articulation   Correct _____   Incorrect _____

Total assessment:

Maxillary denture

1	2	3	4	5

Poor   Excellent

Mandibular denture

1	2	3	4	5

Poor   Excellent

Clinical data (use numerical code below)

Facial expression: Changed _____   Unchanged _____

Lips: Thin _____   Full _____   Short _____   Long _____   Tense _____   Active _____

Resorption   Slight U _____   Uneven U _____   Extensive U _____

L _____   L _____   L _____

Ridge relation: Normal _____   Protruded _____   Retruded _____

Floor of mouth: Favorable _____   Unfavorable _____

Border tissue: Attachments Maxillary _____   Mandibular _____

Oral mucosa: Upper   1. _____   2. _____   3. _____   4. _____

Lower   1. _____   2. _____   3. _____   4. _____

Resiliency of   Upper   1. _____   2. _____   3. _____   4. _____   5. _____

mucosa: Lower   1. _____   2. _____   3. _____   4. _____   5. _____

Undercuts: Upper _____   Lower _____

Tongue: Favorable _____   Unfavorable _____

Saliva: Serious _____   Mucous _____

Throat form: Favorable _____   Unfavorable _____

Radiographic assessment _____

Explain preprosthetic surgical treatment (if recommended) _____
_____

Prognosis explained to patient: probable outcome of treatment and adjustment period _____
_____

Probable future treatment necessary _____
_____

Clinical instructor _____

Code:

Oral mucosa

1. Clinically normal—no signs of inflammation, no granulation
2. Local inflammation—cases with red or small inflamed regions in otherwise normal tissue
3. Diffuse reddening—diffuse hyperemia with practically a smooth surface
   Slight trauma induces hemorrhage
4. Granulated—denture-bearing mucosa degenerates into a nodular, usually greatly hyperemic surface

Resiliency of denture supporting alveolar process

1. Firm—mucosa taut over bone
2. Slight mobility of most ridges—localized
3. Slight mobility of most ridges—generalized
4. Half or more of ridge height is mobile—localized
5. Half or more of ridge height is mobile—generalized

Fig. 4-2. For legend, see opposite page.

REMOVABLE PROSTHODONTIC EXAMINATION FORM

Patient_____Chart No._____

1. Cornel Medical Index results

    Last page_____Section I_____Total_____
    Interview results (agree-disagree) with CMI
    results

2. Previous denture experience
    Type Years Reason for replacement
          Worn (Problems and/or criticism)

    ☐ Additional comments on back

3. Evaluation of current dentures
    (S = Satisfactory, U = Unsatisfactory)
    Speech_____ Esthetics_____
    Occlusion_____
    Extension_____
    Retention_____
    ☐ Additional comments on back, including
       specific patient request(s) for change

4. Habits with current dentures
    Tongue_____ Clenching or bruxing_____
    Dentures worn at night_____

5. Mouth opening (large-small-medium)

6. Arch size
    Maxillary (large-medium-small)
    Mandibular (large-medium-small)

7. Contour of ridge—in cross section
                    Anterior   Posterior
    Max. (U-V-bulbous-flat) (U-V-bulbous-flat)
    Mand. (U-V-bulbous-flat) (U-V-bulbous-flat)

8. Contour of vault (flat-high-U)

9. Contour of soft palate
    (favorable-unfavorable)

10. Maxillary posterior palatal seal area
     Width (wide-narrow-average)
     Displaceability (marked-average-slight)

11. Torus palatinus (present-absent)

12. Torus mandibularis (present-absent)

13. Resorption
     Maxillary (slight-moderate-severe)
     Mandibular (slight-moderate-severe)

14. Mucosa (thickness and resilience)
     Outline areas of 2a, 2b, or 3 type mucosa

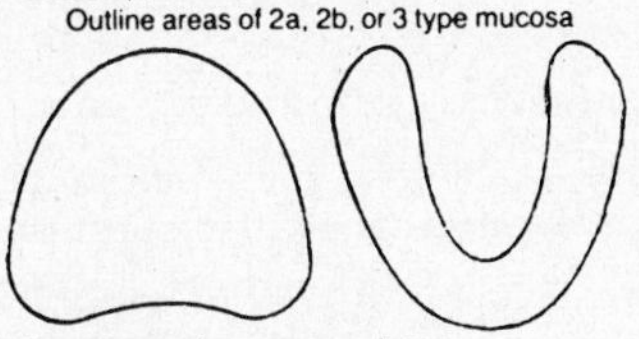

15. Appearance of mucous membrane
     Inflamed (I)
     Hyperplastic: Epulis (E)
                    Papillary (P)
                    Other (O)
     Hyperkeratosis (H)

16. Vestibular depth (note freni)   Where
     Maxillary   (adequate-inadequate) _____
     Mandibular (adequate-inadequate) _____

17. Inter-arch space (adequate-inadequate)
     Comment:

18. Tuberosity (favorable-unfavorable)
     Comment

19. Space between coronoid process and tuberosity
     (adequate-restricted-inadequate)
20. Maxillo-mandibular relation
     (normal-retrognathic-prognathous)
     Posterior (normal-crossbite)
21. Tongue position (normal-posterior)
22. Saliva
     Quantity (normal-excessive-minimum)
23. Radiographic examination
     Impacted teeth . . . .
     Root tips . . . .
     Foreign objects . . . .
     Radiolucent areas . . . .
     Other . . . .
     (Note: If negative, write "Neg.")

24. Corrective surgery indicated:

25. Prognosis (good-fair-poor*)
     Reason(s)-(refer to numbers)

*Patient informed of poor prognosis_____
                                    Instructor

Examination complete_____
                    Instructor   Date

· 3-2444

Fig. 4-2. Two examples of a diagnostic chart. The type of record used is less important than the fact that the dentist records all the features that will enhance the judgment-making process.

Many different types of examination records are being used by dentists for edentulous patients. An example of one is shown in Fig. 4-2. Other record forms can be used equally well. Some of these are more complicated than the example shown, and some are less detailed. Some dentists prefer to write out the conditions they observe and to dictate their observations to their assistant at the same time. This procedure has certain advantages: (1) the records made by the dentist can be less detailed than those being recorded by the dental assistant, (2) patients are made aware of the facts of their own dental problems and of the conditions in their mouth in a single operation, and (3) the dental assistant is made aware of the necessary variations from a basic time schedule for complete denture service.

Remember that the type of record system used is less important than the fact that a record system is used in the course of making a diagnosis.

General observations affecting diagnosis

Age. The age of the patient has a definite bearing on diagnosis for complete dentures. A young person will be more adaptable to new situations such as new dentures than an older person. The facility for learning and coordination appears to diminish with age (Landt, 1976), probably as a result of progressive atrophy of elements of the cerebral cortex. The oral and facial tissues become progressively less elastic and resilient as a person grows older, and they become more easily injured by the necessary manipulation for making impressions and other records.

With advancing age, people have more difficulty in adapting to new situations and learning new skills. This increases their problems in learning how to use their new teeth. Older patients also have a reduced coordination, which complicates the problems faced by dentists who provide complete denture service. If the patient has a hearing loss along with advancing age, the communication of instructions becomes more difficult.

The characteristic loss of tissue tone with age makes the problems of tooth arrangement and positioning more difficult than they would have been when the patient was younger.

Although these conditions should be recognized by the dentist, it is not always wise to discuss them in detail with patients because of the psychologic effect. Many patients know of the changes in their physical condition and ability, but they may resent being told about them. Instead, the dentist should recognize the conditions, make allowance for them in the scheduling by allocating more time to certain critical steps in the procedures, and adjust the fees to cover the extra time the treatment will require.

General health. The general health of the patient may or may not be correlated with the patient's age. Poor health may cause the physiologic age of the patient to be far beyond the chronologic age. The effects are the same. Poor health causes the same kinds of problems as advanced age, and corresponding changes in procedures and scheduling are necessary.

The general health of patients can be estimated by observation of their posture and gait when they enter the dental operatory. However, these judgments may be incorrect, and further information is essential. This additional information can be obtained by use of a health questionnaire, by questioning of the patients, or by consultation with their physicians.

Questions relating to the health of the patient must be carefully worded so as to avoid arousing a feeling of distrust in the mind of the patient or stirring up resentment at the dentist's impertinence. The questions should be dignified and professional in character and tone. They should stimulate the patient to volunteer the information that is essential for the dentist to know.

It is relatively simple to get patients to talk about their health if the questioning is done in a strictly professional manner. After the usual general conversation mentioned in Chapter 3, it is logical to ask, How is your general health? or How have you been feeling? Most of the time, the responses to these questions will not be very revealing, but sometimes they will open the floodgates and an extensive story of bad health will come out. Much of what will be said is of no real concern to the prosthodontic treatment, but some of it will be. It is at this time, particularly, that dentists must be good, careful, and sympathetic listeners. Their attitude at this time can build the confidence that is essential for successful treatment.

Responses to the questions, Are you taking any medicines? or What medicines are you taking? will tell the dentist much more than the previous leading questions. For example, if patients say they are taking chlordiazepoxide (Librium), diazepam (Valium), or some other tranquilizer, the dentist will know there is some nervous tension involved that may be a real problem during denture construction or in adaptation to the new prostheses. The medicines being taken can also indicate possible personal problems of the patient, which later can be reflected in criticism of the prosthetic treatment. The patient's marital problems or loss of family members can cause problems for the dentist that are more easily handled if the psychologic trauma faced by the patient is known. The existence of diabetes, hypertension, heart problems, allergies, chronic diseases, and other disorders should be known by the dentist so that the procedures can be altered if necessary and the dentist can be prepared for possible emergencies. Patients taking hormones, digitalis, nitroglycerin, and other drugs have special problems that can affect construction procedures and cause difficulties after the dentures have been completed.

It is important that these health problems be recognized *before* treatment is started so that the difficulties they may cause will not be considered as excuses when troubles do arise. Certainly, consultation with the patient's physician should be obtained before certain surgical procedures are prescribed. If the patient's health is endangered by the surgical shortening of a tuberosity, for example, the prosthodontic procedures should be altered to avoid the dangers, even though the result might not be as satisfactory.

Social training. The life-style or social training of patients must be considered when the diagnosis is made. Some people will expect more of their new dentures than others, and the expectations of the patient must be determined before a treatment plan is proposed. Some people will be concerned only about their ability to eat and their comfort, whereas others will want their new teeth to defy detection by their family, friends, and associates. Some will accept whatever is done without question, but others will insist on the impossible. Some will be concerned about their appearance and others will not, probably because they do not know what can be done. Some patients will want no change whatever in the appearance of their new teeth from the appearance of the dentures they have been wearing. Others will wish to have their face lifted and all the lines and wrinkles removed by their new teeth, even though to do this would give them a grotesque appearance. They want the "bloodless face-lifting" and the "wrinkle removers" though it is clearly impossible to turn the physiologic clock back 20 years or so, just because the patient desires it (Fig. 4-3). Instead, the new dentures should be planned to restore the dignity and harmony of the mouth region with the conditions found in the rest of the face. These special problems must be determined and recognized by *both* the patient and the dentist before any treatment is started.

Patients' complaints. Patients must be given the opportunity to tell what problems they had with the old dentures. The reason for this is the guidance the dentist may receive from the complaints about the area of greatest concern to the patient. Is it comfort, ability to eat, difficulty with speech, looseness, gagging? Is it the attitude of friends and relatives or the appearance of their teeth or their face? When this is known, the dentist will know which parts of the procedures will be most critical, how to overcome the difficulty if possible, and thus how to adjust the time schedule and fee properly.

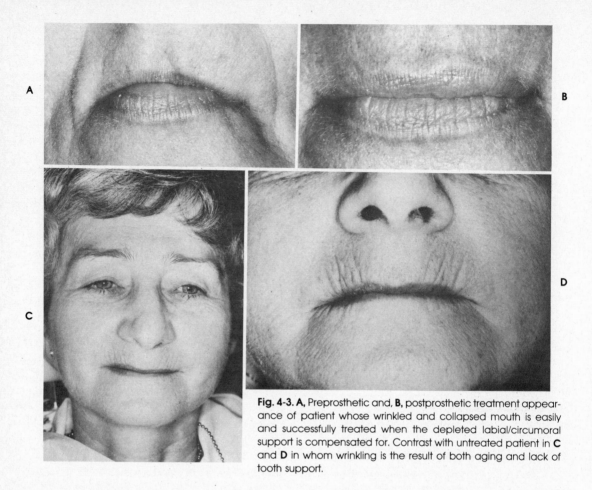

Fig. 4-3. A, Preprosthetic and, **B,** postprosthetic treatment appearance of patient whose wrinkled and collapsed mouth is easily and successfully treated when the depleted labial/circumoral support is compensated for. Contrast with untreated patient in **C** and **D** in whom wrinkling is the result of both aging and lack of tooth support.

If the chief concern is appearance, the dentist should make a personal assessment for comparison with that of the patient. In other words, is the patient's judgment correct or is it misdirected? To make an assessment, the dentist should observe the color and size of the teeth on the existing dentures and determine their harmony, or lack of it, with the patient's face and features. The basic position of the teeth should be observed, along with the amount of teeth that is exposed when the patient talks and smiles. The dentist should judge whether the irregularities of the teeth are natural or unlikely to be found in natural teeth.

Lip support. If the tissue around the mouth has

wrinkles (Fig. 4-3, *C* and *D*) and the rest of the face does not, significant improvement can be expected. If the existing anterior teeth are set too far lingually or palatally, the lips will lack the necessary support, and plans can be made to bring the new teeth further forward and thus provide the necessary support to help eliminate the wrinkles. If the wrinkles, especially the vertical lines in the lower half of the lip, are longstanding, they will not disappear at once and patients should be warned about this. Also, they should be told that for a short time their mouth might appear to them to be too full because of the sudden change. The real danger insofar as the dentist is concerned is that too much support for the lips might be provided in an attempt to eliminate the vertical lines in the upper lip. Extra time will be needed at the try-in of the wax dentures and should be planned for.

Questions about the prominance of the natural upper anterior teeth may reveal that surgery was done when the teeth were removed—"to get rid of the buck teeth I never liked." Attempts to reduce the horizontal overlap of anterior teeth by setting the teeth back "under the ridge" and by surgery usually lead to a lack of lip support that produces the vertical lines as tissue tone deteriorates later in life.

Lip thickness. Patients with thin lips present special problems. Any slight change in the labiolingual tooth position makes an immediate change in the lip contour. This can be so critical that even overlapping of teeth may distort the surface of the lip. Both the arch form and the individual tooth positions are involved. Thick lips give the dentist a little more opportunity for variations in the arch form and individual tooth arrangement before the changes are obvious in the lip contour.

Lip length. Patients with short upper lips will expose all the upper anterior teeth and much of the labial flange of the denture base as well. This means that special attention and care must be given to the color and form of the denture base.

Lip fullness. The fullness of the lip is directly related to the support it gets from the mucosa or denture base and the teeth in back of it. Lip fullness should not be confused with lip thickness, which involves the intrinsic structure of the lip. An existing denture with an excessively thick labial flange could make the lip appear to be too full, rather than displaced. The problem with lip fullness is in the patient's reaction to changes. If the existing dentures have the teeth set too far palatally, the patient may feel that the new and corrected tooth arrangement makes the lip too full.

Profile and contour of features. Observation of the facial profile gives an indication of the relative size of the upper and lower jaws and of the

vertical jaw relations. A receding chin and convex profile mean that the upper jaw is larger than the lower, and the occlusion will have a characteristic Class II disharmony in the centric position (Fig. 4-4, *A* and *B*).

If the chin is prominent, the profile will be concave, and the occlusion will have a characteristic Class III disharmony (Fig. 4-4, *C* and *D*), unless the appearance is created because the vertical separation of the jaws is too small. This reduced occlusal vertical dimension can result from loss of bone from the basal seats or from errors in the construction of the existing dentures. If the latter have occurred, improvement in the patient's appearance can be expected. If the variation from an ideal straight profile was developmental, only restoration of the profile similar to the one with natural teeth present can be expected.

Tone of facial tissues. A close inspection of the skin of the face will reveal the tone of the facial tissues. This is important because two factors affect tissue tone. First, the age and health of the patient influence the intrinsic structures of the facial tissues. These must be accepted as two of the conditions under which the dentist must work, unless the patient's general health can be improved. The tone of facial tissues may indicate limitations on what might be done to improve the patient's facial contours. A face that has poor tissue tone, with loose or wrinkled tissues throughout, cannot be made to appear youthful by new dentures. Second, poor tissue tone may be the result of inadequate support by the intraoral structures. This can be improved by new dentures if the existing ones are inadequate. The arch form and placement and the denture base contours are the keys to supplying adequate, but not excessive, support for facial tissues. It should be remembered, however, that the facial tissues around the mouth should be supported only to their original positions and that the tone of the skin should be comparable throughout the face.

Vertical face length. General observation of the patient's face while in conversation or while

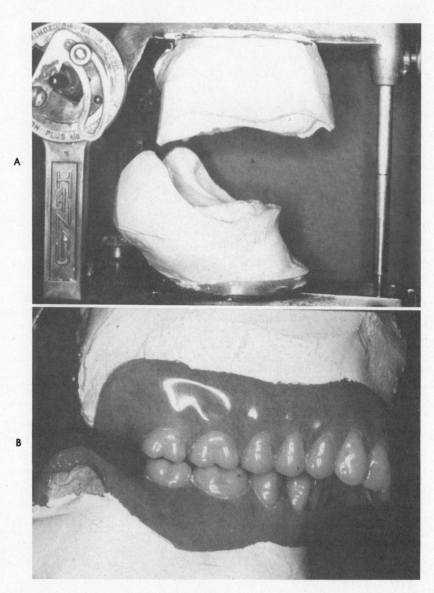

Fig. 4-4. A and **B,** Upper jaw is much larger than lower one. Since teeth must be correctly related to each of the residual ridges, large horizontal overlap is necessary.

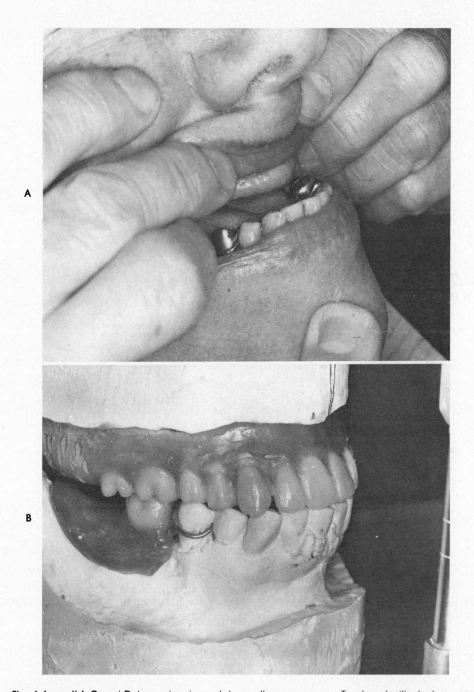

Fig. 4-4, cont'd. C and **D,** Lower jaw is much larger than upper one. Treatment with dentures can modify appearance of Class III disharmony.

the esthetic possibilities and limitations are considered should be directed to the length of the patient's face. This dimension is directly related to the vertical height of the dentures. If the dentures permit the jaws to close too far when the teeth are in contact, the muscles of mastication and facial expression are affected, and the tone of the facial tissues in the lower third of the face is not maintained. A judgment made at this time (i.e., during the examination) may be more effective than one made while new teeth are being constructed. A general appearance of the chin being too intimate with the nose can be apparent with the old dentures in place, and this should be observed.

Some patients may suggest that the occlusal vertical dimension be increased to eliminate wrinkles around the mouth. Care should be taken to avoid excessive denture height for these people. Usually, the cause of the wrinkles is a lack of anteroposterior support for the lips, and the dentist should not be led into using the patient's judgment in this regard. Misunderstandings regarding vertical jaw relations and vertical face length can consume much construction time later if the problems are not recognized.

Oral health

The health of the oral tissues should be thoroughly studied as soon as the existing dentures are removed from the mouth. The reason for doing this at once is that the dentist may be able to distinguish between damage being caused by the old dentures and damage from underlying conditions that may be observed. Superficial inflammation caused by the dentures may disappear quickly, but the results of long-term irritation by dentures will cause more lasting problems for both dentist and patient. To decide on the best treatment, one should observe, palpate, and evaluate many conditions.

Color of the mucosa. The color of the mucosa will reveal much information about its health. The differences in appearance between a healthy pink mucosa and red inflamed tissue are

apparent. The problem is how to get all the oral mucosa into a healthy state. The solution will be different in different patients because of the differences in the causes of the inflammation and the length of time the tissues have been irritated. Some tissues will recover with simple rest by keeping the dentures out of the mouth; others will require the use of tissue-conditioning resins inside existing or treatment dentures. Still others will require surgery of the mouth to make them as healthy as possible.

Regardless of the problem and its treatment, however, the oral tissues *must* be healthy before impressions for new dentures are made. To fail to see that the tissues are healthy is to invite trouble from a continuing inflammation or from new dentures that become loose because the inflammation disappears after the new dentures are in service. The treatment plan and schedule must provide for the necessary procedures to be carried out and for complete recovery of the tissues from the preparatory treatment used.

Abrasions. Abrasions, cuts, or other sore spots may be found in any location under the basal seats of the existing dentures or at the borders. They may be the result of overextended or underextended borders, or malocclusion may cause them. At the time of the examination the causes should be removed to allow the tissues an opportunity to heal before impressions are made.

Pathosis. Many types of pathologic lesions may be found in the oral cavity. These may be lesions of the mucous membrane or of tissues under it. The lesions may be in the bone or glandular tissue, the soft palate, hard palate, cheeks, tongue, the floor of the mouth, or the throat. Like mechanical cuts and abrasions, pathologic lesions should be diagnosed and treated before impressions are made. Among the more common lesions found in the mouths of edentulous patients are pseudoepitheliomatous hyperplasia, papillary hyperplasia, aphthous ulcers, lichen planus, hyperkeratosis and leukoplakia, and epulis fissuratum.

Other lesions may be more serious. These are

lumps and ulcers that may be evidence of malignancies. They may be found in the floor of the mouth and on the tongue, throat, and palate. If they are not detected, serious consequences can result for the patient and for the dentist. If suspicious lesions are found, adequate steps must be carried out to determine the precise cause. These include biopsy and referral for further tests. Oral malignancies are most common in people who are old enough to be likely to need complete dentures, but they may occur in people of all ages. Dentists' obligations in the area of health do not end when the last teeth are gone. Instead, they become more important.

Hard and soft areas in the maxillary basal seat

Each basal seat has some areas that are harder than others, and these should be located so that the dentures can be planned to distribute occlusal and limiting forces where they should be. This consideration is discussed in detail in Chapter 7, but the observations are made at the time of the examination. Some of the hard areas such as the torus palatinus should be relieved of pressure from the denture. Likewise, soft areas such as the incisive papilla should be protected from pressure that would impinge on the blood vessels and nerves that lie under it.

An ideal basal seat for a maxillary denture is one that has a more or less uniform layer of soft tissue over the bone. The ideal layer of tissue is one that is quite firm, but still slightly resilient. When the tissue covering the bone is too thin, it will be easily damaged by the pressure from the denture and will be more difficult to fit with the denture base. When the tissue is too thick, it will be too soft and will permit the denture to move more than it should when under occlusal pressure.

The maxillary tuberosities are often enlarged with movable fibrous tissue. Obviously, freely movable soft tissues will not provide as good support for the denture as would firm ones. It may be desirable to remove large fibrous tuberosities if they are movable, even though they may not interfere with the location of the occlu-

sal plane (Chapter 6). See Figs. 3-9 and 3-10.

An even more hazardous condition affecting stability and support for maxillary dentures is the hyperplastic or flabby maxillary ridge. This large mass of easily movable and displaceable tissue occupies the space formerly occupied by the residual alveolar (bony) ridge. It may extend from one tuberosity to the other, or it may be only in the anterior part of the maxillary arch. The best treatment for this condition is to remove it by surgery. The foundation for the denture will appear to be smaller, but in fact, it is not. The bone is the same after surgery and is more effective in its support of the mucosa that supports the denture.

When the patient who has this condition is examined for dentures, other factors must also be considered in the decision to remove the hyperplastic tissue. If the patient's general physical health is not good, if his or her age is such that the physical tolerance is low, or if there is a recent history of a number of general surgical operations, it may be wise to alter the impression procedure and avoid or postpone further oral surgery. In this situation it is important that the patient understand that the dentist is using an alternate procedure that is more difficult than the usual one and that the results may not be as good as might be expected from the regular procedure. The dentist is choosing the lesser of two evils in a bad situation.

Whether the hyperplastic tissue is surgically removed, the maxillary bones will be smaller than before the hyperplasia developed. This inevitably produces unfavorable leverages on the maxillary denture base and more difficulty in developing occlusal harmony. These factors must be recognized at the time the diagnosis is made so that time adjustments can be made in the treatment schedule and in the fee to be quoted to the patient for the denture service.

One other hard area found in some patients is the zygomatic process of the maxillary bone as it crosses the buccal vestibule on each side. When the top of the buccal vestibule is palpated in the molar region, this bony process may be observed to be low in relation to the crest of the residual ridge. When the soft tissue is thin over the zygomatic process, the denture may tend to rock over these hard areas on each side and thus be loosened. This difficulty can be anticipated when the mouth is examined, and the correction is simple when the cause is known.

Torus palatinus. A torus palatinus is a bony enlargement found at the midline of the hard palate. It is not found in all patients, and it varies in size from that of a small pea to a huge enlargement that may even fill the palate to the level of the occlusal plane. The palatine tori are covered with a thin layer of soft tissue, and consequently they are very hard. In fact, they are much less resilient than the fibrous tissues on the crest of the residual ridge, which provide the primary support for the maxillary denture. Therefore the torus palatinus must be relieved from pressure from the denture, or it may be removed by surgery (Chapter 6).

Generally surgery to remove a torus palatinus should be avoided, but if the torus is so large that it extends beyond the vibrating line and over part of the soft palate, it should be removed or reduced in size. When the torus extends too far back, it may interfere with the development of a posterior palatal seal (Fig. 6-7).

Palatine tori are easily relieved of pressure by placement of sheet of lead of appropriate thickness over it on the cast when the denture is processed. The size of the relief will coincide with the size of the convexity in the hard palate. The thickness of the relief will vary with the relative hardness of the torus, which is usually harder in larger tori.

Adhesions. Adhesions between the residual ridge and the cheek may occur in either the maxillary or mandibular basal seats. Usually, a notch or notches in the impression and in the denture base will accommodate these adhesions, but if they attach too close to the crest of the residual ridge, it is best to remove them before the impression is made. When they are "clipped" or removed, a stent must be used to keep the soft tissue parts separated while heal-

ing occurs. Otherwise, the cut surfaces will grow together again, and the situation will be worse than before the surgery.

Hard and soft areas in the mandibular basal seat

The hard areas in the mandibular basal seat are either favorable (as on a broad residual ridge crest) or unfavorable (as a torus mandibularis, a series of hard sharp points, or a sharp bony ridge). Each of these must be handled in a different way.

The torus mandibularis is a bony bulge or knob found on the lingual side of some mandibular alveolar ridges in the region of the premolar teeth. Mandibular tori form while the teeth are present and stay there after the teeth are lost unless they are removed. They range in size from a small pea to half a hazelnut or larger. They occur singly or in rows just above the floor of the mouth (Fig. 4-5). They are usually removed long before impressions for complete dentures are made. They are thinly covered by soft tissue, which means that this tissue is more sensitive to pressure from dentures than the other tissue of the basal seat.

The torus itself has a thin covering of cortical bone, and the interior of the torus is made up of cancellous bone. When the cortical bone is removed, pressure from a denture would be against cancellous bone unless there was adequate healing time for a new cortical plate to be formed. This takes from 2 to 6 months.

It is practically impossible to provide relief for mandibular tori inside a denture. The tori are too close to the floor of the mouth, and so attempts to take pressure off the tori will break the border seal that the mandibular denture should have. However, some mandibular tori can be accommodated by carefully planned relief of the denture.

Two other hard areas are of practical significance. These are of hard points of attachment of the mentalis muscles that exist near the crest of badly resorbed residual ridges. These hard "bumps" can be relieved by modification of the

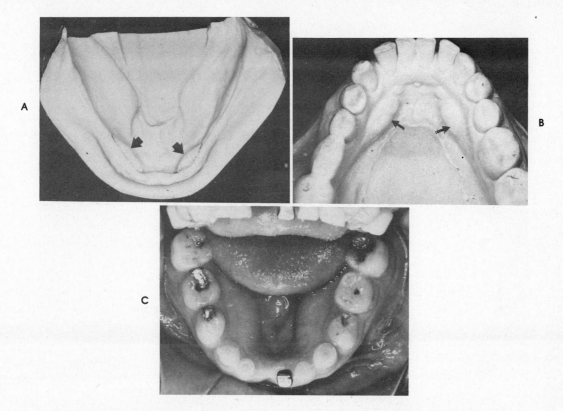

Fig. 4-5. Examples of mandibular tori. **A** and **B,** Average size; **C,** extremely large. See also Fig. 9-15.

denture bases. No surgery to reduce them is indicated.

The crest of the residual mandibular ridge is a relatively hard area as compared with the tissue covering the broad area of the buccal shelf, provided that unfavorable resorption has not occurred. The buccal shelf is on the body of the mandible between the buccal frenum and the retromolar pad and between the residual ridge crest and the external oblique line. It has a good cortical bone surface, but it also has a covering of the suctorial pad and the inferior attachment of the buccinator muscle, as well as free gingiva on top of it. These soft tissues are more easily displace than those found on the crest of the residual ridge unless there has been severe bony ridge resorption.

Diagnostic procedures should be used to determine the relative thickness of these soft tissues and the condition of the residual ridge itself. Radiographs are essential for making these determinations.

The soft areas include the retromolar pad, which is both soft and easily displaceable. The pad cannot supply support for the denture, but it must be covered by the denture if a border seal is to be maintained. It should not be displaced from its normal relaxed position, since some movable structures enter or pass through it. These include the buccinator muscle, the superior constrictor of the pharynx, and the pterygomandibular raphe. The structure of the retromolar pad also includes fibers from the temporal tendon and some mucous glands. When the diagnosis is made, plans should include full coverage of the retromolar pads.

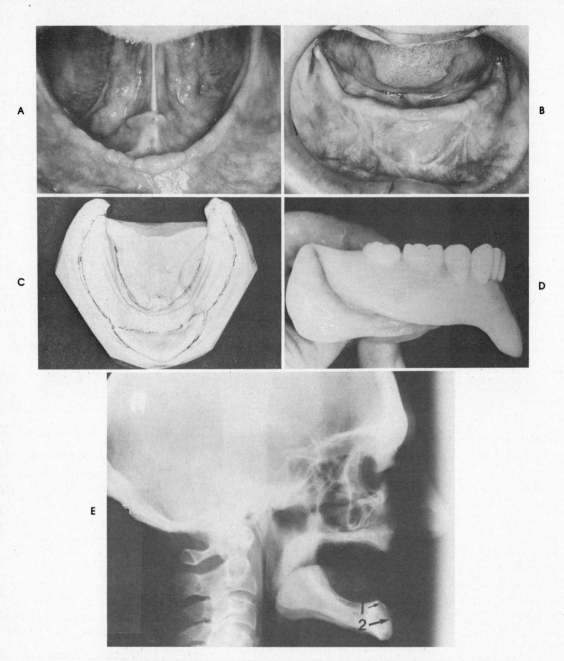

Fig. 4-6. A, Residual ridge consists of flabby, cordlike, soft-tissue crest. Attached mucosa is limited and mobile. In **B** to **D** a similar clinical situation was treated surgically, and the new labial sulcus can now be filled by a significant labial denture extension. **E,** This occurs because the mentalis muscle origin has been several at *1,* and the labial sulcus depth is now at *2.*

Fibrous cordlike ridges. Some patients with severely resorbed mandibles have cordlike, soft-tissue ridge crests (Fig. 4-6, *A*). These are fibrous tissue and usually extend from one retromolar pad to the other. These soft-tissue ridges are easily displaced labially, buccally, or lingually, and they do not supply stability or support for dentures. They must not be displaced when impressions are made, since they will be painful when the dentures are worn and they would tend to lift the denture when the teeth are not in contact.

Surgery could improve this situation by removing the movable tissue, but this has its hazards as well. In many patients, the surgical removal of a fibrous ridge crest detaches the mucosa from the mandible, so that the mucous membrane over the residual ridge can be pulled forward by the lip and backward by the tongue. This is disastrous, and is of course avoided by the oral surgeon's combining the tissue "trim" with a vestibuloplasty procedure (Fig. 4-6, *B* to *E*).

Absence of tuberosities and loss of pterygomaxillary notch

Advanced bone resorption or excessive surgical reduction of the tuberosity area can lead to absence of one or both tuberosities. Such a morphologic feature is frequently accompanied by obliteration of the pterygomaxillary notch area, which is essential for ensuring the maximum breadth to the posterior palatal seal of the denture. When this is encountered, the patient should be informed, since the maxillary denture will not be as resistant to posterior downward dislodgment when incising takes place. Our oral surgical colleagues can sometimes improve the area for the prosthesis by creating a localized vestibuloplasty.

Biomechanical considerations

A number of biomechanical factors influence the choice of methods to be used and the difficulties that will be encountered in providing complete denture service. These must be recog-nized even though not much can be done to eliminate the causes of problems. Instead, it is necessary to make alterations in the technical procedures that help to reduce the adverse effects of the unfavorable conditions.

Arch size. The size of the mandible and the maxillae determines the ultimate support available for complete dentures. Large jaws provide more support than small jaws, and the difference is directly proportional to their sizes. Therefore a patient with small jawbones should not expect to put as much closing force on the dentures as a person with large jawbones.

The size of the maxillae and mandible is also involved in the margin for error in impression making. If the jaws are small, the impressions must be as accurate as possible because a small error would be relatively larger than the same error in an impression of a large mouth. This is not to say that impressions of large jaws should not be as accurate as those of small jaws. Instead, impression requirements for small jaws are more critical than those for large ones.

Disharmony in jaw sizes. Some patients have large maxillary jaws and small mandibular jaws, and some have the opposite disharmony with the mandibular jaw being larger than the maxillary one. These conditions arise from genetic factors and from improper growth and development. When the natural teeth were present, these patients had severe malocclusions, which may or may not have been treated by orthodontists. The replacement of teeth for people who had Class II or Class III malocclusions presents some special problems. The artificial teeth should occupy the same basic positions as the natural teeth, and this requires that the occlusion must be planned in relation to the disharmony. The modifications from an ideal occlusion to a crossbite occlusion or one with an excessive horizontal overlap of the upper teeth over the lower teeth will require time to develop. These difficulties should be recognized and anticipated when the diagnosis is made.

Ridge form. The cross-section contour of the ridge has an important influence on the selection of the impression procedure. Resorption of the residual ridge after the removal of teeth makes radical changes in its crosssection form. When the teeth are first removed, the ridge is broad at its occlusal surface, but as resorption occurs, the residual ridge becomes progressively narrower and shorter. The ideal ridge has a broad top and parallel sides. As the ridge becomes narrower, it becomes sharper and consequently is unable to withstand as much force as a broader ridge.

When the mandibular ridge is sharp and has sharp bone spicules, it is best to use a selective pressure impression (that is, one which selectively "unloads" the ridge crest area) so that more of the occlusal force is placed on the cortical bone of the buccal shelf on either side of the sharp crest of the ridge.

When the sharp ridge has disappeared, it is best to use an impression procedure that will distribute occlusal forces more evenly. A minimum pressure procedure is best in this situation.

When severe undercuts exist after the teeth have been removed, some surgical alteration may be necessary. However, this should be avoided if possible. The undercuts may not be as severe as they seem because of the resiliency of the mucosa. Occasionally an elastic impression material such as Thiokol or silicone rubber will overcome the difficulty caused by the undercuts.

Ridge relations. The ridge relations change as shrinkage occurs. Therefore the amount of resorption that has occurred after teeth have been lost affects this relationship (see Fig. 2-18).

The bones of the upper jaw (the maxillae) resorb primarily from the occlusal surface and the buccal and labial surfaces. This means that the upper residual ridge becomes shorter and that the maxillary arch becomes narrower from side to side and shorter anteroposteriorly.

The lower jaw (the mandibular ridge) resorbs primarily from the occlusal surface. As this occurs, the mandibular residual ridges in the posterior part of the mouth become progressively farther apart. It appears as though the mandibular arch becomes broader while the maxillary arch becomes narrower. The mandible changes in this way because the inferior border of the mandible is broader from one side of the jaw to the other than the occlusal part of the mandible. The cross-section skrinkage in the molar region is downward and outward. The cross-section shrinkage in the anterior region, at first is downward and backward. Then as shrinkage continues, the anterior part of the basal seat for the mandibular denture moves forward.

These changes must be noted at the time of the examination to plan for the resultant problems of leverage, occlusion, and tooth position for esthetics.

Arch shape. The shape of the residual arch, when observed from the occlusal surface, should be noted to anticipate, in a general way, the form of the teeth to be used and to estimate the relative development of the lower third of the face. This can be a guide to the arrangement of the teeth. If the arches are asymmetrical, some problems of tooth arrangement and occlusion can be anticipated.

Sagittal profile of residual ridge. Closely related to the factor of parallelism of residual ridges is the problem of the upward slope of the distal part of the mandibular residual ridge. In making the intraoral examination, the mandibular residual ridge should be observed by palpation to determine the location where the ridge slopes up toward the retromolar pad and the ramus. This is important because occlusal contacts immediately above the incline at the back part of the residual ridge will cause a complete denture to skid forward. Plans must be made to avoid this kind of dislodging force on mandibular dentures. Unfavorable ridge slopes are not often found in recent extraction situations, but they are common in mouths of patients whose posterior teeth have been out a long time.

Shape of the palatal vault. Palatal vaults vary considerably from patient to patient. The most favorable vault form is one that has a medium depth, with a well-defined incline of the rugae area in the anterior part of the palate.

A flat palatal vault can present some difficulties if the bone in the anterior region is severely resorbed. The problem in this situation is one of insufficient resistance to a forward movement of the maxillary denture. Such a loss of stability will cause a loss of retention of the denture, especially during masticatory function. Dentures in a mouth with a flat palatal vault can resist removal by a direct downward pull, but they can be easily dislodged by a laterally or anteriorly directed force or by a rotating force. Therefore particular attention must be paid to balancing the occlusion.

A high, narrow, V-shaped vault is also unfavorable for the retention of dentures. The tighter the denture presses against the sides of the palatal vault, the faster the denture will loosen and slip out of place. In most mouths with a V-shaped vault, the residual ridges also are V-shaped in cross section. Thus the problem is complicated. The solution involves the development of the border seal, border thickness, and shape of the polished surfaces so that the cheeks and buccinator muscles can automatically perfect the border seal and mechanically aid in the retention of the denture. The necessary additional time and care should be planned for at the time of the examination.

Muscular development. The muscular development of the tongue, cheeks, and lips is a significant factor influencing impression making and the ability of patients to use their dentures after they have been completed. The tongue can be very troublesome if it is overly large or small.

Tongues seem to become larger and more powerful if patients have been wearing loose or otherwise inadequate dentures. Apparently the tongue is used by these patients to hold their upper dentures up, and others even masticate their food by pushing it against the roof of the mouth with the tongue. Patients who have worn a complete upper denture against eight or ten lower anterior teeth are especially prone to develop these habits. Also, when lower molar teeth have been missing for some time, the tongue tends to fill the space vacated by the teeth, and often the sublingual glands are forced over the crest of the residual ridge into the place to be occupied by the denture. This must be recognized at the time of the examination so that adequate time can be scheduled to handle a difficult situation (Fig. 4-7).

A small tongue will cause difficulty for the patient wearing a complete mandibular denture. Usually the small tongues will drop back away from the lower anterior teeth and thus break the border seal. Proper training can help

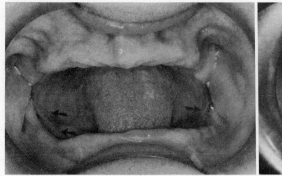
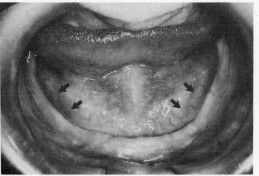

Fig. 4-7. A and **B,** Large tongue and sublingual glands occupy some of space necessary for denture. was necessary to push tongue and glands aside with a finger to get tray in position to make impression, as well as to seat denture. Usually, a reduction in lingual flange dimensions is required.

patients to learn where they should carry their tongue for the best results. Time should be allotted for this training at each step of the construction procedures. If the training is to be effective, it must be done while the dentures are being made rather than after they are completed.

Saliva. The amount and consistency of saliva will affect the stability and retention of dentures and the comfort with which patients can wear them.

An excess of saliva will complicate impression making and be an annoyance to patients. This is usually much worse when dentures are new. The new dentures may feel like foreign objects, which they are, and this does stimulate the flow of saliva. In time, the feeling and the flow of saliva will decrease. Patients will need assurance about this.

A lack of saliva, xerostomia, presents some more serious problems. Moisture is necessary for the usual factors of retention to act, and if saliva is absent, there is the possibility of reduced retention for dentures. Furthermore, the absence of saliva often causes the cheeks and lips to stick to the denture base in an uncomfortable manner. Petroleum jelly applied over the surface of the denture can alleviate the latter problem.

A saliva that is thick and ropy can cause problems. It is made up of heavy secretions of mucus formed from the palatal glands under the maxillary denture. The very thickness of the mucus is often sufficient to force the dentures out of their correct position. The thick saliva also complicates impression making by forming voids in the impression surface while the impression material sets. Thick, ropy saliva is also a factor in causing patients to gag while impressions are made and after the new dentures are installed. The palatal surface should be wiped free of saliva before the final impression is made, and the mucous glands should be massaged with a small piece of gauze just before the final impression is made to eliminate as much of the mucus as possible.

Ideally, there should be a moderate flow of serous type of saliva, and this seems to be the situation most frequently found.

Cheeks and lips. The muscles in the cheeks and lips have a critical function in successful use of dentures. The denture flanges must be properly shaped so that they can aid in maintaining the dentures in place without conscious effort on the part of the patient. This involves the development of the proper arch form and tooth positions as well as the shape of the polished surfaces and the thickness of the denture borders.

Patients with very thick cheeks may present severe technical problems during impression making and jaw relation recording. Thick cheeks often do not allow easy manipulations at the proper time for border molding of the impression materials or for manipulation of the mandible into the desired position for certain jaw relation records.

Muscle tonus. The tone of the facial and muscle tissues is critical to several steps of denture construction. If the tonus is too tense, the cheek and lip manipulations are difficult, if the tissue tone is too poor, the lips and cheeks may be too easily displaced by the dentures. Either too firm or too weak a tissue tone is unfavorable, and this means that extra time will be needed to overcome the difficulties.

Muscular control. Good muscular control and coordination are essential to the effective wearing of complete dentures. For example, if tongue movements are used for border molding the lingual flanges of a mandibular impression, the timing, direction, and amount of movement are critical to the success of the border molding. If the tongue movement is too slow, too fast, too little, too great, or to the wrong direction, the effort is wasted, and more time is required to complete the operation successfully.

To make an observation of muscular control, the patient is asked to open the mouth about half way and then to put the tongue into the right cheek and into the left cheek, to stick it out, and to put it up and back inside the mouth. The ability, or lack of ability, of the patient to do these things on demand will be apparent, and the work schedule can be modified accordingly.

Jaw movements. The ability, or lack of ability, of the patient to move the mandible to the right place at the right time will reveal problems in making jaw relation records before they are attempted. If patients cannot move the mandible in the direction they are instructed to, problems of recording jaw relations can be expected. This will affect the scheduling of treatment appointments.

Temporomandibular joint problems. Patients presenting with one or more of the following symptoms are usually considered to be suffering from mandibular or temporomandibular joint dysfunction. The definitional symptoms include (1) pain and tenderness in the region of muscles of mastication and temporomandibular joints, (2) sounds during condylar movements, and (3) limitations of mandibular movement (Zarb and Speck, 1979). Quite logically the temporomandibular joints should be healthy before new dentures are made. Unhealthy temporomandibular joints complicate the registration of jaw relation records and sometimes even preclude them completely. Centric relation depends on both structural and functional harmony of osseous structures, the intra-articular tissue, and the capsular ligaments if it is to be a functional position. If these specifications cannot be fulfilled, the patient will not have a centric relation or for that matter provide the dentist with a recordable one (Gilboe, 1983), hence the importance of the routine evaluation of a patient's temporomandibular function as an integral part of complete denture treatment. If symptoms are present, they must be treated. The treatment usually takes the form of a soft diet, improvement in fit and occlusion of the prosthesis, recovery of overt loss of vertical dimension of occlusion in the old prosthesis, and prescription of appropriate medication where necessary. Simple but accurate explanation of the dysfunction, its multifactional etiology, and its consequences, treatment, and prognosis should also be provided for the patient. Furthermore when there is reason to believe that organic joint pathosis exists, radiographs of the temporomandibular joints should be taken.

Gagging

A patient's protective gag reflex can compromise a dental treatment plan if the reflex is an active one. The exaggerated gag reflex, though not common, can frustrate both patient and dentist. A thorough history and oral examination will reveal the presence of such a reflex early in the patient-dentist relationship. The dentist can then assess the possible cause of the problem as being attributable to iatrogenic factors, organic disturbances, anatomic anomalies, biomechanical inadequacies of existing prostheses, or psychological factors (Conny and Tedesco, 1983). Effective management of the gagging problem tends to be based on experience and anecdote, with combinations of clinical techniques, prosthodontic management, medication, and psychologist referral being regarded as the most successful approaches. Usually, reassurance and kind handling of the patient prove to be useful therapeutic adjuncts. However it has to be conceded that some gaggers need the services of trained specialists, and the dentist should be vigilant about seeking such help for his or her patients.

DEVELOPMENT OF THE TREATMENT PLAN

After all the indicated observations have been made, it is time to develop the treatment plan and to inform the patient about it. The decisions are based on an analysis of the information collected during the diagnosis.

The dentist should review each item in relation to its effect on procedures that might be used and in relation to the amount of time the item will require during and after the treatment. The amount of time is important because it will determine the estimate of the cost of the treatment to the patient. In this regard, certain minimum costs to the dentist in time and money are unavoidable, and the unfavorable factors found in the examination will add to the dentist's costs.

Once the methods, procedures, materials, and time requirements are known, a fairly accurate estimate of the cost to the patient will be known. Only after all these factors have been considered should the dentist discuss the proposed treatment or fees with the patient.

REFERENCES

Bolender, C.L., Swoope, C.C., and Smith, D.E.: The Cornell Medical Index as a prognostic aid for complete denture patients, J. Prosthet. Dent. **22**:20-29, 1969.

Conny, D.T., and Tedesco, L.A.: The gagging problem in prosthodontic treatment. Part I: Identification and causes; Part II: Patient management, J. Prosthet. Dent. **49**:601,757, 1983.

Gilboe, D.B.: Centric relation as the treatment position, J. Prosthet. Dent. **50**:685, 1983.

Landt, H.: Oral recognition of forms and oral muscular coordination ability in dentulous subjects of various ages, Svensk Tandlak. Tidskr. **69**(supp. 5), 1976.

Levitt, E.E.: The psychology of anxiety, London, 1971, Paladin Books.

Nairn, R.I., and Brunello, D.L.: The relationship of denture complaints and the level of neuroticism, Dent. Pract. **21**:156-157, 1971.

Zarb, G.A., and Speck, J.E.: The treatment of mandibular dysfunction. In Zarb, G.A., and Carlsson, G.E., editors: Temporomandibular joint function and dysfunction, St. Louis, 1979, The C.V. Mosby Co.

5

Communicating with the patient

Not all the problems of diagnosis and treatment of edentulous patients are mechanical or biologic. A major problem involves informing the patient about the conditions observed during the course of the examination and about the importance of these conditions for the final result of treatment.

The things that are said to the patient after the general observations and the radiographic, digital, and visual examinations have been made will affect the reactions of the patient to any proposed treatment. They will also affect the reaction of the patient to the treatment after it is completed.

Perhaps the best way to inform patients about various observations that have been made is to dictate these observations to an assistant at the time they are made. This has two desirable effects. First, such dictation tells the patient that the dentist is seeing specific conditions existing in the mouth of the one who is most concerned or affected by them—the patient. The procedure is therefore more than an observation that there are no teeth and that the patient needs new dentures. Second, it tells the patient in a dignified and formal manner of conditions that may or may not affect the success of treatment. In most instances, patients will not know the significance of each dictated statement, but if they are curious and ask, they should be told the meaning and importance of the condition they inquire about. It will not be necessary to discuss every item of diagnosis in detail with the patient, but questions should be answered simply and truthfully. For example, the dentist may say, "The mental foramen is on top of the ridge on the left side," and the patient may reply, "What does that mean?" An answer should be given, such as the following. "This means that I will have to keep pressure off the nerve and blood vessels that pass through that opening in the bone or relieve it of pressure when the denture is completed. Pressure on the mental nerve that passes through the mental foramen can cause pain or numbness in the lip on that side. Did you ever have that experience with your old dentures?" If patients have experienced such discomfort, they will understand the problem, but more important, they will know that the dentist is making a thorough examination and knows what he is doing. Consequently, confidence is established, and it is not likely that more than a few specific questions will be asked by most patients.

AVOID DISCUSSIONS OF EXISTING DENTURES

Many patients will ask their new dentist to evaluate or criticize their existing dentures. This should be avoided. It is especially important that dentures made by other dentists not be discussed. The primary reason is that you should make your own diagnosis, and you cannot do this as well if you try to judge the existing dentures before you know all the facts.

If patients insist on talking about existing dentures or previous dentists, simply listen and say nothing for a while, and then say that you want to make your own diagnosis. The reaction of patients at this time is critical because it will give a good indication of their mental attitude.

INFORM THE PATIENT ABOUT THE TREATMENT PLAN

Assuming that the dictation to the assistant has pointed out to the patient many of the factors involved in making the treatment plan, the decisions regarding technical procedures can be dictated to the assistant and also recorded on the patient's record card by the dentist.

The first discussion will have to be about the procedures necessary for preparing the mouth for dentures. These may include the amount of time the existing dentures must be kept out of the mouth before impressions are made or other preparatory procedures (discussed in detail in Chapter 6).

Construction decisions such as the types of tray, impression materials, impression, jaw relation records, teeth to be used, and base material can be tentatively specified to the assistant so that the patient can hear the comments. Of particular importance is the request for the allowance of extra time to be scheduled for operations where it is needed. For example, if conditions indicate that more time than usual will be required for making impressions, the assistant is told to allow that extra time in arranging the schedule of appointments. If the esthetic requirements will be difficult to satisfy, the assistant is told to allow extra time at the try-in appointment.

By instructing the assistant to allow time to meet individual conditions, the dentist automatically informs the patient of the problems without making a big issue out of them. At this time, it is best to avoid specific mention of the problems and, instead, to place the emphasis on the time needed for solving them. This will reassure the patient.

Some decisions must be made that involve patients' choices. These include the possible use of metal bases or soft liners for the new dentures. For obvious reasons, these special bases involve greater costs than bases made of a single material such as acrylic resin.

Some patients will prefer a metal base in the maxillary denture because of its conduction of heat and cold to the hard palate. Since the laboratory procedures involved in making these bases are more expensive, there should be a logical difference in the fee for the denture, and the patient can make the choice.

Soft linings for complete dentures likewise are more expensive to produce than all-resin bases. The cost of time to the dentist is the same as for bases made entirely of hard resins. So the difference in cost to the patient should be the difference in laboratory costs to produce the denture with a soft lining. The dentist should not recommend the soft-lined denture unless there is a special indication for its use and then only if adequate space is available within the denture for its use. The patient can make the final choice regarding the use of soft liners *provided* that the dentist sees some value to the patient in their use.

SUMMARY OF DIAGNOSTIC FINDINGS

A brief oral summary of the findings determined during the examination should be made to the patient, and the possibilities and limitations of the proposed treatment should be explained. This summary should be made in simple language so that the chance for misunderstanding by the patient will be minimal. The prognosis should be factual as far as can be determined, and it should be conservative and yet encouraging.

ECONOMICS OF PROSTHODONTIC SERVICE

It is only after the diagnosis is complete and the treatment plan has been made that a fee for complete denture service can be determined. A uniform or standard fee for dentures is totally unrealistic. The conditions in patients' mouths vary so much that a fixed fee for this service would be unfair to the patient in some cases and unfair to the dentist in others. The patient who has favorable ridges and jaw relations and a favorable mental attitude will require less time to treat than one who has unfavorable conditions. Therefore with a standard fee the patient with uncomplicated conditions would, in effect, be paying for the cost of treating the patient with more complicated problems. This is unfair to all concerned. The fee should be determined on an individual basis for each patient according to the time and difficulties involved in the treatment.

There is, however, a basic cost to each dentist for the production of complete denture service that is based on the minimum time it takes to render the service. This cost must include the time spent in diagnosis, treatment planning, basic treatment procedures, installation of the dentures, and their adjustment after the dentures have been completed. The time spent in these activities will vary with the difficulties presented by the patient. Other costs will include office overhead and maintenance, payroll for office assistance, and laboratory service. All these items together establish the actual cost of rendering complete denture service. They represent the basis for the minimum fee for service to any patient, but the fees for patients with difficult problems that will take more time to treat should be greater than the minimum fee. This variation should be based on the amount of time required for the solution of the problems. If the impressions are difficult to make, they will require more of the dentist's time, and this should be reflected in the fee quoted to the patient.

The patient is entitled to know the cost of treatment before it is started. The cost can be estimated with assurance if the diagnosis is thorough and if the treatment plan has been carefully worked out.

When the fee is quoted to the patient, the arrangement for its payment should be explained at the same time. The most satisfactory arrangement is for the fee to be paid in full on the day on which the dentures are placed. If this is not convenient for the patient, the treatment can be postponed until it is convenient. Fortunately, complete denture service is an elective service and can be postponed if necessary.

A failure to make definite arrangements for both the amount of the fee and the method of its payment can lead to misunderstandings and unhappiness. This part of complete denture service is a business arrangement between the dentist and the patient, and it must be handled on a businesslike basis so that good rapport between them can be maintained. Once these details have been agreed on, a series of appointments for providing the service should be made.

6

Improving the patient's denture foundation and ridge relations

Dentures can be no better than their supporting tissue foundations and several conditions in the edentulous mouth should be corrected or treated before the construction of complete dentures. Often patients are not aware that tissues in their mouth have been damaged or deformed by the presence of old prostheses. Other oral conditions may have developed or be present that must be altered to increase the chances for success of the new dentures. The patient must be made cognizant of these problems, and a logical explanation by the dentist, supplemented with radiographs and diagnostic casts, will usually convince the patient of the necessity for the suggested treatment.

The methods of treatment to improve the patient's denture foundation and ridge relations are usually either nonsurgical or surgical in nature, or a combination of both methods.

NONSURGICAL METHODS

Nonsurgical methods of edentulous mouth preparation include (1) rest for denture-supporting tissues, (2) occlusal correction of old prostheses, (3) good nutrition, and (4) conditioning of the patient's musculature.

Rest for denture-supporting tissues. Rest for the denture-supporting tissues can be achieved by removal of the dentures from the mouth for an extended period of time or the use of temporary soft liners. Both procedures allow deformed tissue of the residual ridges to recover normal form. Clinical reports and experience also support the merits of regular finger massage of denture-bearing mucosa, especially of those areas that appear edematous and enlarged.

Lytle (1957, 1959) demonstrated that tissue abuse caused by improper occlusion could be made to disappear and redevelop at will by (1) withholding the faulty dentures from the patients, (2) substituting properly made dentures, and (3) allowing the patient to reuse the faulty dentures with the improper occlusal relations. He showed that it was necessary to allow for recovery of the soft tissues by removing the dentures for 48 to 72 hours before impressions for use in the construction of new dentures could be undertaken. Generally it is not feasible to withhold a patient's dentures for an extended period while the tissues are recovering. Therefore temporary soft liners were developed as tissue treatment or conditioning materials. These soft resins maintain their softness for several days while the tissues recover. Tissue conditioners consist of a polymer powder and an aromatic ester–ethanol mixture (Braden, 1970). These materials have been widely used in dentistry in recent years and provide the dentist with an expanded scope for short-term resolution of patient problems.

The major uses of these tissue-conditioning materials are tissue treatment (Lytle, 1959; Chase, 1961), liners for surgical splints (Frisch and associates, 1968), trial denture base stabilizers, optimal arch form or neutral zone determinants (Wilson and associates, 1966) and functional impression materials (Braden). Clinical experience indicates that these soft liners can also be used as functional impression materials with wide clinical application in refitting complete dentures.

Östlund (1958) showed that denture-bearing tissues demonstrate microscopic evidence of inflammation, even if they appear clinically normal. Consequently, tissue rest for at least 24 hours and the use of the tissue treatment resins are essential preliminaries to each prosthetic appointment. Tissues recover rapidly when the dentures are not worn or when treatment liners are used. The method of achieving optimal health of the denture-bearing tissues is not as important as the result of the tissues being made healthy. Many dentures fail because the impressions or registrations of the relations are made when the tissues are distorted by the old dentures. The same error is frequently commited when dentures are relined without adequate rest or tissue treatment.

Occlusal correction of the old prostheses. An attempt should be made to restore an optimal vertical dimension of occlusion to the dentures presently worn by the patient by using an interim resilient lining material. The latter clinical step enables the dentist to prognosticate the amount of vertical facial support that the patient can tolerate, as well as allowing the presumably deformed tissues of the temporomandibular joints to recover. The decision to create room inside the denture depends on its fit and the condition of the tissues. The tissue treatment material also permits some movement of the denture base so that its position becomes compatible with the existing occlusion, part from allowing displaced tissues to recover their original form. Consequently, ridge relations are improved, and this improvement will facilitate the dentist's eventual relation-registration procedures.

It may also be necessary to correct the extent of tissue coverage by the old denture base so that all usable supporting tissue will be included in the treatment. This can be easily achieved by use of one of the resin border-molding materials combined with a tissue conditioner.

Good nutrition. A good nutritional program must be emphasized for each edentulous patient. This is especially important for the geriatric patient whose metabolic and masticatory efficiency have decreased (see Chapter 2).

Conditioning of the patient's musculature. The use of jaw exercises can permit relaxation of the muscles of mastication and strengthen their coordination as well as help prepare the patient psychologically for the prosthetic service (Boos,

1959). If, at the initial appointment, the dentist observes that the patient responds with difficulty to instructions for relaxation and coordinated mandibular movement, a program of mandibular exercises may be prescribed. Clinical experience indicates that such a program is usually beneficial and the subsequent clinical appointment stages of registration of jaw relations are facilitated.

SURGICAL METHODS

Frequently, certain conditions of the denture-bearing tissues require edentulous patients to be treated surgically. These conditions are caused by morphologic variations or, more frequently, result from long-term wear of ill-fitting dentures. Surgical alterations or modifications are necessary to improve retention and function of the dentures and to treat residual pathoses. Preprosthetic surgical mouth preparation can be conveniently considered under the following headings:

1. Soft-tissue pathosis that results from the traumatic effects of long-term wear of complete dentures (The resultant hyperplasia of the soft tissues and their treatment have already been described in Section one.)
2. Frenular attachments and pendulous maxillary tuberosities
3. Bony prominences (tori, exostoses), undercuts, spiny ridges, and nonparallel bony ridges
4. Enlargement of denture-bearing areas: vestibuloplasty, ridge augmentation
5. Discrepancies in jaw size
6. Pressure on the mental foramen
7. Prescribing dental implants (Chapter 30)

Frenular attachments and pendulous maxillary tuberosities

Frena, or fibrous bands of tissue attached to the bone of the mandible and maxillae, are frequently superficial to muscle attachments. If the frenum is close to the crest of the bony ridge (Fig. 6-1), it may be difficult to obtain the ideal extension and border of the flange of the denture. The upper labial frenum may be composed of a strong band of fibrous connective tissue that attaches on the lingual side of the crest of the residual ridge. This tissue can be removed surgically. Frena frequently become prominent as a result of reduction of the residual ridges. If muscle fibers are attached close to the crest of the ridge when the frenum is removed, they are usually detached and elevated or depressed to expose the amount of desired ridge height. The frenectomy can be carried out before prosthetic treatment is begun, or it can be done at the time of denture insertion when the new denture can act as a surgical template. The former is preferred because the patient will not have to contend with postoperative discomfort along with adjustment to the dentures.

Pendulous, fibrous maxillary tuberosities (Fig. 6-2) are frequently encountered. They occur unilaterally or bilaterally and may interfere with denture construction by excessive encroachment on or obliteration of the interarch space. Surgical exicision is the treatment of choice (Fig. 6-3), but occasionally maxillary bone must be removed. Care must be used to avoid opening into the maxillary sinus. In those instances in which the sinus dips down into a pneumatized and elongated tuberosity, it may be possible to collapse the sinus floor upward without danger of opening into it. This technique is also employed when a bony undercut exists on the buccal side of the tuberosity and the sinus has pneumatized into this undercut (Fig. 6-4).

Bony prominences, undercuts, spiny ridges, and nonparallel bony ridges

Mandibular tori are usually removed to avoid undercuts and to make possible a border seal beyond them against the floor of the mouth (Fig. 6-5). Usually they occur so close to the floor of the mouth that a border seal cannot be made. On the other hand, maxillary tori are infrequently removed. Satisfactory dentures can be

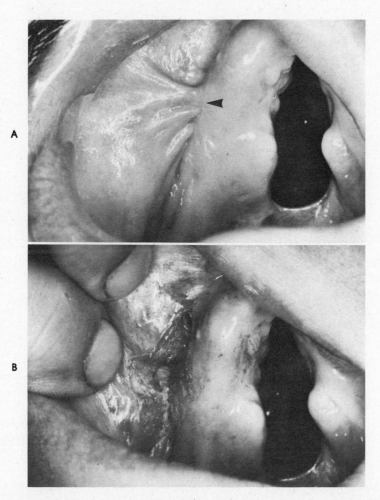

Fig. 6-1. A, Preoperative and, **B,** postoperative views of maxillary buccal frenum *(arrow)* in edentulous patient with unrepaired palatal cleft. Excision of this frenum allowed for optimal extension of denture flange in this area.

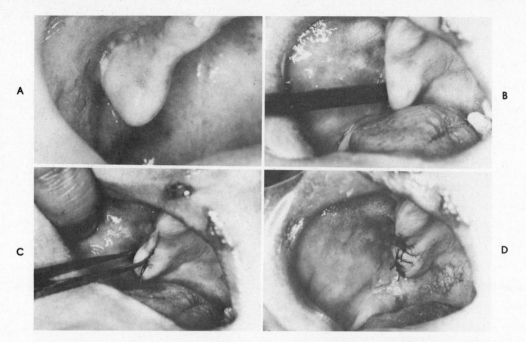

Fig. 6-2. A, Pendulous, fibrous, mobile right maxillary tuberosity that is easily displaced, **B,** Two elliptical incisions undermine fibrous mass, **C,** and allow for approximation of mucosal surfaces, **D,** over a firm bony base.

made over most palatine tori. Specific indications for maxillary tori removal include the following:

1. An extremely large torus that fills the palatal vault and prevents the formation of an adequately extended and stable maxillary denture (Fig. 6-6).
2. An undercut torus that traps food debris, causing a chronic inflammatory condition. Surgical excision is necessary to create optimal oral hygiene.
3. A torus that extends past the junction of the hard and soft palate and prevents the development of an adequate posterior palatal seal (Fig. 6-7).
4. A torus that causes a patient concern because of "cancerphobia."

Bony exostoses may occur on both jaws but are more frequent on the buccal sides of the posterior maxillary segments (Figs. 6-8 and 6-9).

They may create discomfort if covered by a denture and are usually excised. It must be emphasized that routine excision of mandibular exostoses is not recommended (Fig. 6-8 *B*), since all alveolar ridge surgery is accompanied by varied, but frequently dramatic, residual ridge reduction. Frequently, the denture can be relieved to accommodate the exostoses, or a permanent soft liner can be employed.

Sometimes the genial tubercles are extremely prominent as a result of advanced ridge reduction in the anterior part of the body of the mandible (Fig. 6-10). If the activity of the genioglossus muscle has a tendency to displace the lower denture or if the tubercle cannot tolerate the pressure or contact of the denture flange in this area, the genial tubercle is removed and the genioglossus muscle is detached. If it is clinically necessary to deepen the alveololingual sulcus in this area, the genioglossus muscle is sutured to

Text continued on p. 107.

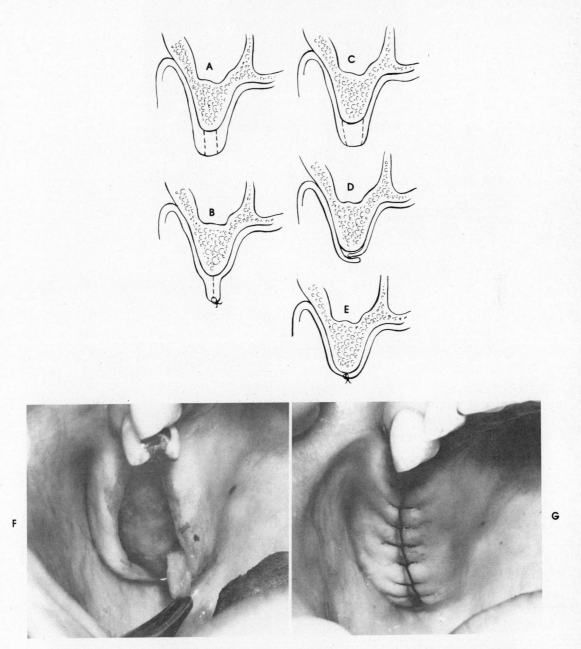

Fig. 6-3. Procedure for reducing vertical height of maxillary tuberosity. **A,** Incisions are made in fibrous tuberosity. **B,** Wedge of fibrous tissue is removed. Tuberosity is less bulky but is still as long vertically as before tissue was removed. **C,** Incisions made just under mucosa permit removal of all unwanted fibrous connective tissue. **D** and **E,** Thin mucosal flaps are fitted, trimmed, and sutured. This technique decreases vertical length of tuberosity. Clinical pictures of diagrammatic items **C** and **E** are shown in **F** and **G.**

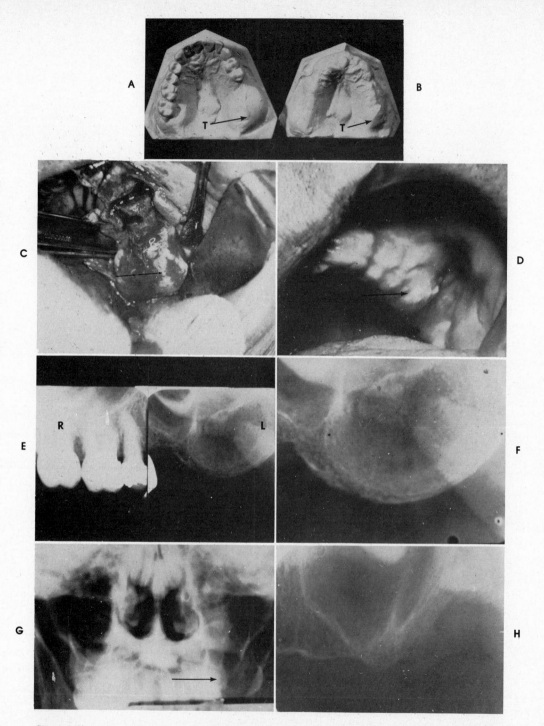

Fig. 6-4. Reduction in size of huge pneumatized tuberosity, *T.* **A,** Preoperative diagnostic cast. **B,** Cast made 2 years after surgery. **C,** Clinical view of enlarged tuberosity. **D,** Tuberosity 2 years after surgery. **E,** Dental radiographs of patient's right and left maxillary molar regions. **F,** Radiograph of enlarged pneumatized tuberosity. **G,** Radiograph showing buccal undercut of pneumatized sinus. **H,** Dental radiograph made 2 years after surgery.

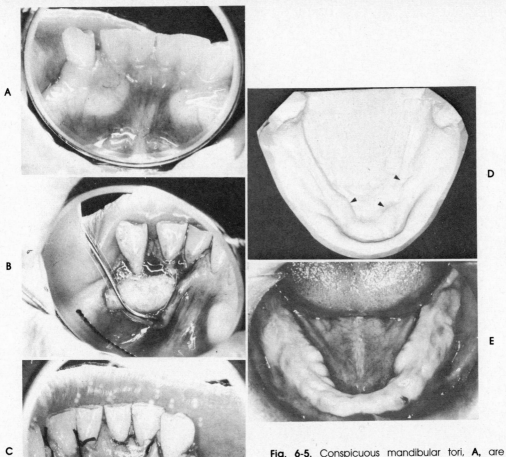

Fig. 6-5. Conspicuous mandibular tori, **A,** are surgically exposed, **B. C,** Mucoperiosteal flap is replaced and sutured interdentally. **D,** Prominent mandibular tori on edentulous cast and, **E,** intraoral view of extensive mandibular tori that must be excised before denture fabrication.

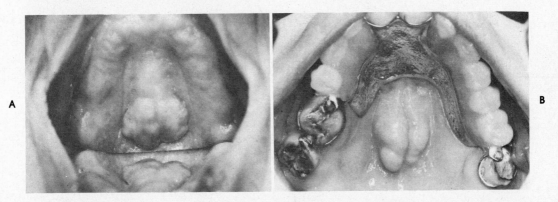

Fig. 6-6. Sheer bulk of this torus will prevent conventional palatal coverage by denture base. **A,** This can frequently be avoided in a partially edentulous mouth by modification of major connector design, **B.**

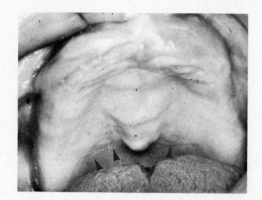

Fig. 6-7. Large maxillary torus that extends distally past a proposed posterior palatal seal area.

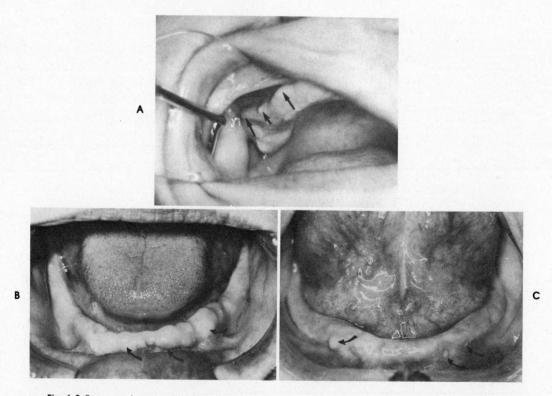

Fig. 6-8. Bony exostoses on right buccal aspect of maxillary residual ridge, **A,** and on labial and buccal aspects of anterior mandibular ridge, **B** and **C.**

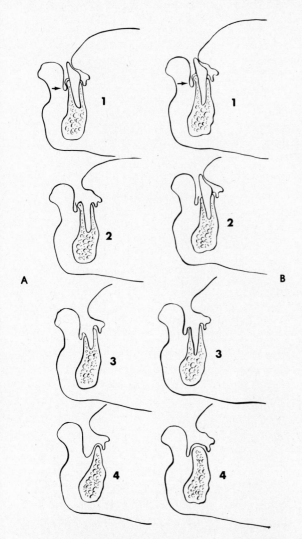

Fig. 6-9. Incorrect, **A,** and correct, **B,** methods for trimming exostosis at crest of alveolar process labial to mandibular incisors. The exostosis should be removed *before* incisor teeth are removed. **A,** Undesirable loss of bone occurs if a labial undercut is trimmed *after* tooth is removed. *1,* Tooth in position. Note labial bony prominence. *2,* Removed tooth leaves an undercut. *3,* Removal of undercut shortens labial plate of bone. *4,* End result is a lingually placed, sharp residual ridge. **B,** Correct method is to remove a labial undercut *before* teeth are removed. This conserves bone and results in a larger and more desirable residual ridge. *1,* Tooth in position, with a labial bony prominence. *2,* Bony prominence is removed, but height of bone is retained. *3,* Tooth is removed. *4,* Resulting residual ridge is favorable.

the geniohyoid muscle below it (see Fig. 6-10).

Residual alveolar ridge undercuts (Fig. 6-11) are rarely excised as a routine part of improving a patient's denture foundations. Usually a complex path of insertion and withdrawal of the prosthesis or careful adjustment of a denture flange enables the dentist to utilize the undercuts for extra stability. Diagnostic casts can be surveyed as a guide in the assessment of the minimal amount of tissue to be removed. Considerable evidence exists that indicts residual ridge surgery as causing excessive bone reduction. This matter is discussed at length in Chapter 26. However, the dentist may comfortably elect to remove a severe undercut that occurs opposite the lingual side of mandibular second and third molars and is tender to palpation (Fig. 6-12). Such an undercut is caused by a sharp mylohyoid ridge, which is usually covered by very thin mucosa. When painless undercuts occur in this area, they can be employed usefully to achieve added stability with a lower denture (Fig. 6-13). The path of insertion in such a situation is altered to allow for distal initial placing of the lingual flanges with a downward and forward final seating movement.

Enlargement of denture-bearing area: vestibuloplasty

The reduction of alveolar ridge size is frequently accompanied by an apparent encroachment of muscle attachments onto the crest of the ridge. These so-called high (mandible) or low (maxilla) attachments serve to reduce the denture-bearing area available and to undermine denture stability. The anterior part of the body of the mandible is the site most frequently involved: the labial sulcus is virtually obliterated, and the mentalis muscle attachments appear to "migrate" to the crest of the residual ridge (Fig. 6-14). This usually results in the dentist arranging the teeth more lingually than the position of the former anterior teeth. Such lingual crowding (Chapter 14) may not be tolerated by the patient and when the absent sulcus is accom-

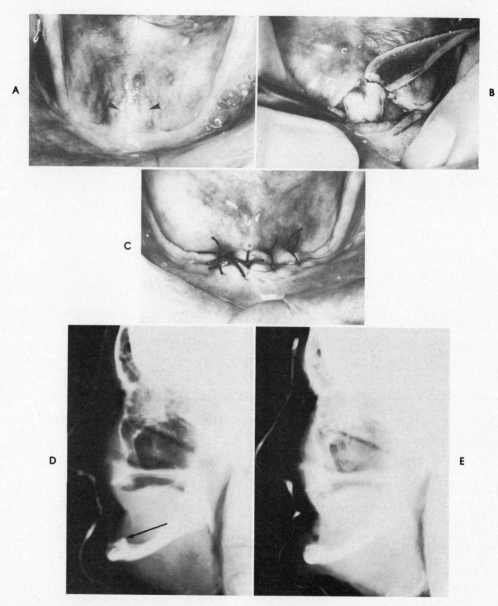

Fig. 6-10. Prominent, painful superior genial tubercle, **A,** is surgically exposed, **B,** and excised, **C. D** and **E,** Cephalometric radiographs showing thinness of mandible. **D,** Superior genial tubercle *(arrow)* is higher than crest of bony ridge. Notice extreme interarch distance at rest position. **E,** After genial tubercle had been removed.

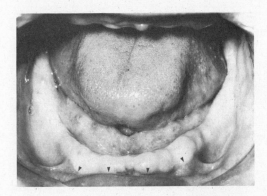

Fig. 6-11. Anterior mandibular alveolar ridge undercuts. Such undercuts are rarely excised and can even enhance denture stability.

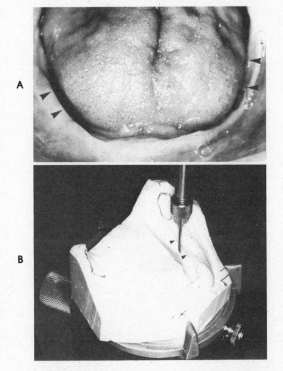

Fig. 6-12. Undercuts frequently occur in lingual side of mandibular second and third molar regions. Occasionally they are very tender, and sharp mylohyoid ridge of bone must be excised, **A.** In **B,** a surveyor is used to emphasize undercut that such a ridge can create.

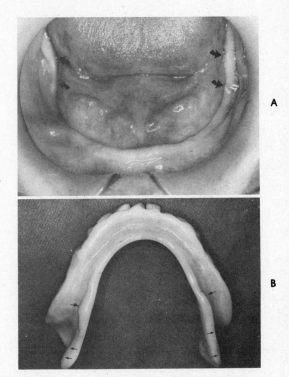

Fig. 6-13. Posterior mandibular lingual undercuts occur frequently and can be used to enhance mandibular denture stability.

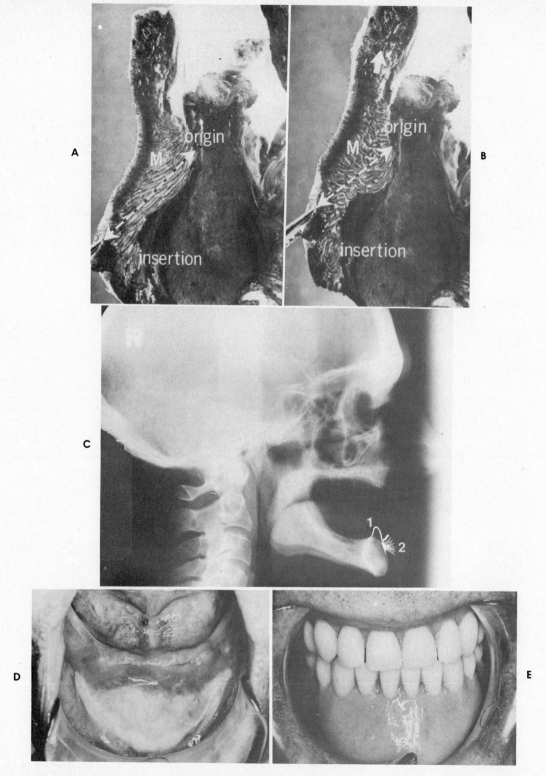

Fig. 6-14. For legend, see opposite page.

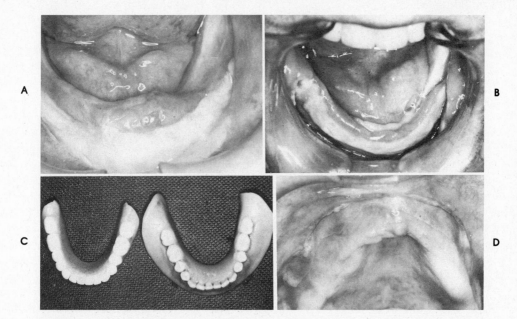

Fig. 6-15. A and **B,** Deepened facial mandibular sulcus with skin graft in place. Current procedures do *not* aim at achieving such a wide area of operation. **C,** Mandibular dentures before and after sulcus deepening are compared. **D,** Maxillary vestibuloplasty.

panied by little or no attached alveolar mucosa in this area, it is virtually impossible for a lower denture to be retained. Myoplasties accompanied by sulcus deepening have been carried out in attempts to improve denture retention function. With this operation the oral surgeon detaches the origin of muscles on either the labial or lingual side, or both sides, of the edentulous residual ridges. This enables the prosthodontist to increase the vertical extensions of the denture flanges. When horizontal bony shelving

is present in the mentalis muscle region, the surgical procedure is less successful and its relative efficacy is attributable to the modification of the powerful mentalis muscle's activity.

In recent years close cooperation between the two involved disciplines has resulted in a clearer understanding of what the surgical intervention should achieve. A wide and deep sulcus is not essential for success (Fig. 6-15, *A* and *B*), and the vestibuloplasty can be restricted to the interpremolar region, since the buccinator mus-

Fig. 6-14. Sagittal sections through lower lip and anterior part of mandible show space available for labial flange and effect of action of mentalis muscle, *M,* on this space, **A** and **B.** The muscle has its origin on the bone and its insertion in the skin. Contraction of muscle lifts lip and reduces space available for flange of denture. In **C,** a lateral cephalogram shows contour of residual alveolar ridge immediately after tooth extraction, *1,* and the origin of the mentalis muscle (simulated in *2*). When *1* resorbs to its present level, relative locale of origin of this muscle now obliterates labial sulcus. **D** and **E,** Mandibular vestibuloplasty provides for dramatic increase in labial flange extension. (**A** and **B** courtesy Dr. A.L. Martone.)

cles are not the major cause of the problem (Fig. 6-14, *D* and *E*) as emphasized by Quayle (1979). Displacement of the mentalis muscle and adjacent muscle slips allow for the production of a looser lower lip, along with a wound margin low down in the sulcus and an increase in both stability and depth of the labial flange. The situation varies in the maxillae, where a muscle comparable to the action of the mentalis in its unstabilizing potential is not encountered. A broader vestibuloplasty is indicated here.

Although lingual vestibuloplasties can provide for a major denture dimensional increase, the procedure *is* traumatic, particularly in frail and elderly patients, and therefore not frequently recommended. The long-standing clinical impression that free skin grafts lose resiliency and develop nuisance crinkling was confirmed by Moller and Jolst. Skin grafts tend to have a noticeable increase in parakeratosis with subsequent clinical sogginess. Furthermore, they seem to exhibit poor cohesion and adhesion compared with mucosa. Whenever possible, mucosal grafts are preferred.

Current research has aimed at providing substitutes for homologous grafts. Heterologous collagen grafts have been used as a biological dressing, and the denuded areas are quickly covered by normal mucous membrane. It appears that collagen xenografts may prove to be suitable alternatives for split skin or mucosal grafts (Mitchell, 1983). The use of acrylic resin templates or the modified previous denture to support vestibuloplasty in the mandible is essential. These templates must be fastened to the mandible with circummandibular wires for 1 week. Carefully designed splints will reduce inflammation, reduce postoperative scarring, and maintain muscles in the desired position, thereby improving the result. Björlin and associates (1967) investigated the effect of vestibular extension surgery in the anterior region of the mandible on muscle activity and prosthesis retention. The electromyographic activity of the mentalis and inferior orbicularis muscles was shown to undergo very slight changes despite the mentalis muscle being severed completely from its origin in the mandible. This was presumed to be caused by the mentalis muscle having a new origin in the lower lip, with mainly the same activity pattern.

One other result of excessive alveolar bone loss or reduction is the obliteration of the hamular notch. This anatomic cul-de-sac with its potential for displacement makes it an important part of the posterior palatal seal of the maxillary denture. Its absence can severely undermine retention of the denture, and a small localized deepening of the sulcus in this area is then indicated. The patient's old denture or a surgical template is employed after the surgery to help retain the patency of the newly formed sulcus, or notch.

Ridge augmentation. For many years surgeons have attempted to restore mandibular bulk by placing onlay bone grafts from the iliac or ribs source above or below the mandible. Unfortunately, follow-up reports suggest that the result generally leaves much to be desired in respect to ridge height. Current research in the area of alveolar ridge deficiencies and nonresorbable all plastic materials indicates some optimism (Kent and others, 1982) for this approach. However, longitudinal studies in several treatment centers must be analyzed before such an approach is accepted as an integral part of preprosthetic surgical strategies. Other methods of dimensional increase of the mandible by means of a "visor" and "sandwich" osteotomy have also been proposed. The report by de Koomen et al. suggests optimism for the procedure, although a cautious approach is recommended because it is a formidalbe procedure for some patients.

Discrepancies in jaw size

The recent advances in surgical techniques of mandibular osteotomy have enabled the oral surgeon to create optimal jaw relations for prosthetic patients who have discrepancies in jaw size. The prognathic patient frequently places an excessive amount of stress and unfavorable leverages on the maxillary basal seat. This may cause excessive reduction of the maxillary residual ridge. Such a condition is even more conspicuous when some mandibular teeth are still present. A mandibular osteotomy in such situations can create a more favorable arch alignment and improve cosmetic appearance as well (Fig. 6-16). However, changes in the soft tissues of the face tend to be accentuated by such a procedure as evidenced by both patients in Fig. 6-16. Usually an adjunctive face-lifting procedure in this type of patient produces impressive results.

Pressure on the mental foramen

When the resorption of bone of the mandible has been extreme, the mental foramen may open near or directly at the crest of the residual

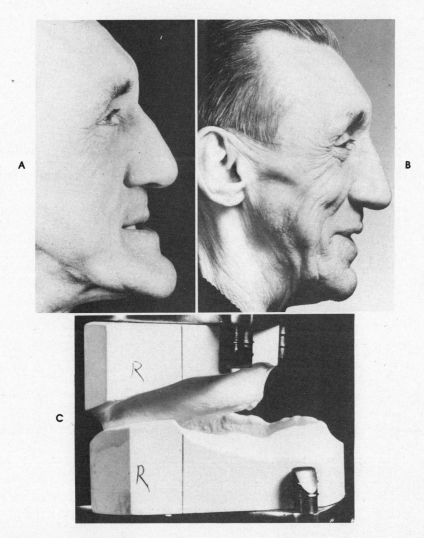

Fig. 6-16. A, Preoperative and, **B,** postoperative views of a male patient who underwent a mandibular osteotomy. **C,** Preoperative diagnostic cast.

Continued.

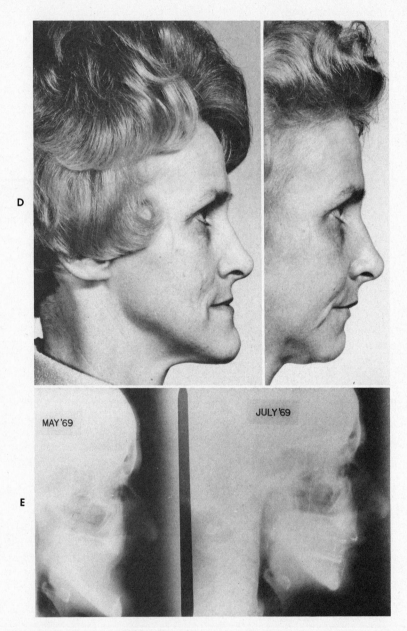

MAY '69

JULY '69

Fig. 6-16, cont'd. D and **E,** Preoperative and postoperative profiles and cephalometric views of a female patient treated in similar manner. (Courtesy Dr. P. Smylski.)

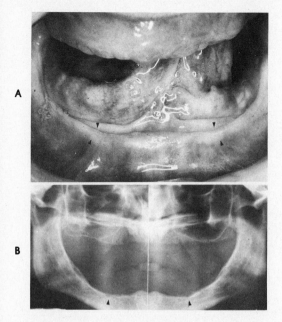

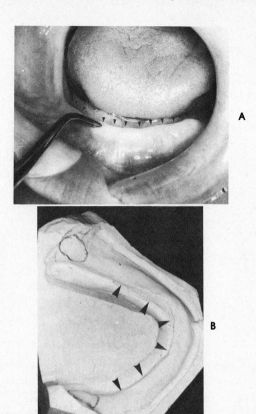

Fig. 6-17. A, Intraoral and, **B,** radiographic views of an edentulous patient's mandible with superficially placed mental foramina secondary to extensive residual ridge reduction. The foramina are usually quite palpable in such situations.

Fig. 6-18. A, Slender knife-edge mandibular alveolar ridge is covered by thin, nonresilient mucosa. **B,** Working cast in which knife-edged character of ridge is conspicuous *(arrows.)*

bony process (Fig. 6-17). When this happens, the bony margins of the mental foramen are usually more dense and resistant to resorption than the bone anterior or posterior to the foramen is. This causes the margins of the mental foramen to extend and to have very sharp edges 2 to 3 mm higher than the surrounding mandibular bone. When such a condition exists, pressure from the denture against the mental nerve exiting from the foramen and over this sharp bony edge will cause pain. Also, pressure against the sharp bone will cause pain because the oral mucosa is pinched between the sharp bony margin of the mental foramen and the denture. The most suitable way of managing this is to alter the denture so that the pressure does not exist. However, in some instances it may be necessary to trim the bone and relieve the mental nerve from pressure. One relieves pressure on the mental nerve by increasing the opening of the

mental foramen downward toward the inferior border of the body of the mandible. Such a change permits the mental nerve to exit from the bone at a point lower than it had previously. This should take pressure off the nerve.

Occasionally the anterior part of the residual ridges may become so resorbed that it is extremely thin labiolingually, and it may have a sharp knife-edge with small spicules of bone protruding from it (Fig. 6-18). Careful denture relief in these areas frequently overcomes this problem. If, however, constant irritation develops as a result of the soft tissue being pinched between the denture and the bone, the spicules and the knife-edged ridge must be reduced.

A lack of parallelism between the maxillary and mandibular ridges can be encountered and, on occasion, may have to be repaired surgically. This lack of parallelism may be caused by a lack of trimming of the tuberosity and ridge behind the last maxillary tooth when it is removed or result from jaw defects, unequal ridge reduction, and abnormalities of growth and development. Most clinicians favor parallel ridges for their denture foundations, since the resultant forces generated are directed in a way that tends to seat the denture rather than dislodge it. Also, the height of the occlusal plane of the upper denture can be elevated posteriorly to improve the denture esthetically. Virtually all the surgical procedures described necessitate the use of a surgical template. The patient's old dentures can usually be modified with a soft treatment resin to function as such. The use of a lined template protects the operated area from trauma and enables the patients to continue wearing their dentures. All the surgical interventions mentioned in this chapter must be considered in the context of their potential effects on residual ridge resorption. It must be underscored that extensive surgical preparation of the edentulous mouth is rarely necessary and that any required surgical procedure should be as conservative as possible.

REFERENCES

Björlin, G., Palmquist, J., and Ahlgren, J.: Muscle activity and denture retention after vestibular extension surgery, Odontol. Revy **18**:179-190, 1967.

Boos, R.H.: Preparation and conditioning of patients for prosthetic treatment, J. Prosthet. Dent. **9**:4-10, 1959.

Braden, M.: Tissue conditioners. I. Composition and structure, J. Dent. Res. **49**:145-148, 1970.

Chase, W.W.: Tissue conditioning utilizing dynamic adaptive stress, J. Prosthet. Dent. **11**:804-815, 1961.

de Koomen, H.A., Stoelinga, P.J.W., Tideman, H., and Huybers, J.M.: Interposed bone-graft augmentation of the atrophic mandible, J. Maxillofac. Surg. **7**:129, 1979.

Frisch, J., Levin, M.P., and Bhaskar, S.N.: Clinical study of fungal growth on tissue conditioners, J. Am. Dent. Assoc. **76**:591-592, 1968.

Kent, J.N., Quinn, J.H., Zide, M.F., et al.: Correction of alveolar ridge deficiencies with nonresorbable hydroxylapatite, J. Am. Dent. Assoc. **105**:993-1001, 1982.

Lytle, R.B.: The management of abused oral tissues in complete denture construction, J. Prosthet. Dent. **7**:27-42, 1957.

Lytle, R.B.: Complete denture construction based on a study of the deformation of the underlying soft tissues, J. Prosthet. Dent. **9**:539-551, 1959.

Mitchell, R.: A new biological dressing for areas denuded of mucous membrane, Br. Dent. J. **155**:346-348, 1983.

Møller, J.F., and Jolst, O.: A histologic follow-up study of free autogenous skin grafts to the alveolar ridge in humans, Int. J. Oral Surg. **1**:283, 1972.

Östlund, S.G.: Effect of complete dentures on the gum tissues; a histological and histopathological investigation, Acta Odontol. Scand. **16**:1-36, 1958.

Quayle, A.A.: The atrophic mandible: aspects of technique in lower labial sulcoplasty, Br. J. Oral Surg. **16**:169-178, 1979.

Wilson, H.J., Tomlin, H.R., and Osborne, J.: Tissue conditioners and functional impression materials, Br. Dent. J. **121**:9-16, 1966.

SECTION THREE

Rehabilitation of edentulous patients

7

Biologic considerations of maxillary impressions

Complete dentures are artificial substitutes for living tissues that have been lost. The dentures must replace the form of the living tissues as closely as possible. Most importantly, the dentures must function in harmony with the remaining tissues that both support and surround them. For this harmony of living tissues and nonliving material (dentures) to coexist for reasonable periods of time, the dentist must fully understand both the macroscopic and microscopic anatomy of the supporting and limiting structures of the dentures. The clinical application of this knowledge determines (1) the selective placement of forces by the denture bases upon the supporting tissues and (2) the form of the denture borders that will be harmonious with the normal function of the limiting structures that surround them. Both the proper placement of selective pressures by the denture base and the form of its borders are developed during preliminary and final impression procedures.

MACROSCOPIC ANATOMY OF SUPPORTING STRUCTURES

The foundation for dentures is called the basal seat, and it is made up of bone that is covered by mucous membrane—mucosa and submucosa. In the submucosa are the vessels that carry the blood supply to the basal seat and the nerves that innervate it. The microscopic anatomy of the basal seat is discussed later in this chapter. The macroscopic structures involved in supporting maxillary dentures are considered first.

Each type of tissue found in the oral cavity has its own characteristic ability to resist external forces. This is important to the maintenance of health of the tissues of the basal seat and to the stability and support of dentures. For example, nature has placed fibrous connective tissue in places where external forces are applied, and these tissues are firmly attached to the bone underneath. Glandular tissues, on the other hand, are not found in locations where external forces are to be applied. Therefore the distribution of forces applied to the basal seat by dentures should be planned in relation to the types of tissues found in various parts of the basal seat.

Support for the maxillary denture

The ultimate support for a maxillary denture is the bone of the two maxillae and the palatine bone. The palatine processes of the maxillae are joined together at the midline in the median suture (Figs. 7-1 and 7-2). The two palatine processes of the maxillae and the palatine bone form the foundation for the hard palate and provide considerable support for the denture. But more importantly, they support soft tissues that increase the surface areas of the basal seat.

A cross section of the hard palate readily shows that the palate is bone covered by tissues of varying depths. A study of these sections further reveals how important it is to employ an impression technique that equalizes the pressure distribution. The center of the palate may be very hard because the layer of soft tissues

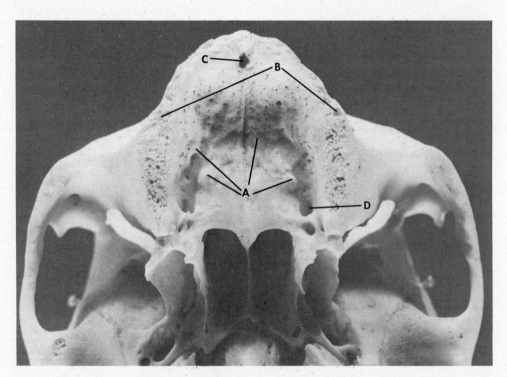

Fig. 7-1. Bone of the maxillae and the palatine bone provide support for upper denture. Individual differences in form determine how forces should be directed to these bones during function with complete dentures. *A,* Spiny projections that would irritate tissues under a denture; *B,* rough and irregular bone of maxillary ridge, *C,* Incisive foramen, *D,* Greater palatine foramen.

covering the bone in the region of the median palatal suture is extremely thin. If the hard palate is less resilient than the soft tissues (submucosa) covering the residual ridges, it should be relieved to prevent a tendency of the denture to rock or the development of soreness in this region when vertical forces are applied to the teeth. The relief for the median palatal suture and its overlying raphe can be developed in the impression or denture-processing procedure or after the denture has been completed. These alternatives are discussed in Chapter 8. The various regions in the mouth to which special responsibilities of stress distribution have been assigned may be seen in Fig. 7-3.

The alveolar processes develop as the teeth are formed and erupt. The maxillary deciduous, or primary, teeth develop in the maxillae, and the process stimulates the alveolar processes to grow. This kind of development continues as the permanent teeth are formed, also in the alveolar processes. The alveolar process then supports the natural teeth. The socket that surrounds the root of each natural tooth is the alveolus, and the bony ridge that supports the teeth is the alveolar ridge. The bony process that remains after teeth have been lost is the residual alveolar ridge, which also includes the mucous membrane that covers the bone. The thickness of the soft tissues covering the bone is different in different parts of the maxillary basal seat (Plates 7-1 to 7-4). The nature and relative thickness of the soft tissues

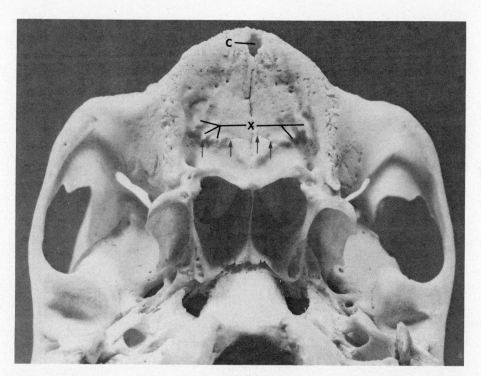

Fig. 7-2. Notice junction of the two palatine processes of maxillae and palatine bone *(arrows)*. X, Sharp bony spines present in palate are covered with soft tissue; these spines frequently are the obscure cause of soreness under denture pressure. Because of increased resorption of residual alveolar ridge, the incisive foramen, C, is nearer crest of ridge than incisive foramen in Fig. 7-1. The location of incisive papilla (covering incisive foramen) in relation to crest of ridge is guide to amount of resorption that has occurred.

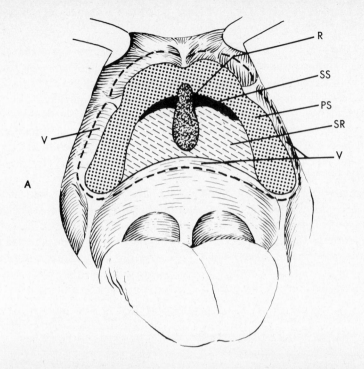

A

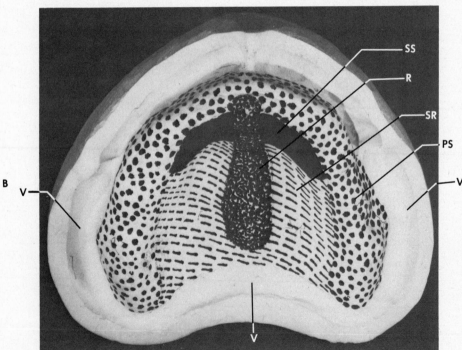

B

Fig. 7-3. A, Various areas of primary function of maxillary basal seat are indicated on edentulous upper jaw. *PS,* Primary stress-bearing area; *SS,* secondary stress-bearing area; *SR,* secondary retentive area; *R,* relief area; *V,* valve seal area. **B,** Various areas of primary function of maxillary basal seat are indicated on a cast. *PS,* Primary stress-bearing area; *SS,* secondary stress-bearing area; *SR,* secondary retentive area; *R,* relief area; *V,* valve seal area.

in different parts of the basal seat will determine the amount of support these tissues can provide for a denture.

Residual ridge

The shape and size of the alveolar ridges change when the natural teeth are removed. The alveoli are now merely holes in the jawbone, which begin to fill up with new bone, but at the same time the bone around the margins of the tooth sockets begins to shrink away. This shrinkage or resorption is rapid at first, but it will continue at a reduced rate throughout life.

The resorption of the alveolar process will cause the foundation for the maxillary denture to become smaller and otherwise change its shape.

If a denture is made soon after the teeth are removed, the apparent foundation could be large, but it could also be tender to pressure. This is the result of incomplete healing and a lack of cortical bone over the crest of the residual alveolar ridge.

If the teeth have been out for many years, the size of the residual ridge may be quite small, and the crest of the ridge may lack a smooth cortical bone surface under the mucosa. There may be large nutrient canals and sharp bony spicules (Figs. 7-1 and 7-5). These conditions would cause unfavorable leverages to develop or limit the amount of pressure that could be applied on a denture without creating pain or tenderness.

Stress-bearing areas

The residual ridge is considered to be the primary stress-bearing area in the upper jaw (Fig. 7-3). The crest of the residual alveolar ridge (after healing from the surgery) is covered with a layer of fibrous connective tissue, which is most favorable for supporting the denture because of its firmness and position. The artificial teeth will be placed near this ridge so that leverage will be minimal under the circumstances.

The rugae area is considered to be the secondary stress-bearing area in the upper jaw, since it can resist the forward movement of the denture.

The rugae are irregularly shaped rolls of soft tissue in the anterior part of the palate. They serve no function, but for the sake of the patient's comfort they should not be distorted in an impression technique, since rebounding distorted tissue tends to unseat the denture. In the rugae area the palate is set at an angle to the occlusal plane of the residual ridges and is rather thinly covered by soft tissues (Fig. 7-3).

The third area of special concern is the glandular region on either side of the midline in the posterior part of the hard palate. This region should be covered by the denture so that it can aid in retention, but it should not be expected to provide support for the denture. The mucous glands in this region should not be subjected to significant occlusal forces from dentures since such subjection could interfere with their function. The mucous glands are relatively thick, and they cover the blood vessels and nerves coursing forward in the palate from the greater palatine foramen. These vessels and nerves anastomose with vessels and nerves passing through the nasopalatine canal and into the region of the basal seat at the incisive papilla.

Incisive papilla

The incisive papilla covers the incisive foramen and is located on the median line immediately behind and between the central incisors (see Fig. 7-6). Its position varies in the mouths of different patients (Figs. 7-1 to 7-5). It is located on the center of the ridge after resorption has occurred in mouths that have been edentulous for a long time.

The incisive papilla covers the incisive foramen, the opening of the nasopalatine canal, which carries the nasopalatine vessels and nerve. Relief for the incisive papilla should be provided in every denture to avoid any possible interference with the blood and nerve supply (Plate 7-4).

Posterior palatine area

The posterior palatine foramina are so thickly covered by soft tissue that they do not need to

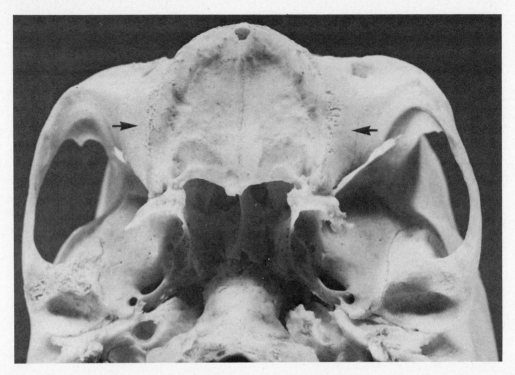

Fig. 7-4. Zygomatic process *(arrows)* is close to crest of residual alveolar ridge in molar region because of excessive amount of bone resorption of alveolar ridge. The zygomatic process is thinly covered by mucous membrane and may likely require relief of the denture border to prevent or eliminate soreness.

be relieved except in extreme cases of resorption. A study of the bony portions of the palate reveals many sharp spines, which are a source of trouble in ridges with extreme resorption and loss of the palatal glands. These bony spines are difficult to locate when they are covered by soft tissues of the palate (Fig. 7-1).

Bone of the basal seat

The configuration of the bone that forms the basal seat for the maxillary denture varies considerably with each patient. Factors that influence the form and size of the supporting bone of the basal seat include (1) its original size and consistency, (2) the patient's general health and resistance, (3) forces developed by the surrounding musculature, (4) severity and location of periodontal disease, (5) forces accruing from the wearing of dental restorations, (6) surgery at the time of removal of the teeth, and (7) the relative length of time different parts of the jaws have been edentulous. Important components of the bone of the basal seat for the maxillary denture that will be described include the incisive foramen, the zygomatic process, the maxillary tuberosity, sharp spiny processes, and the torus palatinus. The pterygomaxillary (hamular) notch is discussed under macroscopic anatomy of limiting structures.

Incisive foramen. The incisive foramen is located in the palate on the median line at the lingual gingiva of the anterior teeth and comes nearer to the crest of the ridge as resorption progresses (Figs. 7-1 and 7-2). Relief for the incisive

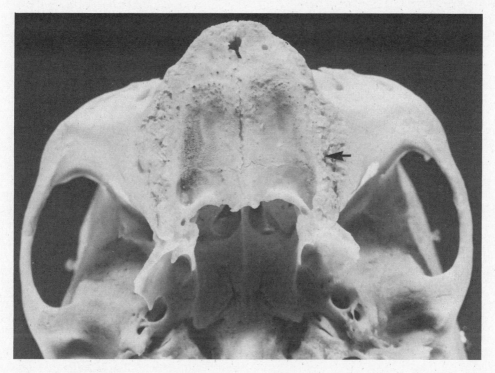

Fig. 7-5. Notice rough and irregular bone on crest of residual alveolar ridge, particularly the left maxillary tuberosity *(arrow).*

foramen should be provided in the denture to prevent impingement on the nasopalatine nerves and blood vessels as they pass through the incisive foramen. The location of the incisive papilla gives an indication as to the amount of resorption of the residual ridge and thus is an aid in determining vertical dimension and the proper position of the teeth.

Zygomatic process. The zygomatic, or malar, process, which is located opposite the first molar region, is one of the hard areas found in mouths that have been edentulous for a long time (Fig. 7-4). Some dentures require relief over this area to aid retention and prevent soreness of the underlying tissues.

Maxillary tuberosity. The tuberosity region of the maxilla often hangs abnormally low because when the maxillary posterior teeth are retained after the mandibular molars have been lost and not replaced, the maxillary teeth extrude, bringing the process with them. Often the low-hanging tuberosity is complicated by an excess of fibrous connective tissue (Fig. 3-10). This excess soft tissue can prevent the proper location of the occlusal plane if it is not removed. In addition, rough and irregular bone could cause irritation from the denture base (Fig. 7-5).

Sharp spiny processes. Frequently there are sharp spiny processes on the maxillary and palatal bones, deeply covered with soft tissue (Figs. 7-1 and 7-2). However, in patients with considerable resorption of the residual alveolar ridge, these sharp spines irritate the soft tissues left between them and the denture base. The canal leading from the posterior palatine foramina often has a sharp spiny overhanging edge, which may cut and irritate the palatal soft tissues overlying it as a result of pressures transmitted from the maxillary denture (Fig. 7-1).

Torus palatinus

A hard bony enlargement that occurs in the midline of the roof of the mouth is called a torus palatinus (Figs. 6-6 and 6-7). This condition occurs in about 20% of the population. One type is almost entirely soft tissue and is loose and flabby; the other type has a thin layer of mucosal tissue covering the bone. The extent of the torus can be determined by palpation, and an arbitrary relief shape that disregards the extent of the hard area should not be used. Such a relief shape may rob the denture of a part of its bearing area and support (Fig. 6-6). The relief provided in the palate should conform accurately to the shape of the hard area. Generally, the more convex the hard area, the more relief will be required.

MACROSCOPIC ANATOMY OF LIMITING STRUCTURES

The functional anatomy of the mouth determines the extent of the basal surface of dentures. The denture base should include the maximum surface possible within the limits of the health and function of the tissues it covers and contacts. This means that dentures should be made in such a way that they cover all the available basal seat tissues without causing soreness at the denture borders and without interfering with the action of any of the structures they contact or that surround the denture.

To follow the basic principle of impression making—extend the impression to cover the maximum area possible within the limits of the health and function of the tissues of the basal seat—a thorough knowledge of the functional anatomy of the basal seat and its limiting structures is essential. The anatomy to be considered is the anatomy in function, rather than descriptive anatomy. Certain definite anatomic limita-

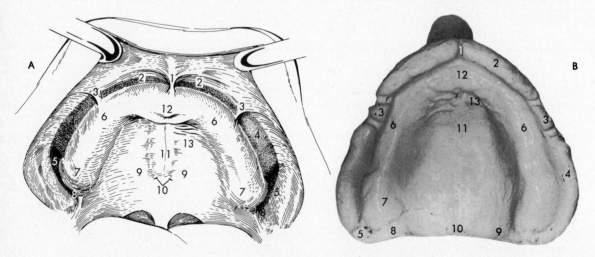

Fig. 7-6. Correlation of anatomic landmarks. **A,** Intraoral drawing of maxillary arch. *1,* Labial frenum; *2,* labial vestibule; *3,* buccal frenum; *4,* buccal vestibule; *5,* coronoid bulge; *6,* residual alveolar ridge; *7,* maxillary tuberosity; *8,* hamular notch; *9,* posterior palatal seal region; *10,* foveae palatinae; *11,* median palatine raphe; *12,* incisive papilla; *13,* rugae region. **B,** Maxillary final impression showing the corresponding denture landmarks: *1,* Labial notch; *2,* labial flange; *3,* buccal notch; *4,* buccal flange; *5,* coronoid contour; *6,* alveolar groove; *7,* maxillary tubercular fossa; *8,* pterygomaxillary seal; *9,* posterior palatal seal; *10,* foveae palatinae; *11,* median palatine groove; *12,* incisive fossa; *13,* rugae. (From Martone, A.L.: J. Prosthet. Dent. **13:**4, 1963.)

tions for dentures exist in both jaws. Their details vary from patient to patient, but the location and function of the various structures are basically the same for all edentulous patients.

The limiting structures of the maxillary basal seat can be analyzed in different regions (Fig. 7-6). The anterior region extends from one buccal frenum to the other on the labial side of the maxillary ridge and is called the labial vestibular space. In this region three objectives are apparent. First, the impression must supply sufficient support to the upper lip to restore the relaxed contour (or appearance) of the lip. This means that the thickness of the labial flange of the upper tray and the final impression must be developed according to the amount of bone that

has been lost from the labial side of the ridge. Second, the labial flange of the impression must have sufficient height to reach to the reflecting mucous membrane of the labial vestibular space without distorting it. Third, there must be no interference of the labial flange with the action of the lip in function.

Labial frenum

The maxillary labial frenum is a fold of mucous membrane at the median line. The labial frenum contains no muscle and has no action of its own. This band of tissue starts superiorly in a fan shape and converges as it descends to its terminal attachment to the labial side of the ridge (Fig. 7-7, A). The labial notch in the labial flange

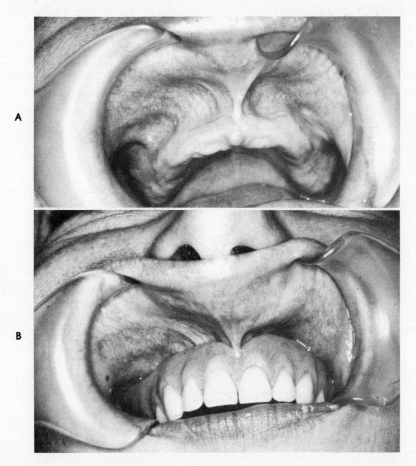

A

B

Fig. 7-7. A, Broad maxillary labial frenum. **B,** Labial flange must fit snugly around labial frenum.

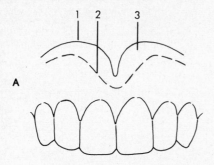
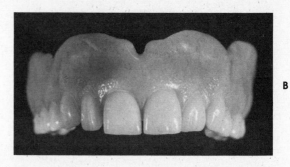

Fig. 7-8. Maxillary labial flange. **A,** *1,* Correct contour of labial flange; *2,* incorrect contour of denture border; *3,* tissue that should have been covered. **B,** Properly formed labial notch and labial flange in a complete denture.

of the denture must be just wide enough and just deep enough to allow the frenum to pass through it without manipulation of the lip (Fig. 7-7, *B*). This fact should be taken into consideration in the relief for this attachment. The denture borders should not only be cut lower but also have less thickness adjacent to the labial notch in the border of the denture. A shallow bead can be formed in the denture base around the notch to help perfect the seal.

Orbicularis oris muscle

The orbicularis oris muscle is the main muscle of the lips, and it lies in front of and rests upon the labial flange and teeth of a denture. Its tone depends on the support it receives from the thickness of the labial flange and the position of the arch of teeth.

The fibers of the orbicularis oris pass horizontally through the lips and anastomose with fibers of the buccinator muscle (see Fig. 7-29). Since these muscle fibers run in the direction they do, the orbicularis oris muscle has only an indirect effect on the extent of an impression and the denture base. This muscle and its action are discussed in more detail in Chapter 19.

Buccal frenum

The denture border between the labial frenum and the buccal frenum is known as the labial flange (Fig. 7-8). The buccal frenum is some-

times a single fold of mucous membrane, sometimes double, and, in some mouths, broad and fan shaped. The buccal frenum requires more clearance for its action than the labial frenum. The caninus (levator anguli oris) muscle attaches beneath the buccal frenum and affects the position of the frenum. The orbicularis oris muscle pulls the buccal frenum forward, and the buccinator muscle pulls it backward. The buccal notch in the denture must be broad enough to allow this movement of the buccal frenum (Fig. 7-9). The border of the denture should be functionally molded to fit exactly the depth and width of this frenum when it is in function, being moved by the three muscles that are associated with it (orbicularis oris, buccinator, and caninus muscles). The buccal frenum is part of the continuous band of tissue going from the maxilla through the modiolus in the corner of the mouth to the buccal frenum on the mandible. Inadequate provision for the buccal frenum or excess thickness of the flange distal to the buccal notch can cause dislodgment of the denture when the cheeks are moved posteriorly as in a broad smile.

Buccal vestibule

The buccal vestibule is opposite the tuberosity and extends from the buccal frenum to the hamular, or pterygomaxillary, notch (Fig. 7-6, *A, 4*). This space between the ridge and the

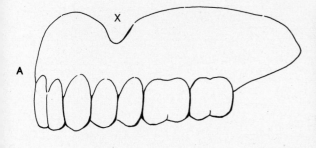 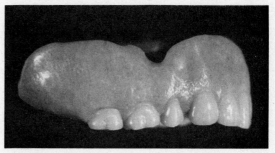

Fig. 7-9. Maxillary buccal notch. **A,** Denture border contour, *X,* in region of buccal frenum. The buccal frenum moves posteriorly as a result of action of buccinator muscle and anteriorly from forward movement of modiolus and corner of mouth. **B,** Properly formed buccal notch in an upper complete denture. The size and form of the notch varies with the individual patient.

cheek in the buccal vestibule is available for the buccal flange of the maxillary denture, which should fill but not overfill it. However, the size of the buccal vestibule varies with the contraction of the buccinator muscle, the position of the mandible, and the amount of bone lost from the maxilla. The thickness of the distal end of the buccal flange of the denture must be adjusted to accommodate the ramus and coronoid process and the masseter muscle as they function. As the mandible moves forward or to the opposite side, the width of the buccal vestibule is reduced. When the masseter muscle contracts under heavy closing pressures, it also reduces the size of the space available for the distal end of the buccal flange. The extent of the buccal vestibule can be deceiving because the ramus obscures it when the mouth is wide open during examination. Therefore it should be examined with the mouth as nearly closed as possible. This space usually is higher than any other part of the border (Fig. 7-10). The size and shape of the posterior part of the buccal vestibule are altered by the lateral movements of the mandible. The distal end of the flange must not be too thick or the ramus will push the denture out of place during opening or lateral movements of the mandible.

Distal to the buccal frenum, the zygomatic process is often unyielding and needs relief (Fig. 7-4).

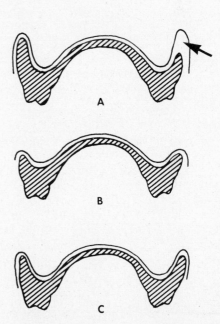

Fig. 7-10. Buccal vestibule. **A,** High buccal vestibule; **B,** low buccal vestibule; **C,** medium height of buccal vestibule. *Arrow,* Space improperly filled by denture base with a consequent loss of tissue coverage and border seal.

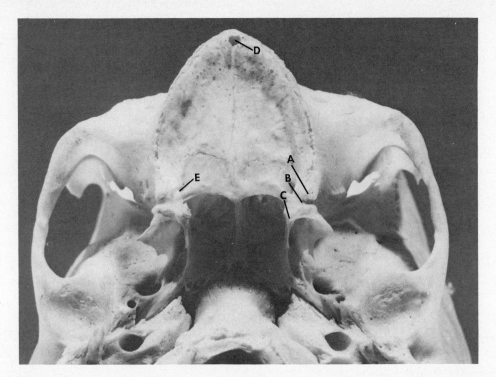

Fig. 7-11. *A,* Maxillary tuberosity; *B,* pterygomaxillary (hamular) notch; *C,* hamular process of pterygoid plate; *D,* incisive foramen; *E,* greater palatine foramen.

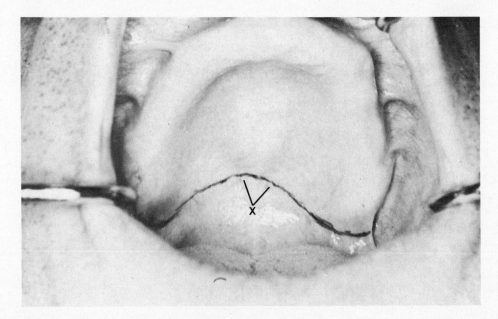

Fig. 7-12. Vibrating line indicated by indelible marks. Notice foveae palatinae, *X,* just posterior to vibrating line in midline region of soft palate.

Pterygomaxillary (hamular) notch

The hamular notch is situated between the tuberosity of the maxilla and the hamulus of the medial pterygoid plate (Fig. 7-11). This notch is used as a boundary of the posterior border of the maxillary denture back of the tuberosity. The posterior palatal seal is placed through the center of the deep part of the hamular notch, since no muscle or ligament is present at a level to prevent the placement of extra pressure.

Palatine fovea region

The foveae palatinae (Figs. 7-12 and 7-24) are indentations near the midline of the palate that are formed by a coalescence of several mucous gland ducts. The foveae are close to the vibrating line and are always in soft tissue, which makes them an ideal guide for the location of the posterior border of the denture.

Vibrating line of the palate

The vibrating line is an imaginary line drawn across the palate that marks the beginning of motion in the soft palate when the patient says "ah." It is a line extending from one pterygomaxillary notch to the other. At the midline it usually passes about 2 mm in front of the foveae palatinae (Fig. 7-12). The vibrating line is not to be confused with the junction of the hard and soft palates, since the vibrating line is always on the soft palate. This is not a well-defined line and should be described as an area rather than as a line. The direction of the vibrating line usually varies according to the shape of the palate (Fig. 7-13). The higher the vault, the more abrupt and forward the vibrating line. In a mouth with a flat vault, the vibrating line is usually father posterior and has a gradual curvature, affording a broader posterior palatal seal area.

The distal end of the upper denture must extend at least to the vibrating line. In most instances, the denture should end 1 or 2 mm posterior of the vibrating line. However, when the anterior teeth are to be placed well anterior to the residual ridge, it may be possible to extend the denture farther posteriorly, provided

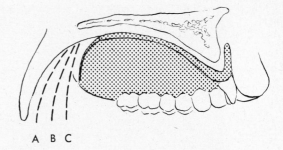

Fig. 7-13. *A,* Type of soft palate form that allows a broad posterior palatal seal area; *B,* type of soft palate form that allows a medium width of posterior palatal seal area; *C,* type of soft palate form that has a very narrow posterior palatal seal area.

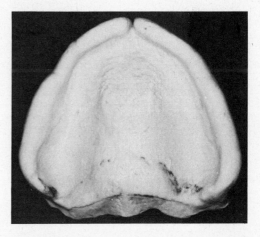

Fig. 7-14. Posterior palatal seal on tray displaces tissue across palate on both sides of vibrating line to form posterior palatal seal on denture.

that the patient can tolerate it. The denture must cover the tuberosities and extend into the pterygomaxillary or hamular notches (Fig. 7-14). Overextension at the hamular notches will not be tolerated because of pressure on the pterygoid hamulus and interference with the pterygomandibular raphe, which extends from the hamulus to the top inside back corner of the retromolar pad. When the mouth is opened wide, the pterygomandibular raphe is pulled forward (Fig.

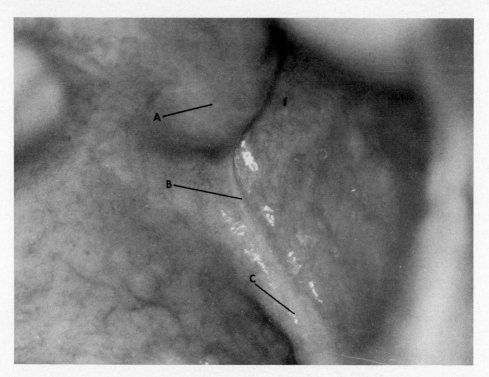

Fig. 7-15. Pterygomandibular raphe pulls forward when mouth is opened wide. *A,* Maxillary tuberosity; *B,* pterygomandibular raphe; *C,* retromolar pad.

7-15). If the denture is too long at these places, the mucous membrane covering the raphe will be injured by the denture.

MICROSCOPIC ANATOMY*

The clinical procedures used in making impressions are directly related to gross anatomic structures of the oral cavity and their function. However, the response of the individual cellular components that make up the basal seat determines the ultimate success of the dentures in terms of preservation of the residual ridges and comfort to the patient. Thus a constant awareness of the microscopic anatomy of the mucous membrane and bone that form the residual ridge

is essential in the development of border form and length and in selective placement of pressures on the basal seat during impression procedures.

Histologic nature of soft tissue and bone

The bones of the upper and lower edentulous jaws are covered with soft tissue, and the oral cavity is lined with soft tissue known as mucous membrane. The denture bases rest on the mucous membrane, which serves as a cushion between the bases and the supporting bone. The mucous membrane is composed of two layers, the mucosa and the submucosa.

The mucosa in the oral cavity is formed by stratified squamous epithelium, which is often keratinized on its outer surface, and a subjacent narrow layer of connective tissue known as the lamina propria.

*We wish to acknowledge the assistance of Dr. Steve Kolas, Professor, Department of Oral Pathology, Medical College of Georgia School of Dentistry, Augusta.

The submucosa is formed by connective tissue that varies in character from dense to loose areolar tissue and also varies considerably in its width or thickness, depending on its location in the mouth. The submucosa may contain glandular, fat, or muscle cells and transmits the blood and nerve supply to the mucosa. When the mucous membrane is attached to bone, the attachment occurs between the submucosa and the periosteal covering of the bone.

The nature of the mucous membrane in different parts of the mouth varies between patients and within the same patient. The keratinized layer of the epithelium (stratum corneum) may be totally absent in some instances and extremely thick in others. The presence of dentures in the mouth does not always have the same effect on the amount of keratinization in different patients.

Although the importance of the mucosa (epithelium and lamina propria) from a health standpoint cannot be neglected, the thickness and consistency of the submucosa are largely responsible for the support that the soft tissues (mucous membrane) afford the dentures, since in most instances the submucosa makes up the bulk of the mucous membrane.

In the healthy mouth, the submucosa is firmly attached to the periosteum of the underlying bone of the residual ridge and will usually successfully withstand the pressures of dentures. When the submucosal layer is thin over the bone, the soft tissue will be nonresilient, and small movements of the dentures will tend to break the retentive seal. When the submucosal layer is loosely attached to the periosteum of the residual ridge or is inflamed or edematous (excess fluid present), the tissue is easily displaceable, and the stability and support of the dentures are adversely affected. The impression procedure often requires modification to accommodate to these variations in the submucosa.

The histologic nature of the bone in different parts of the residual ridge also varies between patients and within the same patient. The amount and location of resorption can often be difficult or impossible to predict. Normally certain parts of the bone of the jaws are made up of compact bone, as opposed to spongy or trabeculated bone. Impression procedures should take advantage of these differences. A knowledge of the normal microscopic anatomy of the oral cavity can be the key to effective biologic impression procedures.

Classification of oral mucosa

Most classifications divide the oral mucosa into three categories, depending on its location in the mouth: the masticatory mucosa, the lining mucosa, and the specialized mucosa.

In the edentulous patient the masticatory mucosa covers (1) the crest of the residual ridge, including the residual attached gingiva that is firmly attached to the supporting bone, and (2) the hard palate. Masticatory mucosa is characterized by a well-defined keratinized layer on its outermost surface that is subject to changes in thickness depending on whether dentures are worn and on the clinical acceptability of the dentures.

The lining mucosa is generally found covering the mucous membrane in the oral cavity that is not firmly attached to the periosteum of the bone. The lining mucosa forms the covering of the lips and cheeks, the vestibular spaces, the alveololingual sulcus, the soft palate, the ventral surface of the tongue, and the unattached gingiva found on the slopes of the residual ridges. Lining mucosa is normally devoid of a keratinized layer and is freely movable with the tissues to which it is attached because of the elastic nature of the lamina propria.

The specialized mucosa covers the dorsal surface of the tongue. This mucosal covering is keratinized and includes the specialized papillae on the upper surface of the tongue.

Microscopic anatomy of supporting tissues

The microscopic anatomy of the supporting tissues of the upper impression is described for the crest of the residual ridge, the slopes of the residual ridge, and the palatal tissues.

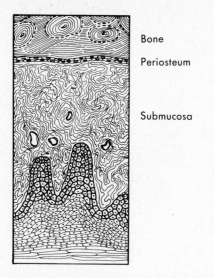

Bone

Periosteum

Submucosa

Fig. 7-16. Histologic drawing of mucous membrane covering crest of residual ridge. Notice that submucosal layer is sufficiently thick to provide resiliency for support of complete dentures and that bone covering crest of upper residual ridge is often compact in nature. Thus crest of residual ridge is primary stress-bearing area for upper denture.

The mucous membrane covering the crest of the upper residual ridge in the healthy mouth is firmly attached to the periosteum of the bone of the maxillae by the connective tissue of the submucosa (Fig. 7-16). The stratified squamous epithelium is thickly keratinized. The submucosa is devoid of fat or glandular cells or edema but is characterized by dense collagenous fibers that are contiguous with the lamina propria. The submucosal layer, though relatively thin in comparison with other parts of the mouth, is still sufficiently thick to provide adequate resiliency for primary support of the upper denture. The mucous membrane covering the crest of the edentulous ridge is comparable to the attached gingiva in the dentulous mouth, except that the submucosal layer in the edentulous mouth is usually thicker than that found in the attached gingiva of the dentulous mouth.

The outer surface of the bone in the region of the crest of the upper residual ridge may be compact in nature, being made up of haversian

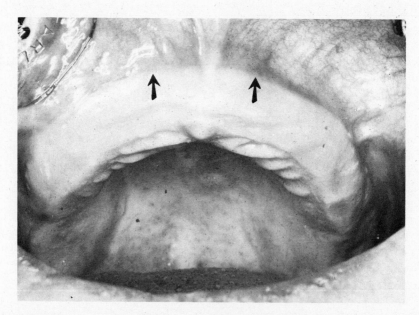

Fig. 7-17. *Arrows,* Line of demarcation between attached and unattached residual mucous membrane. Residual attached mucous membrane is desirable for support of complete dentures. Notice prominent incisive papillae anteriorly at center of residual alveolar ridge. It overlies the incisive foramen.

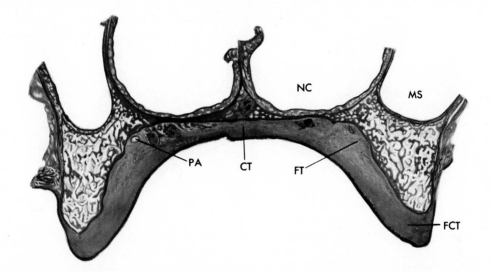

Plate 7-1. Buccolingual section in region of maxillary first molar. *NC,* Nasal cavity; *MS,* maxillary sinus; *FCT,* fibrous connective tissue on crest of ridge; *FT,* fat tissue; *PA,* palatine artery; *CT,* connective tissue. (Courtesy E.C. Pendleton.)

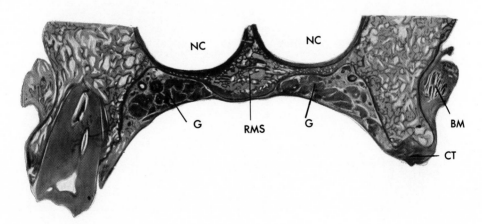

Plate 7-2. Frontal section through maxillae in third molar region. *NC,* Nasal cavity; *BM,* buccinator muscle; *CT,* fibrous connective tissue; *G,* mucous glands; *RMS,* ridge of maxillary suture. (Courtesy E.C. Pendleton.)

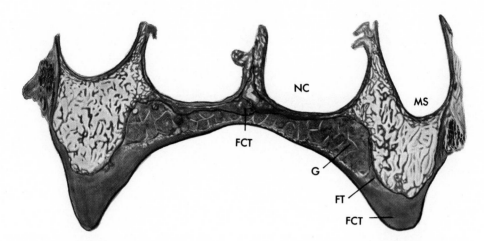

Plate 7-3. Buccolingual section through region of maxillary third molar. *NC,* Nasal cavity; *MS,* maxillary sinus; *FCT,* fibrous connective tissue on crest of ridge and over maxillary suture; *FT,* fat tissue; *G,* glands of palate. (Courtesy E.C. Pendleton.)

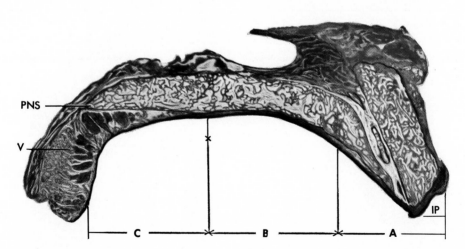

Plate 7-4. Sagittal section through median line of edentulous maxillae. *A,* Area of maxillary ridge and incisive foramen; *B,* hard palate; *C,* soft palate; *IP,* incisive papilla; *X,* crest of ridge of maxillary suture; *PNS,* posterior nasal spine; *V,* velum. (Courtesy E.C. Pendleton.)

systems. This compact bone, in combination with the tightly attached mucous membrane, makes the crest of the upper residual ridge histologically best able to provide primary support for the upper denture. Impression procedures should take advantage of the nature of this tissue when one provides for additional stress to be placed on the crest of the ridge of the upper jaw during the making of the final impression.

As the mucous membrane extends from the crest along the slope of the upper residual ridge to the reflection, it tends to lose its firm attachment to the underlying bone. This change marks the end of the residual attached mucous membrane (Fig. 7-17). The more loosely attached mucous membrane in this region has a nonkeratinized or slightly keratinized epithelium, and the submucosa contains loose connective tissue and elastic fibers. This loosely attached tissue will not withstand the forces of mastication or other stress transmitted through the denture bases and the firmly attached mucous mem-

brane over the crest of the ridge. Less stress is placed on the movable tissue of the slope of the ridge during the making of the final impression because the final impression material in that region is closer to the escapeways (border of the impression tray) than the impression material over the crest of the ridge (Fig. 7-18). This fact is in accord with the principle that in a semiconfined container, the impression material farthest from the escapeways is under the greatest pressure.

The soft tissue covering the hard palate varies considerably in consistency and thickness in different locations even though the epithelium is keratinized throughout. Anterolaterally, the submucosa of the hard palate contains adipose tissue (Fig. 7-19) and posterolaterally the submucosa contains glandular tissue (Fig. 7-20). These tissues should be recorded in a resting condition because when they are displaced in the final impression, they tend to return to normal form within the completed denture base,

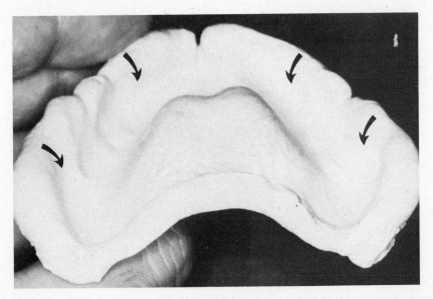

Fig. 7-18. Impression material near borders of impression tray *(arrows)* can flow out of the tray relatively easily during making of final impression. Thus less pressures are placed on tissues near borders of impression than on those near crest of ridge during making of final impression. This is desirable because of histologic nature of the tissue.

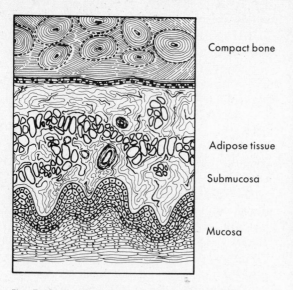

Compact bone

Adipose tissue

Submucosa

Mucosa

Fig. 7-19. Histologic drawing of mucous membrane in anterolateral part of hard palate. Notice that submucosa contains a relatively large quantity of adipose tissue.

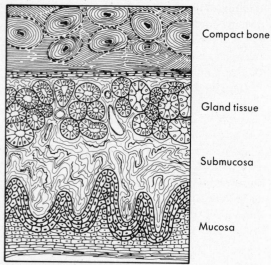

Compact bone

Gland tissue

Submucosa

Mucosa

Fig. 7-20. Histologic drawing of mucous membrane in posterolateral aspects of hard palate. Notice abundance of glandular tissue found in mucous membrane.

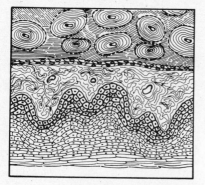

Compact bone

Submucosa

Mucosa

Fig. 7-21. Histologic drawing of mucous membrane covering median palatal suture. The submucosal layer is thin or may be practically nonexistent, making this part of mouth unsuitable for support of upper denture.

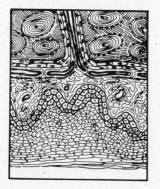

Compact bone

Nasopalatine vessel and nerve

Submucosa

Mucosa

Fig. 7-22. Histologic drawing of region of incisive papilla showing nasal palatine vessels and nerves contained in submucosa. The histologic nature of papilla makes it essential that proper relief be provided in completed denture.

creating an unseating force on the denture or causing soreness in the patient's mouth. Proper relief of the final impression tray aids in recording these tissues in an undistorted form. In addition, the secretions from the palatal glands can be an important factor in the selection of the final impression material.

The submucosa in the region of the median palatal suture of the maxillary bones is extremely thin. The mucosal layer is practically in contact with the underlying bone (Fig. 7-21). For this reason, the soft tissue covering the median palatal suture is nonresilient. Little or no stress can be placed in this region during the making of the final impression or in the completed denture. Otherwise, the denture will tend to rock over the center of the palate when vertical forces are applied to the teeth. In addition, this part of the mouth is highly sensitive, and excess pressure can create excruciating pain. Proper relief in the impression tray or the completed denture is essential for accommodation of the histologic nature of this tissue.

A histologic section through the incisive papilla and the nasopalatine canal would reveal that the submucosa contains the nasopalatine vessels and nerves (Fig. 7-22). Relief should be provided for the incisive papilla in both the final impression and the completed denture to prevent pressure on the nasopalatine vessels and nerves.

Microscopic anatomy of limiting structures

The microscopic anatomy of the limiting tissues of the upper denture will be described for the vestibular spaces, the hamular notches, and the posterior palatal seal area in the region of the vibrating line.

A histologic section of the mucous membrane lining the vestibular spaces depicts a relatively thin epithelium that is nonkeratinized. The submucosal layer is thick and contains large amounts of loose areolar tissue and elastic fibers (Fig. 7-23). The nature of the submucosa in the vestibular spaces makes this tissue easily movable. For this reason, the labial or buccal flanges of the upper impression can easily be overextended or underextended. A knowledge of the size of the space in the vestibule that is available for dentures is the key for proper determination of the length and form of the flange. The procedures for molding the borders of an impression that simulate natural muscle activity in the lips and cheeks are important in the development of properly formed flanges that will be in harmony with the histologic limitations of these tissues.

The submucosa in the region of the vibrating line on the soft palate contains glandular tissue similar to that in the submucosa in the posterolateral part of the hard palate (Fig. 7-24). However, because the soft palate does not rest directly on bone, the tissue for a few millimeters on either side of the vibrating line can be repo-

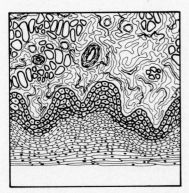

Adipose tissue

Elastic fibers

Submucosa

Mucosa

Fig. 7-23. Histologic drawing of mucous membrane lining vestibular spaces. the loose areolar tissue and elastic fibers in submucosal layer permit a relatively large degree of movement of the tissues at the reflection.

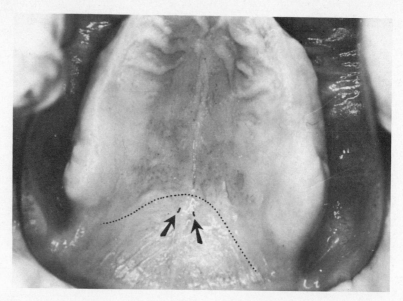

Fig. 7-24. *Dotted line,* Approximate location of vibrating line, which is the first point of movement of soft palate in relation to hard palate. *Arrows* point to faveae palatinae, which have been accentuated by black marks. Note that reflections posteriorly follow curvature of the maxillary tuberosities and blend into hamular notches. This anatomic form should be reflected in form of the borders of the impression.

sitioned in a controlled manner in the impression procedure to improve the posterior palatal seal. The secretion of palatal glands during the making of final impressions can affect the choice of the final impression material.

The submucosa of the mucous membrane contained within the hamular notch, the space between the posterior part of the maxillary tuberosity and the pterygoid hamulus, is thick and made up of loose or areolar tissue (Fig. 7-25). Additional pressure can also be placed on this tissue at the center of the notch to complete the posterior palatal seal. Space is provided in the final impression tray except in the region of the vibrating line and through the hamular notches before the final impression is made. Thus the tray itself contacts the soft tissue in this region when the impression is made (Fig. 7-26). In this manner, additional pressure by the denture can be placed on these palatal tissues because the histologic nature of the mucous

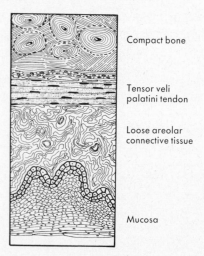

Compact bone

Tensor veli palatini tendon

Loose areolar connective tissue

Mucosa

Fig. 7-25. Histologic drawing of mucous membrane in hamular notch. The loose areolar connective tissue in submucosal layer can be displaced without trauma by the complete denture to improve posterior palatal seal.

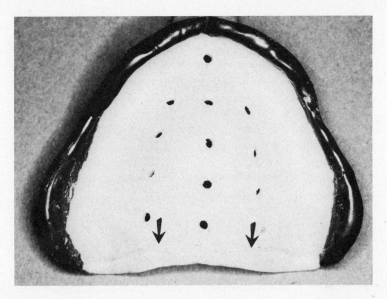

Fig. 7-26. Posterior part of impression tray *(arrows)* contacts and displaces soft tissue in region of vibrating line and hamular notches during making of final impression to develop posterior palatal seal. Space has been provided throughout the rest of the tray for final impression material.

membrane allows it to be displaced without trauma.

CLINICAL CONSIDERATIONS OF MICROSCOPIC ANATOMY

A knowledge of the microscopic anatomy of the oral mucous membrane has direct clinical implications for dentists and directly affects their success when they treat edentulous patients.

Histologic studies of the effect of wearing dentures on the keratinization of the mucosa of the crest of the residual ridges and the palate have produced conflicting results. However, most studies indicate that wearing dentures does not seem to be harmful to the epithelium even though keratinization is reduced in thickness and the stratum corneum is thinner in patients who wear them. Cytologic studies indicate that increased amounts of keratinized material are present in edentulous ridges when the clinical

quality of the dentures is good, an indication that goodfitting dentures may be important in maintaining the normal histologic condition of the mouth. Stimulation of the mucosa of the residual ridge through toothbrush physiotherapy also increases the presence of keratinized material. Histologically, removing the dentures from the mouth for 6 to 8 hours a day, preferably during periods of sleep, allows keratinization to increase and the signs of inflammation, often found in the submucosa when dentures are worn, are dramatically reduced.

The aging process can be held accountable for a number of important unfavorable histologic changes in the oral mucous membrane. Nerves in the mucous membrane of the residual ridges in elderly edentulous patients are greatly reduced, and those present are mostly confined to the lamina propria adjacent to the underlying bone. Alveolar and gingival arteries show signs of sclerosis. Age also plays a major role in the ability of the oral mucous membrane to recover from compression loading caused by pressures from the denture base. In the child or young person, recovery of deformed mucosa occurs in terms of seconds, whereas in the elderly person it may require hours or eventually result in irreversible changes. The immediate changes in the form of the supporting mucous membrane by pressures from the denture base seriously compromise correction of the occlusion of dentures in the patient's mouth or correction of parts of final impressions by addition of impression material directly to the defect rather than a remaking of the total impression.

Cross-sectional anatomy of the maxillae

A study of the soft and hard tissues of the edentulous mouth in cross section reveals many important facts in relation to complete denture construction. The idea is all too prevalent that the bony contours of the ridge are covered with a more or less uniform thickness of soft tissue. The vast difference in depth of tissue in different parts of the palate may not be abnormal. A comparison of the bony outline with the soft-tissue

outline will usually show a moderate amount of fibrous connective tissue over the crest of the ridge and an increasing depth of glandular tissue toward the higher portion of the vault, with a decreasing amount of submucosal tissue over the median suture of the maxillary bones. This tissue has (1) a layer of epithelium, (2) a layer of fibrous and loose connective tissue, (3) a layer of glandular tissue, and (4) periosteum that attaches these tissues to the bone (see Plates 7-1 to 7-4, facing p. 134).

RELATED ANATOMIC STRUCTURES
Muscles

Muscles of the soft palate. The muscles of the soft palate are the levator veli palatini, tensor veli palatini, musculus uvulae, glossopalatinus, and pharyngopalatinus (Figs. 7-27 and 7-28).

The wall of the soft palate is formed principally by the pharyngopalatinus muscle, with fibers of the glossopalatinus intermingling. The levator and tensor veli palatini are attaching muscles that affect the movement of the soft palate. The posterior border of the maxillary denture, which forms the posterior palatal seal, rests on the soft

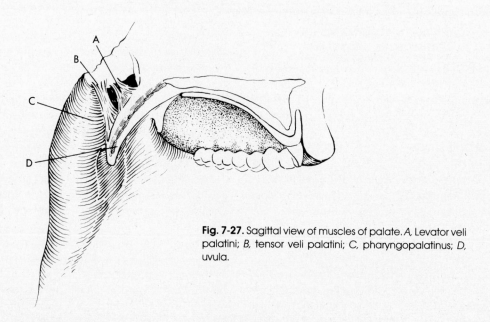

Fig. 7-27. Sagittal view of muscles of palate. *A,* Levator veli palatini; *B,* tensor veli palatini; *C,* pharyngopalatinus; *D,* uvula.

palate as far posteriorly as the vibrating line or else the place where the soft palate becomes movable. The function of these muscles is not impaired if the denture border is not carried too far posteriorly.

Muscles of the pharynx. The muscles of the pharynx are the constrictor superior, constrictor medius, constrictor inferior, stylopharyngeus, salpingopharyngeus, and pharyngopalatinus.

The superior constrictor is a muscle of the kinetic chain involved in the act of swallowing (Fig. 7-29). It is separated from the buccinator muscle by the pterygomandibular raphe just after the buccinator muscle swings into the inner surface of the ramus. The superior constrictor muscle forms the side wall of the throat.

Muscles of the tongue. The muscles of the tongue are divided into two groups, the intrinsic and extrinsic muscles. The intrinsic muscles (Fig. 7-30) are the superior longitudinal, inferior longitudinal, transverse, and vertical muscles. The extrinsic muscles (Fig. 7-31) are the genioglossus, hyoglossus, chondroglossus, styloglossus, and glossopalatinus.

Nerve and blood supply

The maxillary denture foundation gets its blood supply from the descending palatine artery and from the posterior superior alveolar artery. The mandible is supplied by the inferior alveolar artery and by the inferior alveolar artery and by its branches: the incisive, mental, lin-

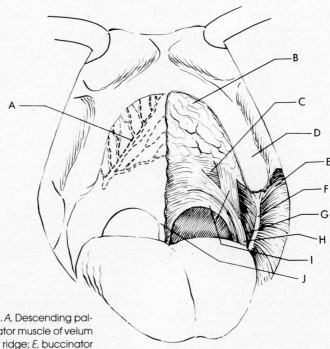

Fig. 7-28. Diagram of an open mouth. *A,* Descending palatine artery; *B,* mucous glands; *C,* levator muscle of velum palatinum; *D,* upper residual alveolar ridge; *E,* buccinator muscle; *F,* pterygomandibular raphe; *G,* superior constrictor muscle; *H,* glossopalatine muscle; *I,* pharyngopalatinus muscle; *J,* uvula.

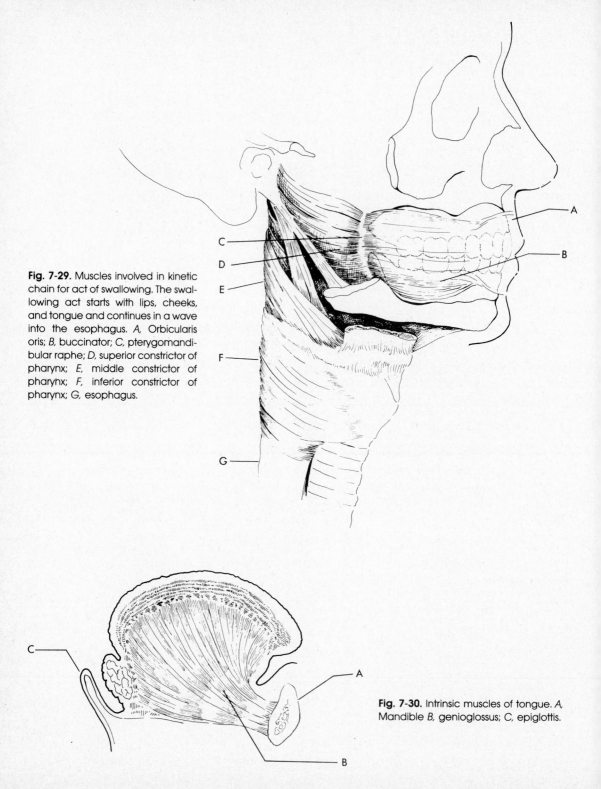

Fig. 7-29. Muscles involved in kinetic chain for act of swallowing. The swallowing act starts with lips, cheeks, and tongue and continues in a wave into the esophagus. *A,* Orbicularis oris; *B,* buccinator; *C,* pterygomandibular raphe; *D,* superior constrictor of pharynx; *E,* middle constrictor of pharynx; *F,* inferior constrictor of pharynx; *G,* esophagus.

Fig. 7-30. Intrinsic muscles of tongue. *A,* Mandible *B,* genioglossus; *C,* epiglottis.

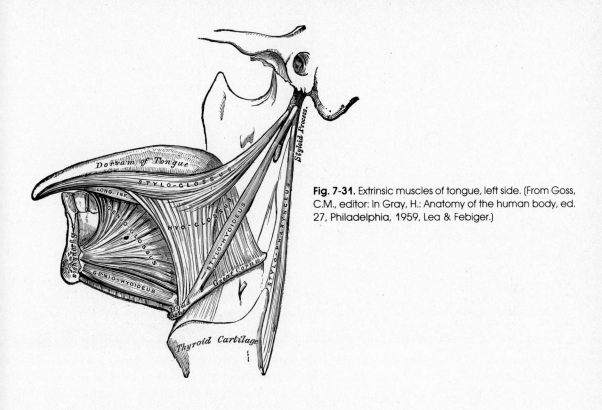

Fig. 7-31. Extrinsic muscles of tongue, left side. (From Goss, C.M., editor: In Gray, H.: Anatomy of the human body, ed. 27, Philadelphia, 1959, Lea & Febiger.)

gual, and mylohyoid. The tongue is supplied by the lingual artery.

The innervation of the maxillary area is supplied by the nasopalatine, anterior palatine, middle palatine, and inferior nasal nerves on the palatal side. On the buccal side the region is supplied by the posterior superior alveolar branch, middle superior alveolar branch, and anterior superior alveolar branch of the maxillary nerve.

The mandibular region is supplied by the inferior alveolar nerve and its branches: the mylohyoid, dental, incisive, and mental.

The buccinator (long buccal) nerve supplies the buccinator muscle, vestibule, and cheek.

The anterior two thirds of the tongue is supplied by the lingual nerve, and the posterior one third is supplied by the glossopharyngeal nerve.

8

Maxillary impression procedures

The capability of the mucous membrane of the basal seat to withstand stress from the denture base varies greatly because of the histologic makeup of different parts of the residual ridge. For example, the crest of the healthy maxillary residual ridge is often designated as a primary stress bearing area for dentures because the submucosa is formed by a layer of thick fibrous connective tissue that is attached firmly to compact bone. This combination provides favorable support for the denture. On the other hand, the much thinner nonresilient mucous membrane and underlying bone of the median palatal suture often requires relief for the denture base. Because of these variations, impressions of edentulous ridges must selectively place pressures on the mucous membrane and bone in amounts that are compatible with the histologic tolerances of the supporting tissues for each patient. When this important biologic principle is violated, dentures lose retention, stability, and support; create soreness; or cause resorption of the underlying bone. It becomes obvious that for successful treatment to occur the dentist must (1) understand the histology and pathology of the living tissues that make up the basal seat and (2) use a clinical technique in making impressions that selectively distributes pressures to the basal seat to meet the needs of each edentulous patient.

PRINCIPLES AND OBJECTIVES OF
IMPRESSION MAKING

Impression techniques, methods, and materials of choice are constantly changing, but underlying principles and fundamentals remain constant. Sensational claims for techniques and materials are misleading because results cannot always be spectacular. There are, in fact, many thousands of combinations of conditions in which results are unpredictable.

Impression techniques and materials should be selected on the basis of biologic factors. Techniques too often follow shortcuts, perhaps to satisfy the patient's desire for immediate results, without a consideration of the future destruction that such procedures may induce.

An impression is a record of the negative form of the tissues of the oral cavity that make up the basal seat of the denture. An impression is made to make a cast that is a positive replica of the shape and size of the same oral tissues. The five objectives of an impression are to provide retention, stability, and support for the denture, provide esthetics for the lips, and at the same time maintain the health of the oral tissues.

Retention for a denture is its resistance to removal in a direction opposite that of its insertion. It is the quality inherent in a denture that resists the force of gravity, the adhesiveness of foods, and the forces associated with the opening of the jaws. Retention is the means by which dentures are held in position in the mouth. When the soft tissues over the bones are displaced under pressure, the denture bases may lose their retention because of the change in adaptation of the basal surface of the denture to its basal seat.

The *stability* of a denture is the quality of a denture to be firm, steady, and constant in position when forces are applied to it. Stability refers especially to resistance against horizontal movement and forces that tend to alter the relationship between the denture base and its supporting foundation in a horizontal or rotatory direction. The size and form of the basal seat, the quality of the final impressions, the form of the polished surfaces, and the proper location and arrangement of the arificial teeth play a major role in the stability of the dentures (Figs. 8-1 and 8-2).

Dentures *support* is the resistance to vertical components of mastication and to occlusal or other forces applied in a direction toward the basal seat. Support is provided by the maxillary and the mandibular bones and their covering of mucosal tissues. It is enhanced by selective

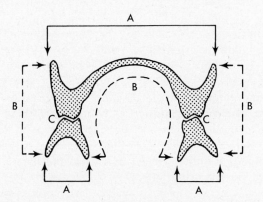

Fig. 8-1. Dentures have three surfaces. *A,* Impression or basal surfaces that are fitted to basal seats; *B,* polished surfaces that are contoured so that they will support and contact the cheeks, lips, and tongue; *C,* occlusal surfaces that must fit occlusal surfaces of opposing denture.

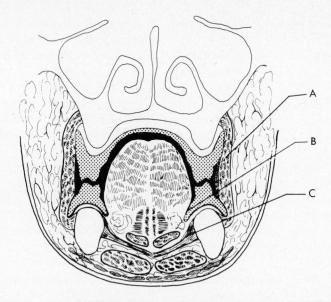

Fig. 8-2. Schematic frontal section. Dentures properly fill available denture space. *A,* Buccinator muscle; *B,* lingual flange and border are placed under tongue; *C,* mylohyoid muscle. Notice that polished surfaces of both upper and lower dentures are shaped so that action of tongue and cheeks tends to seat rather than unseat dentures. If posterior artificial teeth are too wide buccolingually, the form of the dentures will be changed, and tongue and cheeks will tend to unseat the dentures.

placement of pressures that are in harmony with the resiliency of the tissues that make up the basal seat (see Fig. 7-3).

Impression procedures must adhere to biologic principles dictated by the anatomy (gross and microscopic) and the physiology of the edentulous mouth. These principles were discussed in Chapter 7. The following essential, biologically related principles should be incorporated in any impression procedure. Most of these principles enhance the retention, stability, and support of a denture, which are all interrelated.

1. The impression is extended to include all of the basal seat within the limits of the health and functions of the supporting and limiting tissues.
2. The borders are in harmony with the anatomic and physiologic limitations of the oral structures.
3. A physiologic type of border-molding procedure is performed by the dentist or by the patient under the guidance of the dentist.
4. Proper space for the selected final impression material is provided within the impression tray.
5. Selective pressure is placed on the basal seat during the making of the final impression.
6. The impression can be removed from the mouth without damage to the mucous membrane of the residual ridge.
7. A guiding mechanism is provided for correct positioning of the impression tray in the mouth.
8. The tray and final impression are made of dimensionally stable materials.
9. The external shape of the final impression is similar to the external form of the completed denture.

The two most important factors in making satisfactory impressions for complete dentures are a properly formed and accurately fitting final impression tray and proper positioning of the final impression tray on the basal seat in the mouth.

FACTORS OF RETENTION OF DENTURES

A number of forces and factors combine to retain complete dentures in position in the mouth. Not all these factors act at the same time. Instead, some act only when they are needed to meet or resist a certain dislodging force.

Adhesion

Adhesion is the physical attraction of unlike molecules for each other. Adhesion acts when saliva wets and sticks to the basal surface of dentures and, at the same time, to the mucous membrane of the basal seat. The effectiveness of adhesion depends on the close adaptation of the denture base to the supporting tissues and the fluidity of the saliva. A watery saliva is quite effective, provided that the denture base material can be "wetted." Some denture base materials allow water (or saliva) to stick to them and spread out in a thin layer. These materials have greater potential for being retained by adhesion than materials that cause drops of water to form over their surfaces.

Adhesion of saliva to the mucous membrane is no problem because the saliva "wets" it very effectively.

Thick, ropy saliva adheres well to both the denture base and to mucosa, but since much of this type of saliva is produced by the palatal glands under the maxillary basal seat, it builds up and literally pushes the denture out of position. The force of adhesion still acts on both surfaces, but the hydraulic pressure produced by the thick mucus secretions may overpower it.

Adhesion is also the molecular attraction between the surfaces of unlike bodies in contact. This type of adhesion is observed between denture bases and the mucous membranes of patients with xerostomia. The denture base materials seem to stick to the dry mucous membrane of the basal seat and of the cheeks and lips. Such adhesion is not very affective for retaining dentures, and it is annoying to patients when it sticks the denture base to the cheeks and lips. A mouthwash of Cepacol and glycerin can be helpful in this situation.

The amount of retention supplied by adhesion is directly proportional to the area covered by the denture. Patients with small jaws (basal seats) cannot expect retention by adhesion to be as effective as patients with large jaws can. Thus the dentures (and hence the impressions) must be extended to the limits of the health and function of the oral tissues if the dentures are to have their maximum adhesion and retention.

Cohesion

Cohesion is the physical attraction of like molecules for each other. It is a retentive force because it occurs in the layer of saliva between the denture base and the mucosa. It is effective in direct proportion to the area covered by the denture, if other factors are equal. Since saliva is a liquid, the layer of saliva must be thin if it is to be effective for retention. Therefore the adaptation of the denture base to the mucosa must be as close as possible.

Interfacial surface tension

Interfacial surface tension is the tension, or resistance to separation, possessed by the film of liquid between two well-adapted surfaces. Interfacial surface tension is found in the thin film of saliva between the denture base and the mucosa of the basal seat. It is quite similar in its action to cohesion and to capillary attraction, or capillarity. It is also effective in direct proportion to the size of the basal surface of dentures, if other things are equal. One of the requirements for its retentive value is minimal distortion or displacement of the soft tissues by the impression and, of course, the denture. A perfect fit is essential.

Capillary attraction, or capillarity

Capillary attraction, or capillarity, is a force (developed because of surface tension) that causes the surface to a liquid to become elevated or depressed when it is in contact with a solid. Capillary attraction causes a liquid to rise in a capillary tube, since surface tension tends to form a round surface on the liquid. When the adaptation of the denture base to the mucosa on which it rests is sufficently close, the space filled with a thin film of saliva acts like a capillary tube and helps to retain the denture. This force, like the others, is directly proportional to the area of the basal seat covered by the denture base.

Atmospheric pressure

Atmospheric pressure operates as a retentive force when dislodging forces are applied to dentures. Some have called it "suction" because it is a resistance to the removal of dentures from their basal seat, but there is no suction, or negative pressure, except when another force is applied. Atmospheric pressure itself is supplied by the weight of the atmosphere, and it amounts to 14.7 lb/in^2. This means that the retentive force supplied by atmospheric pressure is directly proportional to the area covered by the denture base. For atmospheric pressure to be effective, the denture must have a perfect seal around its entire border. Atmospheric pressure is an *emergency* retentive force. If the other retentive forces are being overpowered, the atmospheric pressure may be able to keep the denture in position. Suction alone applied to the soft tissues of the oral cavity for even a small period of time would cause serious damage to the health of the soft tissues under negative pressure.

Oral and facial musculature

The oral and facial musculature can supply supplementary retentive forces, provided that (1) the teeth are positioned in the neutral zone between the cheeks and the tongue and (2) the polished surfaces of the dentures are properly shaped. This is not to say that patients must hold their teeth in place by conscious effort but only that the shape of the buccal and lingual flanges must make it possible for the musculature to automatically fit against the denture and reinforce the border seal of each denture (Figs. 8-1 and 8-2). If the buccal flanges of the maxillary denture slope up and out from the occlusal surfaces of the teeth and if the buccal flanges of the mandibular denture slope down and out from the occlusal plane, the contraction of the buccinator muscles will tend to seat both dentures on their basal seats.

The lingual surfaces of the lingual flanges should slope toward the center of the mouth so that the tongue can fit against them and perfect the border seal on the lingual side of the denture. The base of the tongue is guided on top of the lingual flange by the lingual side of the distal end of the lingual flange, which turns laterally toward the ramus. This part of the denture also helps to perfect the border seal at the back end of mandibular dentures. All this reinforcement is automatic, without conscious effort on the part of the patient.

The base of the tongue serves also as an emergency retentive force for some patients. It rises up at the back and presses against the distal border of the maxillary denture during incision of food by the anterior teeth. This is done without conscious effort when the experienced denture wearer bites into an apple or sandwich or other food. It is seldom that a patient needs to be told how to do this. For the oral and facial musculature to be most effective in providing retention for complete dentures, the following conditions must be met: (1) denture bases must be properly extended to cover the maximum area possible without interfering with the health and function of the structures that surround the denture, (2) the occlusal plane must be at the correct level, and (3) the arch form of the teeth must be in the neutral zone between the tongue and cheeks.

HEALTH OF BASAL SEAT TISSUES

It is essential that the oral tissues be healthy before impressions are made. A careful diagnosis will reveal pathosis in the oral cavities of a startling number of edentulous patients who wear dentures. In a study of responses to variations in denture techniques, 41 of 64 edentulous denture-wearing patients selected from the general population required special treatment to restore abused oral tissues to a healthy condition. Oral lesions and their causes must be treated before impressions are considered. Simple observation of the oral mucosa provides important information about the health of the tissues. Some conditions require immediate attention before impressions are made, such as the following:

1. *Inflammation of the mucosa*. Because of the nature of inflammation, the soft tissues are not their natural size. The swelling, which is a characteristic result of inflammation from either trauma or disease changes the gross form of the surface to be recorded in the impression. All inflammation must be eliminated before the new impressions are made, or the new dentures will not fit the tissues after they are no longer distorted by the swelling. Treatment is accomplished by surgery or proper medication or by keeping the old dentures out of the mouth until the tissues are healthy. Soft resin treatment (tissue-conditioning) materials may be used in the old dentures to reduce the period in which the dentures must be left out of the mouth (Chapter 6). However, the old dentures must be kept out of the mouth at least 24 hours before the impressions are made.

2. *Distortion of denture-foundation tissues*. The denture that the patient is wearing may appear to have good retention and stability, but at the same time it may not fit the true form of the oral structures. In such a situation, the denture had molded the soft tissues to its own shape. This molding could have progressed slowly over a period of time, and the patient's resistance could have been such that little or no inflammation occurred in the process. The distortion of the oral tissues can be corrected when the old dentures are left out of the mouth for 1, 2, or more days before the impressions are made. A combination of leaving the dentures out and the use of conditioning materials that allow tissues to assume more normal form within

the confines of the denture base can be an effective treatment. Some patients will object to leaving their dentures out of the mouth, but their objections can be overcome by careful explanation, insistence by the dentist, use of conditioning material, and selection of a convenient time for scheduling of their appointments.

3. *Excessive amounts of hyperplastic tissue*. Since the maxillae and the mandible (the bones) are the real foundations for dentures, their soft tissue covering must be firm. Excessive amounts of movable soft tissue will permit the dentures to move in relation to the bone, and there will result many types of difficulties, such as looseness, tipping, malocclusion of the dentures, and difficulty in recording jaw relations accurately. The treatment is by finger massage on a daily prescribed basis or by surgical removal of the hyperplastic tissue, followed by sufficient time for complete healing. The apparent ridge size will be reduced by this procedure, but the real foundation will be the same size and much more effective (Chapter 6).

4. *Insufficient space between the upper and lower ridges*. Usually the insufficient space is found in the tuberosity region (Fig. 8-3). It may be caused by an excessive amount of fibrous connective tissue covering the tuberosity (Fig. 3-10), which will be disclosed by dental radiographs. Intraoral radiographs on small dental films are more effective than panoramic radiographs for this purpose (Chapter 6). Mounted diagnostic casts will disclose potential interference by the excess fibrous tissue over the tuberosities with the correct location of the occlusal plane. This determination should be made before the impressions are started. Excess fibrous tissue should be removed surgically, and time should be allowed for complete healing before impressions are made.

IMPRESSIONS FOR EDENTULOUS PATIENTS

Impressions are made with many types of materials and techniques. Some materials are more fluid than others before they harden or set. The softer materials displace soft tissues less

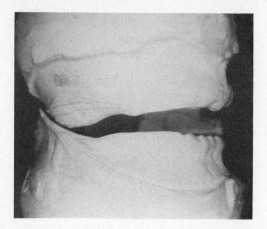

Fig. 8-3. Lack of maxillomandibular space as a result of tooth and bone migration; maxillary posterior teeth were unopposed by mandibular posterior teeth. Lower line on maxillary tuberosity of cast indicates level of soft tissue, and upper line the level of bone that must be removed to create adequate space for denture bases.

and require less force in their molding than materials that flow more sluggishly. These variations in the working properties of materials make it possible to devise many types of techniques for controlling the position and shape of the oral tissues. Some techniques are intended to record the shape of the tissues with a minimum of displacement; others are intended to displace the border tissues to a predetermined extent. Still other techniques are devised to obtain the advantages of placement or control of the border tissues with a minimal displacement of the tissues under the denture. The choice is made by the dentist on the basis of the oral conditions, concept of the function of the tissues surrounding the denture, and ability to handle the available impression materials.

Impression trays

Regardless of the type of impression being made, the tray in which it is made is the most important part of the impression. If the tray is too large, it will distort the tissues around the borders of the impression and will pull the soft tissues under the impression away from the bone. If the tray is too small, the border tissues will collapse inward onto the residual ridge. This would reduce the support for the denture and prevent the proper support of the lips by the denture flange.

A properly formed tray can carry the impression material to the mouth and control it without distorting the soft tissues that surround it. An improperly formed tray will make impossible the registration of the true negative form of the basal seat tissues on which the denture must rest. The tray must not distort or displace the tissues and structures that are to fit against the borders and polished surfaces of the denture.

The design of trays must be related to the impression material to be used. If the impression material is to be modeling compound, there must be sufficient space between the tray and the soft tissue to allow for adequate bulk of material and to allow the sluggish-flowing material to move into the desired relationship with the basal seat and border tissues.

If the impression material is to be a zinc oxide–eugenol paste, which flows readily, the tray must fit more accurately than for plaster of paris, which is free-flowing but more viscid. Consequently, these free-flowing materials must be used in trays made especially for each patient. These "individual" or "custom" trays are made of different materials with borders that can be adjusted so that they control the movable soft tissues around the impression but do not distort them. At the same time, space is provided inside the tray so that the shape of the tissues covering the residual alveolar ridge may be recorded with minimal or selective displacement.

The second most important part of the impression is the proper positioning of the final impression tray on the basal seat in the mouth. One can best accomplish this by using guiding factors incorporated into the tray and by practicing proper placement of the tray in the mouth before actually making the final impression.

Final impression materials

Many different types of materials have been used successfully for making final impressions.

Plaster of paris, zinc oxide–eugenol paste, irreversible hydrocolloid, silicone, polysulfide rubber, polyether, and tissue-conditioning material have been used for this purpose. Each has its advantages and its disadvantages.

The setting time of plaster of paris must be accelerated and is often modified so that its molding time will be increased. It absorbs some of the mucous secretions from the palate while it sets, but requires the use of a separating medium before the cast is formed in it. Plaster of paris has enough body to support itself up to 1.5 mm beyond the border of a tray.

Zinc oxide–eugenol paste records accurate surface detail and does not require a separating medium. It does not absorb the mucous secretions that are produced in the palate, and these secretions can cause defects in the palatal part of the impression. The borders of the tray must be accurately formed because the material is so fluid. The borders of the tray should be adjusted so that they reach to within 1 mm of the reflecting tissues.

The irreversible hydrocolloids record accurate detail if they are properly controlled and confined, and they do not require the use of a separating medium. They do not absorb the mucous secretions from the palate, and these secretions produce defects in the palatal part of the impression. Also, these materials lose moisture and consequently change their size so rapidly that the casts must be poured into them immediately or the record will be distorted. The

weight of the artificial stone of the cast may be sufficient to distort the borders of the impressions, and removal of the impressions from the mouth without distortion presents some difficulties.

Tissue-conditioning materials have been shown to be sufficiently accurate for making final impressions. They are resilient and continue to flow under stress for periods of up to 24 hours. They are useful for making functional impressions that record the basal seat and border tissues in their functional state. Although the composition of individual conditioning materials is not available, reports indicate that the liquids contain carboxylic esters or ethanol. The powders are acrylic resin polymers.

The silicone, polysulfide rubber, and polyether impression materials can record the shape of the soft tissues accurately if they are adequately supported by an accurately fitted tray. The polysulfide rubbers must be closely confined to the soft tissues, or they will produce an inaccurate impression. They are particularly useful for making impressions of thin high mandibular ridges with soft-tissue undercuts. The elasticity of the rubber and its tear strength, which is higher than silicone or polysulfide materials, allow the impression to be removed from the cast without fracture of the delicate ridge on the cast. The polyether impression materials have sufficient body to make up discrepancies between tray borders and the reflecting vestibular tissues of up to 4 or 5 mm, they can be shaped by the fingers, and they are accurate in reproducing detail. Since these materials are opaque, it is more difficult to detect pressure spots in the impressions than it is with other impression materials. Pressure spots are places where the tray shows through the impression material, and they indicate a displacement of tissues by pressure from the tray.

Impression techniques

Three techniques are described in this chapter. The first technique involves making a preliminary impression in a stock metal tray using

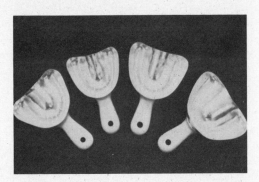

Fig. 8-4. Selection of different sizes of properly designed stock metal trays for maxillary impressions.

alginate (irreversible hydrocolloid) impression material. The final impression is made in a border-molded special tray. The second technique involves the use of a polyether impression procedure for a one-step border-molding technique. The third technique uses a preliminary modeling compound tray made from an impression in an oversize stock metal tray. The modeling compound tray is border molded and prepared, and the final impression is made in it.

First technique—border-molded special tray

The same diagnostic and treatment-planning procedures are followed for each patient regardless of the impression technique. Proper preparation of the oral tissues is essential and is completed as described previously.

Preliminary impression. The space available in the mouth for the upper impression is studied carefully by observation of the width and height of the vestibular spaces when the mouth is held partway open and the upper lip is held *slightly* outward and downward.

An edentulous stock metal tray that is approximately ¼ inch (6 mm) larger than the outside surface of the upper residual ridge is selected (Fig. 8-4). The dentist places the tray in the mouth and initially positions it by centering the labial notch of the tray over the labial frenum (Fig. 8-5, A). The dentist observes the posterior

extent of the tray in relation to the posterior palatal seal area by maintaining the tray in this proper anteroposterior position and then dropping the handle downward to permit visual inspection. Posteriorly, the tray must include both the hamular notches and the vibrating line (Fig. 8-5, B).

The borders of the stock tray are lined with a strip of soft boxing wax so that a rim is created to help confine the alginate (irreversible hydrocolloid) impression material (Fig. 8-5, C). The tray is placed back into position in the mouth. The wax across the posterior border of the tray is adapted to the tissue of the posterior palatal seal area by careful elevation of the tray in this region with the anterior part of the tray in the proper position (Fig. 8-6, A). Again the borders of the tray are observed visually in relation to the limiting anatomic structures (Fig. 8-6, B and C). The objective is to obtain a preliminary impression that is slightly overextended around the borders.

Before making the preliminary impression, the dentist should practice placing the preliminary tray into position on the upper residual ridge. The tray is positioned by first centering it below the upper residual ridge. The upper lip is elevated with the left hand, and the tray is carried upward into position with the labial frenum used as a centering guide. When the tray is located properly anteriorly, the index fingers are placed in the first molar region on each side of the tray, and with alternating pressure the tray is seated upward until the wax across the posterior part of the tray comes into contact with the tissue in the posterior palatal seal area. The fingers of one hand are shifted into the middle of the palate of the tray, and border-molding procedures are carried out with the other hand.

The tissue surface and borders of the metal tray, including the rim of wax, are painted with an adhesive material to make certain that the irreversible hydrocolloid adheres to the tray. The irreversible hydrocolloid is mixed according to instructions provided by the manufacturer. The impression material is placed into the tray

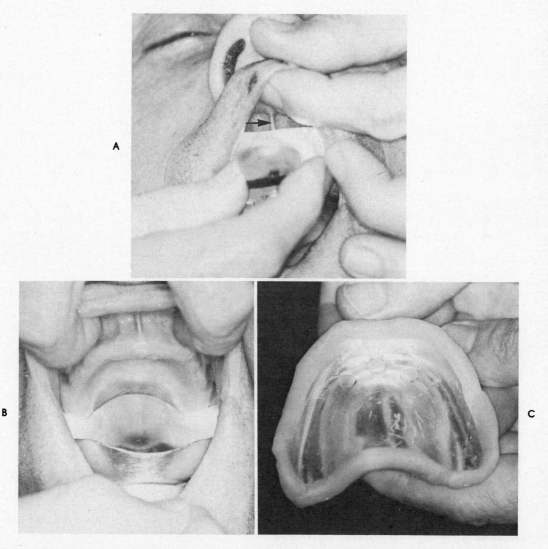

Fig. 8-5. Stock metal tray must be the proper size and be correctly positioned in mouth. **A,** Tray is inserted into the mouth and is centered by positioning of labial notch over labial frenum *(arrow).* **B,** Tray covers the hamular notches and vibrating line posteriorly. **C,** Strip of boxing wax lines borders of stock tray.

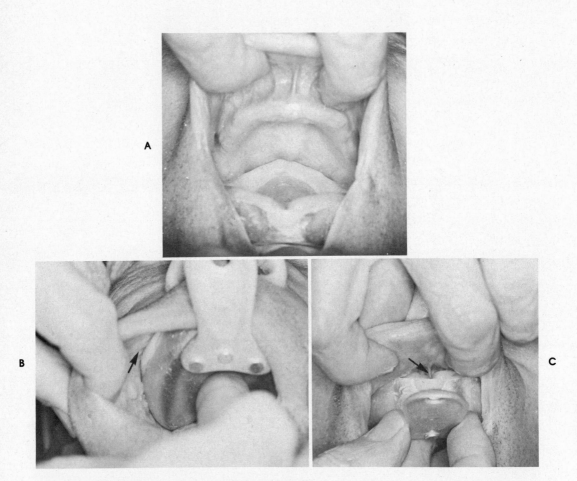

Fig. 8-6. A, Wax across posterior border of tray is adapted to tissue of posterior palatal seal area. **B,** Space for buccal frenum is provided in notch formed by wax lining the stock tray *(arrow).* **C,** Space for labial frenum is provided in notch formed by wax lining the stock tray *(arrow).*

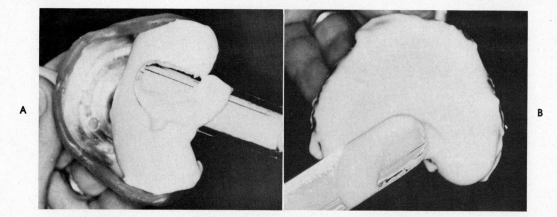

Fig. 8-7. A, Impression material is placed into tray from posterior border. **B,** Impression material is evenly distributed throughout tray, with care taken to prevent trapping of air within material.

and evenly distributed to fill the metal tray to the level of its borders (Fig. 8-7). A small amount of irreversible hydrocolloid is placed in the area of the rugae of the hard palate to help prevent air being trapped in this part of the preliminary impression (Fig. 8-8, *A*), and the loaded tray is positioned in the mouth in a manner similar to that during the practice sessions (Fig. 8-8, *B* to *D*). The impression tray is left in the mouth for 1 minute after the initial set of irreversible hydrocolloid. The impression is removed from the mouth in one motion and inspected to be certain that all the basal seat is included (Fig. 8-8, *E*).

Making the final impression tray. The cast is poured in artificial stone, and the outline for the wax spacer is drawn in pencil on the cast (Fig. 8-9, *A*). The wax spacer will provide space in the tray for the final impression material. The posterior palatal seal area on the cast is not covered with the wax spacer. In this manner the completed final impression tray will contact the upper residual ridge across the posterior palatal seal, and additional stress can be placed here during the making of the final impression. In addition, this part of the tray will act as a guiding stop to help position the tray properly on the residual ridge during the impression procedure.

Baseplate wax approximately 1 mm in thickness is placed on the cast as designated by the previously drawn outline (Fig. 8-9, *B*).

A self-curing acrylic resin tray material is mixed and uniformly adapted over the cast so that the tray will be approximately 2 to 3 mm in thickness (Fig. 8-9, *C*). A resin handle is attached in the anterior region of the tray to facilitate removal of the final impression. The handle is positioned in the approximate position of the upper anterior teeth so that it will not distort the upper lip when the tray is in position in the mouth (Fig. 8-9, *D*).

Preparing the final impression tray. When the acrylic resin final impression tray is removed from the preliminary cast, the wax spacer is left inside the tray. The spacer allows the tray to be properly positioned in the mouth during border-molding procedures (Fig. 8-10, *A*).

Border molding is the process by which the shape of the borders of the tray is made to conform accurately to the contours of the buccal and labial vestibules. This is often erroneously referred to as muscle trimming.

Border molding is accomplished by the manipulation of the border tissues against a moldable impression material that is properly supported and controlled by a tray. The amount

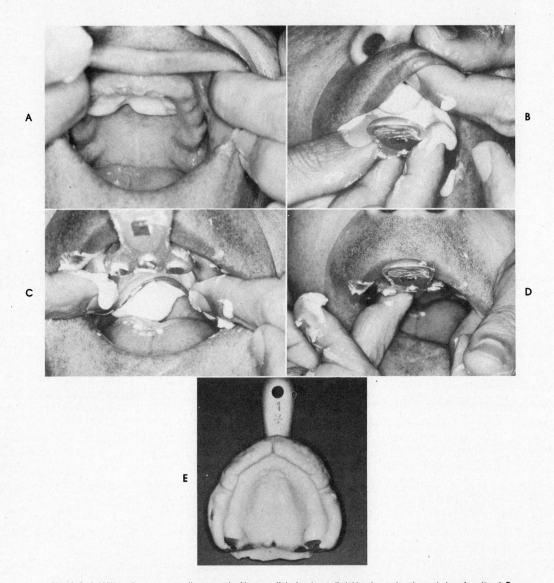

Fig. 8-8. A, With a finger, a small amount of irreversible hydrocolloid is placed onto palate of patient. **B,** Tray containing impression material is carried to position anteriorly by observation of labial frenum in relation to labial notch of tray. **C,** Tray is seated posteriorly by index fingers in first molar region. **D,** Tray is held steadily in position until irreversible hydrocolloid impression material has set. Notice position of finger on palatal part of tray. **E,** All of the basal seat is included in preliminary impression.

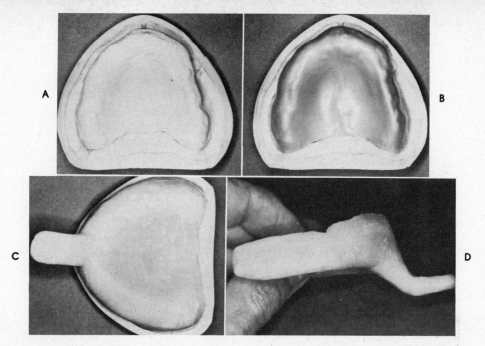

Fig. 8-9. A, Outline for wax spacer drawn in pencil on cast that was poured in preliminary impression. **B,** Relief wax covers basal seat area except for labial and buccal reflections and posterior palatal seal area. The reflections are not covered, so that proper length and width of borders of impression tray will be maintained as determined by preliminary impression or as desired. **C,** Final impression tray of self-curing acrylic resin and approximately 2 to 3 mm in thickness. **D,** Handle on final upper tray should not interfere with normal position of upper lip during making of final impression.

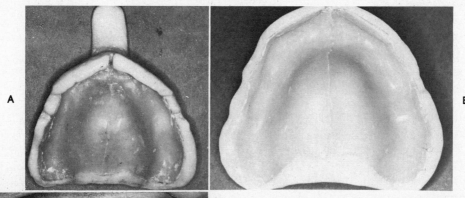

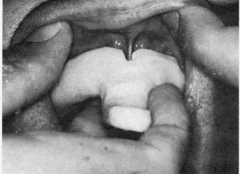

Fig. 8-10. A, Final impression tray covers entire basal seat area. Borders of tray have not been molded to be in harmony with physiologically limiting oral structures and must be corrected. Wax spacer has been left inside tray so that tray can be properly positioned in mouth during border-molding procedures. **B,** Borders of tray are reduced so that modeling compound can be added for border-molding procedures. **C,** Notice that space has been created between borders of tray and reflection.

of support supplied by the tray and the amount of force exerted through the tissues vary according to the resistance or viscosity of the impression material.

After the available space for denture flanges is again checked in the patient's mouth, the buccal and labial flanges of the impression tray are marked in pencil and reduced until they are short of the reflections (Fig. 8-10, *B* and *C*).

Stick modeling compound is added in sections to the shortened borders of the resin tray; then the compound is heated with the flame from an alcohol air torch, tempered, and molded in the mouth to a form that is in harmony with the physiologic action of the limiting anatomic structures. The tray is carefully removed from the mouth, and the modeling compound border is chilled in ice water. The border molding is accomplished in the anterior region when the upper lip is elevated and extended out, downward, and inward (Fig. 8-11, *A* and *B*). In the region of the buccal frenum, the cheek is elevated and then pulled outward, downward, and inward and moved backward and forward to simulate movement of the upper buccal frenum. Posteriorly, the buccal flange is border molded when the cheek is extended outward, downward, and inward (Fig. 8-11, *C* to *E*).

The posterior palatal seal is formed through both hamular (pterygomaxillary) notches and across the palate over the vibrating line. The vibrating line is observed in the patient's mouth as the patient says a series of short "ahs," and the hamular notches are palpated. The posterior border of the impression tray is marked with indelible pencil, the palatal tissues are dried quickly, the tray is placed in the mouth, and the patient is asked to say "ah." The tray is removed from the mouth, and the mark transferred from the tray to the mouth is compared with the vibrating line and the hamular notches (Fig. 8-12, *A* and *B*). The tray must contain both hamular notches and extend approximately 2 mm posterior to the vibrating line. Should the tray be underextended, the length is corrected by the addition of modeling compound. A strip of low-fusing modeling compound is traced on the impression over the vibrating line and through the hamular notches. The compound is chilled and then heated with the alcohol torch, tempered, and seated in the mouth under pressure. The added material will spread out on either side of the vibrating line and form a raised strip across the distal end of the impression (Fig. 8-12, *C*). This procedure will enhance the posterior palatal seal, which has the three functions of (1) slightly displacing the soft tissues at the distal end of the denture to enhance the posterior border seal, (2) serving as a guide for positioning the tray properly for making the final impression, and (3) preventing excess impression material from running down the patient's throat (Fig. 8-12, *C*).

After the border-molding procedure is completed, the modeling compound forming the labial and buccal borders of the tray is reduced approximately 1 mm to make space for the final impression material. The spacer wax is removed from the inside of the final impression tray for the same reason. Space must be provided inside the tray for the final impression material. If this is not provided, pressure spots will form in the impression. Pressure spots are regions where the tray displaces the soft tissues to be recorded in the impression. These regions of extra pressure would tend to dislodge the denture when it is completed and to interfere with the health of the tissues with which they would come into contact. Holes are placed in the palate of the impression tray with a No. 6 round bur to provide escapeways for the final impression material (Fig. 8-12, *D*). The holes provide relief during the making of the final upper impression for the median palatal raphe and in the anterolateral and posterolateral regions of the hard palate.

Making the final upper impression. The soft tissues in the mouth must be rested and healthy before the final impression is made. To allow for final tissue recovery, the patient *must* leave the old dentures out of the mouth a minimum of 24 hours before the making of the final impression.

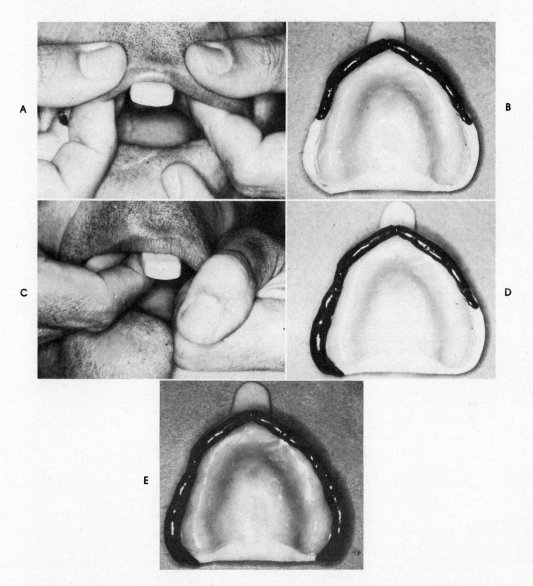

Fig. 8-11. A, Procedure of border molding in anterior region by moving upper lip outward, downward, and inward. **B,** Modeling compound border molded anteriorly. **C,** Buccal flange is border molded by moving cheek outward, downward, inward, and backward and forward. **D,** Properly molded border of left buccal flange. **E,** Completed labial and buccal borders. Notice that wax spacer has been kept inside tray during the border-molding procedures.

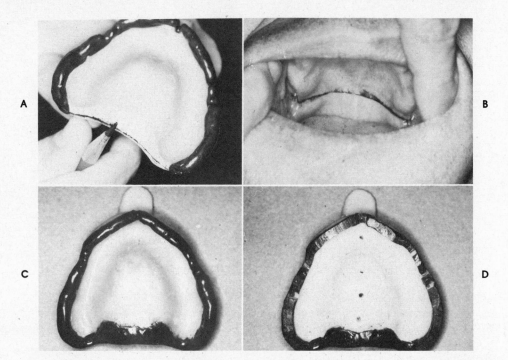

Fig. 8-12. A, Posterior border of impression tray is marked with indelible pencil to determine extent of the tray onto soft palate in patient's mouth. **B,** Line has been transferred to patient's mouth and indicates that tray includes vibrating line and both hamular notches posteriorly. **C,** Modeling compound has been added to posterior border of upper final impression tray to enhance posterior palatal seal. Wax spacer is still in place inside tray. **D,** Labial and buccal borders of tray have been reduced approximately 1 mm for final impression material. Wax spacer has been removed, and holes have been placed in tray to selectively relieve pressure during making of final impression. Posterior palatal seal has been left intact.

Positioning the tray properly in the patient's mouth for the final upper impression is essential for a successful result and can be a difficult procedure. The sequence of steps to be followed requires practice by the dentist for each patient but will help ensure the proper placement of the tray. The practice procedures are performed step by step without final impression material in the tray. First, the dentist centers the tray as it is carried to position on the upper residual ridge by observing the labial frenum going into proper relation to the labial notch (Fig. 8-13, A). When the frenum is within 1 to 2 mm of being in place in the notch, the index fingers of each hand are

shifted to the first molar region, and with alternating pressure being used the tray is carried upward—without displacement of the front end of the tray downward—until the posterior palatal seal of the tray fits properly into the hamular notches and across the palate (Fig. 8-13, B). Then the tray is held in position with a finger placed in the palate immediately anterior to the posterior palatal seal (Fig. 8-13, C). The practice procedure with the empty final impression tray is repeated until the dentist feels confident of the proper position of the tray in the mouth.

The final impression material is mixed accord-

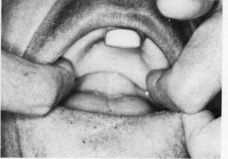

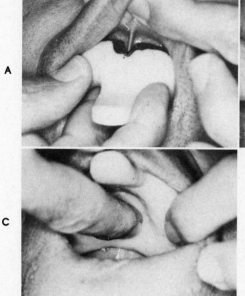

Fig. 8-13. A, During the practice procedures, the tray is centered in mouth when labial frenum is guided into labial notch. B, Tray is carried upward posteriorly until posterior palatal seal can be observed and felt to contact posterior palatal seal area in the patient's mouth. C, Tray is held in position with a finger placed immediately anterior to posterior palatal seal.

ing to the manufacturer's directions and uniformly distributed within the final impression tray. The amount of materials used and the spatulation time should be as uniform as possible from mix to mix. This uniformity is essential if the dentist is to become familiar with the working properties of the materials he uses. All borders must be covered. Excess impression material is allowed to run out the posterior border of the tray before the tray is placed into the mouth (Fig. 8-14, A). An additional small amount of impression material is placed in the center of the palate of the tray to help prevent air being trapped in this part of the final impression (Fig. 8-14, B). The final impression tray is positioned in the mouth in a manner similar to that used during the practice sessions (Fig. 8-14, C to E).

Border-molding procedures are performed in the posterior regions on both sides first and then in the anterior region (Fig. 8-15, A to C).

When the final impression material has com-

pletely set, the cheeks and upper lip are elevated above the borders of the impression to introduce air between the soft tissue at the reflection and the border of the impression. While the lip is elevated, the dentist removes the impression from the mouth by grasping the handle of the tray and gently working the tray downward and forward in the direction of the labial inclination of the residual ridge (Fig. 8-15, D).

The impression is inspected for acceptability (Fig. 8-15, E). Should the impression need to be remade, and often this will be true, the impression material is removed, with particular care in the region of the modeling compound at the borders.

Remaking final impressions. Often final impressions must be made over. Assuming that the tray was properly formed, faulty positioning of the tray is the most frequent reason that a final impression must be remade. A number of reasons for remaking final impressions are described in Chapter 10.

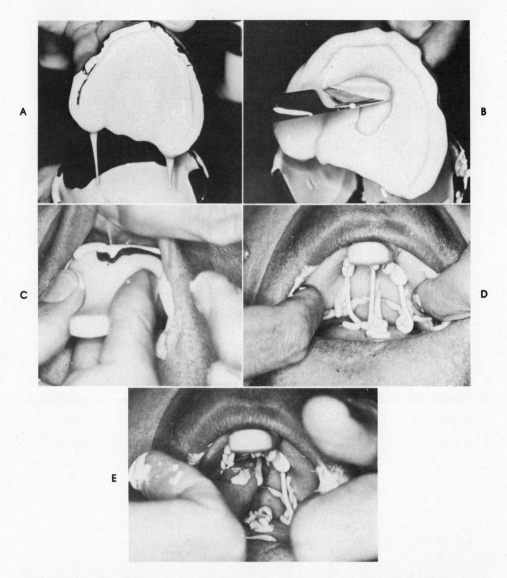

Fig. 8-14. A, Final impression material is distributed uniformly within final impression tray, with the excess being allowed to run out posterior border of tray. **B,** Small amount of impression material added to center of tray reduces possibility of trapping air in this part of final impression. **C,** Final impression tray is positioned anteriorly by centering of labial notch in relation to labial frenum. **D,** Posterior palatal seal is guided into position through hamular notches and in region of vibrating line by placement of pressure alternately on either side with fingers in first molar region of tray. **E,** Final impression is held in position by a finger placed immediately anterior to the posterior palatal seal.

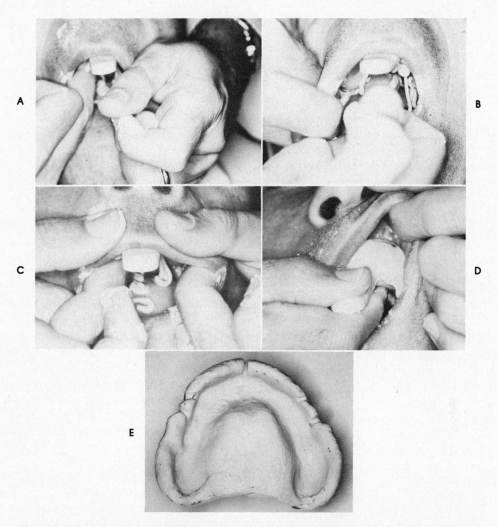

Fig. 8-15. A, One molds left posterior border of final impression by extending cheek outward, downward, and inward and moving it backward and forward in region of the buccal frenum. **B,** Right posterior border of final impression is molded by same procedures. Upper lip is properly supported by impression tray during making of final impression. **C,** One molds anterior border of final impression by moving upper lip downward and inward with thumbs. No side-to-side movement of upper lip is desirable during this procedures. **D,** Upper lip is elevated, and the anterior handle is used to remove the final upper impression. **E,** Acceptable final upper impression. Borders are in harmony with available space in patient's mouth. There are no undesirable pressure spots. Impression shows evidence that tissues forming posterior palatal seal area have been placed in a manner that will enhance seal at posterior border.

Pouring the cast. A technique for boxing the impression and pouring the cast is described in Chapter 10.

Second technique—one-step border-molded tray*

A material that will allow simultaneous moldings of all borders has two general advantages: (1) the number of insertions of the trays for maxillary and mandibular border molding are reduced to two, a great time and motion advantage; and (2) development of all borders simultaneously avoids propagation of errors caused by a mistake in one section affecting the border contours in another section.

The requirements of a material to be used for simultaneous molding of all borders are that it should (1) have sufficient body to allow it to remain in position on the borders during loading of the tray, (2) allow some preshaping of the form of the borders without adhering to the fingers, (3) have a setting time of 3 to 5 minutes, (4) retain adequate flow while the tray is seated in the mouth, (5) allow finger placement of the material into deficient parts after the tray is seated, (6) not cause excessive displacement of the tissues of the vestibule, and (7) be readily trimmed and shaped so that excess material can be carved and the borders shaped before the final impression is made.

Hard acrylic resin and silicone materials have been used for this purpose, and both have serious deficiencies. Hard resins have a long setting time, do not attain proper consistency immediately after mixing, which requires a waiting time before insertion, and are difficult to trim. Also, if insertion is delayed too long, overextension will result. Heavy-bodied silicone materials do not allow preshaping, placement into deficient spaces with a finger after insertion, and are difficult to trim after setting.

Polyether impression materials* meet all the requirements previously listed. They can be shaped with a moist finger in or outside the mouth and can be trimmed with a scalpel or a bur.

The following procedure is a technique that utilizes polyether impression materials for border molding. It significantly reduces the time required for making impressions and also reduces the amount of motion used by the dentist, thus reducing the psychologic stresses of a busy practice.

Constructing autopolymerizing acrylic resin impression tray

1. Make a preliminary upper impression, and pour the cast as described in the first technique (p. 152).
2. Construct an autopolymerizing acrylic resin final impression tray on the relieved preliminary cast as in the first technique (p. 155).
3. Reduce the borders of the impression tray until they are 2 mm underextended and confirm the extension of the posterior palatal border (Fig. 8-12, *A* and *B*). Leave the relief wax in the impression tray (Fig. 8-16).

Border molding the maxillary tray

1. Place adhesive for polyether impressions on the borders of the tray. Cover 6 mm inside the borders and 3 mm outside the borders.
2. Express a 3-inch strip of polyether material from the large tube onto a large mixing pad. Next, express 2½ inches of catalyst from the small tube. The reason for using less catalyst than recommended is to provide sufficient working time to complete the border molding.
3. Thoroughly mix the material for 30 to 45 seconds using a metal spatula.
4. Position the polyether material on the borders, making certain a minimum width of 6 mm exists on the inner portion (Figs. 8-17 and 8-18).

---

*Smith, D.E., Toolson, L.B., Bolender, C.L., and Lord, J.L.: One-step border molding of complete denture impressions using a polyether impression material, J. Prosthet. Dent. **41:**347, 1979.

*Impregum, Premier Dental Products Co., Philadelphia, Pa.

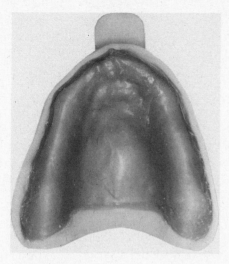

Fig. 8-16. The borders of the acrylic resin tray have been reduced. The relief wax remains inside the impression tray. Notice that the relief wax does not cover the borders or the posterior palatal seal area of the tray.

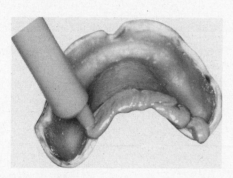

Fig. 8-17. The polyether material is placed across the posterior palatal seal area.

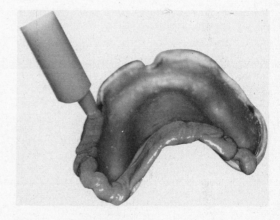

Fig. 8-18. The polyether material is continued around the borders of the impression tray until all have been covered.

5. Quickly preshape the material to proper contours with fingers moistened in cold water.
6. Place the impression tray in the mouth as described in the first technique, making certain to retract the lips sufficiently to avoid scraping the material from the borders (Fig. 8-13).
7. Inspect all borders to make certain that impression material is present in the vestibule. If there is a deficient space, transfer some material from an adjacent site

with a finger moistened in the patient's saliva.
8. Border mold as described in the first technique (Fig. 8-15).
9. Remove the tray when the impression material is set. The material is set when no permanent indentation results when the fingernail is intruded into it.
10. Examine the border molding and determine if it is adequate (Fig. 8-19). The contour of the borders should be rounded. Any deficient sites can be corrected with

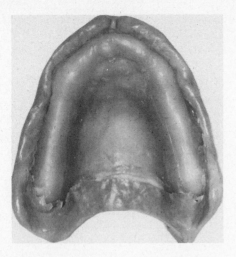

Fig. 8-19. Border molding has been completed, including the posterior palatal seal area. Notice that the relief wax is still in the impression tray.

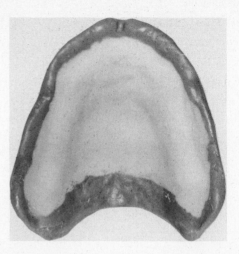

Fig. 8-20. The relief wax has been removed from the tray and polyether material has been removed from undercuts. The impression tray is ready for the final impression.

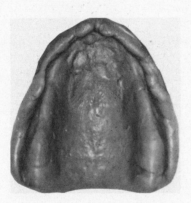

Fig. 8-21. The completed final impression, using the one-step border-molded tray.

a small mix of polyether material or with a small addition of impression compound that will adhere to set polyether materials. Overextensions are readily detected because the tray will protrude through the polyether border molding.

Preparation of the maxillary tray to secure the final impression

1. Reduce borders on the tray that protrude through the polyether material because they indicate overextension or pressure spots. Use a denture bur for these reductions.

2. Remove any material that extends internally within the tray more than 6 mm. A scalpel works best for this step.
3. Remove the relief wax (Fig. 8-20). Heating the wax in warm water makes removal easier.
4. Reduce the polyether material where it extends into an undercut with a denture bur to allow the tray to go into place easily.
5. Remove any excess material that has flowed onto the external portion of the tray away from the borders.

6. Reduce the thickness of the labial flange to approximately 2.5 to 3 mm from one buccal frenum to the other.
7. Remove a small amount (approximately 0.25 mm) of material from borders that have not been previously adjusted. This includes the inner portion, the border, and the outer surface to allow space for a thin film of final impression material.
8. Make the final impression in silicone, metallic oxide paste, or rubber base impression material (Fig. 8-21). Use an appropriate adhesive on the impression surface of the tray when using the silicone material.

Third technique—border-molded modeling compound tray

Maxillary impression procedure. The requirements of maxillary impressions can be satisfied when a preliminary modeling compound impression is made in a stock metal tray and this impression is converted into a tray. The objectives of the preliminary impression are to obtain a record of the approximate shape of the basal seat and to have sufficient bulk in it so that a tray can be made from it. For these reasons the preliminary impression is made in a stock tray that is oversize for the maxillary arch (Fig. 8-4).

Knife trimming. The preliminary impression is removed from the stock tray after being thoroughly chilled in ice water. Modeling compound can be added if necessary to form the minimal thickness of 6 mm over the palatal and ridge surfaces.

Knife trimming is done with a very sharp knife. The objectives of knife trimming are to shape the preliminary impression as nearly as possible into the shape of the denture to be constructed. The labial flange is carved so it is at least 2 mm thick at the border. This is necessary to provide adequate support for the final impression material. If shrinkage of the anterior part of the residual ridge has been excessive, the thickness of the labial flange is made proportionately greater.

The buccal flanges of the preliminary impression are carved so that they will fill the space in each buccal vestibule between the residual ridge and cheek without overfilling it. The distal end of the buccal flange must be thin enough to allow the ramus to move forward and inward as the mandible is moved into various eccentric positions. The more accurately the height and width of the spaces available are judged, the more accurately the knife trimming can be done and the less border molding will be required (Fig. 8-22).

Impression of palatal surface. One can make the form of the impression of the palatal and ridge surface more nearly accurate by heating the entire impression surface of an ice-cold knife-trimmed preliminary impression and, after tempering, forcing the softened surface against the palatal and residual ridge tissues. The cold (and therefore hard) surface of the preliminary impression serves as a tray to carry the softened interior layer of modeling compound against the soft tissues. This procedure will eliminate distortion and will record details of form that were not recorded in the preliminary impression (Fig. 8-22).

Border molding. The modeling compound borders are made moldable to a depth no greater than 2 mm by heat from an alcohol blowtorch. If the material is underheated, the modeling compound will not be soft enough to mold. If it is overheated, the entire flange may collapse. One molds the modeling compound in the buccal vestibules by grasping the cheek between the thumb and forefinger and pulling it out, down, forward, backward, and in. The same procedure is carried out on a section of the border of a similar size that includes the buccal frenum. The labial border of the flange is molded in a similar manner, except that the lip is not moved from side to side (Fig. 8-23).

Distobuccal angles of buccal flange. Since the width of the distal end of the buccal vestibule varies with the position of the mandible and since the buccal vestibule must be filled within the limits of health and function, the distobuccal

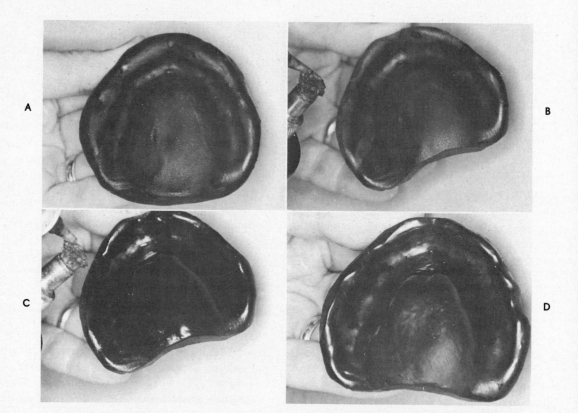

Fig. 8-22. A, The modeling compound preliminary impression has been removed from stock metal tray. Notice bulk of material. **B,** Tray has been reduced to proper form by knife trimming. **C,** Entire inside of impression is heated to a depth of 2 mm. Notice shiny appearance of softened modeling compound. **D,** Readapted basal surface of impression. Notice increase in detail of impression of palate and residual ridge (compare with **A**).

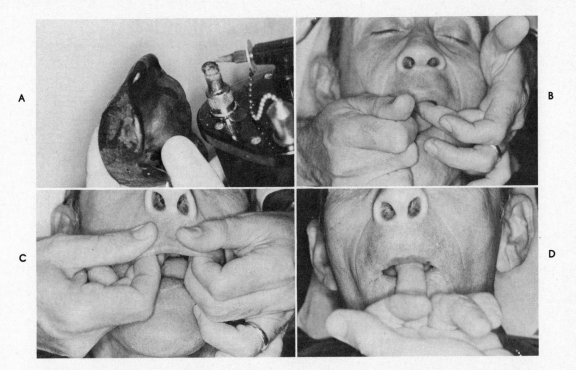

Fig. 8-23. A, Border of buccal flange is heated to a 1.5 to 2 mm depth. **B,** Border is molded in mouth to fill buccal vestibule without being overfilled. Cheek is pulled outward, downward, inward, and forward and backward in region of buccal frenum. **C,** Lip is drawn down over labial flange by dentist or by patient, **D,** to mold softened compound.

ends of both buccal flanges must be border molded. One molds the border by softening the modeling compound on both sides at these places on the tray. Then the patient is directed to move the lower jaw from side to side, causing the mandibular rami to push the soft tissues of the cheek against the soft material. Thus space for the mandible to move will be provided.

Posterior palatal seal. The posterior palatal seal is formed through both hamular (pterygo-maxillary) notches and across the palate over the vibrating line. The procedure is performed in the same manner as that described for the first technique by the addition of low-fusing compound across the posterior border of the modeling compound tray (Fig. 8-24). When properly formed, the eventual posterior palatal seal will

be about 1 mm thick and about 4 mm wide. The excess extending beyond the impression is removed (Fig. 8-24).

Making space in the tray. Space must be provided inside the tray for the final impression material. For this reason, the entire inside of the modeling compound impression, except the posterior palatal seal, is scraped away to a depth of at least 1 mm. Another 0.5 to 1 mm of material is removed on the impression surface that covers the median palatal raphe to provide relief for this unyielding tissue.

The buccal and labial borders of the modeling compound impression are shortened 1.5 mm so that the final impression material can form the borders as well as the inside of the impression. By this means, minute errors in the molding of

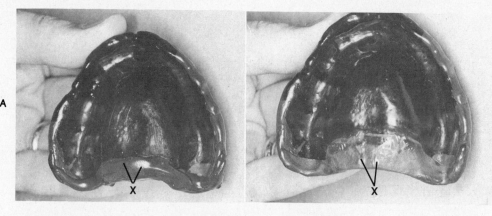

Fig. 8-24. A, Buccal and labial borders have been molded to fill the available vestibular spaces and do not interfere with function of upper lip or cheeks. Green stick modeling compound, *X,* has been traced onto distal end of palatal surface and up distal edge of buccal flange. The green compound is chilled in ice water and then softened with an alcohol torch before it is placed into mouth. Compound tray is placed in mouth with pressure applied at distal end of impression. **B,** Green modeling compound has formed the posterior palatal seal area on impression. *X,* Impression of the foveae palatinae.

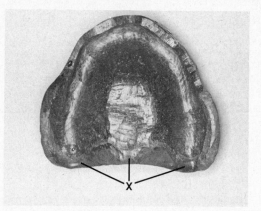

Fig. 8-25. Basal surface of completed modeling compound impression is reduced to a depth of 1 mm except at the posterior palatal seal. Borders of buccal and labial flanges are shortened 1.5 mm. Completed modeling compound tray is ready for making final impression. Posterior palatal seal, *X,* is left intact to help guide tray in place in mouth when the final impression is made and to increase seal at posterior border of impression.

the modeling compound borders can be eliminated (Fig. 8-25).

Final impression. The final impression material is mixed according to the manufacturer's directions and spread evenly in excess throughout the entire inside surface of the tray.

The loaded impression tray is carried to the mouth. The labial notch of the tray is aligned with the labial frenum as the tray is carried partway to position. Then the two index fingers are placed on the occlusal surface of the tray in the

molar region, and slight alternate forward and backward (rotational) movements are produced as the tray is pushed gently to its final position (Fig. 8-26). The contact of the posterior palatal seal with the palate and with the buccal sides of the hamular notches affords the guidance necessary for final seating of the tray. After the tray has been floated almost to position, a finger is placed in the center of the palate directly under the posterior palatal seal and the tray is pushed upward to its final position (Fig. 8-26).

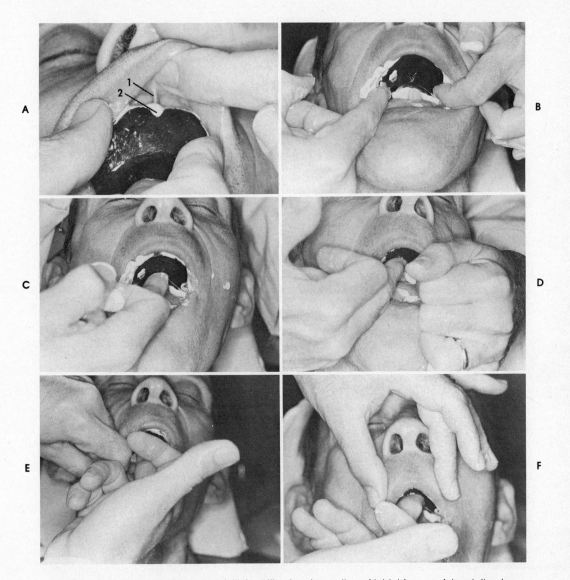

Fig. 8-26. A, Tray is guided to proper initial position by observation of labial frenum, *1,* in relation to labial notch, *2.* **B,** Tray is floated to place by alternate forward and backward rotation of index fingers placed on occlusal surface of tray in molar region. **C,** Tray is stabilized with middle finger at distal end of impression. **D** and **E,** Plaster in buccal vestibules is molded when cheek is grasped with thumb and forefinger and is lifted outward, downward, and inward and then is moved forward and backward. **F,** Plaster at labial border is molded when lip is moved downward and inward.

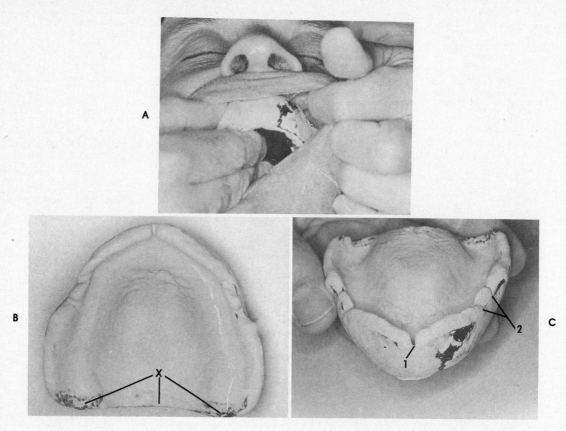

Fig. 8-27. A, To remove impression, left index finger raises cheek while right thumb and finger grasp impression and tip its left back corner downward. **B,** Completed final impression made by use of a modified plaster of paris. Notice that posterior palatal seal, *X,* shows through final impression material. **C,** Notice labial notch, *1,* and buccal notch, *2.*

Border molding the final impression. While one finger holds the tray in position, the thumb and forefinger of the other hand grasp the cheek and move it gently forward, backward, downward, and inward. The same procedure is followed on the opposite side. Then the lip is lifted and pulled gently outward and downward (Fig. 8-26). The lip is released, and the patient is directed to pull the lip down over the front teeth using the action of the lip itself.

Removal of impression. After the final impression material has set, the impression can be removed. The thumb of one hand is placed at the border of the impression in the premolar region, and the index finger of the same hand is placed on the occlusal surface of the tray just under the thumb. While the impression is grasped between the finger and thumb, the index finger of the other hand raises the cheek on the opposite side. This will allow air to get under the impression when the distobuccal corner of the impression on the second side is tipped downward (Fig. 8-27). If the impression does not loosen by this procedure, the patient is directed to blow with the lips closed and to puff out the cheeks to force air under the impression.

Inspection of impression. The impression should have no pressure spots or places where the tray material shows through the impression material except at the posterior palatal seal. The posterior palatal seal should be thinly covered by the impression material (Fig. 8-27). The border tissues should be recorded entirely in the final impression material, and there should be no voids in this part of the impression.

If pressure spots exist, those places should be relieved further by removal of tray material. Then all the impression material should be removed, and a new final impression should be made.

9

Biologic considerations of mandibular impressions

Biologic considerations for mandibular impressions are similar in many ways to those for maxillary impressions, and yet there are many dissimularities. The basal seat of the mandible is different in form and size from the basal seat of the maxillae. The submucosa in some parts of the mandibular basal seat contains anatomic structures that are different from those found in the upper jaw. In addition, the nature of the supporting bone on the crest of the residual ridge usually differs between the two jaws. These differences are often sufficient to require major variations in impression procedures for the mandible and maxillae. The presence of the tongue and its individual size, form, and activity complicates the impression procedures for lower dentures and the patient's ability to learn to manage them. The clinical application of the biology of the supporting and limiting structures will enable the dentist to unravel what is sometimes called the "mystery of the lower denture" and successfully provide prosthodontic treatment for edentulous patients.

The same fundamental principles are involved in the support of a mandibular denture as are involved in support for maxillary dentures (Chpater 7). The denture bases must be extended to cover the maximum area possible without interfering with the health or function of the tissues, whose support is derived from bone. The support for the mandibular denture is supplied by the body of the mandible.

The total area of usable support from the mandible is less than it is from the maxillae. This means that the mandible is less capable of resisting occlusal forces than the maxillae and that much care is essential if the available support is to be used to advantage.

SEQUELAE TO THE LOSS OF TEETH

When the teeth are removed from the mandible, the alveolar tooth sockets will tend to fill with new bone, but the bone of the alveolar process will start resorbing. This means that the bony foundation for the mandibular dentures becomes shorter vertically and narrower buccol-

ingually. In this manner the bony foundation for the basal seat becomes progressively less favorable as a support for the denture. The bony crest of the residual ridge becomes narrower and sharper. Often, sharp bone spicules remain and can cause tenderness when pressure is applied by a denture.

The total width of the bony foundation and mandibular basal seat becomes greater in the molar region as resorption continues. The reason is that the width of the inferior border of the mandible from side to side is greater than the width of the mandible at the alveolar process from side to side (Figs. 9-1 and 9-2).

Other changes occur on the occlusal surface of the bone. The shrinkage of the alveolar process

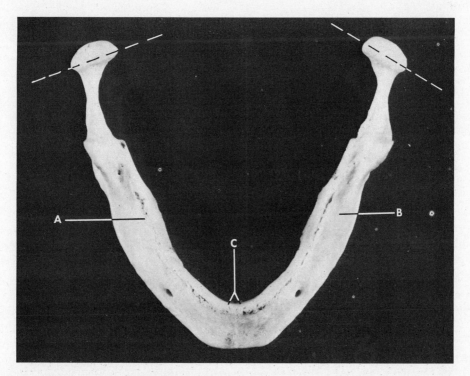

Fig. 9-1. After removal of teeth, resorption of alveolar process causes bony support for mandibular denture (residual alveolar ridge) to become more narrow buccolingually and reduced in height. *A,* Crest of residual alveolar ridge—cancellous bone. *B,* Buccal shelf—compact bone. *C,* Genial tubercles. Notice that buccolingual long axis of condyles of this mandible, if extended posteriorly, would meet in region of foramen magnum.

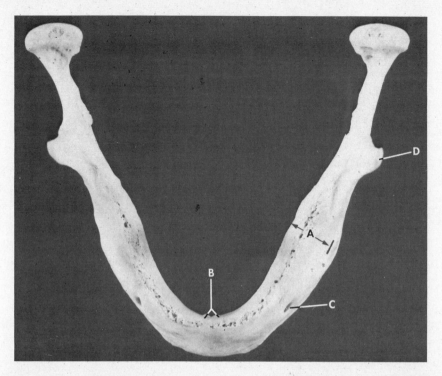

Fig. 9-2. Continued resorption of residual alveolar ridge, depending on shape of mandible and nature of resorption, often results in a mandibular basal seat, A, that becomes wider and increases in size. This change occurs because as resorption causes crest of residual alveolar ridge to move more inferiorly, width of mandible from side to side becomes greater than width of alveolar process at time the teeth were removed. A, Width of basal seat; B, genial tubercle; C, mental foramen; D, coronoid process.

in the anterior region moves the residual bony ridge lingually at first. Then as resorption continues, this bony foundation may move progressively further forward (see Fig. 19-5). Bone loss in this region often continues on the mandible below the level of the alveolar process.

Resorption of the alveolar process often develops occlusal contours of residual ridges that make them become curved from a low level anteriorly to a high level posteriorly when viewed from the side (Fig. 9-3). These conditions can cause severe problems of denture stability, which must be considered in impression making and in occlusion.

Dentures must be made for people who have these unfavorable conditions. This means that the impressions must be made in such a way that maximum advantage is gained from each part of the support from the basal seat.

MACROSCOPIC ANATOMY OF SUPPORTING STRUCTURES

Support for the lower denture is provided by the mandible (the bone) and the soft tissues overlying it. Some parts of the mandible are more favorable for this function than others, and pressures must be applied to the bone through the soft tissues according to the ability of the tissues and different parts of the bone to resist the stresses of occlusion.

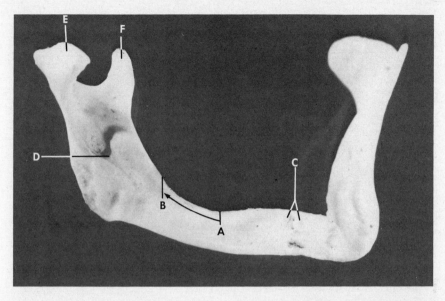

Fig. 9-3. Nature of bony resorption has caused an anteroposterior curvature in bone of basal seat when mandible is viewed from side (*A to B*). Such inclinations of residual alveolar ridge create problems in maintaining stability of mandibular dentures. Artificial teeth should not be placed over this incline (*A to B*). *C,* Genial tubercles; *D,* mandibular foramen: *E,* condyle; *F,* coronoid process.

Crest of residual ridge

The crest of the residual alveolar ridge is covered by fibrous connective tissue, but in many mouths the underlying bone is cancellous and without a good cortical bony plate covering it (Fig. 9-4). The fibrous connective tissue closely attached to the bone is favorable for resisting externally applied forces, such as those from a denture. However, if the underlying bone is cancellous, this advantage is mostly lost.

Buccal flange area and buccal shelf

The area between the mandibular buccal frenum and the anterior edge of the masseter muscle is known as the buccal shelf or buccal flange area. It is bounded medially by the crest of the residual ridge, anteriorly by the buccal frenum, laterally by the external oblique line, and distally by the retromolar pad (Fig. 9-5). The buccal shelf may be very wide and is at right angles to the direction of vertical occlusal forces. For that

reason it offers excellent resistance to those forces. Some buccinator muscle fibers are located under the buccal flange because the mandibular attachment of this muscle is close to the crest of the ridge in the molar region. This attachment is dissimilar to other muscle insertions in that the fibers run anteroposteriorly paralleling the bone and the denture does not resist the contracting force of the muscle (Fig. 9-6). The inferior part of the muscle is attached in the buccal shelf of the mandible. For this reason the contraction of this muscle does not lift the lower denture. The buccal shelf is the principal bearing surface of the mandibular denture and takes the occlusal load off the sharp narrow crest of the residual alveolar ridge that so many edentulous mandibles present (Fig. 9-6). The buccal shelf is covered with good smooth cortical bone, which is usually at right angles to the occlusal plane (Fig. 9-7).

These relative conditions vary from patient to

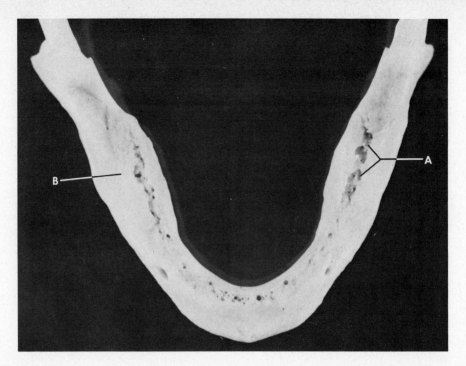

Fig. 9-4. Crest of residual alveolar ridge is formed of spongy or cancellous bone. Porous nature and roughness of this bone, particularly in molar region, *A,* make it unsuitable as a primary stress-bearing area for mandibular denture. For this reason the buccal shelf, *B* (see Figs. 9-5 and 9-7) most often becomes the primary stress-bearing area for lower denture.

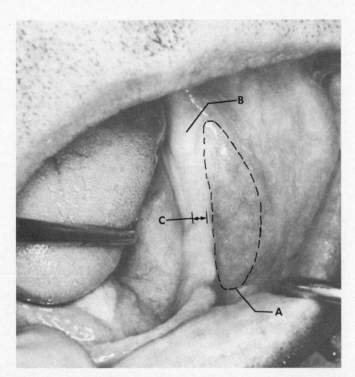

Fig. 9-5. Buccal shelf (within the dotted line) in patient's mouth extends from, *A,* buccal frenum anteriorly to, *B,* retromolar pad posteriorly, and, *C,* from the external oblique line laterally to the crest of residual alveolar ridge medially.

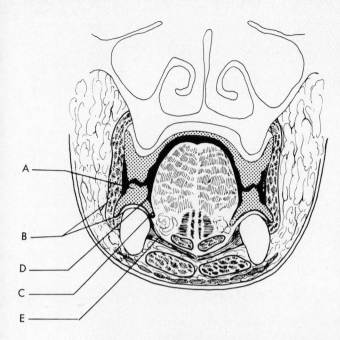

Fig. 9-6. Scheme showing cross section of mandible, tongue, and cheeks with the denture in place. *A,* Cross section of denture with polished surface contours that will aid muscles to press denture in place instead of displacing it. *B,* Buccinator muscle. Notice that attachment of muscle goes under buccal flange area to a point near crest of ridge. *C,* Lingual flange area. Notice how this flange extends away from bony contour of mandible and is out under the tongue to aid in seating denture in place. *D,* Lingual polished surface contour provides space for tongue and places rather than displaces denture. *E,* Mylohyoid muscle contracts during swallowing and should not be impinged on.

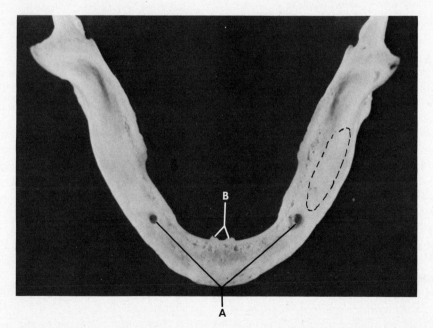

Fig. 9-7. Buccal shelf is outlined by dotted line on mandible and is formed by smooth compact bone. The buccal shelf, by both the nature of the bone and its position at right angles to the denture base, affords the primary support for lower denture. The crest of this residual ridge should not be used as a primary stress-bearing area. Notice that mental foramina, *A,* are on crest of residual ridge in this badly resorbed residual alveolar ridge. The mental vessels and nerves must be provided relief from impingement by denture base. Notice difference between location of mental foramina in this illustration and the more usual position seen in Figs. 9-1 and 9-2. *B,* Genial tubercles.

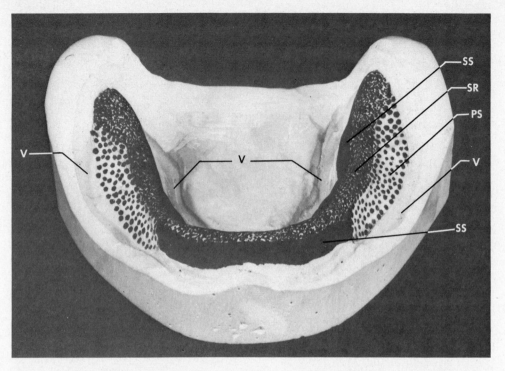

Figs. 9-8. Cast showing distribution of force in a selective pressure impression procedure. *PS,* Primary stress-bearing area—buccal shelf; *SS,* secondary stress-bearing area slopes of the residual ridge; *SR,* secondary relief area when crest of residual ridge is sharp, thin, and unfavorable; *V,* valve seal area.

patient, and so a choice as to the best distribution of pressures on the mandibular basal seat must be made. If the residual bony ridge is unfavorable, that is, if it is sharp, spiny, or full of nutrient canals, the masticatory pressures should be transferred to the buccal shelf. Otherwise, the residual ridge can help carry the load effectively. The accuracy of the diagnosis and the skill with which the impressions are made will determine the effectiveness of the distribution of pressure to selected parts of the basal seat (Fig. 9-8). The requirements of mandibular impressions can be fulfilled by a selective pressure technique.

Flat mandibular ridges

On the labial surface of the anterior region of the mandible several muscles show a proximity to the crest of the ridge, especially in badly resorbed ridges. This proximity accounts for the short flanges necessary in this region. These muscles should not be impinged on because their action is nearly at right angles to the flange. Many edentulous mandibles are extremely flat because of the loss of the cortical layer of bone (Fig. 9-7). The surface is weakened and changed in form by the more rapid resorption of the cancellous portion of the mandible. The bearing surface often becomes concave, allowing the attaching structures, especially on the lingual side of the ridge, to fall over onto the ridge surface. Such conditions require placement of these tissues by the impression. Such treatment can gradually reestablish a suitable bearing surface. The crest of these greatly resorbed ridges is often at the level of the mental foramina, and the

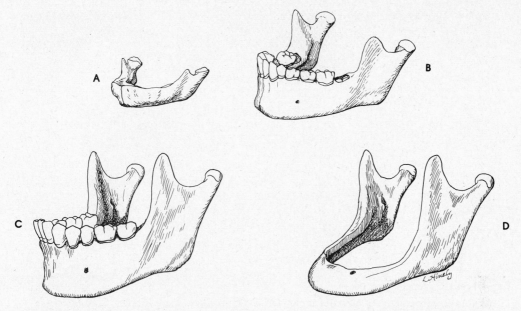

Fig. 9-9. Mandible in four stages of development. **A,** At birth. Notice absence of condyle. **B,** At 8 years of age. **C,** In adult life. **D,** Edentulous mandible.

nerves and blood vessels are impinged on easily unless the area is palpated and relieved on the impression (Fig. 9-7).

Bone of basal seat

The configuration of the bone that forms the basal seat for the mandibular denture varies considerably with each patient. Factors that influence the form of the supporting bone of the basal seat were listed previously in Chapter 7. Important variations of the bone of the basal seat for the mandibular denture include stages of change in the mandible, sharp mylohyoid ridge, mental foramen area resorption, insufficient space between the mandible and the tuberosity, low mandibular ridges, direction of resorption of ridges, and torus mandibularis.

Stages of change in mandible. Fig. 9-9 shows the mandible at various stages. The final illustration shows the mandible fully developed with the loss of the alveolar process down to a point opposite the mental foramen. As the alveolar

process is progressively lost, the attaching structures converge so that the supporting surface of the denture becomes more and more limited.

Mylohyoid ridge. The soft tissues often hide the sharpness of the mylohyoid ridge, which can be found by palpation. The shape and inclination of the mylohyoid ridge varies greatly among edentulous patients.

In Fig. 9-10 are diagrams illustrating cross sections of the mandible to show the inclination of the mylohyoid ridge and the level of the mylohyoid muscle in the variuos parts of the mandible from the incisal region through the third molar region. Note the various levels of the mylohyoid muscle as it extends posteriorly along the mylohyoid ridge from the symphysis of the mandible. Anteriorly the muscle attaches close to the inferior border of the mandible, and posteriorly it may be flush with the superior surface of the residual ridge. Fig. 9-11 depicts what would be considered a desirable form of the mylohyoid ridge for an edentulous patient,

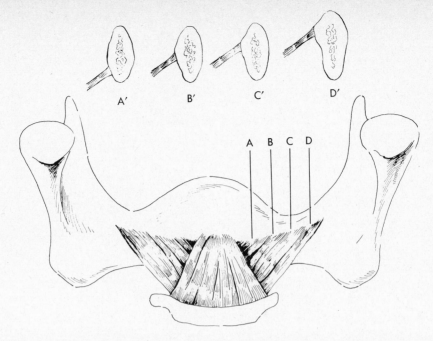

Fig. 9-10. Diagrams showing relationship of mylohyoid muscle in various regions. *A',* Cross section in canine region, *A. B',* Cross section in premolar region, *B. C',* Cross section in first molar region, *C. D',* Cross section of third molar region, *D,* showing mylohyoid ridge approaching the level of crest of residual alveolar ridge. Angle of posterior part of lingual flange of denture in molar region is affected by angle of mylohyoid muscle. Anteriorly, only the length of the flange is affected by mylohyoid muscle.

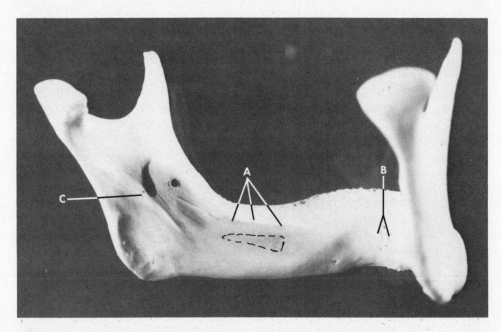

Fig. 9-11. An edentulous mandible with moderate undercut beneath mylohyoid ridge, *A.* Denture base cannot be extended into this relatively slight undercut *(dotted line)* because mylohyoid muscle, attaching to the ridge, moves outward and upward during contraction. Notice location of genial tubercles, *B,* midway between superior and inferior borders of mandible on lingual surface anteriorly. *C,* Mandibular foramen.

whereas the mylohyoid ridges in Fig. 9-12 are bulbous, irregular, and severely undercut. Extremely thin, sharp mylohyoid ridges are seen in Fig. 9-13 and illustrate another source of aggravation and soreness for edentulous patients.

Mental foramen area resorption. The mental foramina on or near the crest of the residual ridge of greatly resorbed mandibles result in an impingement on the mental nerves and blood vessels if relief is not provided in the denture base (Fig. 9-7). Pressure on the mental nerve can cause numbness in the lower lip.

Insufficient space between the mandible and the tuberosity. The maxillary sinus enlarges throughout life if it is not restricted by natural teeth or dentures, thus moving the tuberosity downward. The angle of the mandible is frequently made more obtuse by the early loss of the posterior teeth and the retention of the anterior teeth. Removal of the posterior support destroys the necessary counterbalance against the muscle pull at the angle of the mandible. This straightening of the mandible reduces the maxillomandibular space in the posterior region and is the cause of difficulty in obtainment of

sufficient space for the teeth and denture bases. The lack of space causes many denture failures.

Low mandibular ridges. Frequently the mandibular-supporting area is depressed rather than elevated because of the difference in the rate of resorption of cortical bone and cancellous bone. Lingually, on these greatly resorbed mandibles the bone has shrunk down to the level of the attachments of the structures in the floor of the mouth. This makes the lingual flange of the denture more difficult to adapt.

Direction of resorption of ridges. The maxillae resorb upward and inward to become progressively smaller because of the direction and inclination of the roots of the teeth and the alveolar process. Consequently, the longer the maxillae have been edentulous, the smaller is their bearing area. The opposite is true of the mandible, which inclines outward and becomes progressively wider according to its edentulous age. This progressive change of the mandible and maxillae in the edentulous state makes many patients appear to be prognathic (Fig. 9-14).

Torus mandibularis. The torus mandibularis is a bony prominence usually found in the region

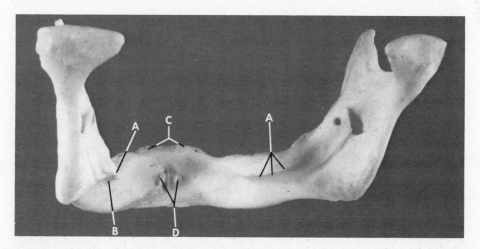

Fig. 9-12. Edentulous mandible with bulbous, irregular, bony mylohyoid ridges, *A,* that are severely undercut, *B,* and cannot be used for securing retention. Notice bony projection anteriorly on crest of residual alveolar ridge, *C,* and genial tubercles, *D.*

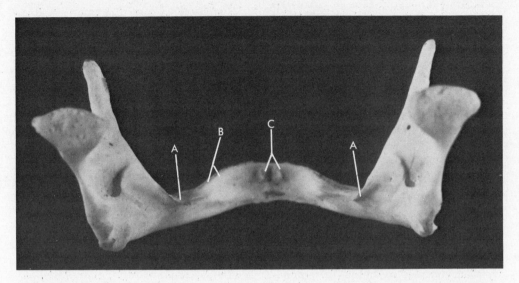

Fig. 9-13. Edentulous mandible with flat residual alveolar ridge. Sharpness of mylohyoid ridges, *A*, is knifelike on both sides and is at level of crest of ridge. The spiny roughness anteriorly on residual alveolar ridge, *B*, cannot be detected when it is covered with mucous membrane. Location of roughness is usually indicated by a band of narrow fibrous tissue along center of ridge. Relief is provided in impression and finished denture. Notice that genial tubercles, *C*, are almost at crest of residual alveolar ridge anteriorly, an indication of the severe resorption that has occurred.

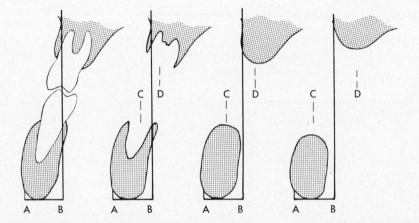

Fig. 9-14. Progressive resorption of maxillary and mandibular ridges, showing how maxilla becomes narrower and mandible wider. Lines *AB* represent the same distance from outer border of mandible to a point on maxilla; lines *C* and *D* represent the center of the ridge. Notice how the distance between *C* and *D* becomes progressively greater as mandible and maxilla are resorbed.

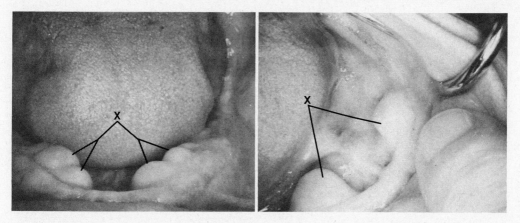

Fig. 9-15. Torus mandibularis, *X*. Surgical reduction is necessary to develop seal for mandibular denture satisfactorily.

between the first and second premolars, midway between the soft tissue of the floor of the mouth and the crest of the alveolar process. In edentulous mouths in which considerable resorption has taken place, the superior border of this prominence may be flush with the crest of the residual ridge on the lingual side. Its size varies from that of a pea to that of a hazelnut (Fig. 9-15). The cause for its occurrence is not known, but it is sometimes coincident with a bulbous torus palatinus. The torus mandibularis is covered by an extremely thin layer of mucous membrane and for that reason may be irritated by slight movements of the denture base. It should be removed surgically if relief cannot be provided for it inside the denture without breaking the border seal.

MACROSCOPIC ANATOMY OF LIMITING STRUCTURES

Mandibular dentures should be extended as far as possible within the limits of health and function of the tissues and structures that support and surround them. This is the same principle that governs the extent of maxillary dentures, but it is more complicated to apply to mandibular dentures than to maxillary dentures. The reason is that the structures on the lingual side of the mandible must be considered as well as those around the labial and buccal surfaces of the denture. The structures on the lingual side of the mandible are more complicated to control than those on the buccal and labial sides. The problem is the greater range of their movement and speed of their actions.

Buccal and labial border anatomy

The underlying structures around the border of complete dentures vary according to the location. This fact is overlooked constantly and is a reason why the possible maximum mandibular denture coverage is seldom attained. If a careful study is made and used, the size of the mandibular denture may be larger than might be expected. Mandibular dentures should be wide back of the buccal frenum and narrow in the anterior labial region. The mandibular labial frenum contains a band of fibrous connective tissue that helps to attach the orbicularis oris; therefore the frenum is quite sensitive and active and must be carefully fitted to maintain a seal without causing soreness (Fig. 9-16).

The part of the denture that extends between the labial frenum (labial notch) and the buccal frenum (buccal notch) is called the mandibular labial flange. This flange is limited in extension

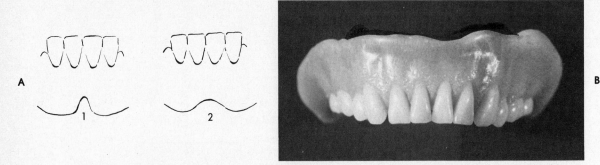

Fig. 9-16. A, Labial notch, *1,* for narrow labial mandibular foramen. *2,* A broad labial notch is often required for the lower denture. **B,** Broadly contoured labial notch is correct for this patient. If the notch is too narrow for function of the labial frenum, soreness will result. If the notch is too broad for the frenum, a loss of seal will result.

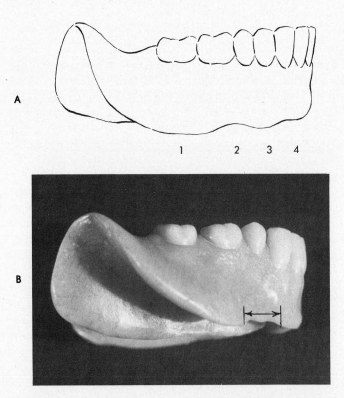

Fig. 9-17. A, Typical contour of labial and buccal borders of mandibular denture. *1,* Broad buccal flange; *2,* mandibular buccal notch for buccal frenum; *3,* mandibular labial flange; *4,* labial notch for labial frenum. **B,** Proper contour of buccal notch *(arrow)* of a lower complete denture. Contours vary somewhat for each patient.

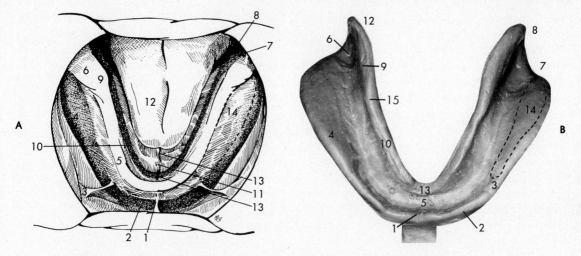

Fig. 9-18. Correlation of anatomic landmarks. **A,** Intraoral drawing of mandibular arch. *1,* Labial frenum; *2,* labial vestibule; *3,* buccal frenum; *4,* buccal vestibule; *5,* residual alveolar ridge; *6,* retromolar pad; *7,* pterygomandibular raphe; *8,* retromylohyoid fossa; *9,* lingual tubercle; *10,* alveololingual sulcus; *11,* submaxillary caruncles; *12,* tongue; *13,* lingual frenum; *14,* buccal shelf; premylohyoid eminence. **B,** Mandibular final impression showing corresponding denture landmarks. *1,* Labial notch; *2,* labial flange; *3,* buccal notch; *4,* buccal flange; *5,* alveolar groove; *6,* retromolar fossa; *7,* pterygomandibular notch; *8,* retromylohyoid eminence; *9,* lingual tubercular fossa; *10,* lingual flange; *12,* inclined plane for tongue; *13,* lingual notch; *14,* buccal flange that fits on buccal shelf; *15,* premylohyoid eminence.

because the fibers of the orbicularis oris and the incisivus labii inferioris muscles run fairly close to the crest of the ridge.

The buccal frenum connects as a continuous band through the modiolus at the corner of the mouth and on up to the buccal frenum attachment on the maxilla (see Fig. 19-6). These fibrous and muscular tissues pull actively across the denture borders, polished surfaces, and teeth. Therefore the denture should be extended less in this region, and the impression must be functionally trimmed to have the maximum seal and yet not so great an extension as to displace the denture when the lip is moved (Fig. 9-17).

The lower lip must be supported to an extent equal to that provided by the natural teeth and their investing structures (Fig. 9-18). The length and thickness of the labial flange in the labial vestibules vary with the amount of tissue that has been lost. The tone of the skin of the lip and

of the orbicularis oris muscle depends on the thickness of the flange and the position of the teeth.

There is no muscle extending from the residual ridge to the lip between the two triangularis muscles, and so the labial flange can be extended in length and thickness to supply the necessary support for the lip (Fig. 9-18).

Buccal vestibule. The buccal vestibule extends from the buccal frenum posteriorly to the outside back corner of the retromolar pad and from the crest of the residual alveolar ridge to the cheek (Fig. 9-18). The buccinator muscle in the cheek extends from the modiolus (anteriorly) to the pterygomandibular raphe (posteriorly). Its lower side attaches in the molar region in the buccal shelf of the mandible (the part of the bone between the residual ridge and the external oblique line). The buccinator muscle action occurs in a horizontal direction, and so it cannot lift the lower denture, even though the buccal flange of a properly extended denture will rest on its inferior attachment.

External oblique ridge and buccal flange. The extension of the mandibular labial and buccal flanges is governed by the same general factors. The impression space in the labial vestibule between the labial and buccal frenums is determined by the turn of the mucolabial fold (the line of flexure of the mucous membrane as it passes from the mandible to the lip and cheeks). The space is not extensive. The buccal flange area, which starts immediately posterior to the buccal frenum and extends to the anterior portion of the masseter muscle, swings wide into the cheek and is nearly at right angles to the biting force, thus providing the lower denture with its greatest surface for resistance to vertical occlusal forces (Fig. 9-19).

The external oblique ridge does not govern the extension of the buccal flange because the resistance or lack of resistance encountered in this region varies widely. The buccal flange may extend to the external oblique ridge, or up onto it, or even over it depending on the location of the mucobuccal fold. However, palpation of the external oblique ridge is a valuable aid or landmark in helping to ascertain the relative amount of resistance or lack of resistance of the border tissues in this region.

The buccal shelf is successfully utilized, despite the fact that the buccinator muscle fibers attach close to the crest of the ridge and the denture rests directly on a considerable portion of this muscle. The bearing of the denture on muscle fibers would not be possible except for the fact that the fibers of the buccinator muscle and its pull when in function are parallel to the border and not at right angles to it, as is the masseter muscle, hence its displacing action is slight. More resistance is encountered in this region when the denture is first inserted than is manifested a few weeks after the patient has worn the completed dentures. Thus it is possible to stretch and place these tissues and create this area, invaluable for biting resistance and stabili-

ty, that is so sorely needed when the residual ridge is sharp or narrow.

Masseter muscle region. The distobuccal corner of the mandibular denture must converge rapidly to avoid displacement because of contracting pressure of the masseter muscle, whose anterior fibers pass outside the buccinator muscle in this region (Fig. 9-20).

When the masseter muscle contracts, it alters the shape and size of the distobuccal end of the lower buccal vestibule. It pushes inward against the buccinator muscle and suctorial pad of the cheek.

The distobuccal border of the mandibular impression encounters the action of the masseter muscle to a greater or less degree, depending on the shape of the madible and the origin of the muscle. If the ramus of the mandible has a perpendicular surface and the origin of the muscle on the zygomatic arch is medialward, the muscle pulls more directly across the distobuccal denture border. Therefore it forces the buccinator muscle and tissues inward, reducing the space in this region. If the opposite is true, greater extension is allowed on the distobuccal portion of the mandibular impression. One can register this masseter muscle pull on the impression by softening the compound with an alcohol flame along the distobuccal border, tempering the compound in warm water, and, after seating the impression in the patient's mouth, exerting a downward pressure by placing the index fingers on the impression in the second premolar region. While this downward pressure is being exerted on the impression by the dentist, the patient is instructed to exert a closing force. These opposing forces will cause the masseter muscle to contract and trim the compound in that area if the relation of the mandible and maxillae causes the masseter muscle to affect the distobuccal border directly. The relative size of the masseter muscle will influence its action on the buccinator muscle. A masseter muscle that is smaller in diameter will have less influence (perhaps none) on the border.

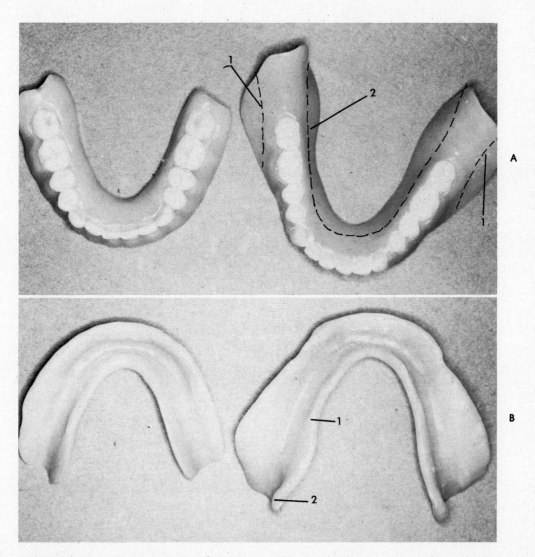

Fig. 9-19. A, External form of new denture *(right)* permits cheek, *1,* and tongue, *2,* to rest on buccal and lingual flanges and help hold denture in place. **B,** Lingual flange slopes toward tongue from *1* to *2* to accommodate for action of mylohyoid muscle. New denture *(right)* takes advantage of all available basal seat to increase retention, stability, and support. The buccal flange immediately posterior to the buccal notch extends outward toward the cheek and provides the greatest surface for resistance of the lower denture to vertical occlusal forces.

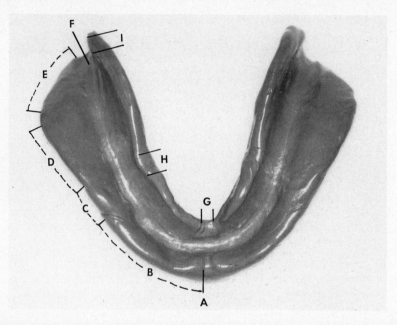

Fig. 9-20. Finished rubber base impression with border outline landmarks. *A,* Mandibular labial notch; *B,* mandibular labial flange; *C,* mandibular buccal notch; *D,* buccal flange; *E,* area influenced by masseter muscle; *F,* retromolar pad area; *G,* lingual notch; *H,* premylohyoid eminence; *1,* retromylohyoid eminence. Note S curve of lingual flanges. Notice also that in molar region lingual flanges slope toward tongue and extend in length below attachment of mylohyoid muscles on mylohyoid ridges in this region. Slope of lingual flange allows mylohyoid muscles to contract and raise the floor of the mouth without displacing lower denture. Length of lingual flange in molar region allows it to reach mucolingual fold in tissue of the floor of the mouth to maintain seal of lower denture. Posterior end of lingual flange turns laterally toward mandible to fit into retromylohyoid fossa. This part of denture guides tongue onto top of lingual flange.

Distal extension of mandibular impression

The distal extent of the mandibular impression is limited by the ramus of the mandible, by the buccinator muscle that crosses from the buccal to the lingual as it attaches to the pterygomandibular raphe and the superior constrictor muscle, and by the sharpness of the lateral bony boundaries of the retromolar fossa, which is formed by a continuation of the internal and external oblique ridges as they ascend the ramus. If the impression is extended onto the ramus, the buccinator muscle and adjacent tissues would be impinged on between the hard denture border and the sharp external oblique ridge. This would not only cause soreness but

also limit the fucntion of the buccinator muscle, which is part of the kinetic chain of swallowing.

The desirable distal extension is slightly to the lingual of these bony prominences and includes the pear-shaped retromolar pad. This tissue forms a splendid soft-tissue seal of the type that is so valuable in carrying out the principles involved in impression sealing.

Retromolar region and pad. The distal end of the mandibular denture region is bounded by the anterior border of the ramus. Thus the denture includes the retromolar pad posteriorly, which defines its posterior limit (Fig. 9-21). The retromolar pad (the triangular soft pad of tissue

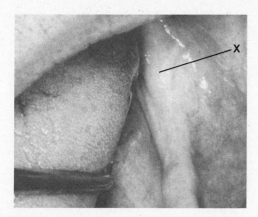

Fig. 9-21. Retromolar pad, X, is posterior landmark for mandibular denture.

at the distal end of the lower ridge) must be covered by the denture to perfect the border seal in this region. It contains some glandular tissue and some fibers of the temporal tendon, but it also has active structures working through it (see Fig. 9-35). Buccinator muscle fibers enter it from the buccal side, and fibers of the superior pharyngeal constrictor of the pharynx enter it from the lingual side. The pterygomandibular raphe enters the pad at its top back inside corner. The actions of these structures limit the extent of the denture and prevent placement of extra pressure on the retromolar pad during impression procedures or by reducing the posterior borders of the pad on the cast.

Lingual border anatomy

The lingual extension on mandibular impressions has been the most abused and misunderstood border region in complete dentures. This misunderstanding is caused by the peculiarities of the tissue under the tongue, which has less direct resistance than that of the labial and buccal borders, and yet it will not tolerate overextension of the lingual flange. Because of their peculiar lack of immediate resistance, these tissues are easily distorted when the impression is being made; yet such extension over a long peri-

od of time will cause tissue soreness or dislodgement of the denture by tongue movement. The lingual border of the mandibular impression is easily carried down along the bony surface of the mandible into the undercut below the mylohyoid ridge, since the mylohyoid muscle is a thin sheet of fibers that in a relaxed state will not resist the impression. However, this extension of the lingual flange under the mylohyoid ridge cannot be tolerated in function without displacing the denture, causing soreness, and limiting the function unless the flange is made parallel with the mylohyoid muscle when it is contracted. Although such a mechanical lock might seem desirable to secure additional retention, it cannot be tolerated because of physiologic factors. Therefore the border tissues in this area must be treated in a distinctly different manner from one involving the usual methods and materials (Figs. 9-10 to 9-12).

Influence and action of the floor of the mouth. An acceptable lingual border that will result in a stable denture can be secured with a proper understanding of the anatomy and function of the floor of the mouth. The mylohyoid muscle arises from the whole length of the mylohyoid line, extending from about 1 cm back of the distal end of the mylohyoid ridge to the lingual anterior portion of the mandible at the symphysis. Medially the fibers join the muscle fibers from the mylohyoid muscles of the opposite side, and posteriorly the fibers continue to the hyoid bone. The muscle lies deep to the sublingual gland and other structures about the region of the second premolar, and so does not affect denture borders in this region except indirectly. However, the posterior part of this muscle in the molar region affects the lingual impression border in swallowing and moving the tongue. Fortunately, the posterior extension of the impression can go beyond the mylohyoid muscle attachment line, since the mucolingual fold is not in that area. For this reason the impression may depart from a stress-bearing area of the lingual surface of the ridge and may be suspended under the tongue in soft tissue on both sides of

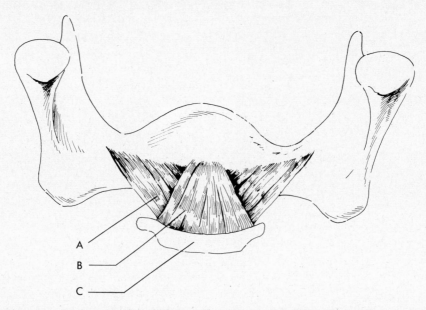

Fig. 9-22. Posterior view showing muscles of the floor of the mouth. *A,* Mylohyoid muscle; *B,* geniohyoid muscle; *C,* hyoid bone. Notice that the mylohyoid muscle is positioned more superiorly on the mandible as its attachment extends posteriorly on the mylohyoid ridge. For this reason, action of the mylohyoid muscle affects the slope of the lingual flange of the impression in the molar region, causing the flange to slope toward the tongue.

the mouth, thus reaching the mucolingual fold of soft tissue for a seal. The distance that these lingual borders can be away from the bony areas will depend on the functional movements of the floor of the mouth and the amount that the residual ridge has resorbed (Figs. 9-6, 9-22, and 9-27).

Mylohyoid muscle and mylohyoid ridge. An extension of the lingual flange well beyond the palpable portion of the mylohyoid ridge, but not into the undercut, has other advantages. One advantage is that the lack of direct pressure on this sharp edge of bone will reduce a possible source of soreness. If the impression is made with pressure on or slightly over this ridge, displacement of the denture and soreness are sure to result from lateral and vertical stresses. On the other hand, if the border stops above the ridge, vertical forces will still cause soreness, and the seal will be broken easily. If the flange is

properly shaped and extended, it will complete the lingual border seal in the retromylohyoid fossa and guide the tongue on top of the flange (Fig. 9-20).

Sublingual gland region. In the premolar region on the lingual side of ridge, the sublingual gland rests above the mylohyoid muscle. When the floor of the mouth is raised, this gland comes quite close to the crest of the ridge, thus preventing the development of a long flange in the anterior part of the lingual flange (Fig. 9-23).

The lingual frenum area is likewise rather shallow, sensitive, and resistant. This frenum should be registered in function because at rest the height of its attachment is deceptive. In function, it often comes quite close to the crest of the ridge, whereas at rest it is much lower (Figs. 9-25 and 9-28).

Direction of the lingual flange. The extension

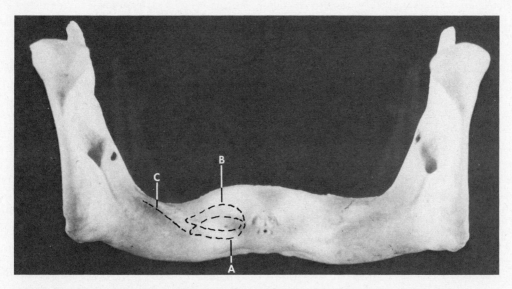

Fig. 9-23. Lingual view of mandible. *A,* Position of sublingual gland in relation to mylohyoid muscle at rest and in a raised position, *B. C,* Mylohyoid line.

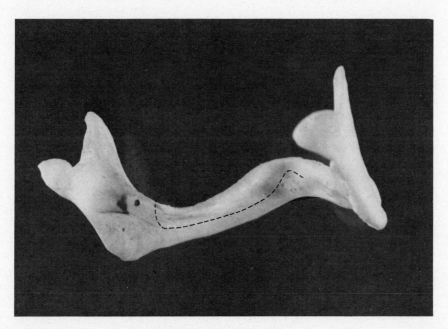

Fig. 9-24. *Dotted line,* Lower border of the lingual flange on the left side. Notice that the flange roughly parallels the lower border of the mandible.

of the lingual flange under the tongue is a concept vastly different from that ending it at the mylohyoid ridges. The lower border of the lingual flange runs parallel with the lower edge of the mandible from the lingual frenum to the posterior end of the denture (Fig. 9-24). This fact makes the flange short in the anterior region and long in the posterior region because the crest of the ridge of the mandible turns up rather sharply as it approaches the ramus (Fig. 9-25). The posterior extension is bounded partially by the action of the glossopalatine muscle, which usually is no farther back than the distal extent of the retromolar pad.

Alveololingual sulcus

The alveololingual sulcus (the space between the residual ridge and the tongue) extends posteriorly from the lingual frenum to the retromylohyoid curtain. Part of this sulcus is available for the lingual flange of the denture.

The alveololingual sulcus can be considered in three regions. The anterior region extends from the lingual frenum to the place where the mylohyoid ridge curves down below the level of the sulcus. At this point, a depression (the premylohyoid fossa) can be palpated, and a corresponding prominence (the premylohyoid eminence, Fig. 9-20, *H*) can be seen on impressions. The premylohyoid fossa results from the concavity of the mandible (as viewed from the above) joining the convexity of the mylohyoid ridge (as viewed from above) (Fig. 9-18).

The lingual border of the impression in this anterior region should extend down to make definite contact with the mucous membrane floor of the mouth when the tip of the tongue touches the upper incisors.

The middle region in the alveololingual sulcus extends from the premylohyoid fossa to the distal end of the mylohyoid ridge (Fig. 9-18). The sulcus curves medially from the body of the mandible. The curvature is caused by the prominence of the mylohyoid ridge. When the mylo-

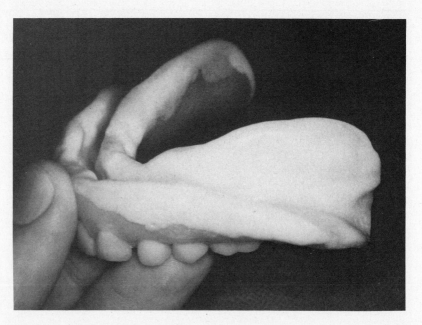

Fig. 9-25. A lower impression made in a lower denture with tissue-conditioning material. Notice that lingual flange is shorter in anterior region than in posterior region.

hyoid muscle and the tongue are relaxed, the muscle drapes back under the mylohyoid ridge. If an impression were made under these conditions, the muscle and other tissues in this region would be trapped under the ridge and buccal to their functioning position when the tongue is placed against the upper incisors. The sublingual gland and submaxillary duct can be pushed down and laterally out of position by resistant impression material. This can be avoided when this part of the lingual flange of the tray is shaped to slope inward toward the tongue and the final impression is made with a very soft impression material. When this part of the lingual flange is made to slope toward the tongue, it can extend below the level of the mylohyoid ridge. Otherwise, the flange must end at the level of the mylohyoid ridge. If the lingual flange slopes toward the tongue and extends below the mylohyoid ridge, the tongue can rest on top of the flange and aid in stabilizing the lower denture on the residual ridge. In addition, the slope of the lingual flange in the molar region provides space for the floor of the mouth to be raised during function (tongue movements and swallowing) without displacing the lower

denture. The seal of the lower denture is maintained during these movements of the floor of the mouth because the lingual flange remains in contact with the mucolingual fold in the alveololingual sulcus (Figs. 9-26 and 9-27).

The third and most posterior region of the alveololingual sulcus is the retromylohyoid space or fossa. It extends from the end of the mylohyoid ridge to the retromylohyoid curtain. It is bounded on the lingual side by the anterior tonsillar pillar, at the distal end by the retromylohyoid curtain and superior constrictor muscle, and on the buccal side by the mylohyoid muscle, the ramus, and the retromolar pad. The superior support for the retromylohyoid curtain is provided by part of the superior pharyngeal constrictor muscle. The actions of this muscle and of the tongue (and their effects on the alveololingual sulcus) determine the posterior limit of the extent of the lingual flange posteriorly.

The denture border should be extended posteriorly to contact the retromylohyoid curtain (the posterior limit of the alveololingual sulcus) when the tip of the tongue is placed against the front part of the upper residual ridge.

The attachment of the mylohyoid muscle

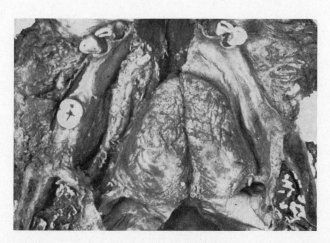

Fig. 9-26. Alveololingual sulcus has an S shape starting at midline. Notice that S shape results from contour of residual ridge and prominence of mylohyoid ridge. The characteristic form is equally apparent on both dissected *(left)* and undissected *(right)* sides.

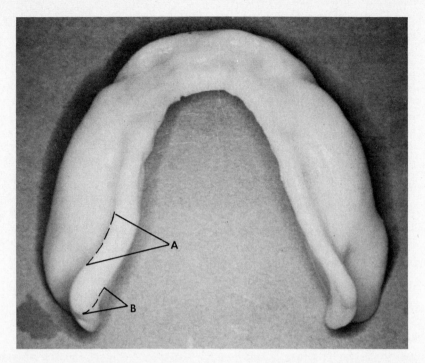

Fig. 9-27. A tissue-conditioning impression illustrates typical S curve of lingual flange. This type of contour permits tissues of the floor of the mouth to function normally. *A,* The slope of the lingual flange toward the tongue in the molar region allows the mylohyoid muscle to contract and raise the floor of the mouth without displacing the denture. *B,* The distal end of the lingual flange turns buccally to fill the retromylohyoid fossa. This part of the flange guides the tongue on top of the lingual flange of the denture.

extends about 1 cm distal to the end of the mylohyoid ridge, which prevents the denture from locking against the bone in this region (Fig. 9-26). However, two objectives are accomplished when the lingual flange is extended into this area. First, the border seal is made continuous from the retromolar pad to the middle region of the alveololingual sulcus, and, second, this part of the flange is shaped so that it will guide the tongue on top of the lingual flange of the denture. Such a contour assists the patient to control the denture without interfering with the functions of the soft tissues. When the flange is developed in this manner, the border of the lingual flange has a typical S curve when viewed from the impression surface (Fig. 9-27).

Lingual frenum and lingual notch. The lingual frenum, that is, the anterior attachment of the tongue, is extremely resistant and active and often wide (Fig. 9-18, *A, 13*). It forms the lingual notch in the lower impression. The denture border needs complete functional trimming so that movements of the lingual frenum will not displace the denture or create soreness of this sensitive band of tissue (Fig. 9-28).

Lingual flange. The lingual flange of the denture occupies the alveololingual sulcus, the space between the residual alveolar ridge and the tongue. The distal end of the alveololingual sulcus ends at the retromylohyoid curtain. This is a curtain of mucous membrane that is supported above by the superior constrictor muscle.

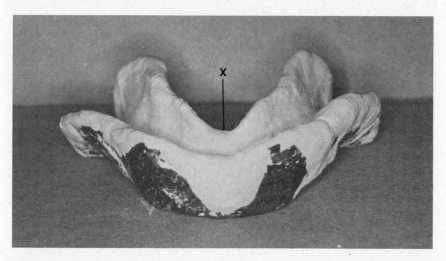

Fig. 9-28. *X,* Lingual notch in completed impression. Lingual notch is usually broad and often is close to crest of ridge.

The retromylohyoid curtain is pulled forward when the tongue is thrust out.

The distal extent of the lingual flange is partly limited by the glossopalatine arch, which is formed in part by the glossopalatine muscle and in part by the lingual extension of the superior constrictor muscle. Moving anteriorly, the lingual flange in the molar region is influenced by the mylohyoid muscle, which attaches to the mylohyoid ridge. The flange extends below and medialward from the mylohyoid ridge to occupy the alveololingual sulcus as limited by the mucolingual fold (the line of flexure of the mucous membrane as it passes from the tongue to the floor of the mouth). This means that the buccal surface of the flange does not rest on mucous membrane in contact with bone, but on soft tissue. The flange leaves the bony attachment at the mylohyoid ridge and slopes inward under the tongue to fill the alveololingual sulcus. Thus there is a space between the flange and the mucous membrane when the mylohyoid muscle is relaxed, but there is contact between the flange and the mucous membrane when the tongue is raised or thrust out (Fig. 9-29). This mucolingual fold is extremely flexible and

mobile because of the type of tissue and the mobility of the entire floor of the mouth. The border tissue on the lingual side of the residual ridge is unlike the border tissue in any other part of the mouth in regard to function and resistance in border molding (Fig. 9-6). It has so little resistance that it is easily distorted and for that reason needs a special type of technique and impression material to record the correct turn of the fold.

The anterior part of the lingual flange over the sublingual gland is usually shallow because of the mobility of the tissues that are controlled indirectly by the mylohyoid muscle. The mylohyoid muscle in this region extends nearly to the inferior border of the mandible, and yet the glandular and other tissues move above it so that only a relatively short flange is usable (Figs. 9-22 and 9-23). The combination of the typical arch form of the lingual side of the body of the mandible, the projection of the mylohyoid ridge toward the tongue, and the retromylohyoid fossa at the distal end of the alveololingual sulcus causes the border of the lingual flange to have a typical S shape when viewed from the impression surface (Fig. 9-20). Starting at the midline,

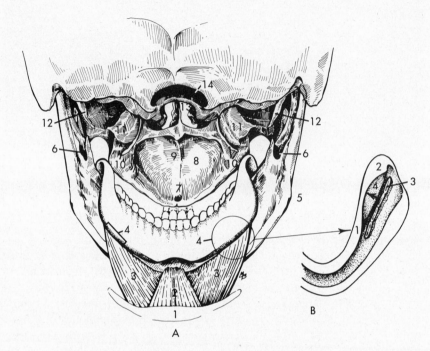

Fig. 9-29. A, Posterior view of skull and lower denture depicting the relationship of the mylohyoid muscle to the lingual flange of the denture. Notice that the attachment of the mylohyoid muscle is inferior to the lingual flange of the denture from the midline of the mandible posteriorly through the premolar region. However, the attachment of the mylohyoid muscle to the mylohyoid ridge in the molar region is superior to the border of the lingual flange *(circle),* and its movement during contraction affects the shape of the lingual flange in the molar region. Labeled structures: *1,* hyoid bone; *2,* geniohyoid muscle; *3,* mylohyoid muscle; *4,* portion of lingual flange *(circle)* covering mylohyoid muscle; *5,* angle of mandible; *6,* mandibular foramen; *7,* incisive fossa; *8,* hard palate; *9,* median palatal suture; *10,* pterygoid hamulus; *11,* lateral pterygoid plate; *12,* styloid process; *13,* nasal septum; *14,* foramen magnum. **B,** Lower denture, inferior view. *1,* Premylohyoid eminence; *2,* retromylohyoid eminence; *3,* mylohyoid muscle (cut section covered by lingual flange of lower denture in molar region); *4,* space in denture for mylohyoid muscle. *Arrow,* Direction mylohyoid muscle moves during contraction. Space in lingual flange allows movement of muscle and overlying floor of the mouth without displacing lower denture or causing soreness of the mucosa in the floor of the mouth.

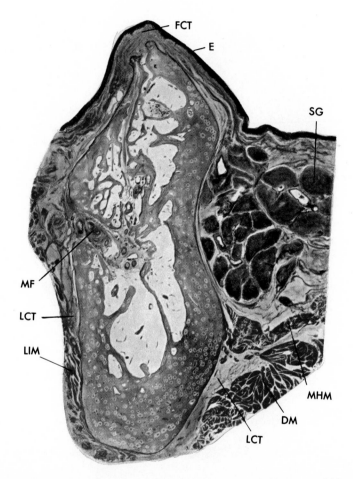

Plate 9-1. Buccolingual section through mandible in region of mental foramen of 80-year-old man. *MHM,* Mylohyoid muscle; *SC,* sublingual gland; *LCT,* loose connective tissue; *E,* oral epithelium; *FCT,* fibrous connective tissue; *MF,* mental foramen; *LIM,* labii inferioris muscle; *DM,* anterior belly of digastric muscle. (From Pendleton, E.C.: J. Am. Dent. Assoc. **21**:488, 1934.)

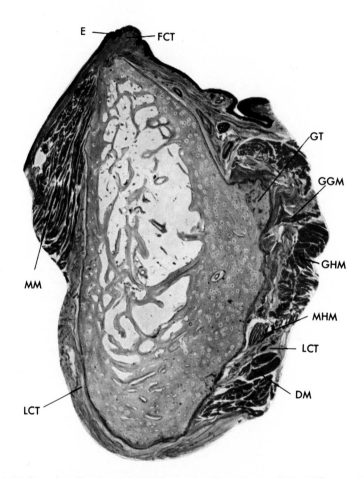

Plate 9-2. Labiolingual section in central incisor region through mandible of 80-year-old man. *DM,* Digastric muscle; *LCT,* loose connective tissue; *MM,* mentalis muscle; *GT,* genial tubercles; *GGM,* genioglossus muscle; *GHM,* geniohyoid muscle; *FCT,* fibrous connective tissue; *MHM,* mylohyoid muscle; *E,* oral epithelium. (From Pendleton, E.C.: J. Am. Dent. Assoc. **21:**488, 1934.)

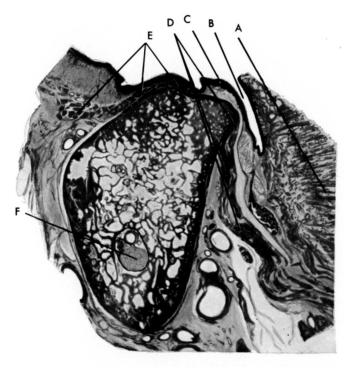

Plate 9-3. Cross section of mandible of a 40-year-old man. This section in region of third molar in a jaw that had remained endentulous for a long time with consequent resorption. Notice that mylohyoid and buccinator muscles almost meet. If denture were to extend only to muscle attachment line, mandibular denture would be of no value because bearing area would be ony a few millimeters wide; however, it is possible to place buccal flange on buccinator muscle and lingual flange on mylohyoid muscle. *A,* Tongue; *B,* space into which lingual flange of denture is placed under tongue away from bony contour of mandible; *C,* epithelium; *D,* mylohyoid muscle; *E,* buccinator muscle; *F,* mandibular canal. (Courtesy C.G. Darlington.)

the flange curves outward, following the curve of the residual ridge. At the premylohyoid fossa, which is located at the front end of the mylohyoid ridge, a premylohyoid eminence forms in the flange. At this point the border of the lingual flange curves away from the body of the mandible to accommodate the mylohyoid muscle when it is contracted or when the tongue is raised. At the distal end of the mylohyoid ridge, the lingual flange turns laterally toward the ramus to fill the retromylohyoid fossa and complete the typical S form. The distal end of the lingual flange is called the retromylohyoid eminence. Its most prominent contour lies medial, posterior, and below the level of the retromolar pad.

MICROSCOPIC ANATOMY*

In Chapter 7 the importance of microscopic anatomy to maxillary impression making, the histologic nature of the soft tissue and bone of the oral cavity, a classification of the oral mucosa, and clinical considerations of oral microscopic anatomy were discussed. A review of this part of Chapter 7 will be helpful at this point because the material is also applicable to considerations for mandibular impressions.

Microscopic anatomy of supporting tissues

The microscopic anatomy of the supporting tissues of the lower impression will be described for the crest of the residual ridge and the buccal shelf.

Crest of the residual ridge. The mucous membrane covering the crest of the lower residual ridge is similar to that of the upper ridge in that in the healthy mouth it is covered by a keratinized layer and is firmly attached by its submucosa to the periosteum of the mandible. The extent of the attachment to the bone varies considerably. In some patients the submucosa is loosely attached to the bone over the entire crest of the residual ridge, and the soft-tissue covering is

quite movable. In a relatively few patients, the submucosa is relatively firmly attached to the bone on both the crest and the slopes of the lower residual ridge. When the soft tissue is movable, it must be carefully registered in its resting position in the final impression. Occasionally surgical procedures are indicated to increase the amount of the "residual attached gingivae." When these tissues become inflamed, the submucosa is edematous, with infiltration of numerous inflammatory cells. Obviously the tissue must be healthy at the time the final impression is made.

The mucous membrane of the crest of the lower residual ridge when securely attached to the underlying bone is histologically capable of providing proper soft-tissue support for the lower denture. However, the underlying bone of the crest of the lower residual ridge is cancellous in nature, being made up of spongy trabeculated bone (Fig. 9-30). Therefore the crest of the lower residual ridge may not be favorable as the

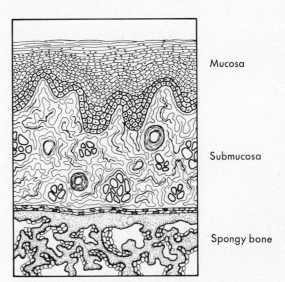

Mucosa

Submucosa

Spongy bone

Fig. 9-30. Histologic drawing of crest of lower residual ridge. Submucosal layer of mucous membrane covering crest may be of adequate thickness and firmly attached to residual ridge. However, bone that forms crest of lower ridge is cancellous, or spongy, in nature. Therefore this part of ridge is generally not used for primary support of lower denture.

*We wish to acknowledge the assistance of Dr. Steve Kolas, Professor, Department of Oral Pathology, Medical College of Georgia School of Dentistry, Augusta.

primary stress-bearing area for the lower denture. The method of providing space in the final impression tray before the final impression is made ensures that proper relief is provided for the crest of the lower residual ridge during the making of the final impression.

Buccal shelf. Anatomically, the buccal shelf is defined as that part of the basal seat that is located posterior to the buccal frenum and extends from the crest of the lower residual ridge to the external oblique ridge (see Fig. 9-5). The mucous membrane covering the buccal shelf is more loosely attached and less keratinized than the mucous membrane covering the crest of the lower residual ridge, and it contains a thicker submucosal layer. Histologically, fibers of the buccinator muscle are found running horizontally in the submucosa immediately overlying the bone.

The mucosa membrane overlying the buccal shelf may not be as suitable histologically to provide primary support for the lower denture as the mucous membrane overlying the crest of the lower residual ridge. However, the bone of the buccal shelf is covered by a layer of compact bone composed of haversian systems (Fig. 9-31).

The nature of this bone plus the horizontal supporting surface provided by the buccal shelf make it the most suitable primary stress-bearing area for the lower denture. The horizontal direction of the fibers of the buccinator muscle allows the denture to rest on this part of the muscle without damage to the muscle or displacement of the denture.

The method of forming the lower final impression tray allows additional load to be placed on the buccal shelf during the making of the final impression (Fig. 9-32). The impression tray comes into direct contact with the mucosa of the buccal shelf, and the soft tissue is slightly displaced as the final impression is made.

Microscopic anatomy of limiting tissues

The microscopic anatomy of the limiting tissues is described for the vestibular spaces, the alveololingual sulcus, and the retromolar pad.

The mucous membrane lining the vestibular spaces and the alveololingual sulcus is quite similar in nature to that lining the vestibular spaces of the upper jaw. The epithelium is thin and nonkeratinized, and the submucosa is formed of loosely arranged connective tissue fibers mixed

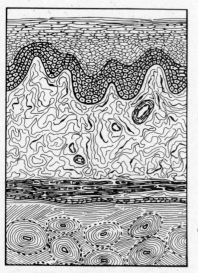

Mucosa

Submucosa

Buccinator muscle

Compact bone

Fig. 9-31. Histologic drawing of buccal shelf of mandible. Bone forming the buccal shelf is compact in nature, in contrast to spongy bone forming crest of lower ridge (Fig. 9-30). The histologic nature of compact bone makes buccal shelf suitable as primary stress-bearing area for lower denture.

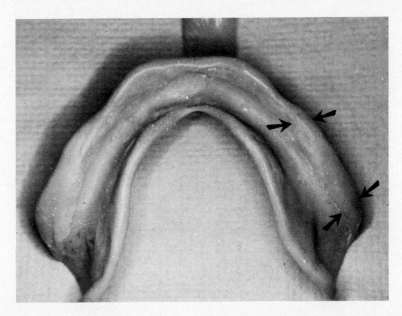

Fig. 9-32. Buccal flanges of final impression tray in region of buccal shelf *(arrows)* are left in direct contact with cast on both sides when tray is made. This part of tray directly contacts mucosa of buccal shelf during making of final impression and places additional load on supporting tissues in these regions. The rest of the tray has been relieved from cast by a wax spacer.

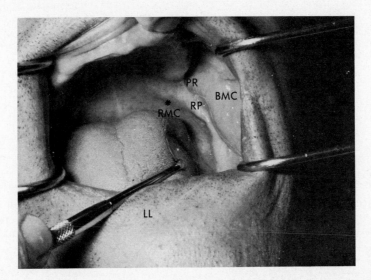

Fig. 9-33. Photograph of mucous membrane lining retromylohyoid fossa, soft palate, retromolar pad, and cheek. *LL,* Lower lip; *RMC,* retromylohyoid curtain, formed by mucous membrane covering superior constrictor muscle; *RP,* retromolar pad; *PR,* pterygomandibular raphe; *BMC,* buccal mucosa of cheek. Retromylohyoid curtain lies at posterior end of alveololingual sulcus and is posterior boundary of retromylohyoid fossa. The *asterisk* indicates location of histologic section shown diagrammatically in Fig. 9-34, *A.*

A

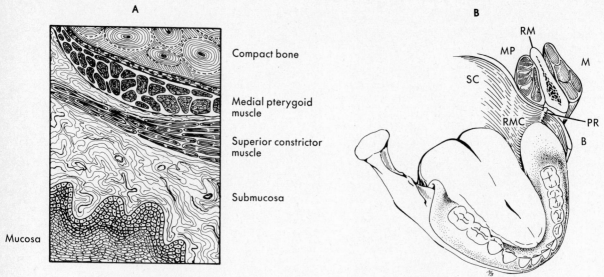

B

Compact bone

Medial pterygoid muscle

Superior constrictor muscle

Submucosa

Mucosa

Fig. 9-34. A, Histologic drawing made posteriorly through retromylohyoid curtain at site of asterisk in Fig. 9-33. Notice superior constrictor muscle and posterior to it medial pterygoid muscle. Contraction of medial pterygoid muscle limits space available for posterior part of lingual flange in retromylohyoid fossa. **B,** Drawing indicates relationship of medial pterygoid muscle to superior constrictor muscle. When the medial pterygoid muscle contracts, it forces the superior constrictor muscle anteriorly, thus limiting the length of the lingual flange in that region. *B,* Buccinator muscle; *M,* masseter muscle; *MP,* medial pterygoid muscle; *PR,* pterygomandibular raphe; *RM,* ramus of mandible; *RMC,* retromylohyoid curtain; *SC,* superior constrictor muscle. Contraction of the medial pterygoid muscle *(MP),* which lies posteriorly to the superior constrictor muscle *(SC),* causes the retromylohyoid curtain *(RMC,* mucosal covering of the superior constrictor muscle) to move anteriorly thus limiting the space in the retromylohyoid fossa for the retromylohyoid eminence at the posterior end of the lingual flange of lower denture.

← LINGUAL   BUCCAL →

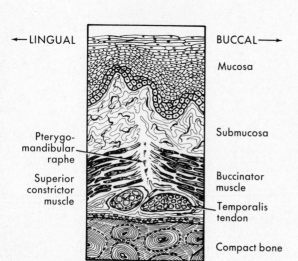

Mucosa

Submucosa

Pterygo-
mandibular
raphe

Superior
constrictor
muscle

Buccinator
muscle

Temporalis
tendon

Compact bone

Fig. 9-35. Vertical histologic drawing through posterior part of retromolar pad shows fibers of buccinator muscle laterally and of superior constrictor muscle medially, which join to form pterygomandibular raphe. Fibers of tendon of temporal muscle lie deep to these structures. Because of histologic makeup of retromolar pad, it should not be displaced during final impression procedures.

with elastic fibers. Thus the mucous membrane lining the vestibules and the alveololingual sulcus is freely movable, which allows for the necessary movements of the lips, cheeks, and tongue. Anteriorly the submucosa of the mucous membrane lining the alveolingual sulcus contains components of the sublingual gland and is attached to the genioglossus muscle. In the molar region, the submucosa attaches to the mylohyoid muscle, and the mucous membrane covering of the retromylohyoid curtain is attached by its submucosa to the superior constrictor muscle. Posterior to the superior constrictor muscle fibers, which run in a horizontal direction, is found the medial pterygoid muscle running in a vertical direction (Figs. 9-33 and 9-34). The length and form of the lingual flange of the lower final impression tray must reflect the physiologic activity of these structures; otherwise their normal movement will be restricted, or they will tend to dislodge the lower denture.

The retromolar pad lies at the posterior end of the crest of the lower residual ridge. Histologically, the mucosa of the pad is composed of a thin, nonkeratinized epithelium, and in addition to loose or areolar tissue, its submucosa contains glandular tissue, fibers of the buccinator and superior constrictor muscles, the pterygomandibular raphe, and the terminal part of the tendon of the temporal muscle (Fig. 9-35). Because of the histologic nature of the retromolar pad, it should be registered in a resting position in the final lower impression.

Cross-sectional anatomy of the mandible

Cross sections of the mandible reveal the proximity of muscle attachments and the lack of a broad bearing surface. The bony contour naturally is much narrower and sharper than the soft-tissue contour. This fact often deceives the dentist as to the width and contour of the bearing surface (Plates 9-1 to 9-3, facing p. 198).

10

Mandibular impression procedures

A survey of dentists who include prosthodontic treatment in their practice would indicate that most of them believe making good mandibular impressions for edentulous patients is far more difficult than making good maxillary impressions. Why should this be true? The difficulty most likely stems from the lack of the dentist's true understanding of the functional anatomy of the structures that determine the length and form of the mandibular lingual flange. These limiting structures of the lingual flanges are directly related to the tongue and the floor of the mouth and their combined movements, which are among the most complex in the body. An understanding of the role that they play can come only from continuing study of their physiology and its clinical application. Both require a concerted effort. The lingual borders of properly molded mandibular impressions are as definite in length and form as the buccal and labial borders of either maxillary or mandibular impressions. Properly formed lingual borders of mandibular impressions do not happen by chance. They require cooperation of the patient to make the proper tongue and jaw movements that create the desirable action of the floor of the mouth for border-molding purposes. They also require time, effort, patience, and a willingness on the part of the dentist to repeat difficult parts of the impression procedure as many times as may be necessary to obtain the desired result. The techniques for making mandibular impressions described in this chapter are based on the clinical application of the tolerances of the supporting structures and the function of the border tissues that make up the basal seat.

CLASSIFICATION OF MANDIBULAR IMPRESSIONS

Mandibular impressions for complete dentures are made in many kinds of materials and by many different techniques. The technique to use for each patient should be selected on the basis of the diagnosis of the basal seat and border tissues.

Impression techniques are classified as (1) pressure, (2) selective pressure, and (3) pressureless impressions. The choice is made on the basis of the objectives for each patient.

Pressure impressions are those made in trays in which no space has been made for the final impression material or those made in a final impression material that has a very sluggish flow, such as modeling compound and wax. These impressions may grip the ridge with sufficient pressure to interfere with the blood supply to the tissues of the basal seat, and eventually the dentures made from them may cause the rapid resorption of the residual ridges. They require great skill to be used without doing damage to the residual ridges.

Selective pressure impressions are those made in trays that have more space in them for the final impression material in some places than in others. The places that have less relief (space between the tray and the tissue to be recorded) will transmit more pressue from the denture in function on favorable parts of the bone such as the buccal shelf, while they transmit less pressure on unfavorable parts of the bone, such as a sharp ridge crest or sharp bone spicules.

The *pressureless impression* is one made with the least possible displacement of soft tissues covering the residual alveolar bone. It is made by providing a large amount of space between the tray and the soft tissues of the basal seat and by using a very fluid type of impression material.

FIRST TECHNIQUE—SELECTIVE PRESSURE MANDIBULAR IMPRESSION—BORDER-MOLDED SPECIAL TRAY

The same principles are incorporated in lower final impression procedures as those for upper impression procedures in Chapter 8. Even though techniques for impressions may vary, the basic principles remain the same.

Making the preliminary impression

The space available in the mouth for the lower impression should be studied carefully to determine the general form, size, and health of the basal seat. Then an edentulous metal stock tray is selected that will provide for approximately ¼-inch (6 mm) bulk of impression material over the entire basal seat area. The patient is asked to raise the tongue slightly as the tray is placed in the mouth to position the tongue in the tongue space of the tray (Fig. 10-1, *A*). Posteriorly the retromolar pads should be covered by the tray, and anteriorly the lingual surface of the labial flange should provide space for the necessary ¼-inch bulk of impression material. The labial and buccal borders of the tray are observed in relation to the limiting anatomic structures. The tray is raised anteriorly for observation of the relation of the lingual flanges to the lingual slope of the lower residual ridge (Fig. 10-1, *B*). The metal lingual flanges are reshaped by bending to allow for the action of the mylohyoid muscle (Fig. 10-1, *C*).

The borders of the tray are lined with a soft boxing wax so that a rim is created within the tray to help confine the alginate (irreversible hydrocolloid) impression material that will be used for the preliminary impression (Fig. 10-2, *A*). The tray is again positioned in the mouth, with the patient's tongue raised slightly, and the borders of the tray are observed in relation to the limiting structures (Fig. 10-2, *B*). The entire basal seat area should be included within the impression surface of the tray so that all supporting tissues for the completed denture will be included in an overextended preliminary impression.

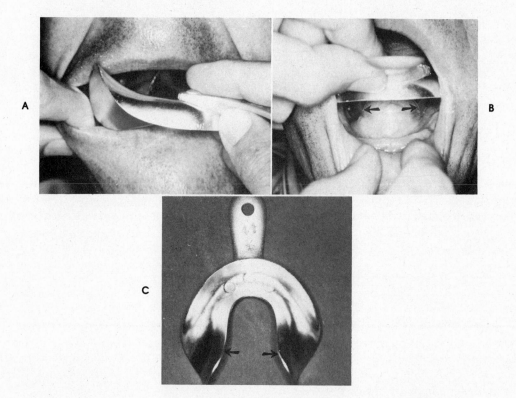

Fig. 10-1. A, Lower stock metal tray is placed into mouth by extension of corner of one side of patient's mouth with index finger or a mouth mirror, with side of tray being placed into opposite corner of mouth, and rotation of tray into position inside mouth. **B,** Lower stock tray is raised anteriorly for observation of whether there is adequate space between lingual flanges of tray *(arrows)* and lingual slope of lower residual ridge to provide for sufficient bulk of impression material. **C,** Lingual flanges of tray slope toward tongue in molar region *(arrows)* to accommodate for action of mylohyoid muscle when it raises the floor of the mouth. Note S shape of lingual flange.

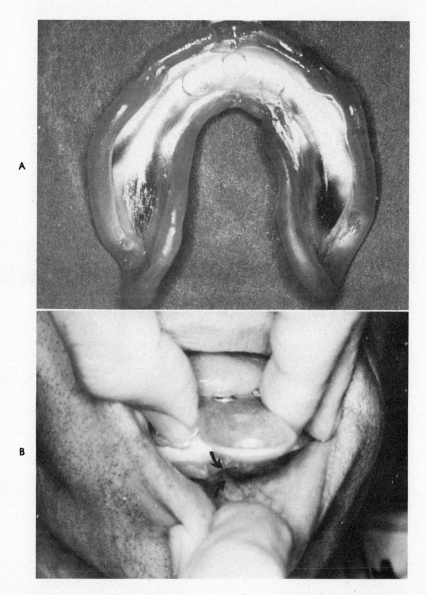

Fig. 10-2. A, Rim of wax helps conform borders of tray to mouth and confines preliminary impression material in tray. **B,** Space is provided for lower labial frenum in boxing wax that lines stock metal tray. *Top arrow* points to labial notch formed in wax, and *bottom arrow* indicates lower labial frenum.

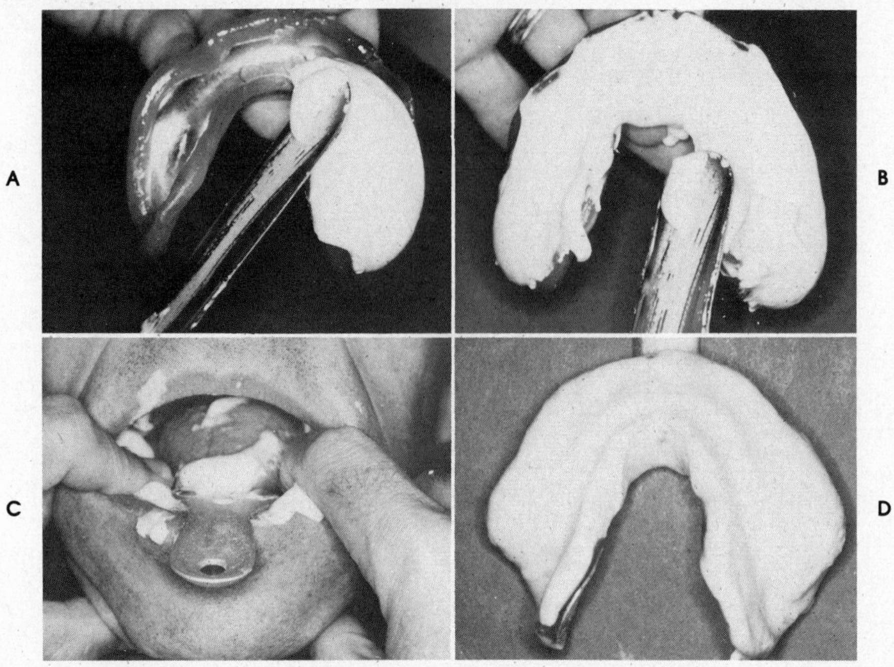

Fig. 10-3. A, Irreversible hydrocolloid impression material is placed into tray so that it moves impression material ahead of itself from one end of tray to the other so that air is not trapped. **B,** Irreversible hydrocolloid impression material is confined in tray by rim of molding wax and is evenly distributed. **C,** Preliminary impression is held in mouth by an index finger from either hand placed on top of tray in region of first molar. Notice position of tongue. **D,** Preliminary impression includes a negative record of all the basal seat area.

The tissue surface and borders of the metal tray, including the rim of wax, are painted with an adhesive material to make certain that the irreversible hydrocolloid impression material adheres well to the tray. The irreversible hydrocolloid is mixed following the directions of the manufacturer. The impression material is loaded into the lower stock tray from the lingual surface and evenly distributed to fill the tray to the level of the borders (Fig. 10-3, *A* and *B*). The tray is centered over the residual ridge, with the tongue raised slightly so that it will be in the tongue space. As the tray is gently seated into position by alternating pressure from an index finger on the top of the tray on either side in the molar region, the patient is asked to let the tongue relax. The tray is held steadily in position for 1 minute after the initial set of the irreversible hydrocolloid impression material (Fig. 10-3, *C*). Then the impression is removed from the mouth in one motion and inspected to be certain that all the basal seat area is included (Fig. 10-3, *D*).

Making the final impression tray

The cast is made of artificial stone poured into the irreversible hydrocolloid impression. The outline for a wax spacer, which will provide space in the tray for the final impression material, is drawn in pencil on the cast (Fig. 10-4, *A*). A wax spacer about 1 mm thick is placed over the crest of the residual ridge and the slopes of the

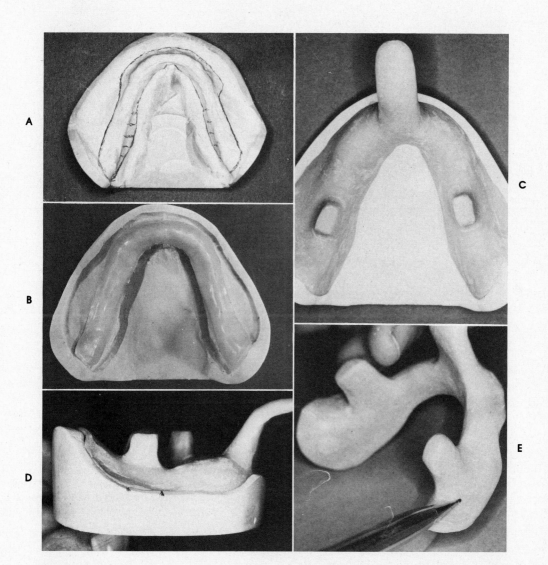

Fig. 10-4. A, Outline form for wax spacer has been drawn on preliminary cast. Notice that buccal shelf on either side of cast is not included in outline form. **B,** Wax spacer has been adapted to cast. Retromylohyoid fossae, buccal shelves, and borders are not covered by wax spacer. **C,** Lower final impression tray is formed on lower cast from self-curing acrylic resin. **D,** Position of posterior handle is indicated by pencil marks on cast. Handle should be located at lowest part of lower residual ridge, usually in first molar region. **E,** External surface of lower impression tray should be similar in form to that of completed denture.

ridge. The buccal shelf on each side and the retromylohyoid spaces on the cast are left uncovered (Fig. 10-4, *B*). Thus the completed final impression tray will contact the mucosa of the region of the buccal shelves and thereby help to correctly position the tray in the mouth and to place additional pressure in this primary stress-bearing area when the final impression is made. Extra wax can be placed over the lingual slopes of the cast below the level of the mylohyoid ridge. This will provide additional space for the action of the mylohyoid muscles when the final impression is made.

Self-curing (cold-curing or autopolymerizing) acrylic resin tray material is mixed and uniformly distributed over the cast so that the final impression tray will be approximately 2 to 3 mm thick. An anterior resin handle is centered over the labial flange in the approximate position of the anterior teeth and shaped so as not to interfere with the position of the lip (Fig. 10-4, *C* and *D*). Two additional handles, one on each side, are placed in the first molar region. These handles are centered over the crest of the residual ridge at its lowest point and are approximately ¾ inch (19 mm) in height. The anterior handle is used to carry the final impression tray into the mouth and position it over the residual ridge. The posterior handles are used as finger rests to complete the placement of the tray on the residual ridge and to stabilize the tray in the correct position with minimal distortion of soft tissues while the final impression material sets. The flanges of the tray should be contoured like the flanges of the completed denture. Thus, while the impression is made, the limiting border tissues will be in a position similar to the one they will be in when the denture is in the mouth (Fig. 10-4, *E*).

Preparing the final impression tray

When the acrylic resin tray is removed from the lower preliminary cast, the wax spacer is left inside the tray (Fig. 10-5, *A*). Retaining the spacer allows the tray to be properly positioned

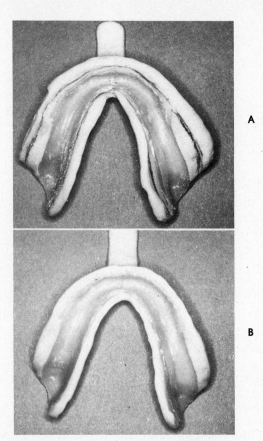

Fig. 10-5. A, Wax spacer is maintained in lower impression tray until border-molding procedures have been completed. Pencil mark indicates approximate amount that tray will be shortened before border-molding procedures. Notice that a part of right buccal flange has already been shortened. **B,** Flanges of final lower impression tray have been reduced so that they will be short of limiting anatomic structures when tray is placed in patient's mouth.

on the lower residual ridge for border-molding procedures.

The available space for the impression is again observed in the patient's mouth and compared with the length and width of the flanges of the final impression tray. The buccal and lingual flanges of the impression tray are marked in pencil and reduced until the borders are short of the limiting anatomic structures (Fig. 10-5, *B*). When possible, observations are made with the modified tray in the mouth to be certain that space is available for the addition of modeling compound.

Border molding labial and buccal flanges. Stick modeling compound is added in sections to the borders of the resin tray, beginning with the labial flange, then the buccal flanges, and finally the lingual flanges. Each section of modeling compound is heated and border molded before the next section is added.

Border molding is accomplished for the labial flange when the lower lip is lifted outward, upward, and inward (Fig. 10-6, *A* and *B*). In the region of the buccal frenum the cheek is lifted outward, upward, inward, backward, and forward to simulate movement of the lower buccal frenum. Posteriorly the buccal flange is border molded when the cheek is moved outward, upward, and inward (Fig. 10-6, *C* to *E*).

Border molding lingual flanges. The lingual flanges are border molded in five steps. First, the length and thickness of the lingual flange in the anterior region are observed with the tray in the mouth in relation to the available space in the alveololingual sulcus as limited by the lingual frenum, the sublingual folds, and the submaxillary caruncles. If space is observed between the lingual border of the tray and the limiting anatomic structures with the tongue slightly raised, more modeling compound is added in this region. If the tray encroaches on the limiting structures, the lingual border is reduced before the border is molded.

When the tray appears to fill the available space in the lingual anterior region, the labial surface of the lingual flange and border of the modeling compound between the premylohyoid eminences are heated and tempered. The tray is placed in the patient's mouth, and the patient is instructed to protrude the tongue (Fig. 10-7, *A*). This movement of the tongue creates functional activity of the anterior part of the floor of the mouth, including the lingual frenum, and deter-

mines the length of the lingual flange of the tray in this region. Both premylohyoid eminences on the tray are usually visible after this procedure, and the length of the lingual flanges on either side of the lingual notch will frequently be symmetrical. This procedure often must be repeated while close observation is maintained on the flange and the space in the mouth.

Second, the compound on the lingual surface of the lingual flange is softened in the anterior region (from premolar to premolar) to a depth of 1 to 2 mm. The tray is placed in the mouth and the patient is asked to push the tongue forcefully against the front part of the palate (Fig. 10-7, *B*). This action causes the base of the tongue to spread out and develops the thickness of the anterior part of the lingual flange (Fig. 10-7, *C*).

The lingual flange will be shorter anteriorly than posteriorly. At the premylohyoid fossa in the canine-premolar region, the flange becomes longer and extends below the level of the mylohyoid line. The lingual flange must slope toward the tongue more or less parallel to the direction of the fibers of the mylohyoid muscle in the molar region.

Third, modeling compound is added to the lingual borders in the molar regions on both sides of the tray between the premylohyoid and the postmylohyoid eminences. The modeling compound is heated and tempered. Then the tray is placed in the patient's mouth, and the patient is asked to protrude the tongue. This procedure develops the slope of the lingual flanges in the molar region to allow for the action of the mylohyoid muscle. In some instances one will need to thicken the lingual flanges by adding modeling compound to the lingual surface so that the buccal surface of the lingual flange can be cut away and sloped toward the tongue. If modeling compound builds up inside the lingual flange in this region as a result of the border-molding process, the excess compound should be removed. This will permit the mylohyoid muscle to function normally and will prevent

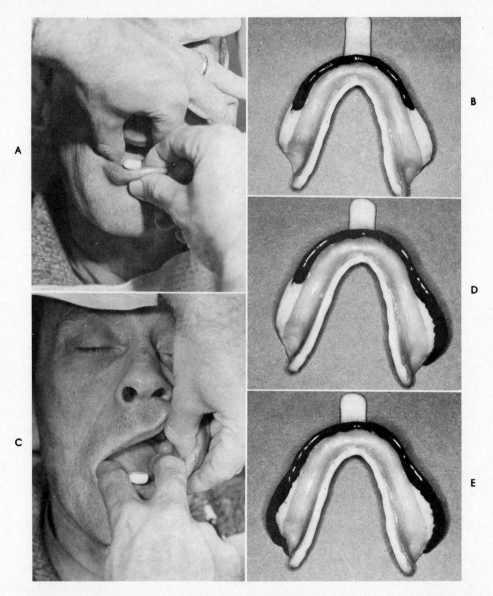

Fig. 10-6. A, Border molding is accomplished in lower anterior region by extension of lower lip outward, upward, and inward. No side-to-side movement of lower lip is necessary in this region during border molding, since the lower labial frenum does not move from side to side during function. **B,** Labial flange of lower final impression tray has been properly border molded in modeling compound. **C,** Posterior flange of lower impression tray is border molded by extension of cheek outward, upward, and inward, and moving of it backward and forward in region of lower buccal frenum. Tray is held in position by the posterior handles. **D,** Left buccal flange has been properly border molded. **E,** Both buccal flanges have been properly border molded. Wax spacer is still in place inside tray.

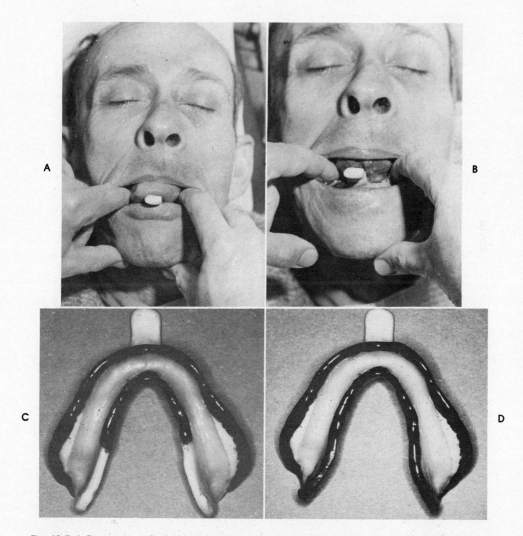

Fig. 10-7. A, Tongue is protruded to regulate length of lingual flange in border-molding procedure. **B,** Tongue is pushed against anterior part of palate to regulate thickness of anterior part of lingual flange. **C,** Anterior part of lingual flange is properly border molded. **D,** Border molding for lower tray is completed. Notice that borders of lingual flange are just as definitely formed as those of labial and buccal flanges. The wax spacer is still in place inside impression tray.

pressure from being applied to the sharp mylohyoid ridge. It is better to have the tray contoured with too much slope toward the tongue in the molar region than with too little, since the final impression material will fill in excess space.

Fourth, the modeling compound on the border of the lingual flange on both sides in the molar region is heated to a depth of 1 to 2 mm. The tray is placed in the mouth, and the patient again protrudes the tongue. The action of the mylohyoid muscle, which raises the floor of the mouth during this movement of the tongue, determines the length of the lingual flanges in the molar region (Fig. 10-7, *D*).

The distal end of the lingual flange is extended about 1 cm distal to the end of the mylohyoid ridge. If this part of the preliminary impression lacks sufficient length, modeling compound is added to it. This part of the lingual flange should be shaped so that it turns laterally toward the ramus below the level of the retromolar pad and mylohyoid ridge.

Fifth, the modeling compound on the distal ends of the lingual flanges is heated, and the tray is placed in the mouth. The patient is instructed to open the mouth and protrude the tongue to activate the superior constrictor muscle that supports the retromylohyoid curtain. Then the patient is asked to close the jaws as the dentist applies downward pressure on the impression tray. The resulting contraction of the medial pterygoid muscle, acting posteriorly on the retromylohyoid curtain, can limit the space available for the border of the impression in the retromylohyoid fossa. Often, modeling compound must be added to the retromylohyoid eminence on the lingual flange of the impression tray so that the eminence will fill the retromylohyoid fossa properly during function of the limiting structures (Fig. 10-7, *D*).

The length and form of the lingual flange should be in harmony with the limiting anatomic structures on completion of the border molding for the distal corner of the lingual flange. With the lower final impression tray in place in the mouth, the patient should be able to wipe the tip of the tongue across the vermillion border of the upper lip without noticeable displacement of the lower tray.

The modeling compound forming the posterior part of the retromolar fossa is heated, the tray is placed in the mouth, and the patient is asked to open the mouth wide. If the tray is too long, a notch will be formed at the posterior medial border of the retromolar fossa, indicating encroachment of the tray on the pterygomandibular raphe. The tray is adjusted accordingly (Fig. 10-7, *D*).

The final tray should be so formed that it can support the cheeks and lips in the same manner as the finished denture is to do. The lingual flange is shaped to facilitate making of the final impression and to guide the tongue into the position it is to occupy in relation to the finished denture. The lingual surface of the lingual flange of the tray should guide the tongue into the same position it will occupy in relation to the finished denture.

The wax spacer is removed from the inside of the tray (Fig. 10-8, *A*). A series of holes about ½ inch (12.5 mm) apart are marked in the center of the alveolar groove and the retromolar fossae of the tray and are cut in the tray with a No. 6 round bur (Fig. 10-8, *B*). The holes provide escapeways for the final impression material and relieve pressure over the crest of the residual ridge and the retromolar pads when the final impression is made. The modeling compound borders of the lower final impression tray are shortened approximately 0.5 to 1 mm to make space for the final impression material (Fig. 10-8, *C*).

Making the final lower impression

Existing dentures must be left out of the mouth for a minimum of 24 hours before the lower final impression is made to allow the tissues of the basal seat to return to health and undistorted form. With proper education, the patient will understand the value of providing this period of rest for the supporting tissues and

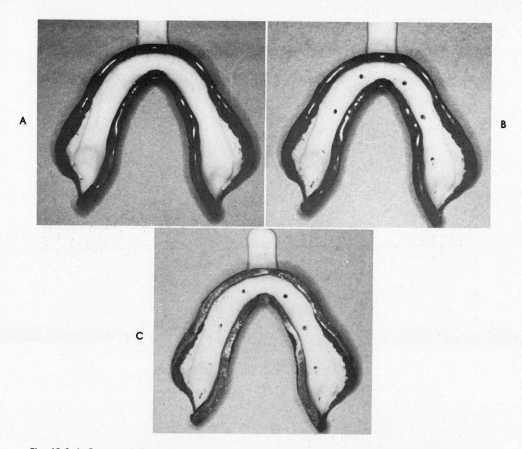

Fig. 10-8. A, On completion of border-molding procedure, wax spacer is removed from tray. **B,** Holes in alveolar groove provide an escapeway for final impression material when final impression is made. **C,** Modeling compound borders have been shortened to provide space for final impression material.

will be willing to comply with this important requirement.

A good final impression cannot be made unless a properly fitting tray is in the correct position on the residual ridge. Therefore the dentist should practice proper positioning of the tray before making the final impression.

Practicing placement of the tray

In the practice procedure the empty lower final impression tray is carried into the mouth with the anterior handle. With the patient's mouth half open, the anterior part of the tray (the part next to the anterior handle) is placed against the left side of the mouth while the right side of the mouth is pulled laterally by the index finger of the left hand or a mouth mirror. Then the tray is rotated in the horizontal plane until it is over the residual ridge.

Note that left-handed dentists will use the opposite hands for each of these operations.

At this time, the patient is asked to slightly raise the tongue. The retromylohyoid eminences are alternatively started to place past the crest of the ridge. It may be necessary to move the tray posteriorly in the mouth beyond its cor-

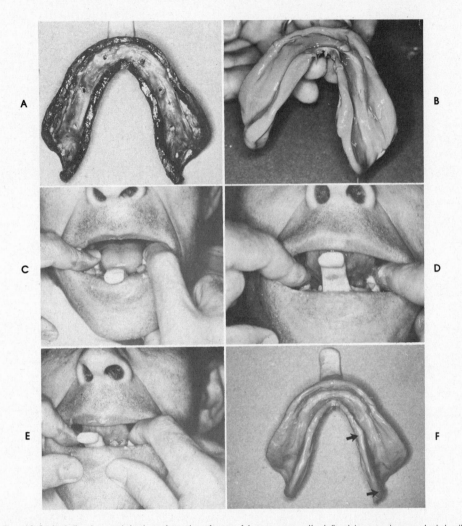

Fig. 10-9. A, Adhesive painted on basal surface of tray ensures that final impression material will adhere to tray. **B,** Final impression material must cover all the basal surface of tray including borders. **C,** Final impression is positioned correctly on lower residual ridge by alternate application of gentle pressure on either side of tray until buccal flanges come into contact with mucosa covering buccal shelf. **D,** Position of tongue under upper lip will cause an action of the floor of the mouth that will border mold lingual flange of lower final impression. **E,** Lower lip and corners of mouth are elevated to complete border-molding procedure in this region. **F,** Final impression indicates that tray has been properly positioned on lower residual ridge and that border-molding procedures have been properly performed. Notice that lingual flange of final impression slopes toward tongue between premylo-hyoid and postmylohyoid eminences *(arrows).*

rect position to initiate this procedure. Then the tray is moved forward and centered and moved downward toward its final position.

The index fingers are placed on top of the posterior handles, and by the alternate application of gentle pressure on either side, the tray is seated until the buccal flanges come into contact with the mucosa covering the buccal shelf. The amount of pressure used will determine the amount of displacement of the soft tissues on the buccal shelf. Heavier pressure will displace the soft tissue more and thus will provide more relief of the tissues over the crest of the ridge. The minimum of tissue displacement, and therefore the minimum pressure, should be the objective unless the crest of the ridge is unfavorable for the support of the denture.

With the tray held steadily and without movement on the residual ridge, the patient is instructed to place the tongue under the upper lip in front of the upper anterior teeth, as if they were present. This position of the tongue actuates the floor of the mouth and border-molds the lingual flange of the impression. The dentist then carefully elevates the lower lip and corners of the mouth with his thumbs to complete the border-molding procedure (Fig. 10-9). The fingers must be held in position on the posterior handles until the impression material has set.

Preparation of the patient

The patient's clothing should be protected by a plastic apron. The patient's face is lubricated with petroleum jelly, and a roll of gauze is placed under the patient's tongue to help keep the mouth dry.

The final impression

An adhesive is painted on the basal surface of the tray. The final impression material is mixed in proper quantities according to the manufacturer's directions and evenly distributed within the tray, with care to make certain that all borders are covered (Fig. 10-9, A and B). The gauze is quickly removed from under the patient's tongue. The final impression tray carrying the impression material is carefully positioned in the mouth and border molded in the manner as planned when practiced (Fig. 10-9, C to E). The tray is held steadily in position for the time specified by the manufacturer until the final impression material is set. Then the completed impression is removed from the mouth and inspected for acceptability (Fig. 10-9, F).

Remaking final impressions

Impression making is not easy if it is done correctly. It requires infinite attention to details and a thorough understanding of the anatomy and physiology of oral tissues if it is to be done with minimal effort. The extra time that may be spent in making impressions not only means the difference between success and failure, but also leads to the expenditure of less time in making adjustments to finished dentures.

Patients should be told that it is often necessary to make more than one impression to correct the tray before a final impression is acceptable. Many impressions must be remade. If the tray was correctly positioned in the mouth, errors in the impression indicate modifications of the tray that are necessary before another impression is made. The tray should *not* be modified unless it was correctly positioned when the impression was made. Errors in one impression must be corrected before the next one is made.

Following are some of the imperfections in an impression that will indicate it must be remade:

1. Incorrect tray position in the mouth
   a. A thick buccal border on one side with a thin corresponding border on the opposite side— indicates that the tray was out of position in the direction of the thick border
   b. A thick lingual border on one side with a thin corresponding border on the opposite side— indicates that the tray had moved toward the thin border

c. Pressure spots on the inside surface of the labial flange—may indicate that the anterior part of the tray was not completely seated on the residual ridge

d. Pressure spots on the anterior part of the lingual flange—may indicate that the lower tray was too far forward in relation to the residual ridge (possibly as a result of anterior movement of the tray when the tongue was extended for border molding)

e. Excess thickness of final impression material in the alveolar groove of the tray or excess length of final impression material on the flange of the tray—may indicate that the tray was not sufficiently seated on that part of the residual ridge

2. Pressure spots on secondary stress-bearing areas (e.g., on the alveolar groove of the lower tray or in the rugae of the upper tray)

3. Voids or discrepancies that are too large to be accurately corrected

4. Incorrect border formation as a result of incorrect border length of the tray

5. Incorrect consistency of the final impression material when the tray was positioned in the mouth

6. Movement of the tray while the final impression material was setting

7. Improper pressure by the posterior palatal seal

Boxing impressions and making the casts

A wax form can be developed around most preliminary and final impressions for complete dentures to give the proper form and simplify making casts. The procedure for developing this form is called *boxing the impression*. Boxing procedures cannot usually be used on impressions made in hydrocolloid materials because the boxing material will not adhere to the impression material or because the impression will be distorted.

A strip of boxing wax is attached all the way around the outside of the impression approximately 1 to 2 mm below the border and sealed to it with a spatula. The boxing wax strip must be

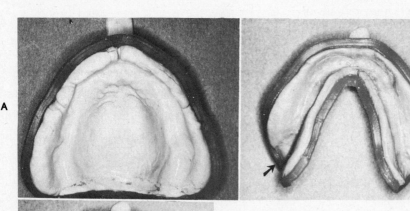

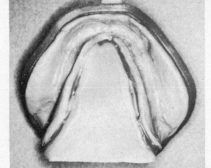

Fig. 10-10. A, Boxing wax has been securely attached just below borders of final upper impression. **B,** Boxing wax extends for its full width at posterior ends of impression *(arrows)* to hold vertical walls of boxing in proper position. **C,** Beeswax tongue-space filler has been securely sealed to boxing wax.

maintained at its full width particularly at the distal ends of the impressions. This will hold the vertical walls of the boxing away from the impressions and provide space for adequate thickness of the cast in these regions (Fig. 10-10, *A* and *B*). The vertical walls of the boxing are made of sheets of beeswax.

The tongue space in the lower impression is filled with a sheet of beeswax that is fitted and attached on the superior surface of the boxing wax. The beeswax tongue space filler is sealed to the boxing wax. The lingual borders of the impression must not be obliterated or disturbed by the beeswax filler or the boxing wax. The beeswax filler should be located just below the lingual border (Fig. 10-10, *C*).

A thin sheet of wax is used for making the vertical walls of the boxing. This may be special boxing wax, or a half sheet of beeswax may be cut lengthwise and used as boxing wax. This boxing wax is attached around the outside of the boxing strip so that it does not alter the borders of the impression. It should extend about ⅜ to ⅝ inch (9 to 15 mm) above the impression so that the base of the cast at its narrowest point will be of this thickness (Fig. 10-11, *A* and *B*). The impression should be supported in a level position by the boxing. The sheet of boxing wax should extend completely around the impression and be sealed to the boxing wax strip to prevent the escape of artificial stone when the stone is poured into the impression. The seal

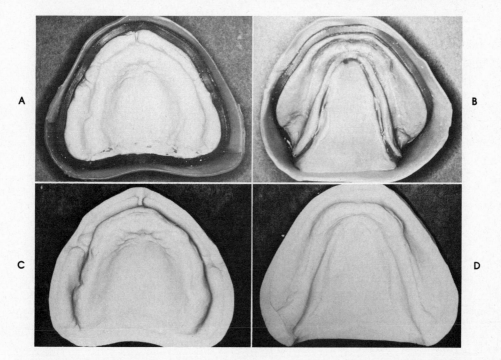

Fig. 10-11. A, Vertical wall of boxing is securely attached to boxing strip. Height of vertical wall will allow base of cast to be from ⅜ to ⅝ inches (9 to 15 mm) in thickness. **B,** Vertical wall of boxing is securely attached to strip of boxing wax and posterior extent of tongue-space filler. Notice that there is adequate space between posterior ends of impression and vertical boxing. **C,** Final upper cast provides an accurate, positive record of basal seat and reflections. The thickness and form of the land of cast will permit easy adaptation of materials used in making occlusion rims. **D,** Lower final cast is formed so that posterior ends of residual ridges are well supported with artificial stone providing needed strength in these regions.

between the boxing wax and the impression can be tested when the impression is held toward the light so that openings are observed. Sufficient space must be available posteriorly between the impression and the boxing to provide for an adequate thickness of the land of the casts distal to the impressions.

If a modified plaster is used as the final impression material, a separating medium must be applied to it and allowed to penetrate into the plaster. Then the impression is soaked in water until all air has been eliminated from the plaster. Just before the cast is to be poured, all excess separating medium is rinsed from the impression, and the excess water is shaken out.

Artificial stone is mixed according to the manufacturer's directions regarding powder and spatulation. Sufficient stone is poured into the boxed impression so that the base of the cast will be from ⅜ to ⅝ inch (9 to 15 mm) in thickness. The artificial stone is allowed to harden for at least 30 minutes before separation.

After the final impression is separated from the cast, the borders of the cast are trimmed so that a ledge of about ⅛ inch (3 mm) remains posteriorly and little or no ledge anteriorly. The cast must be shaped to maintain the form of the borders of the impression and yet be easily accessible for adaptation of the materials to be used for making occlusion rims (Fig. 10-11, C and D).

SECOND TECHNIQUE—SELECTIVE PRESSURE MANDIBULAR IMPRESSION—ONE-STEP BORDER-MOLDED TRAY*
Constructing autopolymerizing acrylic resin impression trays

1. Make a preliminary lower impression and pour the cast as described in the first technique (see p. 205).

*Smith, D.E., Toolson, L.B., Bolender, C.L., and Lord, J.L.: J. Prosthet. Dent. **41:**347, 1979.

2. Construct an auto polymerizing acrylic resin final impression tray on the relieved preliminary lower cast as in the first technique (see p. 208). Leave the relief wax in the tray (Fig. 10-12).
3. Reduce the borders of the tray until they are 2 mm underextended.

Border molding the mandibular tray

1. Prepare the mandibular tray for border molding in a similar manner as described for the maxillary tray (see p. 164).
2. Carefully evaluate the extensions of the tray intraorally.
3. Place adhesive over the borders of the tray.
4. Express a 4-inch strip of polyether material from the large tube and 3½ inches of catalyst from the small tube onto the mixing pad.
5. Thoroughly mix the material for 30 to 45 seconds using a metal spatula.
6. Position the polyether material on the borders. Make sure a minimum width of 6 mm exists on the inner portion (Fig. 10-13). Since approximately twice the length of borders are involved on the lower than on the upper tray, loading must be done with a minimal delay.
7. Place the impression tray in the mouth, making certain to retract the lips sufficiently to avoid scraping the polyether material from the borders.
8. Instruct the patient to elevate the tongue as the tray is seated.
9. Hold the lower lip out so that the excess material can flow labially.
10. Have the patient drop the tongue so that the tip contacts just behind the handle of the tray.
11. Quickly pull both cheeks buccally to make certain the cheek mucosa has not been trapped under the buccal flanges.
12. Complete the border-molding procedures as described in the first technique (Fig. 10-9, C to E).

13. Examine the borders after the material has set to determine if they are adequate (Fig. 10-14). The contour of the borders should be rounded.
14. Prepare the tray as described for the maxillary impression (see p. 166).

15. Make the final impression in silicone, metallic oxide paste, or rubber base impression material (Fig. 10-15). Use an appropriate adhesive on the impression surface of the tray when using the silicone material.

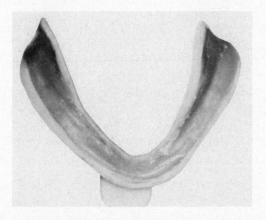

Fig. 10-12. The borders of the acrylic resin tray have been reduced. The relief wax remains in the tray.

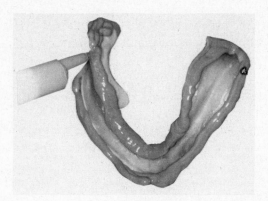

Fig. 10-13. The polyether impression material is placed around the borders of the tray until all have been covered.

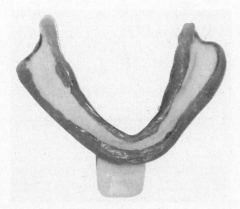

Fig. 10-14. Border molding has been completed. The relief wax has been removed from the tray.

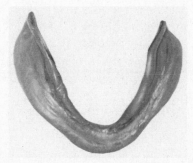

Fig. 10-15. The completed final impression using the one-step border-molded tray.

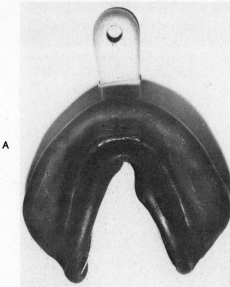

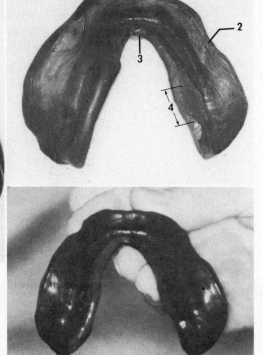

Fig. 10-16. **A,** Preliminary modeling compound impression in stock metal tray. **B,** One half of overextended lower preliminary modeling compound impression has been knife trimmed to approximate size of space available in mouth. Notice provision for labial notch, 1, buccal notch, 2, and lingual notch, 3. Notice also that lingual flange in molar region, 4, has been carved to slope toward tongue. **C,** Basal surface of modeling compound impression has been adapted to basal seat by uniform heating of entire impression surface. Notice that red modeling compound has been added to complete the form and give thickness to the right lingual flange. The borders have not yet been corrected.

THIRD TECHNIQUE—SELECTIVE PRESSURE MANDIBULAR IMPRESSION—MODELING COMPOUND TRAY
Preliminary impression

A preliminary impression is made in black modeling compound in a stock tray. The tray should be large enough for 6 mm of modeling compound between the impression surface and the metal. The preliminary impression should extend beyond the limits of the final impression (Fig. 10-16, *A*).

This impression is removed from the tray and is reinforced on its occlusal surface with a heavy wire. Then it is knife trimmed to approximately the size and shape of the final impression (Fig. 10-16, *B*). Careful observations of the distance from the crest of the residual ridge to the reflecting soft tissues serve as a guide for this trimming. Landmarks such as the impression of the external oblique line of the body of the mandible aid in making these visual measurements. The labial flange is carved to the thickness that will provide adequate support of the lower lip.

The lingual flange is knife trimmed to develop the S curve. If insufficient modeling compound exists on the lingual flange to permit this carving, red modeling compound is added on the lingual side of the lingual flange in the molar region. No modeling compound can be permitted to extend under the mylohyoid ridge. The modeling compound that may form an undercut in the impression under the mylohyoid ridge is carved away to permit the mylohyoid muscle to function normally (Fig. 10-16, *B*).

The distal end of the lingual flange is extended about 1 cm distal to the end of the mylohyoid ridge and is shaped so that it turns laterally toward the ramus below the level of the retromolar pad and mylohyoid ridge. Shaping and carving the lingual flange in this manner will produce the typical S curve in the border of the flange (Fig. 10-16, *B*).

Reshaping impression surface. The impression surface of the carved and chilled preliminary impression is then heated with an alcohol torch, tempered, and inserted into the mouth under pressure. The cold outside surface of the modeling compound impression serves as a tray for carrying, controlling, and confining the softened modeling compound on the impression surface while it is being readapted to the basal seat tissues (Fig. 10-16, *C*). This step may be repeated if necessary after the impression is chilled in ice water.

Border molding buccal and labial flanges. The buccal flanges are molded to fill but not overfill the lower buccal vestibules. The same border-molding procedures are used as were used for forming the buccal flanges of the upper modeling compound tray. A section of the border at a time is heated with an alcohol torch to a depth of 1.5 to 2 mm. Then it is tempered and placed in the mouth, and the cheek is grasped by the thumb and forefinger and is lifted out, up, forward, and back. The sections heated are overlapped so that each section is heated twice. The section including the lower buccal frenum must be molded with particular care in order to develop the buccal notch wide enough to allow clearance for the normal action of the buccal frenum (Fig. 10-17).

The labial flange is molded to provide the proper support for the lip. This flange must be at least 2 mm thick to support the plaster of a plaster impression.

Border molding lingual flanges. The lingual flanges are molded in five steps after having been knife trimmed and after labial and buccal borders are border molded.

First, the edge of the lingual flange is heated from one premylohyoid eminence to the other and is molded by having the tongue thrust out hard (Fig. 10-18, *A*). The premylohyoid eminence on the impression is located on the buccal side of the lingual flange at the position of the premylohyoid fossa. This step in the molding procedure determines the length of the lingual flange from one premolar region to the other.

Second, the *lingual side* of the lingual flange from one premolar region to the other is softened by the alcohol torch, and the tongue is thrust hard against the palate (Fig. 10-18, *B*). The action causes the base of the tongue to spread out and will determine the usable thickness of the anterior part of the lingual flange (see Fig. 10-7, *B*).

Third, the buccal side of the lingual flange from the premylohyoid eminence to the distal end is softened and inserted in the mouth, and the tongue is thrust out hard (Fig. 10-19, *A* and *B*). The *edge* of the flange is not heated in this step to maintain the extension of the border below the level of the mylohyoid ridge. If this procedure forces any modeling compound under the mylohyoid ridge or if the impression of the mylohyoid ridge becomes obvious on the lingual flange, more modeling compound is removed from the buccal side of the flange by knife trimming. This step is repeated until the flange in the molar region slopes toward the tongue and until the impression of the mylohyoid ridge is no longer visible in it.

Fourth, the border of the lingual flange from the premylohyoid eminence to the distal end is softened and border molded by having the tongue thrust out hard (Fig. 10-19, *C*). If this procedure forms an undercut under the mylohyoid ridge, the undercut is removed by knife trimming. Then the border and buccal surface of the lingual flange are reheated and remolded by the tongue thrust out of the mouth. This will determine the usable length and inclination of the flange.

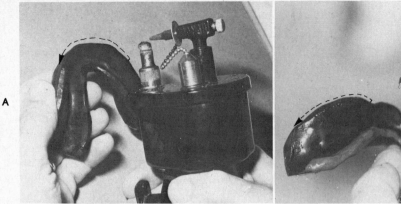

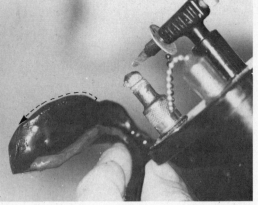

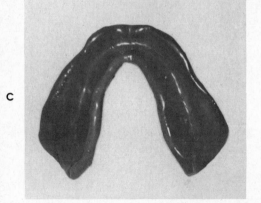

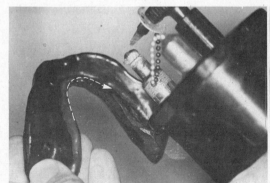

Fig. 10-17. Border molding of buccal and labial flanges is done a section at a time. **A,** Compound that forms edge of labial flange *(dotted line)* is softened to a depth of approximately 1.5 mm. Lower lip is lifted to border mold labial flange (see Fig. 10-6, *A*). **B,** The compound that forms the edge of the buccal flange *(dotted line)* is softened to a depth of 1.5 mm. Cheek is pulled outward, upward, and forward and backward to shape border of right buccal flange. Left buccal flange is shaped by manipulation of cheek in a similar manner (see Fig. 10-6, *C*). **C,** Buccal and labial borders have been molded.

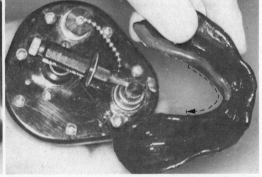

Fig. 10-18. Lingual flange is border molded in five steps that are designed to control amount of change accomplished in each step. **A,** *Step 1.* Edge of lingual flange is softened from premylohyoid eminence to premylohyoid eminence (premolar region to premolar region) *(dotted line)*. Tray is placed in mouth and tongue is thrust out (see Fig. 10-7, *A*). This procedure determines the length of the anterior part of the lingual flange. **B,** *Step 2.* Lingual side of lingual flange is heated from premylohyoid eminence to premylohyoid eminence *(dotted line)*. Tongue is pushed against roof of the mouth causing base of the tongue to spread out (see Fig. 10-7, *B*). This determines thickness of anterior part of lingual flange. (See Fig. 10-20 for description of steps 3 to 5.)

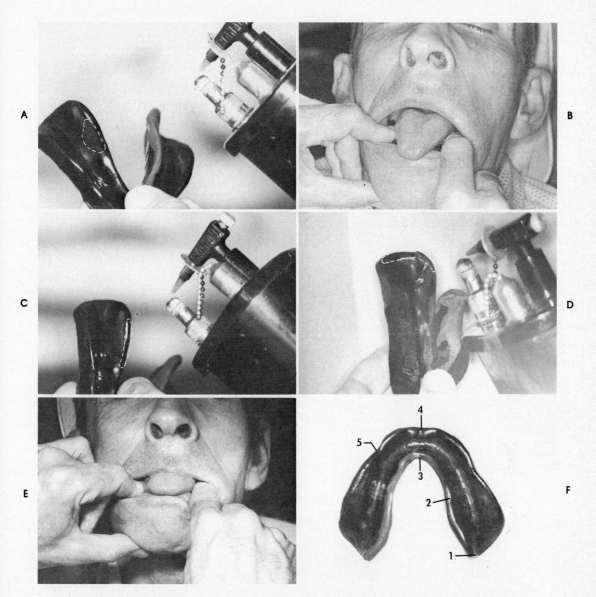

Fig. 10-19. A, Buccal sides of *both* lingual flanges are heated in location of dotted line. **B,** Tongue is thrust out, and action of mylohyoid muscle raising the floor of the mouth determines lingual inclination or slope of lingual flange toward tongue in molar regions. **C,** *Step 4.* Borders of both lingual flanges in molar regions are heated *(at dotted line),* impression is placed in mouth, and tongue is thrust out again. This procedure determines length of lingual flange in molar region. **D,** *Step 5.* Distal ends of both lingual flanges are heated *(at dotted line).* **E,** Tongue is thrust out hard, and patient closes lower jaw against pressure applied by dentist on impression. Resulting action of medial pterygoid muscle on retromylohyoid curtain limits tray in this region. **F,** Completed modeling compound impression. *1,* Postmylohyoid eminence; *2,* premylohyoid eminence; *3,* lingual notch; *4,* labial notch; *5,* buccal notch.

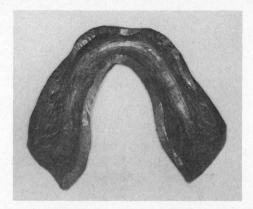

Fig. 10-20. Basal surface of modeling compound tray is reduced 1 mm except from retromylohyoid eminences. Borders are reduced 1.5 mm except at distal end of lingual flange. Completed modeling compound impression has now been converted into a modeling compound tray.

Fifth, the distal end of the preliminary impression from the lower border of the lingual flange to the buccal side of the distal end of the buccal flange is softened (Fig. 10-19, *D*). The impression is placed in the mouth, the tongue is thrust out hard, and the mouth is opened wide and then closed against pressure applied by the dentist on the impression. The tongue thrust determines the distal extent of the lingual flange. The mouth opened wide pulls the pterygomandibular raphe forward against the lingual side of the part of the impression covering the retromolar pad. Thus the pterygomandibular raphe determines the distal extent of the occlusal part of the preliminary impression. Closure of the mouth brings the medial pterygoid muscles as far forward as they would be in function. If they are placed so that they would contact the retromylohyoid curtain under this circumstance, the distal end of the lingual flange will be shortened to accommodate them (Fig. 10-19, *E* and *F*).

Modeling compound tray. The modeling compound impression is converted into a tray by shortening of all its borders 1.5 mm by knife trimming, and 1 mm of modeling compound is scraped from the inside of the impression (Fig. 10-20). The space thus created is available for

the plaster impression material, and it makes possible the elimination of some of the inaccuracies inherent in the modeling compound impression.

At least 1 mm of space is provided over the entire inside of the impression except on the buccal side of the retromylohyoid eminence. No modeling compound is removed from the retromylohyoid eminence. In most instances, it is better to provide a slight excess of space for plaster if there is any doubt about the amount of space being provided for it.

Mandibular preliminary impression

The impression material is mixed according to the manufacturer's directions, is spread uniformly over the prepared surface of the tray in excess, and is carried to the mouth (Fig. 10-21, *A*). The retromylohyoid eminences are placed in position first, and then the tray is centered over the ridge.

Immediately the tips of both index fingers are placed on the occlusal surface of the tray in the molar region and with alternation of pressure from one side to the other, the tray is seated into place. The patient is asked to open the mouth partway and to slowly raise the tongue under the upper lip. Opening the mouth will border mold

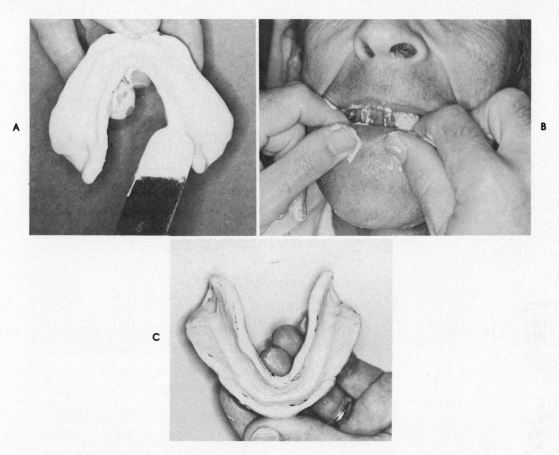

Fig. 10-21. Mandibular preliminary impression. **A,** Impression material is distributed over modeling compound tray. **B,** With tray carrying impression material in position in mouth, patient raises tongue to "touch the upper front teeth" to mold the impression material on borders of lingual flanges. Lip is elevated to mold impression material on labial flange. **C,** Completed impression that will be used to make final impression tray. Labial, buccal, and lingual borders are most important part of this preliminary impression. Final lower impression will selectively place pressure on residual alveolar ridge.

the buccal flange, and raising the tongue will mold the lingual flanges. The lower lip and corners of the mouth are elevated by the thumbs to mold the labial flange and buccal notches (Fig. 10-21, *B*).

When the impression material has set, the impression is removed. The impression should have well-rounded borders all the way around and should have no severe pressure spots (Fig. 10-21, *C*). The tongue space is closed, and a stone cast is poured.

Final impression

Acrylic resin tray. The final impression is made in a zinc oxide–eugenol impression material in a cold curing acrylic resin tray. The tray is made of this material because it can be shaped nearly like the desired final impression, is strong enough to serve the purpose with no more bulk than will be in the finished denture, and will not warp significantly in the process. The final impression tray is made as described for the first technique (see Fig. 10-4). Since this tray has

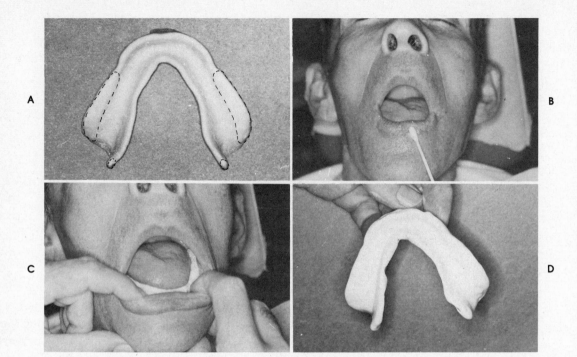

Fig. 10-22. A, Tray is prepared for final impression. Basal surface of tray has not been relieved in regions of buccal shelf or from retromylohyoid eminences *(dotted lines)*. **B,** In preparation for final impression, the skin around mouth is lubricated with petroleum jelly. **C,** A gauze roll is placed under tongue to absorb saliva. It will be removed just before impression is to be made. **D,** Mixed paste is distributed on tray with a spatula.

been border molded, it should be ready for the final impression with only minor adjustments (Fig. 10-22, *A*).

Preparation of the patient. The patient's clothing should be protected by a plastic apron. The patient's face is lubricated with petroleum jelly, and a roll of gauze is placed under the tongue to help keep the mouth dry (Fig. 10-22, *B* and *C*).

Zinc oxide–eugenol impression material. The final mandibular impression can be made in one of the zinc oxide–eugenol impression materials. These are manufactured under different names by many different manufacturers. The essential ingredients are zinc oxide and eugenol, which, when mixed, will form a smooth paste. The paste sets by saponification. The materials are

modified by the manufacturers so that each has a different viscosity and different working properties. This gives dentists a choice of materials to correspond with their impression techniques and working conditions.

Most of these materials are available in collapsible tubes. The extrusion of equal lengths of the two materials from the two tubes onto a mixing pad provides a simple means for measuring the ingredients of a mix. The two ingredients are mixed on the mixing pad according to the manufacturer's directions. Mixing usually requires 60 seconds.

Loading impression tray. The completed mix is spread out in a thin layer on the mixing pad. The tray is grasped by the thumb and forefinger of the left hand, and about one third of the mix is

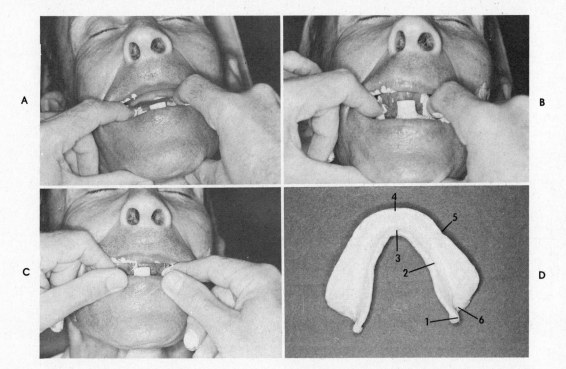

Fig. 10-23. A, Tray carrying final impression material is placed in position in patient's mouth. Amount of pressure exerted on posterior handles will determine amount of displacement of soft tissue on buccal shelf of mandible. This will determine amount of relief given to sharp points of bone on crest of residual ridge. **B,** After 15 seconds, patient is instructed to open the mouth wide and to raise tongue to "touch the upper front teeth." The wide-open position of the mouth molds impression material on buccal and labial borders. Raised tongue molds impression material on lingual borders. **C,** Lip is gently raised to ensure molding of labial borders and in region of buccal notches. **D,** Final zinc oxide–eugenol impression. *1,* Retromylohyoid eminence; *2,* premylohyoid eminence; *3,* lingual notch; *4,* labial notch; *5,* buccal notch; *6,* retromolar fossa.

scraped off the mixing pad onto a spatula. Then starting near the midline, the paste is wiped from the spatula onto the tray on one side. The procedure is repeated to place the paste in the other side of the tray. The remaining paste can be used if necessary to make certain that there is an excess of the material in the tray (Fig. 10-22, *D*). After the impression material is in the tray, the tray is shifted to the right hand and is held by the thumb and forefinger on the anterior handle. When the tray is carried to the mouth, the tray is rotated in such a way that the impression paste does not run out of the tray. To do this, one turns the impression surface down, then up,

then down, then up, and then down again until the tray is inserted into the mouth.

Insertion of tray. The gauze is quickly removed, and the tray is centered in the mouth over the residual ridge.

At this time, the patient is directed to raise the tongue just a little. The distal end of one side (usually the right) of the tray is placed nearly in position in the retromylohyoid space, and the distal end of the other lingual flange is placed nearly in position in its retromylohyoid space. Then the anterior part of the tray is gently pushed down nearly to its eventual position. The relationship of the buccal notch and the buccal frenum on the patient's right side can serve as a guide for this procedure.

At this time, the tray is released completely for a moment as the index fingers are placed on the posterior handles (Fig. 10-23, A). Gentle downward pressure on the posterior handles is used to seat the tray, and the fingers must be held in position until the impression material has set.

Molding borders of final impression. After 15 to 20 seconds the patient is directed to open the mouth wide and to hold it in that position. This will mold the impression material at the labial and buccal borders. Immediately, the patient is directed to place the tip of the tongue against the upper front teeth and to hold it there (Fig. 10-23, B). This will mold the impression material on the lingual flange and borders. The patient must hold this position until the impression material is set. Then, the dentist gently raises the lower lip with his thumbs (Fig. 10-23, C). No other border-molding movements can be permitted, and the patient *must not* press the tongue against the anterior part of the tray. The shape of the tray and the patient's efforts determine the shape of the borders of the impression.

Removal of impression. After the impression material has set to its ultimate hardness, the lower lip is pulled down with the left hand and the front end of the impression is lifted by the finger and thumb of the right hand on the anterior handle. Then the distal end of one side of the impression is unhooked from the retromylohyoid space, after which the other distal end is lifted and the impression is removed from the mouth (Fig. 10-23, D).

The final impression is inspected, and if the impression is acceptable, the cast is poured immediately.

11

Biologic considerations of jaw relations and jaw movements

When the mandible moves as it does in carrying out the functions of mastication and speech, the various movements it makes and the relationships it assumes defy description because of their complexity. However, when the mandible is motionless, definite realtionships to the cranium or the maxillae can be established. Thus one needs to study certain static relationships to understand the motions made by the mandible in function. If we know the potential limits of the motions of the mandible, we will know the confines of the envelope of motion within which it can move.

To understand jaw motions, it is necessary to understand the factors involved in jaw relations.

ANATOMIC FACTORS

All jaw relations are bone-to-bone relations. The mandibular bone has specific relationships to the bones of the cranium. The mandible is connected to the cranium at the two temporomandibular joints by the temporomandibular and capsular ligaments. The sphenomandibular and stylomandibular ligaments also connect the bones in such a way as to limit some motions of the mandible. The masseter, temporal, and medial pterygoid muscles supply the power for pulling the mandible against the maxillae, and the lateral pterygoid muscles connect the mandible to the lateral pterygoid plate in such a way as to act as the steering mechanism for the mandible and act to protrude the jaw or to move it laterally (Fig. 11-9).

The other connection between the upper and lower jaws is through occlusal surfaces of the teeth. For this reason the occlusion of the teeth must be in harmony with the jaw relations when the teeth are in contact.

TEMPOROMANDIBULAR JOINT ARTICULATION

Good prosthodontic treatment bears a direct relation to the structures of the temporomandibular articulation, since occlusion is one of the most important parts of treatment of patients with complete dentures. The temporomandibular joints affect the dentures, and likewise the dentures affect the health and function of the joints. Therefore a knowledge of the interrelationship of the bony structures, tissue resiliency, muscle function, movements of the lips, facial muscles, muscles of mastication, occlusions of the teeth, temporomandibular joints, and overriding mental attitudes seems indispensable for treatment of edentulous patients to qualify as a true health service.

Bony structure

The bony portion of the temporomandibular articulation is made up of the mandibular fossa of the temporal bone and the condyloid process of the mandible.

Mandibular fossa. The fossa is located in front of and below the auditory meatus. It runs forward to the articular eminence, which is at the posterior end of the zygomatic arch. The fossa is approximately 1 inch (2.5 cm) long anteroposteriorly and ¾ inch (19 mm) in width laterally and medially. It runs obliquely from the zygomatic arch medialward, to reach under and behind the auditory meatus. The outer border of the fossa and the bony part of the temporal bone in front of the auditory meatus run parallel; that is, the skull becomes narrower as it approaches the meatus. This converging of the bone accounts for the fact that the condyles project out beyond

the distal part of the fossae and can be felt in the soft tissues in front of the external auditory meatus. The styloid process leaves the temporal bone immediately behind the fossa.

The fossa is divided into two parts by the petrotympanic fissure, through which the anterior tympanic branch of the internal maxillary artery passes. The chorda tympani nerve emerges from the tympanic cavity through a foramen situated at the inner end of the petrotympanic fussure. This foramen is named the iter chordae anterius (canal of Huguier).

Anterior portion. The anterior portion of the fossa is the principal bearing surface upon which the condyle presses through the disk and other structures (Fig. 11-1).

Posterior portion. The posterior portion of the fossa is more nearly perpendicular (Fig. 11-1). The condyle does not bear directly in the fossa because it is separated by the synovial membranes and the articular disk—the meniscus. Too often in the registration of the condylar inclination the erroneous assumption is made that the registration is a reproduction of the bony path, whereas it is a reproduction of the movement created by the condyle sliding with the articular disk over the fossa and the articular eminence. The registration is based on the influence of the bony incline on the meniscus together with the influence of the ligaments and muscle pull.

Condyles. The condyle does not take the shape of the mandibular fossa. It fills it laterally, being approximately ¾ inch (19 mm) wide, but it is less than ½ inch (12.5 mm) in diameter anteroposteriorly and therefore does not fill the fossa to its anteroposterior limits (Fig. 11-2). The outer extremity of the condyle extends ½ inch beyond the bony limits of the meatus, and therefore its movements can be felt in the soft portions of the ear. The shape of condyles varies greatly and so does the direction of the long portion of the condyle if extended medially (Figs. 11-3 and 11-4; see also Fig. 9-1). The lateral extremity of the condyle is nearly flush with the surface of the ramus and projects medialward.

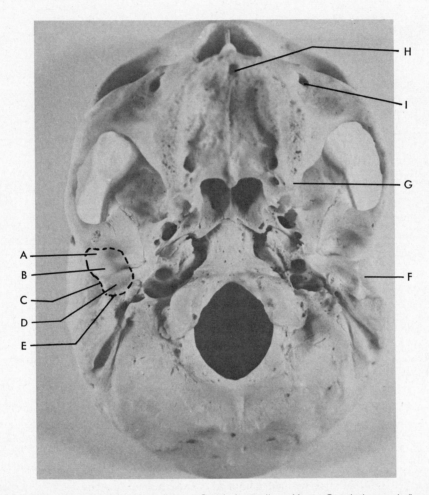

Fig. 11-1. Glenoid fossa. *A,* Articular eminence; *B,* anterior portion of fossa; *C,* petrotympanic fissure; *D,* posterior portion of fossa; *E,* rim of fossa; *F,* external auditory meatus; *G,* pterygomaxillary (hamular) notch; *H,* incisive formen; *I,* infraorbital foramen.

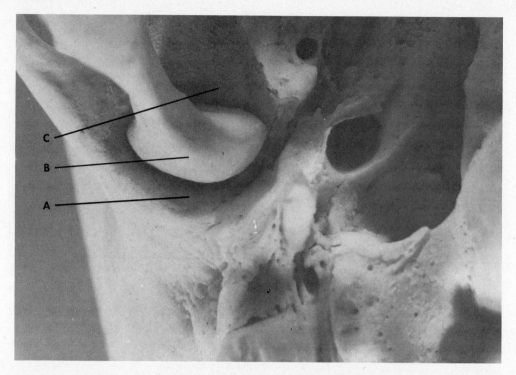

Fig. 11-2. Condyle is in its approximate position in mandibular (glenoid) fossa. Condyle functions through articular disk on slope of articular eminence. Notice that condyle does not fill fossa antero-posteriorly. *A,* Posterior portion of mandibular fossa; *B,* condyle; *C,* articular eminence.

The neck of the condyle is constricted antero-posteriorly and laterally to about one half the size of the maximum dimension of the condyle (Fig. 11-5). The capsular ligament is attached in this constricted area.

Ligaments

The ligaments of the temoromandibular joint are the capsular ligament, the temporomandibular ligament, the sphenomandibular ligament, and the stylomandibular ligament. The function of the ligaments is to limit motion in the joint.

The mandibular fossa is lined by a synovial membrane, which separates the condyle from the fossa. The synovial membrane starts anterior to the condyle, at its full width, and covers it down to the neck posteriorly.

Capsular ligament. The capsular ligament completely envelops the joint. It is attached superiorly to the rim of the mandibular fossa and to the articular eminence. Inferiorly it attaches by enveloping the neck of the condyle. The direction of its fibers is downward and backward.

Temporomandibular ligament. The temporomandibular ligament may be divided into two portions, anterior and posterior. It is attached superiorly to the articular eminence and to the inferior border of the zygomatic arch. Its fibers then run *downward* and *backward* to attach to the outer and posterior border of the upper portion of the ramus. It is a factor in limiting the posterior movement of the condyle by causing the condyle to rotate upward against the disk and fossa.

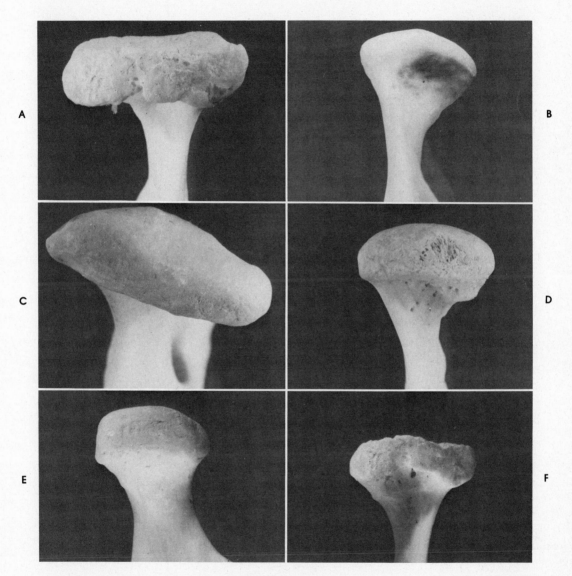

Fig. 11-3. Six condyles (**A** to **F**) from six different edentulous patients are all different in size and form. Notice bony changes on anterior and superior surfaces of condyles **A, D,** and **F**.

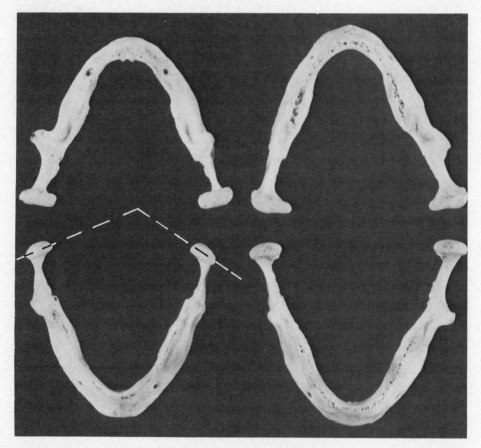

Fig. 11-4. Superior view of four mandibles. If long axes of condyles of mandible *(lower left)* were extended mesiodistally, they would meet posteriorly somewhere in region of anterior part of foramen magnum. However, this would not be true for condyles of the other three mandibles.

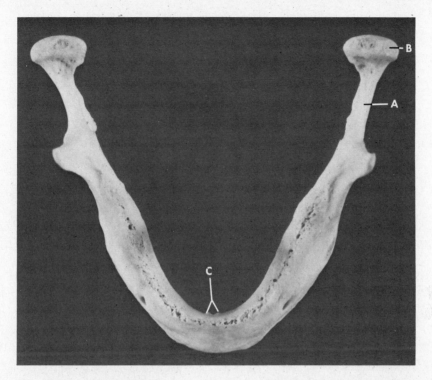

Fig. 11-5. The neck of condyle, A, is considerably constricted in relation to condyle itself, B. Notice cancellous appearance of bone on crest of residual ridge in comparison with compact appearance in region of buccal shelf. C, Genial tubercles.

Sphenomandibular ligament. The sphenomandibular ligament is attached superiorly to the angle spine of the sphenoid bone and runs down on the inner surface of the ramus to attach inferiorly to the lingula of the inferior mandibular foramen.

Stylomandibular ligament. The stylomandibular ligament attaches to the styloid process and to the medial side of the angle of the mandible and at its posterior border.

Articular disk

The articular disk (meniscus) plays a prominent part in the movement of the mandible. It is made up of fibrous connective tissue with collagen fibers running in all directions and providing flexibility. It is situated between the two synovial membranes of the joint. The upper surface of the disk is convex to fit the shape of the fossa. The undersurface is somewhat concave to fit the condyle. This disk extends forward over the articular eminence. The position and movement of the disk are controlled by its attachment to the capsular ligament and, anteriorly, by the tendon of the lateral pterygoid muscle. The lateral pterygoid muscle also attaches along its medial border (Fig. 11-6). The articular disk has very little movement in the first opening movements of the mandible when the condyle merely rotates. However, it has extensive movements when the mandible makes wider opening movements or lateral or protrusive movements. The disk then travels with the condyle (Fig. 11-7) in the healthy joint because it is tightly attached to the lateral and medial poles of the condyle. The disk can move forward and back over the

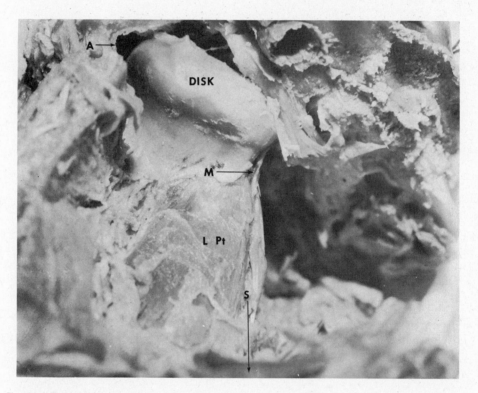

Fig. 11-6. The lateral pterygoid muscle, *L Pt,* and disk from above. Dissection was made from cranium into temporomandibular joint. *A,* Space produced by rotation of mandible, muscle, and disk forward and laterally. *M,* Medial fibers of lateral pterygoid muscle that attach to medial side of disk. *S,* Sagittal plane, with the arrow indicating anterior part of specimen. Notice that lateral pterygoid muscle attaches to mesial side of disk and to neck of condyle as well as to anterior side of disk. (Courtesy Dr. M.R. Porter, Ohio State University College of Dentistry.)

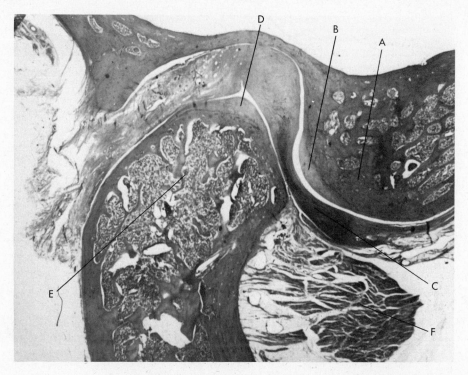

Fig. 11-7. Sagittal section through an adult temporomandibular joint. *A,* Articulating eminence; *B,* fibrous tissue covering eminence; *C,* meniscus; *D,* fibrous tissue covering condyle; *E,* condyle; *F,* lateral pterygoid muscle. (Courtesy Dr. Rudi Melfi, Ohio State University College of Dentistry.)

condyle but cannot move from side to side. The capsule and disk are attached together where they join bone. A number of blood vessels surround the joint but do penetrate within the disk.

Nerve supply

Three nerves innervate the jaw joints. They are the auriculotemporal nerves, the posterior deep temporal nerves, and the masseteric nerves. The auriculotemporal nerves innervate approximately 85% to 90% of the temporomandibular joints.

Muscles

Muscles of mastication. The muscles of mastication include the temporal, the masseter, the medial pterygoid, and the lateral pterygoid mus-

cles. The first three of these are closing muscles, and the fourth is a guiding muscle.

Temporal muscle. The temporal muscle arises on the side of the head from the whole of the temporal fossa and attaches to the tip and the inner and anterior surfaces of the coronoid process of the mandible (see Fig. 11-23). The anterior fibers go down the anterior surface of the coronoid process of the mandible and down the anterior surface of the ramus with some fibers extending into the retromolar pad and nearly as far forward as the third molar. The function of the posterior part of this muscle is to retrude the mandible and brace the condyle during lateral mandibular excursions to the same side. The function of the middle parts is to elevate the mandible into centric position. The temporal muscle does not participate in biting force when the mandible is in protrusion. Therefore the action of this muscle is sometimes used as a test to determine whether the patient is closing in centric relation. When the mandible is in protrusion, no bulging can be felt with the fingers on the side of the head in the region of the temples.

Masseter muscle. The masseter muscle is a thick muscle consisting of two portions, the superficial and the deep. Arising from the zygomatic process of the maxilla and from the zygomatic arch of the zygomatic bone, it is inserted on the outer surface of the ramus and the lateral surface of the coronoid process of the mandible. Its action is almost entirely that of an elevator of the mandible. The deep fibers aid in retruding the mandible from a forward position. The masseter muscle affects the border of the mandibular denture on the distobuccal corner of the buccal flange. Its action pushes the buccinator fibers against the denture border; for this reason the

border must converge rapidly toward the retromolar pad. At the time the preliminary impression is made, while the compound on the border of the impression tray in this region is still soft, considerable downward force should be exerted on the lower jaw by the dentist so that the patient, in attempting to counteract this downward pressure, will cause the masseter muscle to contract, therefore forcing the softened compound away from impingement in this region (Fig. 11-8).

Medial pterygoid muscle. The first portion of the medial pterygoid muscle arises from the medial surface of the lateral pterygoid plate and the palatine bone. The second portion arises from the pyramidal process of the palatine bone and the posterior end of the maxilla. The medial pterygoid is inserted into the lower and posterior surfaces of the ramus and into the medial side of the angle of the mandible (Fig. 11-9). The action of this muscle is mostly that of an eleva-

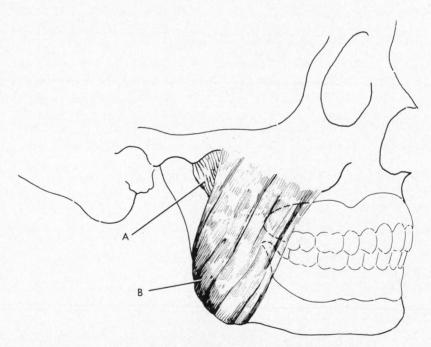

Fig. 11-8. Masseter muscle. The buccal flange contour of a mandibular impression is influenced by anterior fibers of masseter muscle. *A,* Deep portion; *B,* superficial portion.

tor, though it does assist in the lateral and protrusive movements of the mandible.

Lateral pterygoid muscle. The lateral pterygoid muscle arises from two heads, the superior belly from the greater wing of the sphenoid bone and the inferior belly from the lateral pterygoid plate. Its fibers run horizontally backward and laterally. The superior belly attaches mostly to the disk and to the neck of the condyle and the inferior belly to the neck of the condyle (Fig. 11-9). The principal action of the lateral pterygoid muscle is the protrusion of one or both condyles. When only one condyle is protruded, the mandible moves laterally to the opposite side. The lateral pterygoid muscles guide the mandible into lateral or protrusive positions so that food may be engaged by the teeth. The superior belly is active in a stabilizing capacity or fixes the condyle and disk in a specific position during elevation of the mandible. However, it is not a muscle that elevates the mandible.

Muscles of depression. There are three groups of muscles that act to depress the mandible. The suprahyoid muscles (the digastric, geniohyoid, mylohyoid, and stylohyoid) and the platysma act as a group and are the primary movers in the opening of the mandible. The infrahyoid group extends from the hyoid bone to the sternum and acts to stabilize the hyoid bone so that the suprahyoid group can be effective. The third group, the lateral pterygoid muscles, pulls the condyles forward or medialward as the other groups act.

The mylohyoid muscle is the only one of these muscles that affects denture borders. Some of the salient factors regarding this muscle are discussed here (Fig. 11-10). The mylohyoid muscle arises from the inner surface of the mandible on a line extending posteriorly from the symphysis to the distal aspect of the third molar. The area of origin of the muscle on the mandible is known as the mylohyoid ridge. It is close to the crest of

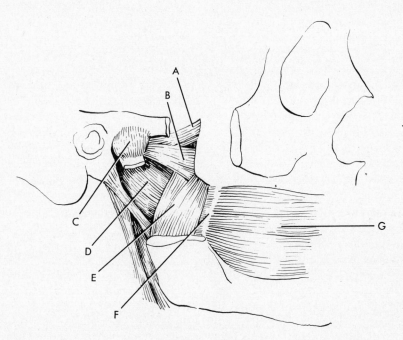

Fig. 11-9. Notice difference in direction of fibers of medial (internal) and lateral (external) pterygoid muscles. *A*, Superior head of lateral pterygoid muscle; *B*, inferior head of lateral pterygoid muscle; *C*, capsule of temporomandibular joint; *D*, superior constrictor muscle; *E*, medial pterygoid muscle; *F*, pterygomandibular raphe; *G*, buccinator muscle.

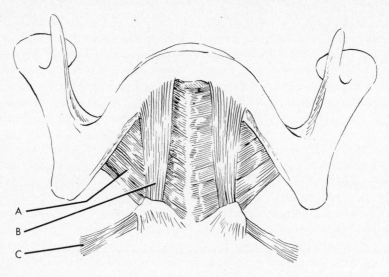

Fig. 11-10. Anteroinferior view of mandible and muscles of the floor of the mouth. *A,* Mylohyoid muscle; *B,* anterior belly of digastric muscle; *C,* posterior belly of digastric muscle.

the alveolar process in the third molar region and then gradually becomes lower as it goes forward until it is near the lower border of the mandible in the anterior portion (see Fig. 9-10). This muscle runs medially and downward and forward to join the opposite mylohyoid muscle at the median line and insert into the anterior cornu of the hyoid bone. The mylohyoid muscle, together with the geniohyoid, forms the muscular floor of the mouth upon which the tongue and other structures rest (see Fig. 9-22). This muscle aids in the opening action of the mandible, but its principal action is that of assisting in the act of swallowing by raising the tongue and the floor of the mouth and elevating the hyoid bone. Consideration of the act of swallowing is extremely important for establishing the stability of the mandibular complete denture. When the mylohyoid muscle is in a tense state, it is pulled away from the mandible; therefore the lingual flange of the denture cannot impinge on this muscle without the denture being displaced at the time of swallowing or raising the tongue.

When the mylohyoid muscle is relaxed, it falls down along the lingual surface of the mandible and even under the mylohyoid ridge in the

molar region. For that reason the impression material can follow incorrectly along the lingual contour of the mandible into the undercut below the mylohyoid ridge. Should the lingual flange of the denture extend into the undercut, it will bind the muscle so that the muscle will be restricted in movement; otherwise, the muscle will cause displacement of the denture when contracted. The resorption of the alveolar process causes a sharpening of the mylohyoid ridge. The resulting sharp ridge with a muscle attaching to it is the source of much soreness because the hard surface of the denture irritates the end fibers of the muscle as a result of an impingement between the sharp ridge and hard denture base (see Fig. 9-13).

CLASSIFICATION OF JAW RELATIONS

Jaw relations are classified into three groups to make them more easily understood: (1) orientation relations, (2) vertical relations, and (3) horizontal relations. Considered in this manner, the relation of the mandible to the maxillae (or cranium) can be accurately determined in three dimensions. Orientation relations establish the references in the cranium. Vertical relations establish the amount of jaw separation allowable for use for dentures, and horizontal jaw relations establish the front-to-back and side-to-side relationships of one jaw to the other. Thus, with specific distances designated in the three dimensions of space, the mandible can be accurately located in relation to the maxillae.

Orientation relations

The orientation relations are those that orient the mandible to the cranium in such a way that, when the mandible is kept in its most posterior position, the mandible can rotate in the sagittal plane around an imaginary transverse axis passing through or near the condyles. The axis can be located when the mandible is in its most posterior position by means of a kinematic face-bow or hinge-bow, or it can be approximated by use of an arbitrary type of face-bow.

Face-bow. The face-bow is a caliper-like device that is used to record the relationship of the jaws to the temporomandibular joints or the opening axis of the jaws and to orient the casts in this same relationship to the opening axis of the articulator. The face-bow is also a convenient instrument for supporting the casts while they are being attached to the articulator.

The face-bow consists of U-shaped frame or assembly that is large enough to extend from the region of the temporomandibular joints to a position 2 to 3 inches (5 to 7.5 cm) in front of the face and wide enough to avoid contact with the sides of the face. The parts that contact the skin over the temporomandibular joints are the condyle rods, and the part that attaches to the occlusion rims is the fork. The fork of the face-bow attaches to the face-bow by means of a locking device. The locking device serves also to support the face-bow, the occlusion rims, and the casts while the casts are being attached to the articulator.

There are two basic types of face-bows: the arbitrary face-bow and the kinematic face-bow, or hinge-bow. The arbitrary face-bow is placed on the face with the condyle rods located approximately over the condyles, and the kinematic face-bow is designed so that the opening

axis of the mandible can be located more accurately (see Fig. 11-16, *B*).

The arbitrary face-bow is the one most used for patients in complete denture techniques. It is considered to be adequate for this purpose. The condyle rods of one commonly used arbitrary face-bow are positioned on a line extending from the outer canthus of the eye to the top of the tragus of the ear and approximately 13 mm in front of the external auditory meatus. This placement of the condyle rods will generally locate them within 5 mm of the true center of the opening axis of the jaws. The condylar rods of another commonly used arbitrary face-bow are designed to fit into the external auditory meatuses. The location of the rods on the articulator approximately compensate for the distance the meatuses are posterior to the transverse opening axis of the mandible.

The fork of the arbitrary face-bow is attached to the maxillary occlusion rim so that the record is one of a simple measurement from the jaws to the approximate axis of the jaws.

The fork of the kinematic face-bow is attached to the mandibular occlusion rim. Then, as the patient retrudes the mandible and opens and closes the jaws, the dentist observes the movement of the points of the condyle rods. The condyle rods of kinematic face-bows have sharp points so that their motion can be observed more accurately. When the points of the condyle rods rotate only and do not translate, the points are on the opening axis of the jaw. At this position the mandible is as far back as it will go and can be considered to be in centric relation for the occlusal vertical relation that has been established.

Since the face-bow is used to orient the casts on the articulator in the same relation to the opening axis of the articulator as the jaws have to the opening axis of the jaws, the face-bow record is not a maxillomandibular relation record. It is a record made for the orientation of the casts to the instrument. However, use of a kinematic face-bow can aid in the recording of centric relation.

The posterior terminal hinge axis of the mandible can be located only when the mandible is in its most posterior position, that is, when the mandible is in centric relation (assuming that the vertical relation of the jaws has been established). The difficulty in attaching the lower occlusion rim to an edentulous mandible so that it does not move in relation to the bone prevents its more extensive use for edentulous patients. The inevitable movement of the recording base in relation to the bone makes the determination of the exact center of the opening axis quite difficult.

Value of the face-bow. Failure to use the face-bow can lead to errors in occlusion of the denture. It is true that the errors may be small if the error in orientation of the casts is small. Likewise, the errors produced by failure to use the face-bow would be negligible if all the

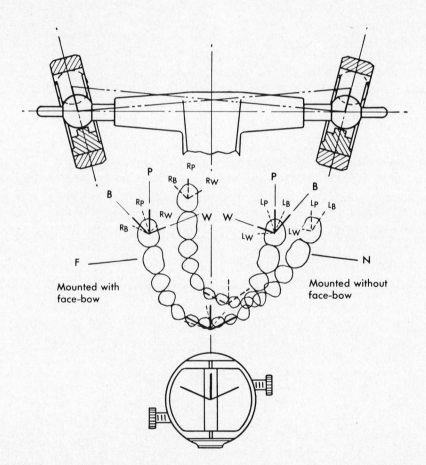

Fig. 11-11. Occlusion and occlusal aspect, with and without face-bow mounting, *B-P-W,* Balancing, protrusive, and working strokes. *F,* Denture mounted with face-bow, showing direction of balancing, protrusive, and working strokes making needle-point tracings in anterior and molar regions. This mounting would coincide with movements in the mouth, and tracings would reflect direction of movements in the mouth. *N,* Denture mounted in articulator without face-bow. The tracings reflect movements of articulator only, and therefore denture would occlude properly only on articulator. When denture *N* is superimposed on denture *F,* tracings of the two dentures *(dotted lines)* do not coincide. Notice that needlepoint tracings of denture *N* are at an incorrect angle and therefore will not coincide with movements of mandible.

interocclusal records were made precisely at the occlusal vertical relation at which the occlusion was to be established and if zero-degree teeth were used. However, if cusp teeth are used or if interocclusal records are made with the teeth out of contact so that the vertical separation of the casts or dentures must be reduced *on the articulator*, the face-bow record is essential. The face-bow transfer allows a more accurate arc of closure on the articulator when the interocclusal records are removed and the articulator is closed. Its use requires little time, and the convenience it provides in the cast-mounting procedure saves that time.

Fig. 11-11 is a schematic drawing of a comparative study of mounting dentures with and without a face-bow.

Fig. 11-12 shows the variations in registration

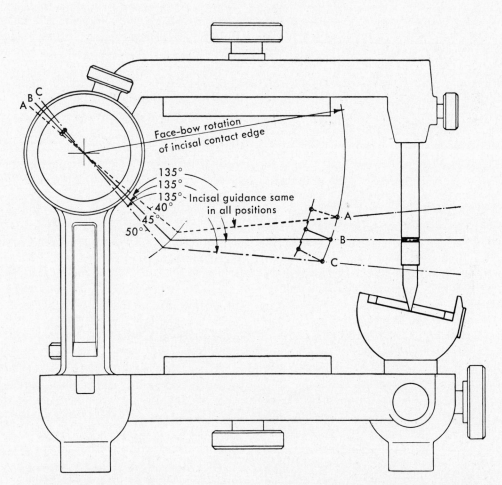

Fig. 11-12. Schematic drawing showing variance of condyle registration on articulator (40, 45, and 50 degrees), which is the result of mounting casts with a face-bow at various heights (*A, B,* and *C*). However, the cast-condylar angle remains the same in all positions, which is 135 degrees. Therefore movement of the cast in relation to condylar inclination is the same in all three positions, which fact makes the height of mounting immaterial.

of condylar guidance on the articulator when the casts are mounted at various heights—the highest mounting at *A*, the intermediate height mounting at *B*, and the lowest mounting at *C*. The cast-condylar angle remains 135 degrees regardless of the height of mounting.

Face-bows such as the Hanau Model C and many others are predicated on an arbitrary location of the opening axis of the mandible. The condyle is not a point, whereas its hinge axis or kinematic center is an exact point. To palpate for the center of the condyle or to set it by arbitrary lines is to use an approximation. However, this method is better than not using a face-bow at all. The approximation works well in complete denture construction, but it produces inaccuracies when wax or plaster is interposed for maxillomandibular records or when fixed or partial dentures are constructed for vertical dimension increase. This difficulty can be removed by use of a kinematic face-bow, which aids in finding the kinematic center of jaw opening.

The Hanau Model C face-bow and most other arbitrary face-bows are adjusted to a point on the face. The point is marked 13 mm forward from the external auditory meatus on a line from the top of the tragus of the ear to the corner of the eye (outer canthus of the eye). Without clamping the condyle rods, the dentist centers the device so that equal readings are obtained on both sides, and the wing nut of the clamp is tightened to hold the face-bow in place on the occlusal fork (see Figs. 15-6 and 15-7).

The Whip Mix face-bow is also an arbitrary face-bow (see Fig. 15-17). The ends of the bow are placed in the external auditory meatus instead of being placed over the condyles. However, when the instrument is attached to the articulator, the transverse axis of the articulator is ⅝ inch (15 mm) anterior to the position of the ends of the face-bow. This distance compensates for the distance between the external auditory meatus and the condyle. Thus the effective result is approximately the same as with other types of arbitrary face-bows.

The kinematic face-bow (see Fig. 11-16, *B*) is

first fastened to the mandibular occlusion rim, and the patient is asked to make simple opening and closing movements with the mandible in its most retruded position (centric position). These movements of the mandible show whether the condyle rods are on the rotational center. If they are not, the points are adjusted during the opening movements until they rotate without any concentric arcing. When the hinge axis center has been determined, it is marked on the face with an indelible pencil. The face-bow is removed from the face-bow fork, and the condyle rods are straightened and made parallel. The face-bow is now used in the regular manner by being fastened into place over the previously determined rotational points. This type of transfer will be exact in the positional relation of the casts and, in addition, will permit a recording medium (wax, zinc oxide–eugenol, plaster) for interocclusal records to be interposed without the usual inaccuracy being produced. This fact is of great advantage in complete dentures, especially when the interarch distance is to be increased or decreased.

Vertical jaw relations

The vertical jaw relations are those established by the amount of separation of the two jaws in a vertical direction under specified conditions. Vertical jaw relations are classified as (1) the vertical relation of occlusion, (2) the vertical relation of rest position, and (3) others. Vertical relations are discussed further in Chapter 12.

The vertical relation of occlusion is established by the natural teeth when they are present and in occlusion. The vertical relation of occlusion of patients with dentures is established by the vertical height of the two dentures when the teeth are in contact. This is the relationship that must be determined for edentulous people so that the teeth in the dentures can be properly related to each other. It has been known as the "occlusal vertical relation," which is a satisfactory designation. It has also been referred to as the "occlusal vertical dimension" and as the "vertical dimension of occlusion."

These terms are incorrect because they fail to designate the reference points where the measurements are made. The terms *occlusal vertical relation* or *vertical relation of occlusion* are more logical and accurate when the vertical relations are thought of as the relationships of one bone to others in space.

The vertical relation of rest position (or physiologic rest position of the mandible) is established by muscles and gravity. It is a postural relationship of the mandible to the maxillae, and the teeth do *not* determine the vertical level of this relationship. The mandible is considered to be in its physiologic rest position when all the muscles that close the jaws and all the muscles that open the jaws are in a state of minimal tonic contraction sufficient only to maintain posture. Since gravity exerts a force on the mandible, this force is added to the force from muscles applied to the mandible, and therefore the position of the head is important when observations of the vertical relation of rest position are made. Specifically, the head must be held in an upright position by the patient and not be supported by a headrest when these observations are made.

The value of the vertical relation of rest position in denture construction is in its use as a guide to the lost vertical relation of occlusion. This is possible because the difference between the occlusal vertical relation and the vertical relation of rest position is the interocclusal distance. The interocclusal distance (formerly referred to as the "free-way space") is the distance or gap existing between the upper and lower teeth when the mandible is in the physiologic rest position. It usually will amount to 2 to 4 mm in a vertical direction if observed at the position of the first premolars.

An interocclusal distance is essential for the health of the periodontal tissues when natural teeth are present. An interocclusal distance is also absolutely essential for complete denture patients. A failure to provide for it in dentures will cause "clicking" of the dentures during speech, soreness of the tissues of the basal seat, and the rapid destruction of the residual alveolar ridges. When denture teeth are in contact without rest for the supporting tissues, except when the mouth is open for speech or eating, the bones of the mandible and maxillae will resorb in an effort to achieve that needed rest.

On the basis of these facts, it can be seen that if the correct vertical relation of rest position can be determined, it is a simple matter to adjust the vertical dimension of the occlusion rims or dentures sufficiently to provide for the necessary interocclusal distance. Then the occlusion can be tentatively established at that reduced distance to establish the vertical relation of occlusion.

Other vertical relations such as the vertical relations of the two jaws when the mouth is half open or wide open are of no significance in the construction of dentures.

Horizontal jaw relations

The horizontal jaw relations are those in a horizontal plane of reference. The basic horizontal relationship is that of centric relation, or centric jaw relation. *Centric relation is the most posterior relation of the mandible to the maxillae at the established vertical relation*. It is a reference relation that must be recognized in any prosthodontic treatment. Horizontal jaw relations are discussed further in Chapter 13.

The other horizontal jaw relations are deviations from centric relation in a horizontal plane. These include the forward protruded relation(s), the right and left lateral relations, and all intermediate relations. These are grouped together as eccentric relations.

All eccentric relations would be in the same horizontal plane as the centric relation, except for the fact that the articulating eminences push the mandibular condyles downward as the mandible is moved forward or laterally. Although the eccentric relations are essentially in the horizontal plane, concurrent changes occur in the vertical relationships between the posterior part of the upper and lower residual alveolar ridges. These changes are in a vertical direction and must be recorded if articulators are to be properly adjusted. These changes are known as the Christiansen phenomenon, and they develop spaces between the upper and lower occlusal surfaces at the posterior end of the occlusion rims or dentures as a result of the downward movement of the condyles as they move forward. If the occlusion of the dentures is to be balanced so that there is a uniform contact between the upper and lower teeth throughout the functional range of jaw movement, the amount of this space must be determined. This may be done by means of interocclusal records, and the articulator can be adjusted accordingly.

MOVEMENTS OF THE MANDIBLE*

Mandibular movements are complex in nature and vary greatly among persons and within each person. Many different mandibular movements occur during mastication, speech, swallowing, respiration, and facial expression. Also, parafunctional movements such as bruxism and clenching may eventually cause pain and pathosis in the structures related to the movement of the jaw. The dentist is the *scientist* who must understand the factors that regulate motion of the jaws. These include contacts of opposing teeth, the anatomy and physiology of the temporomandibular joints, the axes around which the mandible rotates, the actions of the muscles and ligaments, and the neuromuscular integration of all these factors. The dentist is also the *health clinician* who must relate this biologic understanding of mandibular movements to its useful clinical application in the treatment of patients, particularly those who are edentulous.

Practical significance of understanding mandibular movements

A knowledge of mandibular movements is essential for developing tooth forms for dental restorations, understanding occlusion, arranging artificial teeth, treating temporomandibular joint disturbances, preserving periodontal health, and the designing, selection, and adjustment of articulators.

When dental operations involve more than single restorations, most dentists find that restorative procedures can be developed more accurately, conveniently, and quickly on the articulator than in the patient's mouth. The articulator, then, must closely simulate jaw movements within the range of contacts between opposing teeth so that the occlusion planned on the instrument will function properly in the patient's mouth. The degree of success in doing this depends on evoking the desired functional jaw movements in the patient, on accurately recording them and transferring them to the instrument, and on the capabilities of the articulator. Many differences should be expected between the manner in which opposing tooth surfaces make contact on a simple nonadjustable articulator and that during similar movements in the patient's mouth (Fig. 11-13, A). However, fewer differences should be expected during movements of a more fully adjustable articulator (Fig. 11-13, B). The decision whether most adjustments of occlusion in eccentric jaw relations for finished restorations should be made on the articulator or in the patient's mouth will determine the selection of the appropriate articulator for restorative procedures.

Methods of studying mandibular movement

Mandibular, and particularly condylar, activity has been studied for many years by a variety of methods ranging from direct clinical observations to sophisticated electronic instrumentation. In 1889, Luce photographed the reflection of sunlight from beads placed opposite the condyles. Walker, in 1896, used a facial clinometer to measure condylar movements. Bennett, in 1908, traced the pathway of a light positioned opposite the condyle, and Hildebrand recorded condylar movements by roentgen fluoroscopy in 1931. Studies have been conducted using

*We wish to acknowledge the assistance of Jackie G. Weatherred, D.D.S., Ph.D., Coordinator of Physiology for Dentistry, Medical College of Georgia School of Dentistry, Augusta.

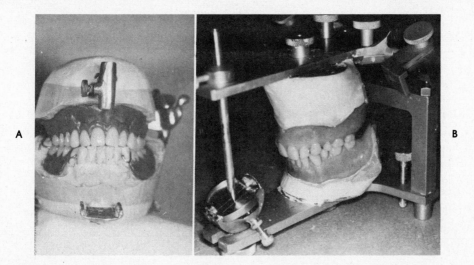

Fig. 11-13. A, This articulator is adjusted by an interocclusal centric relation record and is accurate only for the position at which the record was made. **B,** This articulator is adjusted by a face-bow record, an interocclusal centric relation record, and interocclusal protrusive and lateral records. An occlusion developed on this instrument will function in patient's mouth with fewer discrepancies than an occlusion developed on articulator seen in **A.**

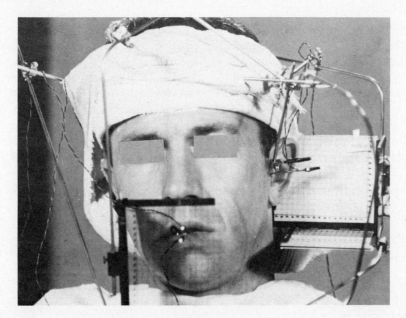

Fig. 11-14. Measurements of mandibular movements can be made when one plots pathway of small lights as recorded by three motion picture cameras simultaneously in frontal, sagittal, and horizontal planes. Grids give an indication of amount of movement of lights. The light at the end of a pin inserted into condyle gives an indication of direction of movement of condyle, and the light facing forward gives an indication of amount of rotation of condyle during mandibular movements.

mechanical and cinematographic techniques, cineradiography, and more recently photoelectric and electromagnetic techniques. Several of these techniques have been coupled with computer analysis to provide valuable information relative to the nature of the mandibular movements. Motion pictures of markers attached to the teeth and others positioned adjacent to the condyles have been made in single planes and with a prism beam splitter. Three-dimensional motion picture photography has depicted movement of markers attached to the teeth and to a pin inserted directly into the condyle (Fig. 11-14). Light-emitting diodes, computer monitored radionuclide tracking, and optical pantography have been used to study mandibular movements. In addition, electronic instruments including a Gnathic Replicator, a Dynamic Duplicator, an ultrasonic probe, and other sensing devices have been computerized and programmed to cause casts of the patient's mouth to move in the same manner as the patient's mandible.

The studies have included the effects of tooth contact on condylar movements, the movement of working and balancing condyles during lateral mandibular excursions, and the presence or absence of opposing tooth contacts during mastication. Mandibular movements have also been studied during mastication, during movement from centric relation to centric occlusion, and during movement from the vertical relation of rest position to the vertical relation of occlusion.

Studies of mandibular movements have revealed important information regarding factors that regulate jaw motion, which in turn have clinical implications in all aspects of occlusion. Through continued research dentists will learn new methods of developing harmony among the factors regulating jaw motion, which will enable them to provide improved dental care for their patients.

Factors that regulate jaw motion

When opposing teeth are in contact and mandibular movements are made, the direction of the movement is controlled by the neuromuscular system as limited by the movement of the two condyles and the guiding influences of the contacting teeth. When the opposing teeth are not in contact and mandibular movements occur, the direction of movement is controlled by the mandibular musculature as limited by condylar movement alone. The condyles and teeth modify only mandibular movements initiated by the neuromuscular system.

Any mandibular movement is the result of the interaction of a number of biologic factors. These include contacts of opposing teeth, the anatomy and physiology of the temporomandibular joints, the rotational axes of the mandible, and the actions of the controlling and moving muscles as directed by the associated neurophysiologic activities. For clarity, the manner in which each of these factors relate to jaw motion are described individually.

Influence of opposing tooth contacts. An important aspect of many jaw movements includes occlusion of opposing teeth. The manner in which the teeth contact is related not only to the occlusal surfaces of the teeth themselves, but also to the muscles, temporomandibular joints, and neurophysiologic components including the patient's mental well-being.

When the patients bring the teeth on complete dentures together in centric or eccentric positions within the functional range of mandibular movements, the occlusal surfaces of the teeth should meet evenly on both sides. In this manner the mandible is not deflected from its normal path of closure nor are the dentures displaced from the residual ridges. In addition, when mandibular movements are made with the opposing teeth on complete dentures in contact, the inclined planes of the teeth should pass over one another smoothly and not disrupt the influences of the condylar guidance posteriorly and the incisal guidance of the teeth anteriorly. Research has shown that condylar movement is not limited solely by the anatomy of the temporomandibular joints but can be influenced by contacts of opposing teeth. Variations in condylar movement have been observed concomitant-

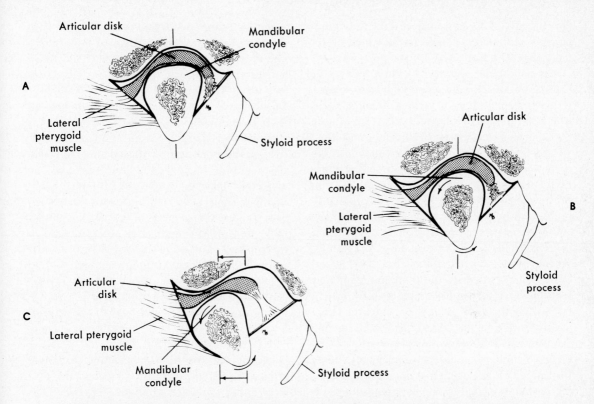

Fig. 11-15. A, Temporomandibular joint is divided into a superior and inferior compartment by articular disk. Condyle is shown diagrammatically (sagittal section) in its most retruded position. Notice
relation of superior surface of condyle to articular disk. Fibers of lateral pterygoid muscle insert at neck
of condyle and through capsular ligament into anterior part of articular disk. **B,** Jaws have been
opened, with mandible in its most retruded position. The rotational movement *(arrows)* has occurred
between superior surface of condyle and inferior surface of articular disk. Notice that no translation of
condyle has occurred during this movement. **C,** Mandible has been moved in a forward position with
an accompanying opening component. The rotation *(arrows)* has occurred between superior surface of condyle and inferior surface of articular disk, just as it did in **B.** However, the forward or
translatory movement has occurred between superior surface of articular disk and inferior surface of
articular eminence. All mandibular translatory movements occur between these two surfaces.

ly as deflective occlusal contacts or steep incisal
guidance from opposing canines change the
pathway of mandibular movement. Thus the
inclined planes of artificial teeth must be so positioned that they are in harmony with the other
factors that regulate jaw motion. A failure to
develop this kind of occlusion can disturb the
stability of complete dentures and cause denture
bases to move on the soft tissues of the residual
ridges.

Influence of the temporomandibular joints.
Each temporomandibular joint is divided into a
superior and inferior compartment by the articular disk, in effect making two joints within each
temporomandibular articulation (Fig. 11-15, *A*).
The basic type of mandibular movement in each
compartment is different. The movement in the
upper compartment is primarily translation, and
in the lower compartment it is primarily rotation. This difference is related to the anatomic

attachments of the articular disk to the lateral surfaces of the condyle and to the lateral pterygoid muscle.

All mandibular motion is either rotation or translation (or a combination of these). A rotational movement is one in which all points within a body describe concentric circles around a common axis. A translatory movement is one in which all points within a body are moving at the same velocity and in the same direction. Rotational movements of the mandible take place in the lower compartment of the temporomandibular joint between the superior surface of the condyle and the inferior surface of the articular disk (Fig. 11-15, B). Translatory, or gliding, movements of the mandible take place in the upper compartment of the temporomandibular joint between the superior surface of the articular disk as it moves with the condyle and the inferior surface of the glenoid fossa. The condyle can translate anteroposteriorly approximately ¾ inch (18 mm). Mandibular movements except the opening and closing movement of the mandible when it is held by the patient or dentist in its most posterior position (posterior terminal hinge movement) are combinations of rotation and translation (Fig. 11-15, C).

Axes of mandibular rotation. Rotational movements of the mandible are made around three axes (transverse, vertical, and sagittal) that move constantly during normal jaw function.

During opening and closing movements, the mandible moves in the sagittal plane around a transverse axis that passes through both condyles (Fig. 11-16, A). The transverse axis can be located when opening and closing movements occur with the mandible in its most posterior position (Fig. 11-16, B). This axis is used to properly orient the maxillary cast on the articulator. The transverse axis moves with the mandible in lateral, protrusive, or lateroprotrusive movements. Thus, if the mandible is in a forward position and opening or closing occurs, the rotation would still take place about the same transverse axis in the lower compartment of the temporomandibular joint. However, since the

mandible cannot be fixed in space in the forward position, the transverse axis would be instantaneous for any given location and would move and tilt with the mandible. (An instantaneous axis is one that operates while the mandible is translating to a series of different positions.)

In a lateral excursion, the mandible rotates around a vertical axis passing through the condyle on the working side (the side toward which the mandible is moved) as the condyle on the opposite (balancing) side moves forward and medially (Fig. 11-16, C). Since it is physiologically impossible to make a lateral mandibular movement with no translation of the condyle on the working side, again the vertical axis is moving and tilting along with the mandible.

During a lateral mandibular movement, the condyle on the balancing side that is moving forward and medially also moves downward because of the slope of the articular eminence. This downward movement of the condyle on the balancing side causes the mandible to rotate around a sagittal axis passing through the condyle on the working side (Fig. 11-16, D). As the condyle on the working side rotates around the vertical axis and translates, the sagittal axis moves in a corresponding manner.

As the mandible moves in a lateral or lateroprotrusive excursion, the downward, forward, and medial movement of the condyle on the balancing side is a form of translation with the movement occurring in the superior compartment of the temporomandibular joint. During these same mandibular excursions, in addition to rotating, the condyle on the working side may also move laterally, anteriorly, posteriorly, upward, or downward. The exact nature of this translatory movement during lateral mandibular excursions is dependent on the movement itself and the anatomic form of the glenoid fossa, the condyle, and the articular disk.

One other important mandibular translatory movement, the direct lateral side shift of the mandible that occurs simultaneously with a lateral mandibular excursion, was first described by Dr. Norman Bennett in 1908 and is called the

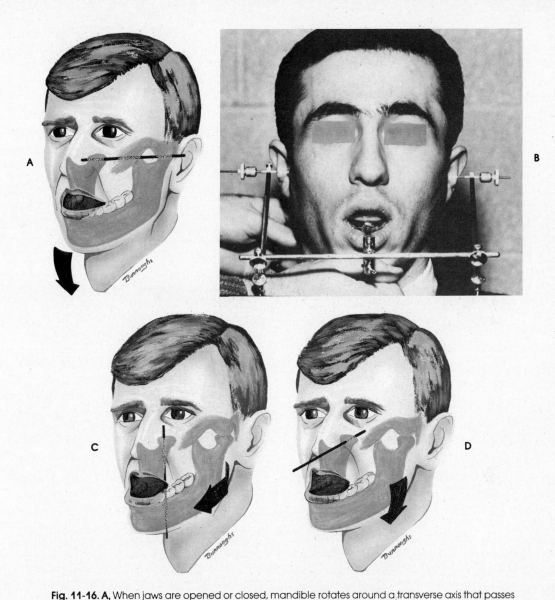

Fig. 11-16. A, When jaws are opened or closed, mandible rotates around a transverse axis that passes through both condyles. No matter where the location of condyles within the temporomandibular joint, the mandible rotates around a transverse axis during opening and closing movements. **B,** Patient makes a series of opening and closing movements with the mandible in its most posterior position in relation to maxillae. The condyle-locating pins are adjusted until they rotate with no arcing component during the retruded opening and closing movements. Thus they indicate location of transverse hinge axis around which mandible is rotating. **C,** When mandible is moved to the right, the left (balancing) condyle moves downward, forward, and inward, with rotation occurring around a vertical axis through the working condyle. **D,** In a right lateral mandibular excursion, there is a downward component of the balancing condyle. During this downward movement, the working condyle rotates around a sagittal axis. (**B** from Hickey, J.C., Allison, M.L., Woelfel, J.B., and Boucher, C.O.: J. Prosthet. Dent. **13:**72-92, 1963.)

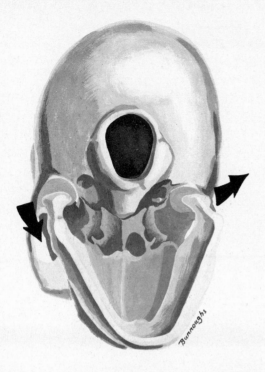

Fig. 11-17. Diagrammatic view of skull from below (inferior view). During a right lateral excursion, the mandible shifts bodily in a lateral direction. This direct lateral movement of mandible (Bennett movement) is a result of a mesial (inward) movement of the balancing condyle *(left arrow),* with a corresponding lateral (outward) movement of the working condyle *(right arrow).*

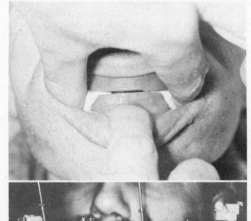

Fig. 11-18. A, Most posterior relation of mandible to maxillae can be transferred from the patient to the articulator by means of an interocclusal centric relation record. Here, a plaster interocclusal centric relation record is made between the occlusion rims. **B,** Relation of mandible to skull during selected mandibular movements can be transferred to articulator with pantographic tracings. Tracings are made by fixed needle points that scribe lines on moving tracing tables attached by means of a clutch to mandible.

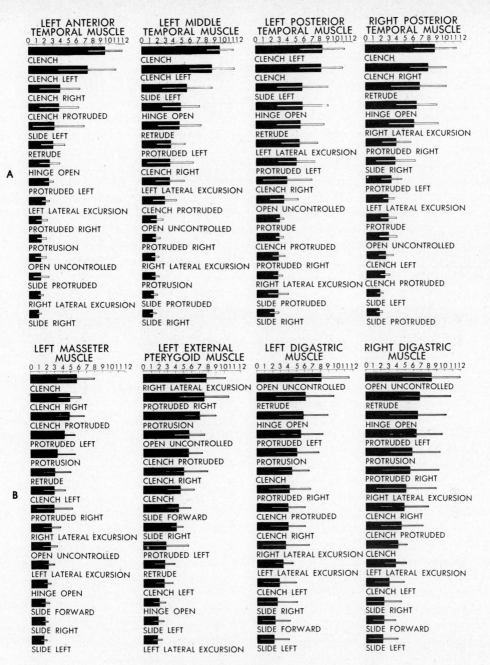

Fig. 11-19. Relative amount of muscle activity in muscles of mastication. The muscles listed at top of charts were measured electromyographically for their activity during various jaw movements as indicated. Each bar indicates the mean of 50 mandibular movements. **A,** Temporal muscles. Notice the relatively large amount of activity of middle and posterior parts of temporal muscles during hinge openings and retrusions of mandible and the reduced activity when mandibular opening was uncontrolled. Posterior parts of temporal muscles brace mandible during lateral excursions to the same side. **B,** Left masseter, left external pterygoid, and digastric muscles. Notice that the external (lateral) pterygoid muscle plays a major role in uncontrolled openings of mandible but has little involvement in hinge openings. On the other hand, the digastric muscles are extremely active in uncontrolled opening, retrusion, and hinge-opening movements of mandible. (From Woelfel, J.B., Hickey, J.C., Stacy, R.W., and Rinear, L: J. Prosthet. Dent. **10:**688-697, 1960.)

Bennett movement. The amount of medial movement of the condyle on the balancing side during the lateral excursion governs the magnitude of the direct lateral slide of the mandible, which can be observed and measured by the movement of the condyle on the working side (Fig. 11-17).

The Bennett movement is an important component of lateral jaw movements for most patients although the amount and timing of the movement varies among persons. Its precise incorporation is more significant when one is restoring the occlusion of dentulous than edentulous patients.

The location of the axes of rotation, the establishment of the horizontal and lateral condylar guidances, and the provision for direct lateral shift of the mandible must be closely approximated on the articulator if it is to adequately simulate jaw movements. This transfer of information from the patient to the articulator requires an understanding of the capabilities and limitations of the articulator and is accomplished by means of accurate interocclusal records or pantographic tracings (Fig. 11-18). In either instance, for edentulous patients the occlusion of the artificial teeth can be perfected better on the articulator than in the mouth because of the movement of the dentures on the basal seat tissues of the residual ridges.

Muscular involvement in jaw motion. The muscles responsible for mandibular motion generally show increased activity during any jaw movement. This increase in activity may be associated with movement of the mandible, fixation of the jaw in a given position, or stabilization of the mandible so that the movement will be smooth and coordinated from one position to another. The activity and interaction of the muscles for a series of jaw movements has been determined by electromyography (Fig. 11-19).

Certain muscles are primarily involved in mandibular movements of particular clinical significance in establishing jaw relations. The role that these muscles play in regulating these mandibular movements are described as follows.

The temporal muscle has a broad, fan-shaped origin on the skull (Fig. 11-20). The muscle fibers that form the posterior part of the temporal muscle run more horizontally than those in the anterior and middle parts. When the posterior fibers contract, they tend to move the mandible posteriorly into centric relation or to hold it in its most posterior position during terminal hinge movement. Thus, when a patient is instructed to "pull your lower jaw back and close on your back teeth" to make a centric relation record or to locate the posterior terminal hinge axis, the temporal muscles and the inframandibular muscles retrude the mandible and maintain it in this most posterior position.

The lateral pterygoid muscles move the mandible forward if acting jointly or to the opposite side when acting individually (Fig. 11-21, *A*). During the conscious effort required by the patient in mandibular terminal hinge opening movements, the lateral pterygoid muscles remain relatively inactive. Meanwhile, the suprahyoid muscles produce the rotary jaw movement around a stationary transverse mandibular hinge axis (Fig. 11-21, *B*). During uncontrolled opening movements, the lateral pterygoid muscles are responsible for the forward movement of the condyles and the mandible. The lateral pterygoid muscles are also responsible for the lateral and protrusive movements of the mandible that are necessary to make eccentric interocclusal records or pantographic tracings used when one is adjusting the horizontal condylar guidances and the lateral condylar guidances (Bennett movement) of the articulator.

The superior belly of the lateral pterygoid muscle acts to fix or stabilize the condyle and disk during elevation of the mandible.

Neuromuscular regulation of mandibular motion. The muscles that move, hold, or stabilize the mandible do so because they receive impulses from the central nervous system. The pathways of the impulses that regulate mandibular motion have been described by Sessle. These impulses may arise at the conscious level

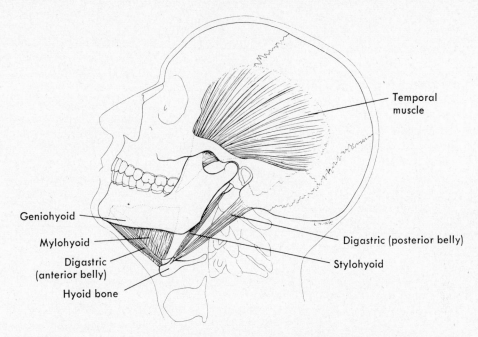

Fig. 11-20. The middle and particularly the posterior parts of temporal muscle contract isotonically (muscle fibers actually shorten during contraction and cause movement of a part) and, in combination with suprahyoid muscles, *position* mandible in centric relation. Then these same muscle groups by contracting isometrically (muscle fibers maintain same length during contraction and fix or hold a part in a particular position) *maintain* mandible in centric relation during making of an interocclusal centric relation record.

and result in voluntary mandibular activity. The impulses may also arise from subconscious levels of the central nervous system as a result of stimulation of oral receptors, muscle receptors, or activity in other parts of the central nervous system. The impulses initiated at the subconscious levels may result in involuntary movements or the modification of voluntary movements. At any one time, the cell body of the motor nerve may be influenced by these various sources to produce inhibition or excitation. When a closing movement is taking place, the neurons to the closing muscles are being excited, and those of the opening muscles are being inhibited. Impulses from the subconscious level, including the reticular activating system, also regulate muscle tone, which plays a primary role in the physiologic rest position of the mandible.

Certain receptors in mucous membranes of the oral cavity can be stimulated by touch, thermal changes, pain, or pressure. Other receptors located principally in the periodontal ligaments, the mandibular muscles, and the mandibular ligaments provide information about the location of the mandible in space and are called proprioceptors (Fig. 11-22). The impulses that are generated by stimulation of these oral receptors travel to the sensory nucleus of the trigeminal nerve or, in the case of the proprioceptors, to the mesencephalic nucleus. From these two nuclei, the impulses can be transmitted (1) by way of the thalamus to the sensorimotor cortex (conscious level) and produce a voluntary change in the position of the mandible, (2) to the motor nucleus of the trigeminal nerve and directly back to the mandibular muscles (in a

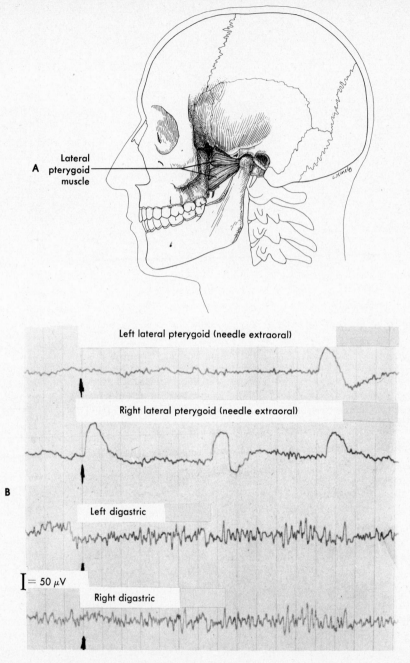

Fig. 11-21. A, Shortening of fibers of lateral pterygoid muscle moves condyle on the same side forward. This muscle also holds or braces condyle and disk in a forward position along articular eminence in certain phases of mastication. Without this action, condyle on balancing side would drop back into fossa as a result of the forces developed by the closing muscles of mastication. **B,** This electromyogram was made during a mandibular hinge or retruded opening movement. *Arrows,* Beginning of the opening movement. Notice that lateral pterygoid muscles maintain their resting pattern while digastric muscles, which are responsible for opening movement, show increased electrical activity. (From Woelfel, J.B., Hickey, J.C., and Rinear, L.: J. Prosthet. Dent. **7:**361-367, 1957.)

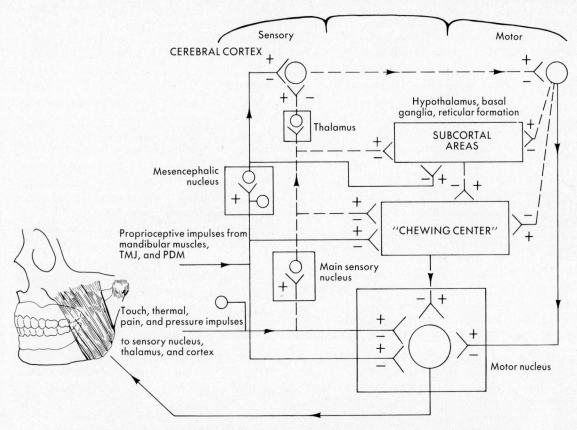

Fig. 11-22. Sensory and central pathways and mechanisms related to chewing and its regulation. Some peripheral sites may influence (+, facilitate; −, inhibit) motoneurons by relatively direct reflex pathways, act on the chewing center itself, or exert their effects by way of their ascending projections to one or more of the higher centers, such as the sensorimotor cerebral cortex, that can regulate motoneuron output relatively directly or via the chewing center. *Broken lines,* Less direct central pathways. (Based on Sessle, B.J.; from Roth, G.I., and Calmes, R., editors: Oral biology, St. Louis, 1981, The C.V. Mosby Co.)

reflex arc), causing involuntary movement of the mandible, or (3) a combination of the first two under the influence of subcortical areas such as the hypothalmus, basal ganglia, reticular formation, and others (Fig. 11-22). The involuntary movement of the mandible away from a source of pain while one is making a jaw relation record or a modification in the physiologic resting position of the mandible because of soreness in the mouth from dentures are examples of this kind of activity.

The loss of receptors located in the periodontal membranes when patients lose their teeth eliminates this source of control in positioning of the mandible for edentulous patients. Such loss of control is an important biologic factor that must be compensated for by construction of complete dentures with centric occlusion in harmony with centric relation. Edentulous patients are no longer able to discern even contacts of opposing teeth or avoid deflective occlusal contacts as they could when they were dentulous.

Therefore it is essential that opposing teeth on complete dentures meet evenly when the jaw is in centric relation and also that they meet evenly whenever the jaw is closed within the normal range of functional activity. This kind of occlusion for complete dentures cannot be established unless the casts are mounted in centric relation on the articulator.

Impulses may also arise in the motor cortex of the brain as a result of voluntary thought. These impulses are transmitted to the motor nucleus and from there to the muscles of mastication, so that the mandible performs the desired activity (Fig. 11-22). Thus patients can be trained to voluntarily make posterior terminal hinge movements of the mandible that can be used by the dentist to locate the transverse hinge axis.

Mastication was formerly believed to be the result of interaction between jaw closing and jaw opening reflexes as influenced by sensory input and conscious control. Recent evidence, however, indicates that mastication is a programmed event residing in a "chewing center" located within the brainstem (probably in the reticular formation of the pons) (Fig. 11-22). The cyclic nature of mastication (jaw opening and closure, tongue protrusion and retrusion) is the result of the action of this central pattern generator (Sessle, 1981). Conscious effort may induce or stop chewing, but it is not required for the continuation of chewing. In a similar manner sensory impulses from the orofacial region may modify the basic cyclic pattern of the chewing center to achieve optimal function (Fig. 11-22). The alteration of chewing characteristics (rate, force, duration) as related to the consistency of a bolus of food is an example of this type of influence. Finally, central influences from areas of the brain associated with other patterned or "learned" behavior, emotion, and stress may inhibit or excite the chewing center.

The cerebellum does not initiate mandibular movement. Rather, it compares information from the motor cortex and other higher centers (signifying the appropriate or intended movement) to the sensory information received from the periphery (signifying actual position and rate of movement). Acting as a feedback control mechanism, the cerebellum sends appropriate signals back to the motor cortex to inhibit agonist muscles and excite antagonist muscles. In this way movement is terminated at the exact point of intention, ensuring a coordinated response from the muscles that are responsible for mandibular function.

The relatively continuous flow of impulses through specific pathways from oral receptors to the central nervous system and back to the regulating musculature establishes memory patterns for the individual patient. Thus patients with natural teeth may subconsciously develop mandibular closing patterns that will bypass deflective occlusal contacts, so that the teeth meet evenly in centric occlusion. However, when memory patterns are disrupted by removal of teeth or placement of new restorations with an occlusion that is not in harmony with the existing mandibular movement pattern, mandibular movements may be significantly altered, causing pain, pathosis, and mental stress.

Clinical understanding of mandibular movement

Parallelogram of forces. From the standpoint of the prosthodontist, the skull presents some interesting facts that need to be taken into consideration. The factor of muscle pull in relation to the direction and strength of each individual muscle used in positioning the mandible after the loss of teeth is an important consideration (Fig. 11-23). The parallelogram of forces can be studied only in relation to the entire skull. The direction of these forces has much to do with the seating or unseating of dentures. The occlusal vertical dimension affects this direction of forces, a fact that makes the positioning of the mandible after the loss of teeth so important. One can understand the relation of the ridges by studying the teeth in the natural occlusion to observe the inclination of the roots and the alveolar process (Figs. 1-11 and 1-12).

A study of the skull as a whole in relation to

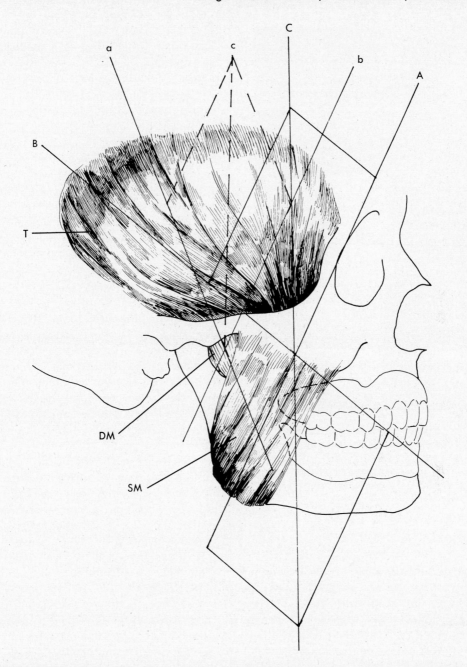

Fig. 11-23. Parallelogram of forces as applied to muscles of mastication. *A,* Direction of force exerted by superficial portion of masseter muscle and by medial pterygoid muscles; *a,* direction of force exerted by deep portion of masseter muscle. *B,* Direction of force exerted by posterior portion of temporal muscle; *b,* direction of force exerted by anterior portion of temporal muscle. *C* and *c,* Direction of resultant forces, that is, the force follows the diagonals of the parallelograms and is exerted in line with long axis of teeth. *T,* Temporal muscle; *DM,* deep portion of masseter muscle; *SM,* superficial portion of masseter muscle.

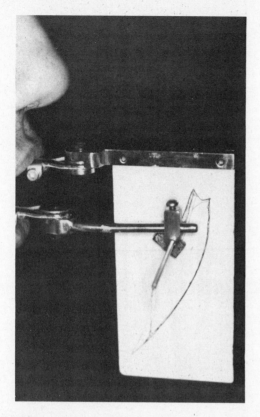

Fig. 11-24. Marker attached by means of a clutch to lower teeth scribes a tracing on plate attached by means of a clutch to upper teeth. Tracing on plate indicates pathway of mandible in sagittal plane. An envelope of motion has been scribed, which indicates extreme limits of mandibular movement in this plane for this particular patient.

the attaching muscles and their consequent pull should reveal the hazard of placing the mandible anterior to its centric position. There is only one true centric relation, and that coincides with the center of muscle pull when the mandible is in its most retruded position in relation to the skull.

Envelope of motion in the sagittal plane. In an explanation of the clinical implications of mandibular movements, it is helpful to define the limits of possible motion and certain mandibular reference positions. Fig. 11-24 shows one method that can be used to record and study mandib-

ular movements. Recent tests indicate that edentulous patients can make reproducible lateral border movements when stabilized baseplates are used to support the pantograph.

Fig. 11-25 shows an envelope of motion (maximum border movements) in the sagittal plane as scribed by a patient. The tracing was made from motion picture film when the pathway of a bead attached to a lower central incisor is plotted. The tracing starts at point *P*, which represents the most protruded position of the mandible with the teeth in contact. As the mandible is moved posteriorly while tooth contact is maintained, the dip in the top line of the tracing occurs as the incisal edges of the upper and lower anterior teeth pass across one another. Point *CO* (centric occlusion) is reached when the opposing posterior teeth are maximally intercuspated. When the mandible is further retruded, as most people with natural teeth can do, the most posterior relation of the mandible to the maxillae is depicted by point *CR* (centric relation). Centric relation and the mandibular position where centric occlusion occurs are two reference positions that are of extreme importance in constructing dental restorations. Single restorations are generally constructed to be in harmony with centric occlusion, that is, with the mandible positioned at point *CO*. Multiple restorations and certainly complete dentures are constructed with their occlusion harmonious with centric relation, that is, with the mandible positioned at point *CR*.

As the teeth separate and jaws open, the mandible moves in its most retruded position from point *CR* (Fig. 11-25), and the patient can continue to open in this retruded position, with no apparent condylar translation, to approximately point *MHO* (maximum hinge-opening position). Any opening beyond *MHO* will force the condyles to move forward and downward from their most posterior position. Line *CR-MHO* represents the posterior terminal hinge movement. This movement is used clinically to locate the transverse hinge axis for the purpose of mounting casts on articulators. The posterior terminal

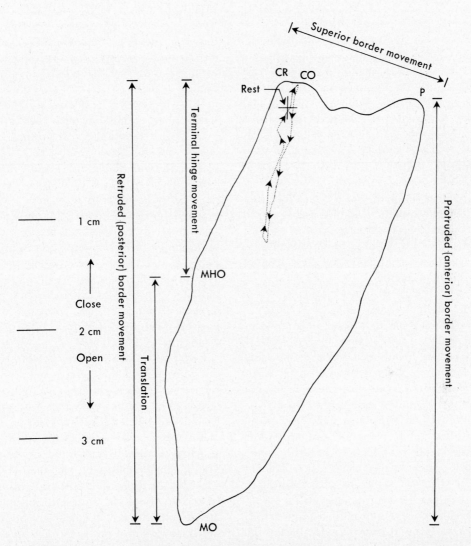

Fig. 11-25. Envelope of mandibular movement in sagittal plane. *P,* Most protruded position of mandible with the teeth in contact; *CO,* centric occlusion; *CR,* centric relation; *MHO,* maximum hinge-opening position; *MO,* point of maximum opening of the jaws; *Rest,* mandibular rest position.

hinge movement and centric relation at the vertical level of tooth contact coincide at point *CR*. This terminal hinge movement can be made only by a conscious effort on the part of the patient.

At approximately point *MHO* (Fig. 11-25) the patient can no longer retain the mandible in the most retruded position, and as further opening occurs, the mandible begins to move forward with translation of the condyles in a forward direction. Obviously, different muscles and impulses come into play. At point *MO* (maximum opening) the jaws are separated as far as possible, and the condyles are in or near their most anterior position in relation to the mandibular fossae. The most forward line on the tracing, running from point *MO* to point *P*, represents the pathway of the mandible as it is moved from its most open position upward in its most protruded position until the teeth contact at *P*, which was the starting point for the tracing of the envelope of motion.

Any mandibular movement observed from the side would fall within this envelope of motion, since it represents all extreme positions into which the mandible can be moved. However, few normal mandibular movements would follow the border tracings; normal mandibular movements would occur somewhere in front of the terminal hinge movement line, *CR-MHO*.

The dotted line beginning with the teeth in centric occlusion at point *CO* and extending downward and then back upward anterior to the path of the posterior terminal hinge movement line *(CR-MHO)* is a tracing of a masticatory cycle viewed in the sagittal plane and superimposed on the envelope of motion (Fig. 11-25). The arrows pointing downward indicate the pathway of the bead attached to the lower central incisor during the opening part of the chewing cycle, and the arrows pointing upward indicate the pathway during the closing part of the chewing cycle. Note that the pathways for the masticating cycle occur anterior to the line representing the terminal hinge movement. This pattern would hold true for most persons with

natural teeth. However, should restorations be constructed so that centric occlusion and centric relation coincide at point *CR*, many of the chewing cycles would terminate at this point. This would apply also to people whose occlusions have been equilibrated for centric relation. The important point to remember, however, is that for edentulous patients the teeth should contact evenly throughout the normal range of function.

When the patient is relaxed and the jaw is in the resting position, obviously the teeth are not in contact. Mandibular rest position normally occurs somewhere downward and slightly forward from point *CR*, as indicated by *Rest* in Fig. 11-25. This position is defined as the habitual postural position of the mandible when the patient is at ease in an upright position. The only muscle activity required at this time is the minimum tonic contraction that is necessary to support the mandible against the force of gravity. The rest position is an important reference position in prosthodontics, particularly for complete denture patients, since it is a guide to reestablishment of the proper vertical relation of occlusion.

Envelope of motion in the frontal plane. The envelope of motion as seen in the frontal plane roughly resembles a shield. Fig. 11-26 shows an envelope of motion scribed by a patient in the frontal plane. The tracing was made from motion picture film when the pathway of a bead attached to a lower central incisor was plotted. The tracing begins with the teeth in centric occlusion at point *CO*. As the mandible is moved to the right with the opposing teeth maintaining contact, the dip in the upper line of the tracing is created as the upper and lower canines pass edge to edge. The mandibular movement is continued as far to the right as possible. Then the opening movement is started and continued with the mandible in the extreme right lateral position until maximum opening occurs at point *MO*.

From *MO* (the position of maximum opening) the mandible is moved in an extreme left lateral

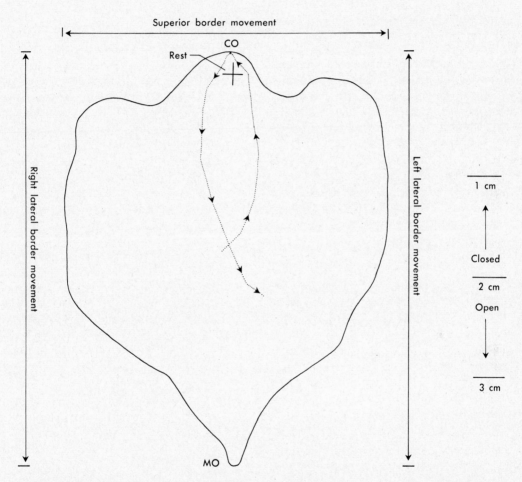

Fig. 11-26. Envelope of mandibular movement in frontal plane. *CO,* Centric occlusion; *MO,* point of maximum opening of the jaws; *Rest,* mandibular rest position.

position as it is closed until the opposing teeth make contact (Fig. 11-26). Then, with the opposing teeth maintaining contact, the mandible is moved from the extreme left lateral position back to where the opposing teeth again contact in centric occlusion, *CO*. The dip in the left side of the superior border movement is made when the upper and lower left canines pass edge to edge.

The dotted line beginning at approximately the middle of the tracing and extending upward (indicated by the upward pointing arrows) represents the upward component of a masticatory cycle as the patient chewed a bolus of food on the left side (Fig. 11-26). The dotted line of the masticatory cycle contacts the superior border of the envelope at point *CO*, indicating that the opposing teeth penetrated the bolus and came into contact with one another. The masticatory cycle moves over to the right when the patient opens from centric occlusion as indicated by the downward dotted line (downward pointing arrows). In the frontal view, the rest position is located slightly downward and to the left for this patient, as indicated by *Rest* in Fig. 11-26.

REFERENCE

Sessle, B.J.: Mastication, swallowing, and related activities. In Roth, G.I. and Calmes, R., editors: Oral biology, St. Louis, 1981, The C.V. Mosby Co.

12

Biologic considerations of vertical jaw relations

ANATOMY AND PHYSIOLOGY OF VERTICAL JAW RELATIONS

The vertical relation of the mandible to the maxillae is established by two things but under different conditions: the mandibular musculature and occlusal stops from the teeth or occlusion rims.

In infants and in edentulous adults the vertical jaw relations are established by the mandibular musculature. This type of vertical relation is known as the vertical relation of rest position. It is assumed only when the muscles that close the jaws and those that open the jaws are in a state of minimal contraction to maintain the posture of the mandible.

The physiologic rest position is a postural position that is controlled by the muscles that open, close, protrude, and retrude the mandible. It is further controlled by the position of the head, which modifies the effect of gravity. If the head is upright, the force of gravity is added to the force applied by the jaw-opening muscles. When the patient is reclining, gravity does not pull the mandible down, and so in observations of the rest position one may find the distance between the jaws to be less than it is when the head is upright. For this reason, the patient's head should be upright and unsupported when observations of physiologic rest position are made.

The second thing that establishes the vertical relation of the mandible to the maxillae is the occlusal stop provided by teeth or occlusion rims. This type of vertical relation is known as the vertical relation of occlusion. The natural teeth establish the occlusal vertical dimension while they are developing and are in place. When a child is young and the teeth are developing, many transient factors are active. These factors are involved with the relative length of the closing and opening mandibular musculature and with the eruptive force of developing teeth.

In the course of a lifetime many things happen to natural teeth. Some are lost, some are abraded so that they lose their clinical crown length, dental caries attacks some of them, and restorations fail to maintain their full clinical crown length. Consequently, even patients who have retained their natural teeth may have a reduced occlusal vertical dimension. The preextraction occlusal vertical relation may not be a reliable indication of the vertical relation to be incorporated in complete dentures. Information about the occlusal vertical relation with natural teeth should not be ignored. Instead, modifications from it should be made as indicated when the information is available.

The masseter, the medial pterygoid, and the temporal muscles are the closing muscles involved in establishing vertical jaw relations. The opening muscles are the inframandibular and suprahyoid muscles including the mylohyoid, geniohyoid, digastric, and platysma muscles. These muscles plus gravity help to control the tonic balance that maintains the physiologic rest position.

The health of the periodontal membranes that support the natural teeth and the health of the mucosa of the basal seat for dentures depend on rest from occlusal forces to maintain their health. For this reason, an interocclusal distance or space between the maxillary and mandibular teeth is essential for the closing muscles, the opening muscles, and gravity to be in balance when the muscles are in a state of minimum ton-

ic contraction. The physiologic rest position allows the supporting tissues and structures to rest. When this rest is not provided by the neuromuscular system, teeth are lost and residual ridges are destroyed. The latter is more immediately critical for complete denture patients than for dentulous patients.

ESTABLISHMENT OF VERTICAL MAXILLOMANDIBULAR RELATIONS FOR COMPLETE DENTURES

The establishment of vertical maxillomandibular relations is a phase of prosthodontic treatment for edentulous patients in which it is difficult to arrive at definite conclusions from a practical viewpoint. The subject has been discussed as the establishment of vertical dimension, but this concept is inadequate because no reference points have been designated. The relationships involved are those in a vertical direction as opposed to those in a horizontal direction, such as centric relation. Studies of growth and development have shown that the rest position of the mandible tends to remain constant for reasonable periods of time. This fact of rest position is important in determination of vertical relation even though the distance between the mandible and the maxillae is advisedly changed.

If the dentist tries to determine the exact vertical relation of occlusion, he is in danger of increasing the interarch distance, which is disastrous because the muscles will not tolerate an *increased* interarch distance as they will a *restored* denture space. The problem of establishing the vertical relations of the jaws is being studied vigorously, and the time may come when this part of the work may be an accurate procedure. Unfortunately, there is no measure that tells the dentist the exact correct point of interarch distance; therefore there is no proof for the most acceptable vertical relation at which occlusion should be established.

Compromises between esthetics and function are often advisable and may be necessary to reduce the known vertical relation of occlusion that has been obtained from preextraction records. Dentures may have favorable esthetics but still may not be comfortable because of excessive leverage from the great amount of maxillomandibular space.

Nature reduces the interarch distance with gradual wear of the natural teeth, usually without damage to the structures concerned. The dentist, attempting to restore youth by restoring the youthful vertical dimension of the face with dentures, is confronted with insurmountable difficulties. The skin, hair, joints, eyes, ears, and all organs of the entire body undergo degenerative changes that are natural and follow nature's scheme of things through the passing of years. Therefore a sacrifice in comfort is often necessary to restore a youthful appearance for the sake of esthetics. Much pressure is brought to bear by many patients trying to stave off old age, and if the dentist succumbs to this pressure, the prognosis will not be favorable.

The greatest danger in this phase of denture construction is an excessive interarch distance because premature striking of teeth causes recurring trauma on the tissues and longer leverage, making the dentures more awkward to manipulate and more easily displaced. The interceptive occlusal contacts may result in clicking of the denture teeth. Extrusion of natural teeth caused by a loss of opposing teeth may bring the alveolar process with it, and closure of part of the interarch space in that region occurs. To get full coverage of the denture bases, an abnormal amount of interarch space is necessary to accommodate the artificial teeth. To bring the vertical dimension of the face back to normal requires surgery; controlled pressure molding of the soft tissue of the maxillary tuberosities, retromolar pads, or soft-tissue irregularities; or reduced denture base coverage. These factors should be studied by mounted diagnostic casts, radiographs, and digital examination before the treatment phase of constructing dentures is started.

Natural teeth provide the occlusal stop that determines the vertical relation of occlusion. When the natural teeth have been lost, there should be adequate space for artificial teeth of the same size. The problem is simplified if the size of the lost natural tooth is known. If there is insufficient space for the denture teeth, the teeth may be larger than the natural teeth or the newly established vertical separation of the two jaws is not great enough.

When an excessive amount of bone has been lost from various causes such as periodontal disease, ill-fitting dentures that have been worn for many years, or partially edentulous mouths (especially all the mandibular posterior teeth), it is possible to reduce the denture space an undesirable amount.

Reduced interarch distance reduces biting force and consequently reduces soreness; therefore it often is used to this end. Narrow knife-edged ridges that cannot be made comfortable in any other manner may be treated by a reduced occlusal vertical dimension to reduce trauma and soreness. However, a reduced interarch distance results in a facial expression that is not desirable, and the vertical dimension of the face should be increased to a point that will be satisfactory and comfortable. With a reduced interarch distance, the lower third of the face is changed because the chin has the appearance of being too close to the nose and too far forward. The lips lose their fullness, and the vermillion borders of the lips are reduced to approximate a line. The corners of the mouth turn down because the orbicularis oris and its attaching muscles are pushed too close to their origin. The reduced vertical relation of occlusion reduces the action of the muscles, with resultant loss of muscle tone. This gives the face an appearance of flabbiness instead of firmness. A reduced interarch distance often results in a crease at the corners of the mouth, which sometimes results in a disease known as *perlèche*.

The reduced interarch distance results in the loss of the cubicle space of the oral cavity. Normally the tongue at rest completely fills the oral cavity; therefore a reduced interarch distance will have a tendency to push the tongue toward the throat, with the result that adjacent tissues will be displaced and encroached on. Encroachment may mean closure or occlusion of the opening of the eustachian tubes, which would interfere with the function of the ear. This may be the cause of much ear discomfort. It has been claimed that impaired hearing has been caused by reduced vertical dimension of the face. However, these claims are difficult to support. One should use caution in large interarch distances by experimenting with a temporary splint over the teeth to test for improvement in hearing or discomfort before the final restorations are made.

Trauma in the region of the temporomandibular fossa may be attributed to a reduced interarch distance of the occlusion. The symptoms of joint involvement often are those of obscure pains and discomfort, clicking sounds, and headaches and neuralgia.

If it is suspected that these various pathologic conditions are attributable to a reduced interarch distance, the dentures should be constructed as treatment dentures. The vertical relation of occlusion should be built up gradually, in successive sets of dentures. Complete restoration of the original occlusal vertical dimension in one set of dentures would likely result in a failure because patients would not be able to accommodate themselves to this great change in so short a period of time.

Methods of determining vertical relation

The methods for determining the vertical maxillomandibular relations can be grouped roughly into two categories. The *mechanical* group of methods includes the use of preextraction records, measurements of various types, parallelism of the ridges, and others. The *physiologic* group of methods includes the use of the physiologic rest position, the swallowing phenomenon, and phonetics as means for determining the facial dimension at which occlusion should be established. The use of esthetics as a guide combines both the mechanical and the physiologic approaches to the problem.

All determinations of the vertical relation must be considered to be tentative until teeth are arranged on the trial bases. At the time of the try-in, observations of phonetics and esthetics can be used as a check against the vertical relation established by mechanical or physiologic means.

Mechanical methods

1. Ridge relation
   a. Distance of incisive papilla from mandibular incisors
   b. Parallelism of the ridges
2. Measurement of former dentures
3. Preextraction records
   a. Profile radiographs
   b. Casts of teeth in occlusion
   c. Facial measurements

Physiologic methods

1. Physiologic rest position
2. Phonetics and esthetics as guides
3. Swallowing threshold
4. Tactile sense

Mechanical methods

Ridge relation. The incisive papilla is used to measure the patient's vertical relation. The incisive papilla is a stable landmark and is changed little by resorption of the residual alveolar ridge. The distance of the incisive papilla from the incisal edge of the mandibular anterior teeth on diagnostic casts averages approximately 4 mm in the natural normal dentition. The incisal edge of the maxillary central incisors is an average of 6 mm below the incisal papilla. Therefore the average vertical overlap of the opposing central incisors is about 2 mm (Fig. 12-1).

Paralleling of the maxillary and mandibular ridges, plus a 5-degree opening in the posterior region as suggested by Sears, often gives a clue to the correct amount of jaw separation. This paralleling is natural because the teeth in normal occlusion leave the residual ridges in the posterior region parallel to each other, provided that there has not been an abnormal amount of change in the alveolar process (Fig. 12-2).

Since the clinical crowns of the anterior and posterior natural teeth have approximately the

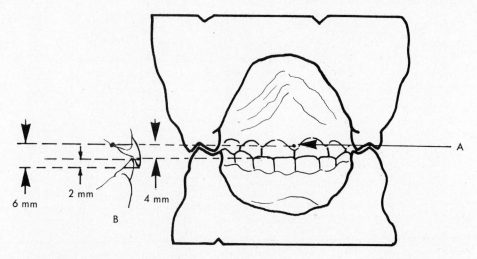

Fig. 12-1. Posterior view of sectioned casts. When teeth are in centric occlusion, incisal edge of mandibular central incisors are 4 mm from incisive papilla, *A. B,* Sagittal view of central incisors shows vertical overlap to be about 2 mm.

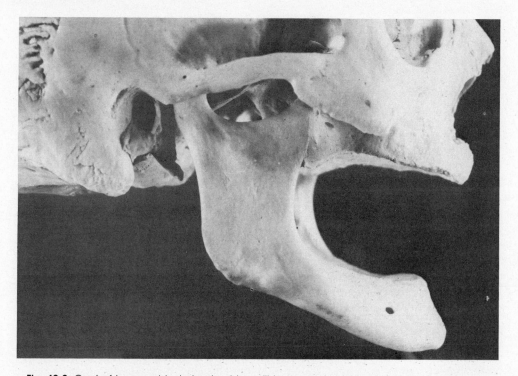

Fig. 12-2. Crest of lower residual alveolar ridge will be approximately parallel with crest of upper residual alveolar ridge when jaws are at position of vertical dimension of occlusion. This relationship provides ideal situation for stability of denture.

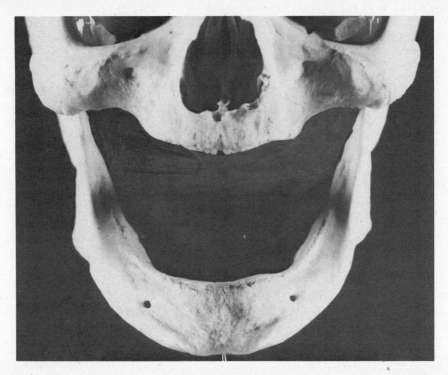

Fig. 12-3. Front view of edentulous skull shows how the mandible has become progressively wider and the maxillae progressively more narrow as resorption continues.

same length, their removal would leave the residual alveolar ridges nearly parallel to each other. This would be ideal from a mechanical standpoint because the dentures would not tend to slide anteriorly or posteriorly. However, in most people the teeth are lost at different times, and so by the time the patients are edentulous, the residual ridges are no longer parallel. If the patient has lost the teeth at irregular intervals or has suffered a great amount of bone loss because of periodontal disease or resorption, the line of the ridges is naturally not parallel. In addition, the edentulous ridges of the mandible and maxillae become progressively different in width (Fig. 12-3).

Measurement of former dentures. Dentures that the patient has been wearing can be measured, and the measurements can be correlated with observations of the patient's face to determine the amount of change required. These measurements are made between the borders of the maxillary and mandibular dentures by means of a Boley gage. Then, if the observations of the patient's face indicate that this distance is too short, a corresponding change can be made in the new dentures.

Preextraction records

Profile radiographs. Profile radiographs of the face may be used, but the problem of establishment of vertical relation of the rest position and enlargement of the image cause some inaccuracies.

Casts of teeth in occlusion. A simple method of recording the vertical overlap relation, as well as the size and shape of the teeth, is through the use of diagnostic casts mounted on an articulator. The casts serve as an indication of the amount of space required between the ridges for teeth of this size.

Facial measurements. Various devices for making facial measurements have been used in many different forms. Devices have been made to record the relation of the head to the central incisors vertically and anteroposteriorly by placement of a face-bow with auditory meatus plugs in position with spectacle suspension. Another method used is to record the distance from the chin to the base of the nose by means of a pair of dividers before the teeth are extracted. Still another method is to use a pair of calipers to find the distance from the undersurface of the chin to the base of the nose.

Physiologic methods

Physiologic rest position tests. Registration of the jaw in physiologic rest position gives an indication to a relatively correct vertical relation. This may not be an exact guide; however, when used with other methods, it will aid in determining the vertical relation of the mandible to the maxillae. A suggested method is to obtain a relaxed state of the patient when the wax occlusion rims are in place, with the trunk upright and the head unsupported. After insertion of the occlusion rims into the patient's mouth, the patient is asked to swallow and let the jaw relax. After relaxation is obvious to the dentist, the lips are carefully parted to see how much space is present between the occlusion rims. The patient must allow the dentist to separate the lips without help or without moving the jaws or lips. This interocclusal distance at the rest position should be between 2 and 4 mm when viewed in the premolar region.

The interarch space and rest position can be measured by indelible dots or adhesive tape on the face. If the difference is greater than 4 mm, the occlusal vertical dimension would be considered too small. If it is less than 2 mm, the occlusal vertical dimension would be assumed to be too great. The occlusion rims are adjusted until the dentist is satisfied with the amount of inter-

arch space (Figs. 12-4 to 12-6). It is essential that an adequate interocclusal distance exist when the mandible is in its physiologic resting position.

Phonetics and esthetics as guides. Phonetic tests of the vertical relation are not so much those of speech sound production as of observations of the relationships of the teeth during speech. The production of the *ch, s,* and *j* sounds brings the anterior teeth very close together. When correctly placed, the lower incisors are moved forward to a position nearly directly under the upper central incisors and almost touching them. If the distance is too large, a vertical dimension of occlusion that is too small may have been established. If the anterior teeth touch when these sounds are made, the vertical dimension of occlusion is probably too great. If the teeth click together during speech, the vertical dimension of occlusion is probably too great.

Esthetics, also, is affected by the vertical relation of the mandible to the maxillae. A study of the skin of the lips as compared with the skin over the other parts of the face is a guide. Normally, the *tone* of the skin should be the same throughout. However, it must be realized that the anteroposterior position of the teeth is at least equally involved with the vertical relation of two jaws in the restoration of skin tone.

The contour of the lips depends on their intrinsic structure and the support supplied behind them. Therefore the dentist must initially contour the labial surfaces of the occlusion rims so that they closely simulate the anteroposterior tooth position and the contour of the base of the denture, which, in turn, must copy those of the natural structures (Fig. 12-7).

If the lips are not supported anteriorly to their correct positions, they will be more nearly vertical than when they were supported by the natural tissues. In such a situation the tendency is to increase the vertical dimension of occlusion to provide support for the lips. This can be disastrous.

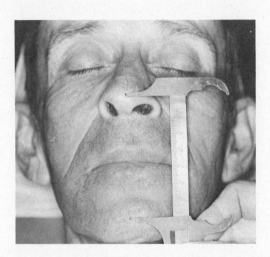

Fig. 12-4. A measurement is made between two points on the face when jaws are at the vertical relation of physiologic rest position.

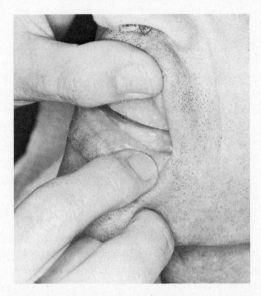

Fig. 12-5. With occlusion rims in mouth and jaws at vertical relation of rest position, interocclusal distance seems satisfactory. Notice the space between the occlusal surfaces of occlusion rims.

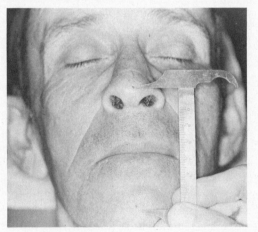

Fig. 12-6. With occlusion rims in contact, distance between the points on the face is 3 to 4 mm less than when the jaws were in the physiologic rest position (see Fig. 12-4).

The esthetic guide to the vertical maxillomandibular relation is, first, the selection of teeth the same size as the natural teeth and, second, the accurate estimation of the amount of tissue lost from the alveolar ridges. The amount of tissue lost can be judged from the dental history and the length of time the teeth have been missing.

Swallowing threshold. The position of the mandible at the beginning of the swallowing act has been used as a guide to the vertical relation. The theory behind this method is that when a person swallows, the teeth come together with a very light contact at the beginning of the swallowing cycle. If denture occlusion is continually missing during swallowing, the vertical dimension of occlusion may be insufficient (too far closed). On this basis, a record of the relation of the two jaws at this point in the swallowing cycle is used as the vertical dimension of occlusion. The technique involves building a cone of soft wax on the lower denture base so that it will contact the upper occlusion rim with the jaws too wide open (see Fig. 13-11). Then the flow of saliva is stimulated by a piece of candy or otherwise. The repeated action of swallowing the saliva will gradually reduce the height of the wax cone to allow the mandible to reach the level of the vertical dimension of occlusion. The length of time this action is carried out and the relative softness of the wax cone will affect the results. We have not found consistency in the final vertical positioning of the mandible by this method.

Tactile sense method. The patient's tactile sense is used as a guide to the determination of the occlusal vertical relation. An adjustable central-bearing screw is attached in the palate of the maxillary denture or occlusion rim, and a central-bearing plate is attached to the mandibular occlusion rim or trial denture base (see Fig. 13-8). The central-bearing screw is adjusted first so it is obviously too long. Then in progressive steps, the screw is adjusted downward until the patient indicates that the jaws are closing too far. The procedure is repeated in the opposite direc-

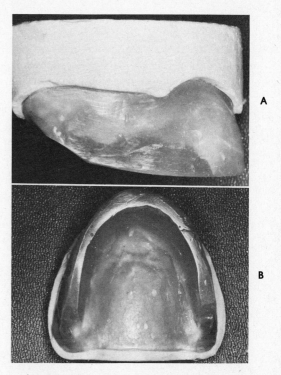

Fig. 12-7. Maxillary occlusion rim is contoured so that its labial surface will be similar to finished denture base and artificial teeth. **A,** Side view. **B,** Occlusal view. Contour and dimensions of neutral zone have been approximated in this occlusion rim. Identical principles are employed in contouring mandibular occlusion rim.

tion until the patient indicates that the "teeth" feel too long. The screw then is adjusted downward until the patient indicates that the length is about right, and the adjustments are reversed alternately until the height of the contact feels right to the patient. The problem with this method relates to the presence of foreign objects in the palate and the tongue space. The final determination must be made at the try-in after the teeth are in position.

Tests of vertical jaws relations with occlusion rims

The vertical separation of the jaws that is established in the mouth with the occlusion rims and mounted on the articulator is the vertical relation of occlusion. This preliminary vertical relationship is established and maintained by the occlusion rims. It precedes the determination of the horizontal jaw relationship and the eventual preliminary centric relation record.

Following are some of the tests that aid the dentist in confirming the correct vertical relation of occlusion with the occlusion rims:

1. Judgment of the overall facial support
2. Visual observation of the amount of space between the rims when the jaws are at rest
3. Measurements between dots on the face when the jaws are at rest and when the occlusion rims are in contact

4. Observations made when sibilant-containing words are pronounced, to ensure that the occlusion rims come close together but do not contact.

The use of these tests enable the dentist to make preliminary and tentative determinations of the vertical dimension of occlusion. The final determination cannot be made by any method until the teeth are set in position in the wax trial dentures, and the vertical dimension is verified in the mouth.

13

Biologic considerations of horizontal jaw relations

The principles of good occlusion apply to both dentulous and edentulous patients. However, different requirements are necessary in the occlusion for complete dentures because artificial teeth are not attached to the bone in the same manner as natural teeth. Thus an occlusion that is physiologically acceptable or desirable for the preservation of the attachment apparatus of natural teeth may not be applicable for complete dentures. To maintain stability of complete dentures, the opposing teeth must meet evenly on both sides of the dental arch when the teeth contact anywhere within the normal functional range of mandibular movement. An occlusion for complete dentures that provides these even contacts can only be developed with centric occlusion in harmony with centric relation.

The centric relation is the most posterior relation of the mandible to the maxillae at the established vertical relation. It is a bone-to-bone relation, and it is classed as a horizontal relation because variations from it (eccentric relations) occur in the horizontal plane. The eccentric relations are either anterior or lateral to centric relation, and those anterior to it are known as protrusive relations.

Centric relation is a reference relation that is constant for each patient, provided that the soft tissue structures in the temporomandibular joints are healthy. Inflammation or swelling within these joints can alter this maxillomandibular relation, but otherwise for clinical purposes it can be considered constant in the healthy patient. Therefore it can be a reference relation with which the desired occlusion can be coordinated.

CONFUSION IN TERMINOLOGY AND CONCEPTS

The term *centric relation* is given a number of different meanings in its clinical application to the development of dental restorations. The use of a single definition is essential to improve communications throughout dentistry.

Centric relation has been defined as (1) the mandibular position that coincides with the median occlusal position, (2) a mandibular position determined by the neuromuscular reflex learned when the primary teeth are in occlusion, (3) the mandibular position that exists when the centers of vertical and lateral motion are in their posterior terminal hinge position, (4) the relationship of the mandible to the maxillae when the mandible is braced during swallowing, (5) a mandibular position synonymous with the physiologic rest position, and (6) a mandibular position synonymous with the position of the mandible during swallowing.

One can eliminate the confusion related to centric relation by accepting one definition: centric relation is the most posterior relation of the mandible to the maxillae at the established vertical relation. All other horizontal mandibular positions are eccentric positions and can be related to centric relation without changing or confusing its meaning.

MUSCLE INVOLVEMENT IN CENTRIC RELATION

Centric relation is not a resting or postural position of the mandible. Contraction of muscles is necessary to move and fix the mandible in this position. However, this neuromuscular activity does not affect the validity of the definition of centric relation.

The anatomic attachments of the posterior and middle parts of the temporal and the suprahyoid muscles (primarily the geniohyoid and digastric) together with electromyographic studies indicate that these muscles move and fix the mandible in its most retruded relation to the maxillae. The temporal, masseter, and medial pterygoid muscles elevate the mandible to a particular vertical relation with the maxillae. The lateral pterygoid muscles show little activity when the mandible is in centric relation (Fig. 13-1).

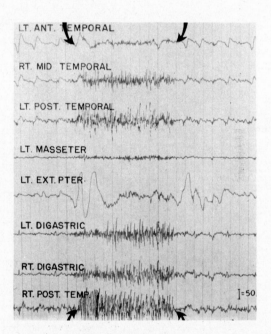

Fig. 13-1. Electromyogram indicates electrical activity recorded from the muscles as labeled, when mandible was moved from resting position into centric relation and from centric relation back to resting position. Increase in both frequency and amplitude of tracings *(arrows)* indicates the time during which mandible was in centric relation. Striking increase in activity from middle and posterior parts of temporal muscles and digastric muscles occurs because these muscles are responsible for positioning and holding mandible in centric relation. Notice that anterior part of temporal muscle, masseter muscle, and external (lateral) pterygoid muscle show little increase above resting activity when mandible is in centric relation.

RELATING CENTRIC RELATION TO CENTRIC OCCLUSION

The understanding of centric relation is complicated by failure to distinguish between centric relation and centric occlusion. This has come about by the incorrect usage of the word *centric* to mean either centric relation or centric occlusion. Centric is an adjective and must be used along with either relation or occlusion to be specific and meaningful. Centric relation is a bone-to-bone relationship, whereas centric occlusion is a relationship of upper and lower teeth to each other (Fig. 13-2). Once centric relation is established, centric occlusion can be built to coincide with it.

Confusion also results from the fact that in many people the centric occlusion of the natural teeth does not coincide with the centric relation of the jaws. This situation could be considered a minor malocclusion that may or may not contribute to damage of the periodontal structures. However, with advancing age and the concurrent loss of recuperative powers by the body tissues, the chances for damage increase. This becomes more acute and more immediately apparent when complete dentures are involved. Centric relation must be accurately recorded so that centric occlusion can be made to coincide with it. The variations in types of occlusion should be limited to eccentric occlusions.

Natural tooth interferences in centric relation initiate impulses and responses that direct the mandible away from deflective occlusal contacts into centric occlusion. Impulses created by closures of the teeth into centric occlusion establish memory patterns that permit the mandible to return to this position, usually without tooth interferences.

When natural teeth are removed, many receptors that initiate impulses resulting in positioning of the mandible are lost or destroyed. Therefore the edentulous patient cannot control mandibular movements or avoid deflective occlusal contacts in centric relation in the same manner as the dentulous patient. Deflective occlusal contacts in centric relation cause movement of denture bases and displacement of the supporting tissues or direct the mandible away from centric relation. Thus centric relation must be recorded for edentulous patients so that centric occlusion can be established in harmony with this position (Fig. 13-3).

RELATING CENTRIC RELATION TO THE HINGE AXIS

The upper cast can be accurately oriented to the opening axis of the articulator by the location of a physiologic transverse hinge axis and a face-bow transfer. The physiologic transverse hinge axis is located by a series of controlled opening and closing movements of the jaws when the

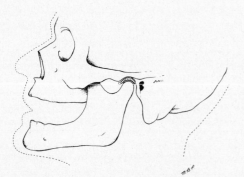

Fig. 13-2. Centric relation is a bone-to-bone relationship. The mandible is in its most retruded relation to maxillae. Centric occlusion should be established in harmony with this position.

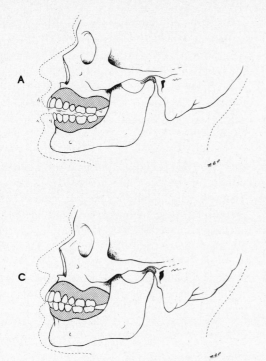
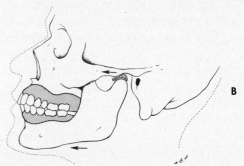

Fig. 13-3. **A,** Centric occlusion is not in harmony with centric relation. When mandible is in centric relation, the opposing teeth do not contact evenly. **B,** Centric occlusion is not in harmony with centric relation. For the opposing teeth to meet evenly as they do in centric occlusion, the mandible must be moved away from centric relation. Notice that condyle has moved forward in the glenoid fossa to permit the opposing teeth to contact evenly. This is not a desirable situation for edentulous patients. **C,** Centric occlusion is in harmony with centric relation. The opposing teeth contact evenly when mandible is in its most retruded relation to maxillae. This is the desirable situation for all edentulous patients.

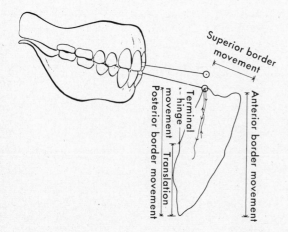

Fig. 13-4. This tracing depicts an envelope of motion scribed in the sagittal plane. Opening and closing the jaws with mandible in its most retruded relation to maxillae (terminal hinge movement) is method used to locate transverse hinge axis. Centric relation is the most retruded relation of mandible to maxillae at a specific vertical relation along pathway of terminal hinge movement. Thus mandible is in its most retruded relation to maxillae for both location of posterior transverse hinge axis and establishment of centric relation. Notice that masticatory cycle (indicated by the arrows pointing upward and downward) terminates with teeth in contact when mandible is in centric relation. (From Hickey, J.C.: Dent. Clin. North Am., pp. 587-600, Nov. 1964.)

mandible is held in its most retruded relation to the maxillae. These mandibular movements are called terminal hinge movements and are that part of the posterior border movement of the mandible which occurs without translation (Fig. 13-4).

As in the determination of the physiologic transverse hinge axis, the mandible is in its most retruded relation to the maxillae when a centric relation record is made. However, the centric relation record is made at an established vertical relation of the jaws corresponding with a specific vertical position of the terminal hinge movement. Therefore, when the upper cast is correctly oriented to the hinge axis of the articulator by an accurate face-bow transfer, the lower cast will also be correctly oriented to the opening axis of the instrument when it is mounted with an accurate centric relation record. This is true because the mandible was in the most retruded relation to the maxillae both for locating the transverse hinge axis and for recording centric relation.

RELATING CENTRIC AND VERTICAL RELATIONS

Many vertical relations are possible between the mandible and the maxillae. However, there is a most retruded relation of the mandible to the maxillae for each vertical relation, and there is a change in the horizontal relation of the *body* of the mandible to the maxillae with each change in the vertical relation. Such a change occurs even though the condyles are maintained in their most retruded position. This most retruded relation is centric relation for that specific vertical relation. A vertical relation of occlusion must be established between the two jaws of the edentulous patient to provide an adequate interocclusal distance and allow the mandibular muscles to function at their optimal physiologic length.

The centric relation record must be made at the established vertical relation of occlusion when an arbitrary face-bow transfer is used to orient the casts to the opening axis of the articulator. This is necessary because the opening

and closing (transverse) axis of rotation of the articulator will be the same as that of the patient only when the casts are mounted with the use of a correctly located physiologic transverse hinge axis. When an arbitrary hinge axis is used, the amount of error that will be introduced by opening or closing the vertical relation of occlusion on the articulator will depend on the relation of the arbitrary location to the true hinge axis and on the amount of change made in the vertical opening of the articulator. Thus, when the centric relation record is made at or very close to the desired vertical relation of occlusion, little or no vertical change (opening or closing) will be necessary on the articulator, and the likelihood of errors from this source will be greatly reduced.

SIGNIFICANCE OF CENTRIC RELATION

The correct registration of centric relation is essential in construction of complete dentures. Many dentures fail because the occlusion is not planned or developed in harmony with this position. The maxillomandibular musculature is so arranged that it is simple for a patient to move his mandible into centric relation. Thus the centric relation can serve as a reference relation for establishing an occlusion. When centric relation and the centric occlusion of natural teeth do not coincide, the periodontal structures around natural teeth are endangered. When centric relation and the centric occlusion of artificial teeth do not coincide, the stability of the denture bases is in jeopardy, and the edentulous patients are subjected to unnecessary pain or discomfort.

The irregular loss of teeth often creates deflective occlusal contacts that guide the mandible into a slightly protrusive or lateral position or both. The muscles, bones, ligaments, teeth, and all related structures grow into a coordinated center for muscular activity. The stability of natural teeth is jeopardized when the mandible is deflected away from centric relation. To change this center for muscular activity is to imperil the stability of the dentures. The edentulous patient does not have the same level of sensitivity of the neuromuscular system as the dentulous patient and cannot learn to avoid the deflective contacts on opposing teeth of complete dentures.

Centric relation is the horizontal reference position that can be routinely assumed by the mandible of edentulous patients under the direction of the dentist. This makes it possible for dentists to verify the relation of casts on the articulator when they are mounted in centric relation. Patients cannot routinely close their teeth into centric occlusion when it is established on the articulator somewhere other than in harmony with centric relation.

Errors in mounting the casts on the articulator may result from incorrect positioning of the occlusion rims in the mouth, unequal pressures on opposite sides of the jaws during the making of interocclusal records, and errors in the mounting procedures. These errors can go undetected when centric relation is not used as the horizontal reference position.

Edentulous patients use centric relation closures in mastication and in other mandibular activities such as swallowing. Therefore the casts must be mounted on the articulator in this position so that the oppoising teeth on complete dentures will meet evenly when the patient closes in centric relation.

Centric relation must be accurately recorded and transferred to the articulator to permit proper adjustments of the condylar guidances for the control of eccentric movements of the instrument. The condylar guidances are adjusted to form a pathway for condylar movement from a beginning point (centric relation) to the position which the eccentric interocclusal records are made. If the beginning point, centric relation, is not recorded, the angulation of the condylar pathway will be incorrect.

An accurate centric relation record properly orients the lower cast to the opening axis of the articulator and orients the centric relation to the hinge axis of the articulator and the mandible. Assuming the maxillary cast to be properly relat-

ed to the hinge axis, an accurate centric relation record will concurrently relate the lower cast to the same hinge axis.

RECORDING CENTRIC RELATION
Conflicting concepts and objectives in recording centric relation

There are two basically different concepts in the making of centric relation records. Each concept has its own objectives.

In one concept, the record should be made with minimal closing pressures so that the tissues supporting the bases will not be displaced while the record is being made. The objective of this concept is for the opposing teeth to touch uniformly and simultaneously at their first contact. The uniform contact of the teeth will not stimulate the patient to clench and relax the closing muscles in periods between mastication.

The second concept is that the records should be made under heavy closing pressure so that the tissues under the recording bases will be displaced while the record is being made. The objective of this concept is to produce the same displacement of the soft tissues as would exist when heavy closing pressures are applied on the dentures. Thus the occlusal forces will be evenly distributed over the supporting residual ridges when the dentures are under heavy occlusal loads. If the distribution of the soft tissues is uneven, however, the teeth would contact unevenly when they first touch. This uneven contact tends to stimulate nervous patients to clench and relax the closing muscles of the jaws, which may cause soreness under the denture bases and changes in the residual ridges.

There is some logic in both concepts, and the dentist must decide which concept will be best for each patient. Regardless of the method selected, the recording technique and the procedures used for testing the occlusion must be based on the objective of the concept chosen. If the minimal closing pressure method is used, the occlusion should be tested at the first contact of the teeth. If the heavy closing pressure method is used, the occlusion should be tested under heavy closing pressure. If centric relation records are made with heavy pressure, it is illogical to expect the teeth to occlude evenly at their first contact. The use of a technique based on minimal closing pressure seems to produce the best result for most patients.

Complications in recording centric relation

Centric relation has been defined as the most retruded unstrained position of the condyles in the glenoid fossae at a given degree of opening. This definition is often misunderstood because the word *unstrained* is taken to mean an absence of anteroposterior strain whereas it should also include absence of a superoinferior strain. This definition is also impossible to use in a practical sense. The condyles are not available for visual observation. The definition given at the beginning of this chapter is more accurate and usable. The structure of the temporomandibular joint is such that it can be displaced downward by uneven pressure between the jaws when records are made and yet the condyles can still be located in their most retruded position. This situation cannot occur on the articulator, and it will result in a deflective occlusal contact that can be the source of instability, soreness, and resorption despite the correctness of the other relations. If the jaws were a hinge, the maxillomandibular relation would then be automatically registered correctly. Unfortunately, the condyles can be easily malpositioned, with resultant difficulties. The basal seats for denture bases made from the best impressions will not withstand the ravages of an incorrect centric relation from any cause.

Centric relation registrations are complicated further in that soft tissues are of varying density. Hanau referred to tissue resiliency as *realeff*, a contraction of "phase *r*esiliency *a*nd *l*ike *eff*ect." This resiliency is present in both the mucosa and tissue of the temporomandibular joints. Thus undue pressure in securing the relation must be avoided to eliminate the possibility of excessive displacement of the soft tissues.

Even though a balanced and equalized registration has been made, this relation is often lost in the cast-mounting procedures and the processing of the dentures. Some of these changes may be unavoidable because of changes in denture base materials during processing. For that reason, it is necessary to reestablish a carefully equalized centric relation after the dentures have been completed.

The theoretical ideal of an equalized occlusal relation is a centric registration made with the same soft-tissue placement that existed when the impressions were made. The objective of this concept is difficult to accomplish with present knowledge. Attempts to record centric relation with minimal closing pressure include the use of soft plaster of paris, zinc oxide–eugenol paste, or carefully softened wax. Maxillomandibular records made in these soft materials that harden in the mouth are reasonably effective.

Retruding the mandible to centric relation

One of the most difficult and most important tasks to accomplish is retruding the mandible to its centric relation. Some of the difficulties are biologic, some psychologic, and some mechanical.

The biologic difficulties arise from the lack of coordination in groups of opposing muscles when the patients are requested to close the jaws in the retruded position. This lack of synchronization between the protruding and the retruding muscles may be caused by habitual eccentric jaw positions adopted by patients to accommodate to malocclusions. For example, a patient having only anterior teeth will have a habit of protruding the jaw and, when asked to retrude it, may find it difficult to do so. In the securing of this retruded position, what may seem like awkwardness on the part of the patient is in fact the difficulty encountered in performing an act consciously that has been merely involuntary for a relatively long period of time.

The psychologic difficulties involve both the

dentist and the patient. The more the dentist becomes irritated over the apparent lack of ability of the patient to retrude the mandible, the more confused the patient becomes and the less likely the patient is to respond to the directions provided by the dentist.

The dentist must be prepared to calmly spend adequate time in securing the centric relation record. This is always one of the most important steps in the construction of complete dentures. Most complete dentures constructed without an accurate centric relation record are doomed to failure. Several methods should be available as aids for the patient to retrude the mandible. One patient might respond to one method and another to a different method. A central-bearing point and plate supported by the recording bases are excellent for exercising a forward and backward jaw movement. They provide the patient with a sliding surface against which to rest the jaws while exercising the mandiblular musculature. Another effective method involves the use of stretch-relax exercises as suggested by Boos. The patient is instructed to open wide and relax, to move the jaw to the right and relax, to move the jaw to the left and relax, and to move the jaw forward and relax in a series of movements four times in each of four sessions a day. The results to be expected are for the patient to be able to follow the dentist's directions in moving the jaw to centric relation and to the desired eccentric relations.

Mechanical difficulties are encountered in the securing of centric relation records because of poorly fitting baseplates. It is essential that the bases on which the centric relation records are made fit perfectly and do not interfere with each other (Fig. 13-5).

The amount of pressure that the patient exerts at the time of registering centric relation is difficult to control. Minimal pressure should be exerted during the registration to avoid displacement of the soft tissues as much as possible. This is obviously difficult to do. If minimal pressure is exerted at the time of this registra-

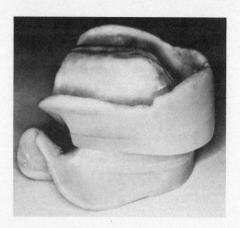

Fig. 13-5. Acrylic resin—lined occlusion rims provide accurately fitting bases for making jaw relation records. Jaw relation records cannot be recorded accurately and transferred to the articulator when the bases do not properly fit on residual ridges.

tion, the jaw relation will be registered with minimal tissue placement, and the denture will have a uniform occlusal contact when the teeth first touch. One side of the mouth might have a thicker layer of soft tissue than the other side, but this would not change the time of first contacts of the teeth. However, under functional loads, the pressures would be unequal as a result of unequal displacement of soft tissue. Patients compensate for this difference by selective placement of food in their mouth. Interocclusal plaster or wax registrations give a better distribution of the placement of soft tissues in all parts of the mouth under minimal pressure than is possible with a record made with a central-bearing point. This is especially true if the tissue depth is uneven and the opposing ridge relation or size is not normal.

Methods for assisting the patient to retrude the mandible. A number of methods are used to assist the patient in retruding the mandible, including the following:

1. Instruct the patient by saying, "Let your jaw relax, pull it back, and close slowly and easily on your back teeth."

2. Instruct the patient by saying, "Get the feeling of pushing your upper jaw out and close your back teeth together."
3. Instruct the patient to protrude and retrude the mandible repeatedly while the patient holds the fingers lightly against the chin.
4. Instruct the patient to turn the tongue backward toward the posterior border of the upper denture.
5. Instruct the patient to tap the occlusion rims or back teeth together repeatedly.
6. Tilt the patient's head back while the various exercises just listed are carried out.
7. Palpate the temporal and masseter muscles to relax them.

The simplest, easiest, and often most effective way of effecting a retrusion of the mandible into centric relation is by verbal instruction to the patient. "Let your lower jaw relax, pull it back, and close on your back teeth" will often get the job done. These instructions must be given in a calm and confident manner. When the patient is responding properly, the dentist should say so. In this manner, the patient's awareness of the desired position is reinforced.

Many patients are not aware of the jaw movements they can make. By getting the feeling of pushing the upper jaw forward, they automatically pull the lower jaw back. Once they have achieved this feeling, it is easy for them to repeat the desired motion.

When the mandible is protruded and retruded with a relaxation each time, the movement into the desired position can be felt by the patient with the patient's own fingers on the chin. The dentist can aid by a slight pressure on the point of the chin. The patient can get an idea of the movement by feeling the dentist's or the dental assistant's chin. This protruding and retruding of the mandible is done repeatedly until the patient is trained in the movement and the dentist can feel the patient's mandible reach its retruded position.

The Boos series of stretch-relax movements (already described) can also be helpful. These stretch-relax exercises will help to get the mandible into the position of centric relation. The dentist soon develops such a sense of touch as to be fairly sure when the mandible is back to the desired position.

When the patient's tongue attempts to reach for the posterior border of the upper denture, the retrusion of the mandible will make the denture border easier to reach. Thus the desired retrusion may be achieved. The problem with this method is the likelihood of displacing the mandibular denture or recording base by the action of the tongue.

Tapping the occlusion rims or back teeth together rapidly and repeatedly is used to help the patient retrude the mandible, since it is believed that the center of muscle pull will gradually work the mandible back. However, it is difficult to record these positions, and a patient can easily tap in a slightly protrusive or lateral position. The results should be checked by other tests.

Often tilting the head backward at the neck will place tension on the inframandibular muscles and tend to pull the mandible to a retruded position. However, it is extremely difficult to obtain registrations with the head in this position because of the awkwardness of insertion and removal of the recording medium and occlusion rims from the mouth when the head is so tilted.

The temporal muscle shows reduced function when the mandible is in a protruded position. For this reason its contraction can be felt when the mandible is in or near its retrusive position and the patient is asked to open and close. Massage or palpation of the masseter and temporal muscles will help patients to relax.

Swallowing may bring the mandible to a retruded position and may be an aid in retruding the mandible to the centric relation. However, a person can swallow when the mandible is not completely retruded. Therefore this method must be verified by another technique.

Methods of recording centric relation

The various methods used for recording centric relation may be classified as static or funtional, and either of these may be extraoral or intraoral techniques.

The static methods are those that involve first placing the mandible in centric relation with the maxillae and then making a record of the relationship of the two occlusion rims to each other. This method has the advantage of causing minimal displacement of the recording bases in relation to the supporting bone. The records in the static class include wax or plaster interocclusal (intraoral) records made with or without a central-bearing point. They may be made with or without intraoral or extraoral tracing devices to indicate the relative position of the two jaws.

The functional methods are those that involve functional activity or movement of the mandible at the time the record is made. These methods have the disadvantage of causing lateral and anteroposterior displacement of the recording bases in relation to the supporting bone while the record is being made. The records in the functional class include the various chew-in techniques such as those suggested by Needles, House, and Essig and Paterson. They also include methods that make use of the function of swallowing for positioning and recording the relative position of the jaws.

Accurate records of centric relation have been made by all the methods in both classes. However, incorrect records also have been made by all the methods in both classes as well.

Extraoral tracings and devices. A needle point tracing made on a tracing table coated with carbon or wax can be used to indicate the relative position of the upper and lower jaws in the horizontal plane (Fig. 13-6, *A*). These tracings are shaped somewhat like a type of architecture known as the Gothic arch and thus are sometimes referred to as Gothic arch tracings. They may also be known as an arrow point tracing.

To make a needle point tracing, one condyle moves forward and inward during a lateral mandibular movement, followed by a movement in

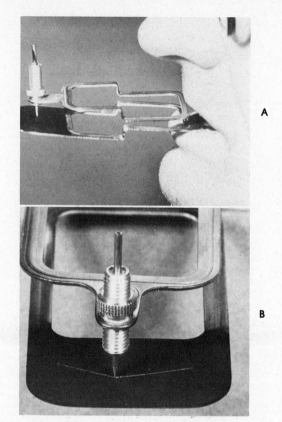

Fig. 13-6. A, Needle point tracing device attached to upper occlusion rim remains fixed during mandibular movement. The lower tracing plate is attached to lower occlusion rim and moves during mandibular movement. The tracing made on lower tracing plate provides an indication of horizontal location of mandible in relation to maxillae. **B,** Needle point tracer is in apex of the tracing, indicating that mandible is in its most retruded relation to maxillae.

the opposite direction with rotation occurring around the opposite condyle. The movements are approximate rotations alternately around the two condyles. These movements cut lines extending to a point representing the most retruded position of both condyles. Therefore, when both condyles are resting in their most retruded positions, the needle point of the tracer will be resting on the apex of the tracing thus created (Fig. 13-6, *B*). A needle point tracing is fundamentally a single representation of the position of the mandible and its movement in the horizontal plane.

Many needle point tracings are not indicative of an exact centric relation because of the roundness of the apex. The lateral movements should be made until the apex is sharp to indicate the true retruded position of the mandible. A dull or rounded apex on a tracing may be caused by the condyles not reaching their most posterior position in the temporomandibular joint or by movement of the recording bases on their basal seats. A rounded apex can be corrected only by repeated manipulation of the mandible from side to side and in a protruded relation to the maxillae. The central–bearing point tracing device affords a sliding table that permits the patient to protrude and retrude the mandible easily while the tracing is made.

One can make a double needle point tracing, one anterior to the other, by increasing or decreasing the vertical dimension at which the tracing is made. With a central-bearing point, one can do this by increasing or decreasing the height of the central–bearing point screw. These two tracings afford an excellent illustration of how the centric position varies at different levels of the occlusal vertical dimension.

The extraoral tracing should be extended a reasonable distance from the recording bases to enlarge the tracing to a size that can be properly evaluated. Tracings made inside the mouth (intraoral) or close to the occlusion rims are often so small that it is difficult to be certain that the apex of the tracing is sharp. Some needle point tracing devices combine the central-bearing point and the needle point tracer into one by having the bearing point cut the tracing on the opposite plate.

Tracing devices that make use of the central-bearing point are placed on and fastened to the baseplates with care being taken to center them laterally and anteroposteriorly so as to have the pressure equally distributed laterally and anteroposteriorly (Fig. 13-7). This is predicated on the assumption that the center of the mandibular

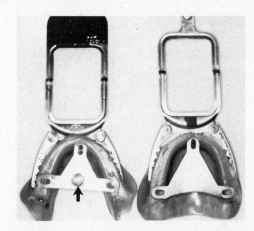

Fig. 13-7. *Right,* Central-bearing plate is centered and attached on the occlusal surface of the upper occlusion rim. *Left,* Central-bearing plate containing the central-bearing point *(arrow)* is centered and attached to the lower occlusion rim. The vertical space between the jaws when occlusion rims and tracing devices are in mouth can be adjusted when the central-bearing point *(arrow)* is raised or lowered.

occlusion rim and the center of the maxillary occlusion rim coincide. However, there is a certain latitude, so that the equalization of pressure is fairly well achieved when the two centers are close to the same point. For this reason, it is a mistake to use a central-bearing point device when the ridge relations are not normal or when there is an excess of soft tissue on the ridges. Likewise, an uneven distribution of soft tissue in different parts of the basal seat can cause errors in a vertical direction, even though the mandible itself is in the correct horizontal position of centric relation.

It is important not to accept any part of the tracing except the apex as an indication of centric relation. When patients chew lightly, they may often close their jaws in eccentric positions. However, patients will pull the mandible to complete retrusion many times under heavy closing pressure exerted during the function of mastication. Therefore, if the dentures are not constructed with centric occlusion in harmony with centric relation, the teeth will not contact evenly when under considerable closing pressure. This uneven or premature contacting is a disturbing factor in the retention and stability of dentures, and it can cause soreness of the tissues supporting the dentures. On the other hand, if centric occlusion is in harmony with centric relation, the patient can function properly with his mandible in all positions under light and heavy chewing pressures.

Extraoral tracings may be used in combination with wax or modeling compound occlusion rims on temporary bases or in combination with a central-bearing point. Extraoral tracings made without a central-bearing point are not considered satisfactory because, although they indicate the correct anteroposterior position of the mandible, they may not record the correct maxillomandibular relation (superoinferior relations of the jaws). It is extremely difficult to maintain equalized pressure on blocks of wax or modeling compound. Therefore there is not much to be gained by securing a tracing without using a central-bearing point.

Intraoral tracing devices. Intraoral tracing devices combine a central-bearing point with a needle point tracing made inside the mouth. The bearing point is sharp, and it makes a tracing on the opposing central-bearing plate (Fig. 13-8). A hole may be drilled in the plate at the apex of the intraoral tracing, or a plastic disk with a hole in it may be placed over the apex of the tracing. The hole or depression is used to ensure that the patient's jaw is in the retruded position while the registration is being recorded with plaster or some such material.

Interocclusal centric relation records. Interocclusal records are made using a recording medium between the occlusion rims, the trial den-

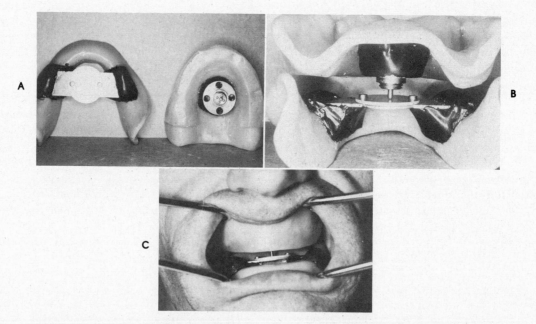

Fig. 13-8. Coble intraoral tracing device. **A,** On the right, the adjustable central-bearing point is attached in palate of upper occlusion rim. On the left, tracing plate is centered in first molar region of lower occlusion rim. **B,** Tracing point is in contact with central-bearing plate as viewed from the posterior aspect of occlusion rims. **C,** Patient is making an intraoral needle point tracing by moving mandible from side to side. Apex of tracing will indicate centric position.

ture bases, or the completed dentures. Materials that are commonly used for interocclusal records include plaster, wax, zinc oxide–eugenol paste, and cold-curing acrylic resins. The patient closes into the recording medium with the lower jaw in its most retruded position and stops the closure at a predetermined vertical relation. Interocclusal records are relatively easy to make, but their success depends on the clinical judgment of the dentist and cooperation between the dentist and the patient. This method is simple because mechanical devices are not used in the patient's mouth and are not attached to the occlusion rims.

Interocclusal registrations are in some respects preferred to registrations using mechanical aids. The earliest registrations of centric relation were generally made with a large mass of wax. This method resulted in many incorrect and inaccurate records. The difficulties in handling wax interocclusal records involve uneven softening and uneven thickness of the recording material and the possible distortion of the record after it is made. Impression plaster, zinc oxide–eugenol paste, acrylic resin, polyether, or silicone can be used as the recording medium. These materials offer little resistance when closure is made into them, their resistance is uniform throughout, and they set hard enough so that the interocclusal records will not be distorted after they set.

The technique for making plaster interocclusal records is quite simple. The patient is comfortably seated upright in the dental chair with the feet flat on the footrest. The head is supported by the headrest to facilitate control of movement of the patient's head, the occlusion rims, and the recording medium.

The thumb and index or middle finger of the dentist's hand are placed between the opposing teeth or occlusion rims. The hand is inverted to cover the eyes of the patient to help control the emotional response of the patient should the concern of the dentist be observed when instructions are not followed properly. The forefinger of the dentist's other hand is placed on the labial surface of the lower anterior teeth or rim to help retain the denture base in position on the residual ridge and to feel the anteroposterior movement of the mandible. As the patient closes the jaws in centric relation, the dentist moves the thumb and finger out of the way, allowing the patient's closing force to maintain both denture bases in position on the residual ridges (Fig. 13-9).

The patient makes sufficient trial closures until both the dentist and the patient are familiar with the procedure. The relationship of the opposing anterior teeth or occlusion rims when the mandible is in centric relation at the desired vertical relation during the trial closure is the dentist's guide to the proper amount of jaw closure when the interocclusal centric relation record is made. Most incorrect centric relation records can be recognized at the time the records are made, but futher checks and tests must be used to detect small errors in the records. One can do this by setting the posterior teeth in centric occlusion on the articulator and observing their occlusion in the mouth.

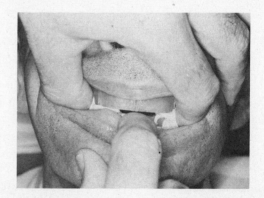

Fig. 13-9. Patient closes jaws into soft plaster to record the most posterior relation of mandible to maxillae. This kind of recording is called a *direct interocclusal centric relation record*. Position of hands when making an interocclusal record permits dentist to make certain that trial denture bases are in proper position on residual ridges, to feel movement of mandible as patient closes jaws together, to help guide mandible during closure, and to cover eyes of the patient.

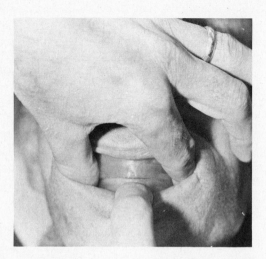

Fig. 13-10. Interocclusal centric relation record is made by adjustment of occlusion rims until they appear to meet evenly when mandible is in its most retruded relation to maxillae and then sealing rims together. This method is unsatisfactory because of unequal displacement of soft tissues of basal seat and uncontrollable movement of occlusion rims.

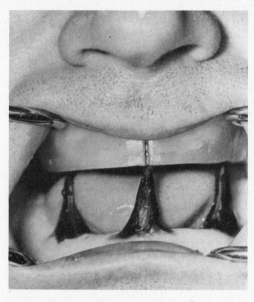

Fig. 13-11. Soft cones of wax attached to mandibular base form an interocclusal record as they are forced against upper occlusion rim during swallowing. Swallowing procedure is supposed to establish both proper vertical and proper horizontal relation of mandible to maxillae.

Other methods of recording centric relation. Some records are made by adjustment of the occlusion rims until they contact fairly evenly in the mouth at the desired vertical relation. Strips of Celluloid or paper placed between the rims are held tight while under closing pressure. If a strip pulls out easily, it indicates less pressure on this side than on the other side. The height of the occlusion rims is reduced at the location of excess pressure or built up at the location of reduced pressure. Such a procedure is most often unsatisfactory.

Another method of obtaining records with wax occlusion rims is to heat the surface of one of the rims and have the patient close into this softened surface to make a new maxillomandibular relation record (Fig. 13-10). This procedure does not remove the errors of unequal pressure.

A great improvement in the method of softening wax rims is deep heating posterior portions of the mandibular wax rim and leaving the anterior portion cold to maintain the predetermined vertical relation to occlusion.

Deep heating sometimes is referred to as pooling. Deep pooling is accomplished by insertion of a hot wax spatula down into the center of the lower occlusion rim, first on one side and then on the other, thus allowing time for the inner hot portion of the wax to soften the outer portion enough so that the outer walls will collapse readily under closing pressure. The maxillary rim is not softened, and thus it will not be affected during its contact with the heated mandibular rim. After the wax has been chilled, the surplus is trimmed away, since it would guide the mandible back into the same relation during subsequent mandibular closures. In other words, the surplus wax would not permit a testing or verification of the centric relation record.

Another method utilizes softened wax placed over the occlusal surfaces of the posterior mandibular teeth. The recording wax is not placed over the anterior teeth because it would tend to cause the patient to protrude the mandible. In this method, the maxillary teeth close into wax instead of wax contacting wax as in other methods. The advantage of this method is that comparatively small surfaces are in contact instead of large flat wax surfaces. A disadvantage is that most often the record must be made at an

increased vertical dimension of occlusion to prevent contact of opposing teeth.

Swallowing procedures and chew-in records are included as physiologic techniques for recording centric relation. In one swallowing technique, soft cones of wax are placed on the lower trial denture base. The wax cones contact the occlusal surface of the upper occlusion rim when the patient swallows. This provides a record of the horizontal relation of the mandible to the maxillae (Fig. 13-11). Unfortunately, the mandibular position recorded by this method is not necessarily consistent with centric relation or repeatable.

14

Recording and transfer bases
and occlusion rims

Dentists should not be exclusively concerned with the vertical forces delivered through the occlusal surfaces of the teeth to the denture-bearing tissues. The horizontal forces exerted on the external surfaces of the dentures are also important and have to be taken into consideration in the making of complete dentures. Fish (1948) described a denture as having three surfaces: the impression surface, the occlusal surface, and the polished surface. All three surfaces are developed independently in complete denture prosthodontics, but they are integrated by the dentist to create a stable, functional, esthetic result. The polished surface of a denture consists of the nonarticulating surfaces of the teeth along with the labial, buccal, lingual, and palatal parts of the denture base material. The design and orientation of this surface is determined by its relationship to the functional role of the tongue, lips, and cheeks (Fig. 14-1, *A* to *C*). The polished surface occupies a position of equilibrium between these groups of muscles and is frequently referred to as the neutral zone (Fig. 14-1, *D*).

Occlusion rims are employed as provisional substitutes for the planned complete dentures and used to record both the neutral zone and maxillomandibular relations. They are made on the stone cast that represents the denture-supporting tissues and consist of a denture base and a wax rim (Fig. 14-2). The denture base, or

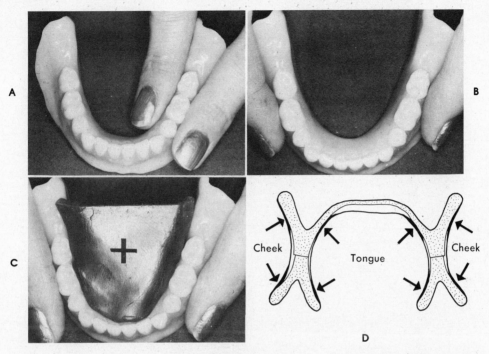

Fig. 14-1. Design and orientation of polished surface of denture is influenced by functional activity of tongue, cheeks, and lips. **A** to **C,** Relative positions of groups of muscles making up tongue, cheeks, and lips is simulated by the fingers. The area marked + in **C** represents a "tongue" made out of wax. **D,** Diagram of direction of muscular activity in a coronal plane drawn through molar region of the two occlusion rims. *Shaded areas,* Neutral zone.

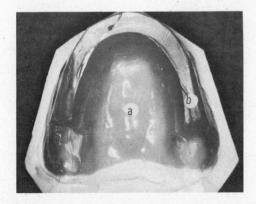

Fig. 14-2. Maxillary occlusion rim. The recording base, *a,* is usually made out of hard baseplate wax or cold-curing resin. The rim, *b,* is made out of wax.

recording base, must be rigid, accurate, and stable. It is referred to as a trial denture base if it is made out of wax or, preferably, autopolymerizing (cold-curing) acrylic resin. Such a denture base will be used at both the registration and try-in appointments. On the other hand, the denture base can be made out of processed acrylic resin, and eventually the selected teeth are processed to it. The rim itself is preferably made out of baseplate wax because of its ease of management and convenience.

TRIAL DENTURE BASE, OR RECORDING BASE

Wax bases are frequently used (Figs. 14-3 and 14-4) and must be reinforced with wire. Sometimes they are lined with a zinc oxide–eugenol

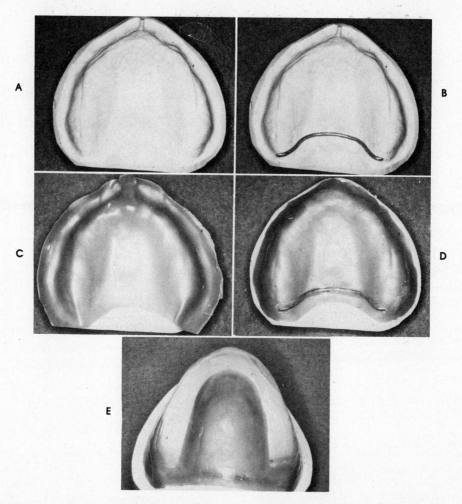

Fig. 14-3. Construction of extra-hard wax occlusion rims. **A,** Maxillary cast has been dusted with talcum powder as a separating medium. **B,** Ten-gauge reinforcement wire is adapted to posterior palatal area to extend through hamular notches, 2 mm in front of vibrating line. **C** and **D,** Sheet of softened baseplate wax is pressed firmly against cast to form recording base. **E,** Roll of softened wax is sealed to this base and contoured to desired arch form. Rim is built to a height slightly greater than total length of teeth and amount of shrinkage of residual alveolar ridge.

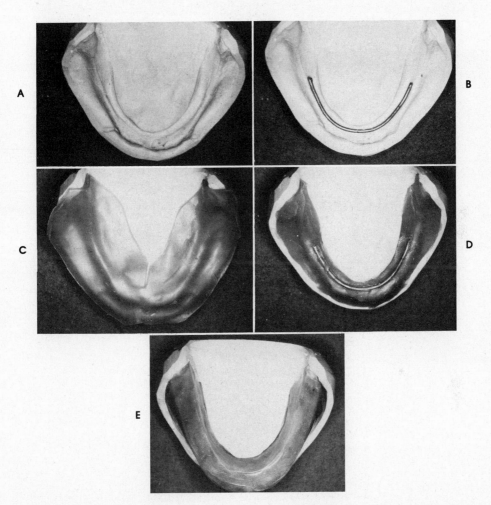

Fig. 14-4. Mandibular cast, **A,** has a reinforcing wire adapted on lingual side of residual ridge. **B** to **D,** Sheet of softened baseplate wax is closely adapted to potential denture-bearing area of cast to form the recording base. **E,** Roll of softened wax is sealed to base and contoured to desired form.

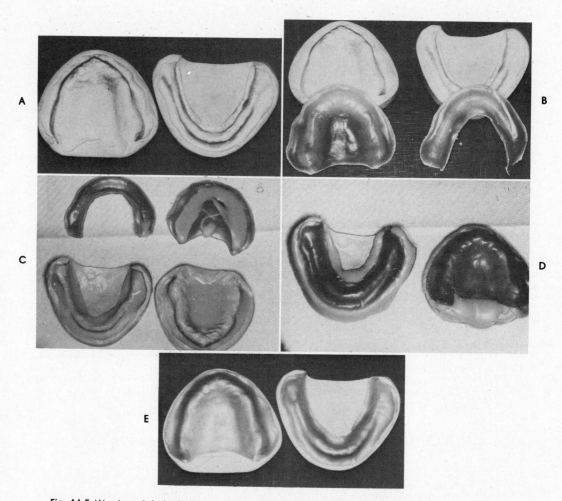

Fig. 14-5. Wax template technique for making a trial denture base. **A,** One prepares master casts by waxing out undercuts and applying a separating medium. **B,** Wax templates are formed and lined with autopolymerizing acrylic resin in **C** and **D.** In **E** the completed (well-fitting and stable) trial base is ready for addition of occlusion rims.

impression paste seated on the cast, to which a separating medium has been applied. These bases may be bulky and brittle, but dentists frequently find them easier to work with when setting up teeth, especially in those situations where a restricted interarch distance exists. Autopolymerizing resin trial denture bases are also extensively used. Undercuts first have to be blocked out on the cast to avoid possible damage, and the resin is molded onto the cast at its doughlike stage. Or a wax template is lined with a cold-curing resin (Fig. 14-5) though a slightly

more time-consuming, autopolymerizing resin base can be made by the "sprinkle-on" method (Fig. 14-6). The monomer and polymer are applied alternately until a relatively even thickness of resin base is achieved. In either case, the casts are placed in hot water in a pressure cooker for 10 minutes under 30 pounds of pressure. This step produces rapid polymerization, and excess monomer is eliminated. Both methods produce a base that is rigid, stable, and easily contoured and polished. Acrylic resin baseplates are excellent bases for making maxillomandibu-

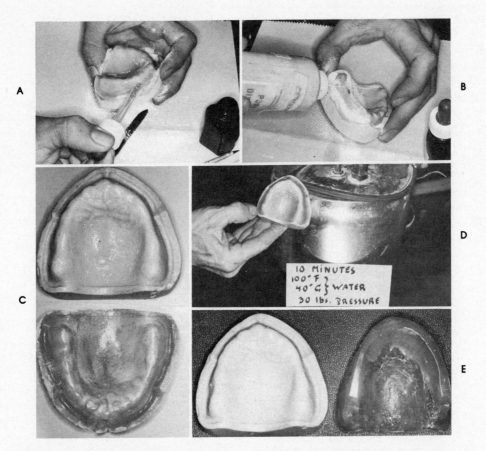

Fig. 14-6. "Sprinkle-on" method of making a resin denture base. **A** and **B,** Monomer and polymer are applied alternately until an evenly thick base is developed, **C. D,** Base and cast are placed in a pressure cooker to complete polymerization. **E,** Denture base is trimmed and polished, and a wax rim is sealed onto it.

lar relation records. They fit accurately and are not easily distorted. Their only disadvantage is that they might take up space that is needed for setting the teeth, necessitating some grinding of the resin base in required areas. They may also be loose because of the necessary blockout of undercuts in the cast. A trial denture base and occlusion rim made of extra-hard baseplate wax is easiest for arranging the teeth (Figs. 14-3 and 14-4). The wax can be softened all the way through to the cast, so that the teeth can be set directly against the cast if necessary. For many patients "hard" baseplate materials must be cut away so that the teeth can be set in their proper places.

The denture base can be processed onto the final cast before the relations-registration appointment. This procedure offers the dentist the advantage of using the base or fitting surface of the completed denture throughout all the patient's clinical appointments. This base may be made of heat-curing, cold-curing, or one of the "pour" type acrylic resins. After the maxillomandibular relations have been confirmed and the set-up completed, the teeth are processed to this base. This is a recommended procedure, but it is more time-consuming and ultimately more expensive.

OCCLUSION RIMS

The occlusion rims can be used to establish (1) the level of the occlusal plane; (2) the arch form, which is related to the activity of the lips, cheeks, and tongue; (3) preliminary jaw relation records, the vertical and horizontal jaw relationships (including tentative facial support), and an estimate of the interocclusal distance. Unfortunately, none of these determinations can be made in a precise scientific way, and most of the knowledge concerning them is theoretical. However, there are several basic principles that have proved to be successful clinically, and these principles can be used to help achieve the objectives enumerated.

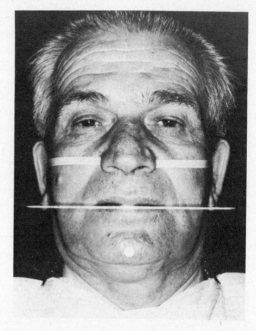

Fig. 14-7. For demonstration purposes, the ala-tragus line on this patient has been "taped on" bilaterally. Occlusal plane is established when wax occlusion rim is made parallel to this line. A Fox plane-guide is generally used for this purpose.

Level of the occlusal plane

Many dentists use a technique wherein the occlusal plane is established on the maxillary occlusion rim. The procedure entails developing the occlusion rim so that the incisal plane is parallel with the interpupillary line and at a height that allows for the length of the natural tooth plus the amount of tissue resorption that has occurred. The length of the upper lip can be a guide if it is of average length. The occlusal plane, posteriorly, is made to parallel the ala-tragus line on the basis of the position of most natural occlusal planes (Fig. 14-7). Then the lower occlusal rim is adjusted to meet evenly with the upper rim and reduced until an adequate interocclusal distance is obtained. This procedure is adequate for many patients and

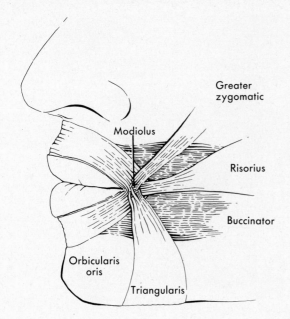

Greater
zygomatic

Modiolus

Risorius

Buccinator

Orbicularis
oris

Triangularis

Fig. 14-8. Diagram of modiolus at corner of the mouth.

usually results in satisfactory dentures. It certainly cannot be regarded as applicable to all patients.

The works of Fish (1948) and Wright (1966) have led to a different approach to occlusal plane determination. Wright described tongue function and its relationship to the occlusal plane and mandibular denture stability. When his work is related to Fish's description of the neutral zone and the activity of the modiolus muscles, a rational and clear guide for occlusal plane determination evolves. The food bolus is triturated while resting on the mandibular occlusal surfaces (occlusal table). This table is an area bounded by the cheek tissues buccally, the tongue lingually, the pterygomandibular raphe and its overlying tissues distally, and the contraction of the corner of the mouth mesially. The mesial boundary is a point where eight muscles meet at the corner of the mouth. The meeting place, called the *modiolus* (Latin, the hub of a wheel), forms a distinct conical prominence at the corner of the mouth (Fig. 14-8). If one puts the thumb inside the

corner of the mouth and the finger outside on the prominence and then the lip and cheek are contracted, the modiolus feels like a knot. The modiolus becomes fixed every time the buccinator contracts, which is a natural accompaniment of all chewing efforts. The modiolus contraction presses the corner of the mouth against the premolars so that the occlusal table is closed in the front. Food is crushed by the premolars and molars does not escape at the corner of the mouth unless seventh nerve damage occurred, as in Bell's palsy.

The practical application of Fish's and Wright's research lies in developing the polished surface of the denture in the occlusion rims and establishing the height of the occlusal plane at this stage. The corners of the mouth are marked on the occlusion rims to provide the dentist and technician with anterior landmarks for the height of the first premolars (Fig. 14-9, *A* to *C*). The retromolar pads are relatively stable posterior landmarks even in patients with advanced ridge reduction. Wright (1966)

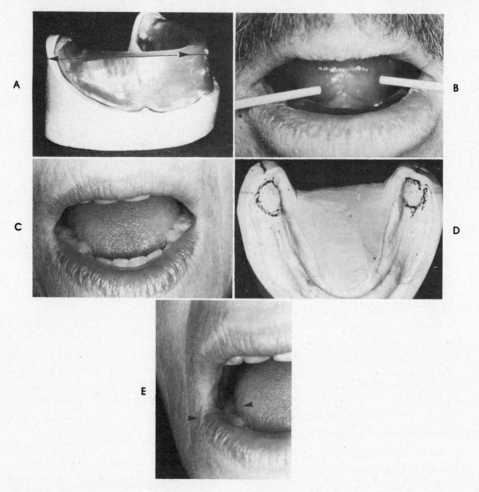

Fig. 14-9. Mandibular occlusion rim, **A,** is trimmed to conform to two pairs of landmarks: the right and left corners of the mouth, **B** and **C,** and two thirds of the way up the retromolar pads, **D.** The wax rim is melted with a hot spatula to the level indicated by arrows in **A.** Mandibular teeth set up to this level, **E,** will conform to tongue, cheeks, and activities of corners of the mouth *(arrows).*

showed that the mandibular first molar is usually at a level corresponding to two thirds of the way up the retromolar pad (Fig. 14-9, *D*). The retromolar pads are circled on the final casts. The land, or edge of the cast, is marked at points two thirds the length of the pad from its anterior border. These points will aid in determining the height of the distal end of the occlusal plane. The anterior and posterior landmarks are joined up when the wax is melted to this level with a

hot spatula. It will be observed that the resultant occlusal plane is almost invariably parallel to the residual alveolar ridges and to the interpupillary line. Its height will conform to tongue, cheek, and corner of the mouth activities (Fig. 14-9, *E*), which will enhance mandibular denture stability. The maxillary occlusion rim is next adjusted to meet evenly with the mandibular rim and reduced until an adequate interocclusal distance is obtained.

The tests that aid the dentist in establishing the correct vertical dimension of occlusion by means of occlusion rims are reviewed in Chapter 13.

Following are the tests most frequently used:

1. Judgment of the overall facial support.

2. Visual observation of space between the rims when the jaws are at rest.

3. Measurements between dots on the face when the jaws are at rest and when the occlusion rims are in contact.

4. Observations made when the *s* sound is enunciated accurately and repeatedly—the average speaking space. This ensures that the occlusion rims come close together but do not contact. It must be emphasized that the interocclusal (interrim), or speaking, space which exists between the posterior teeth when the patient is enunciating *s* sounds is not related to the interocclusal space of rest position. Clinical experience suggests that this space is about 1.5 to 3 mm for most patients. However, patients with Class II occlusions tend to have a larger speaking space (3 to 6 mm), and Class III occlusion patients have a critically small space of about 1 mm (Pound, 1976).

Both tests 1 and 2 are particularly effective if the patient's old dentures are used for comparative purposes. Old dentures can be useful for prognostic purposes, especially if they are used with treatment liners to recover an optimal vertical dimension of occlusion. Old dentures can also have their facial surfaces selectively augmented with a soft wax to assist the dentist in assessment of the required cosmetic support from the dentures' polished surfaces. This is a useful step when the shape of the dental arch form is determined, as it should be, by the dentist.

It is now possible to proceed to the next clinical step and make a preliminary centric relation record. However, the dentist may elect to consider the development of arch forms at this appointment, using the patient's occlusion rims. This step will provide the dentist or technician with even more essential information regarding the horizontal placement of the artificial teeth. Consequently, a discussion of dental arch form will precede the discussion on making centric relation records.

Arch form

Both the width of the occluding surfaces and the contour of the arch form of the occlusion rims should be individually established for each patient to simulate the desired arch form of artificial teeth. Such an analog of the missing teeth and their supporting tissues will enable the dentist or technician to accurately follow instructions for arranging the artificial teeth. This can serve to reduce the amount of time spent with the patient by the dentist at the try-in appointment and allow more time for perfecting the arrangement of the teeth.

Fish (1931) drew the profession's attention to the concept of a neutral zone in complete denture construction. He argued that the natural teeth occupy a zone in complete denture construction. He argued that the natural teeth occupy a zone of equilibrium, with each natural tooth assuming a position that is the resultant of all the various forces acting on it. This is usually a stable position unless actual changes in the dentition occur. When natural teeth are replaced by artificial teeth, it is logical to place the artificial teeth in a position as close as possible to the one previously occupied. The same forces that stabilized the natural teeth can then be used to stabilize the dentures. In the treatment of partially edentulous patients, it is common to find that sufficient natural teeth remain to provide a guide for the positions of the artificial teeth. When the patient is edentulous, it is not always easy to determine where the natural teeth were in realtion to the partially or totally resorbed alveolar ridges. Clinical judgment must be brought to bear on such situations, which are often quite challenging.

Certain types of dentitions are accompanied by specific patterns of soft-tissue behavior. Clinical observation of denture patients suggests that these characteristic types of soft-tissue movements persist into old age and offer a clue to the location of the preexisting natural teeth (Berry and Wilkie, 1964). The best guide to determining and designing the arch form is the consideration of the pattern of bone resorption where the teeth are lost and the utilization of anatomic landmarks that are relatively stable in position.

Clinical experience and reports by Beresin and Schiesser (1978) and, more recently, by Karlsson and Hedegård (1979) confirm that the denture space or neutral zone can be reproduced with only a limited variation that lies within the range of clinical acceptability.

Mandibular arch form. The occlusion rim is designed to conform to the arch form that the dentist judges that the patient had before the natural teeth and alveolar bone were lost. In the lower jaw, a larger proportion of bone loss occurs on the labial side of the anterior residual ridge. The bone loss occurs equally on the buccal and lingual sides of the residual ridge in the premolar region. In the molar region the bone loss appears to be primarily from the lingual side of the ridge because of the cross-section shape of the mandible, which is wider at its inferior border than at the ridge crest. Thus the residual ridge becomes almost invariably more lingually placed in the anterior region and more buccally placed in the posterior region. The occlusion rim is contoured as a guide when the artificial teeth are placed labial to the ridge anteriorly, over the ridge in the premolar region, and slightly lingual to the ridge in the molar region. The curvatures of the occlusion rims, which simulate the arch form of the posterior teeth, follow the curvature of the mandible itself when seen from above. Lines are drawn on the cast to carefully evaluate the arch form. One line is drawn from the lingual side of the retromolar pad and extended anteriorly to a point just lingual to the crest of the ridge in the premolar region. This line aids in positioning the lingual surfaces of the posterior teeth, and it establishes the lingual extent of the occlusion rim (Fig. 14-10). This lin-

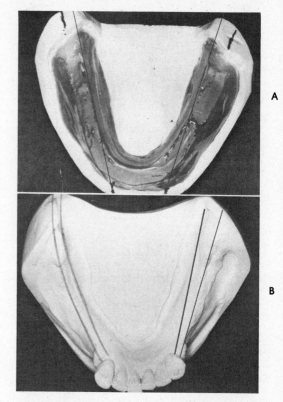

Fig. 14-10. A, Straight line drawn from lingual side of retromolar pad to a point just lingual to the crest of the ridge in premolar region can act as a guide for positioning artificial posterior teeth. **B,** Partially edentulous cast with a straight line on right side and a curved line on left side. Configuration of line depends on curvature of body of mandible.

gual line could be a curved line that is similar to the curvature of the body of the mandible. The anterior part of the occlusion rim is contoured to compensate for the estimated bone loss in this region, and the corners of the mouth are used as guides for determining an approximate location for the canines and first premolars. The experienced dentist learns to visualize the artificial teeth (represented at this state by the contoured rim) as growing out of the alveolar bone and following the curvature of the bone out of which they grew. The end result of this approach is an arch form that is frequently not on the residual ridge. Several techniques using soft waxes (Lott and Levin, 1966), zinc oxide–eugenol impression pastes, and tissue conditioners have been proposed as adjunctive efforts to establish a correct neutral zone for the arch form. In those circumstances in which advanced anterior ridge reduction has been accompanied by mentalis muscle attachment migration to the crest of the ridge, a certain amount of compromise is essential, and the rim is trimmed very thin and placed on, or lingual to, the ridge crest. If this sort of compromise creates an intolerable situation for the patient, surgical labial sulcus deepening in this area may be considered. Some dentists and technicians have subscribed to a tooth-on-the-ridge philosophy, which has seriously undermined efforts for denture stability and esthetics. The concept of a neutral zone in the context of a keen understanding of patterns of alveolar ridge resorption enables the dentist to determine the arch form for the patient receiving treatment.

Maxillary arch form. Bone reduction usually occurs on the labial and buccal areas of the maxillary residual ridge. Consequently, the residual ridge is usually palatal to the original location of the natural teeth. The maxillary teeth should be labial and buccal to the residual ridge if they are to be placed in the neutral zone and occupy the position of their predecessors. Frequently this pattern of bony reduction is ignored, and the dentist ends up with a contracted maxillary arch form that is within the confines of the mandibular arch form. This oversight guarantees inadequate labial support. The incisive papilla appears to occupy a stable locale on the palate, unless it is modified surgically. Clinical experience indicates that the incisal edges of the maxillary central incisors are usually 8 to 10 mm anterior to the center of the incisive papilla. The tips of the canines are also related to the center of the papilla, and a high percentage of canines are ± 1 mm in front of the papilla (Fig. 14-11, A). The papilla is circled, and this landmark is a rough guide in locating the anteroposterior position of the maxillary anterior teeth (Fig. 14-11, B). Watt and Likeman (1974) recently showed

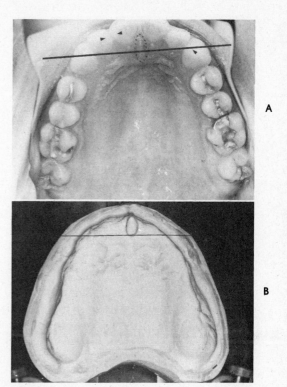

Fig. 14-11. A, Natural dentition in which tips of maxillary canines are frequently ± 1 mm in front of center of incisive papilla *(dotted circle)*. Papilla is circled on edentulous cast, **B,** since it provides a rough guide to position of maxillary canines.

that after the teeth are lost, the canines should be located in a coronal plane passing through the posterior border of the papilla. A patient's old dentures, preextraction photographs, or diagnostic casts and photographs of the patient made before the dentition had deteriorated may be usefully employed at this appointment to assist the dentist not only in his selection of artificial teeth, but also in establishing the optimal labial support for the patient. If the patient has been wearing inadequate dentures, tooth loss will have a pronounced effect on the appearance of the lips and the adjacent tissues. As a result of loss of substance and the reduction in elastic properties, the connective tissue will not pro-

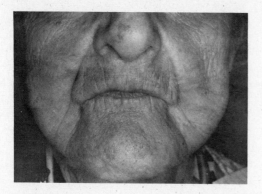

Fig. 14-12. Degenerative skin changes bring about a near continuity between nasolabial fold and corner of the mouth.

vide sufficient resistance to the activities of the orbicularis oris and associated muscles (Lee, 1962). As a consequence the effect of the degenerative changes in the skin become exaggerated, and the lips appear to have aged to a much greater extent than the surrounding parts. The skin becomes roughened, and deep vertical lines appear in the body and margins of the lips. There is a noticeable shortening and thinning of the lips because of a tendency for the lip margins to roll inward. The nasolabial fold changes direction to become almost continuous with the groove at the corner of the mouth, and the lips and cheeks are no longer distinctly separated (Fig. 14-12). Such a loss of well-defined demarcation tends to produce a generally disordered appearance of the lower half of the face (Lee, 1962). At this stage it may be difficult to visualize proper lip support in an attempt to counter the changes described before. However, the experienced dentist will generally use the occlusion rim to achieve the best compromise between neutral zone determination and harmonious labial support. Cheek support is probably not affected as much as lip support by altering labial support, since the buccinator muscle is stretched between the pterygomandibular raphe and the modiolus muscles. It must be remembered that the longer the period of edentulism, the greater will be the loss of the original muscle patterns and the less easily and completely will they be relearned when even the best dentures are provided. The more accurate

the replacement and the sooner it occurs, the easier will be the task of relearning.

The anterior position of the maxillary occlusion rim is modified so that it is gently caressed by the lower lip during pronunciation of the letter f. The rim is usually parallel with the interpupillary line and at a height that allows for the length of the natural tooth plus the amount of assessed bone reduction that has occurred. It is possible, though rather difficult to visualize, to simulate proper length and lip support by contouring the labial aspect of the maxillary occlusion rim. It would be preferable and in fact easier for the dentist to select the anterior teeth for the patient's denture at the examination appointment and set them for proper length and lip support in the occlusion rims. Further characterization of the anterior arrangement can then be done at the patient's next appointment.

Preliminary centric relation record

The preliminary centric relation record is made after the occlusion rims have been contoured, and it is designed to simulate the position that will be occupied by the artificial teeth and tissues of the complete dentures (Fig. 14-13). The occlusion rims are used to establish a preliminary centric relation record and to transfer it by means of a face-bow to a semiadjustable articulator. Once the anterior teeth have been placed in their final positions in the occlusion rim, a record is made of the jaw relation when

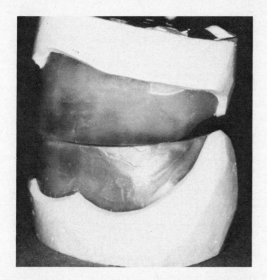

Fig. 14-13. Two occlusion rims have been contoured and adjusted and are now ready to be used for making preliminary centric relation record.

the incisor teeth are in an edge-to-edge position. This record will enable the dentist to adjust the condylar guidances of the articulator.

An articulator is used in complete denture construction to simulate jaw movements for convenience and because of the lack of a solid base in the patient's mouth. The use of a semiadjustable articulator requires that at least four jaw relations be transferred from the patient to the instrument: (1) the relation of the jaws to the opening axis (Chapter 15), (2) the vertical separation of the jaws, (3) the horizontal relation of

the lower to the upper jaw in centric relation, and (4) the relation of the lower jaw to the upper jaw when the mandible is protruded (Chapter 20) so that the incisor teeth are edge to edge. Quite obviously, all these records must be made by the dentist.

The vertical and horizontal relations of the jaws are integral components of the centric relation position of the edentulous patient. The provisional vertical dimension of occlusion is first established, and the horizontal jaw relation record is made at this level.

REFERENCES

Beresin, V.E., and Schiesser, F.J.: The neutral zone in complete and partial dentures, ed. 2, St. Louis, 1978, The C.V. Mosby Co.

Berry, D.C., and Wilkie, J.K.: An approach to dental prosthetics, vol. 2, Pergamon Series on Dentistry, London, 1964, Pergamon Press.

Fish, E.W.: An analysis of the stabilising factors in full denture construction, Br. Dent. J. **52:**559-570, 1931.

Fish, W.: principles of full denture prosthesis, ed. 4, London, 1948, Staples Press, Ltd.

Karlsson, S., and Hedegård, B.: Study of the reproducibility of the functional denture space with a dynamic impression technique, J. Prosthet. Dent. **41:**21-25, 1979.

Lee, J.H.: Dental aesthetics, Bristol, 1962, John Wright & Sons, Ltd.

Lott, F., and Levin, B.: Flange technique: an anatomic and physiologic approach to increased retention, function, comfort, and appearance of denture, J. Prosthet. Dent. **16:**394-413, 1966.

Pound, E.: Controlling anomalies of vertical dimension and speech, J. Prosthet. Dent. **36:**124-135, 1976.

Watt, D.M., and Likeman, P.R.: Morphological changes in the denture bearing area following the extraction of maxillary teeth, Br. Dent. J. **136:**225-235, 1974.

Wright, C.R.: Evaluation of the factors necessary to develop stability in mandibular dentures, J. Prosthet. Dent. **16:**414-430, 1966.

15

Relating the patient to the articulator

The final test for success or failure of complete dentures is made in the patient's mouth. A demonstration of an excellently planned occlusion on the articulator, though an important mechanical entity in itself, is meaningless unless that occlusion functions in the mouth in harmony with the biologic factors that regulate the mandibular activity of the patient.

If it were practical to do so, the patient's mouth would be the best articulator. However, it is mechanically impossible to intraorally perform many of the procedures involved in construction of complete dentures. Furthermore, the dentist must consider the movement of the trial dentures on supporting soft tissues in the mouth and the difficulties posed by the presence of saliva and the patient's ability to cooperate. The convenience of the dentist and dental laboratory technician dictate that an articulator be used.

ARTICULATORS

An articulator is a mechanical device to which maxillary and mandibular casts may be attached, representing the temporomandibular joints and jaw members. Articulators are used to hold casts in one or more positions in relation to each other for the purposes of diagnosis, arrangement of artificial teeth, and development of the occlusal surfaces of fixed restorations. They have been made in hundreds of different designs. The designs of articulators have been based on (1) theories of occlusion, (2) types of records used for their adjustment, and (3) the adjustments of which they are capable. Some articulators are simple with only one function—to hold the casts in centric relation with each other. Most of these consist of a simple hinged device. Other articulators are complex, and some of these require complicated apparatus for transferring records of jaw relationships from the patient's mouth to the articulator. The necessary records may be simple or complex depending on the instrument being adjusted.

Articulators based on theories of occlusion

In the history of articulators, at least three theories of occlusion have been proposed as bases for the inventors' articulator designs. These will be briefly described.

The Bonwill theory of occlusion proposed that the teeth move in relation to each other as guided by the condylar controls and the incisal point. It was known as the theory of the equilateral triangle, in which there was a 4-inch (10 cm) distance between the condyles and between each condyle and the incisor point. The articulator designed by W.G.A. Bonwill is shown in Fig. 15-1. It allows lateral movement, but since the condylar guidances were not adjustable, they permitted movement of the mechanism only in the horizontal plane.

The conical theory of occlusion proposed that the lower teeth move over the surfaces of the upper teeth as over the surface of a cone, with a generating angle of 45 degrees and with the central axis of the cone tipped at a 45-degree angle to the occlusal plane. The Hall Automatic articulator designed by R.E. Hall (Fig. 15-2) is an example of an articulator designed to conform to the conical theory of occlusion. It should be noted that teeth having 45-degree cusps were necessary when dentures were made on this instrument.

The spherical theory of occlusion shows the lower teeth moving over the surface of the

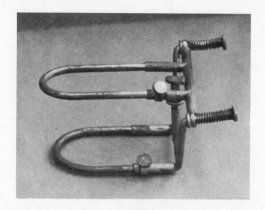

Fig. 15-1. Bonwill articulator.

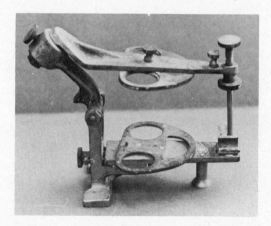

Fig. 15-2. Hall Automatic articulator. Notice steep incisal guidance that makes it necessary to use teeth with high cusps.

upper teeth as over the surface of a sphere with a diameter of 8 inches (20 cm). The center of the sphere is located in the region of the glabella, and the surface of the sphere passes through the glenoid fossae along the articulating eminences or concentric with them. The theory was proposed by G.S. Monson in 1918, and it was based on observations of natural teeth and skulls made by von Spee, a German anatomist. The "Maxillomandibular instrument" (Fig. 15-3), devised by Monson, was based on the spherical theory of occlusion. The Hagman Balancer and one phase

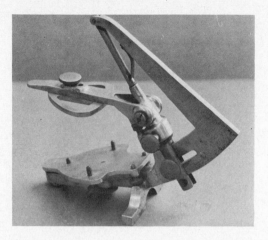

Fig. 15-3. Monson Maxillomandibular instrument.

of the Pankey-Mann occlusal reconstruction technique also have their basis in the spherical theory of occlusion.

The articulators based on theories of occlusion have one common fault: they make no provision for variations from the theoretical relationships that occur in different persons. When the variation of the inclinations of the condylar paths of the two sides of many patients is recognized, the need for variation is apparent. Also, the wide variation of paths of jaw movements between different persons is obvious. These factors make individually variable condylar guidances on articulators essential.

Articulators based on the types of records used for their adjustment

Three general classes of records are used for transferring maxillomandibular relationships from the patient to the articulator: interocclusal records, graphic records, and hinge axis records. Some articulators are designed for use with only one type of record, whereas others use combinations of two or three types of records.

Interocclusal record adjustment. Most articulators in common use today for complete denture construction are adjusted by some kind of interocclusal records. These records may be made in wax, plaster of paris, zinc oxide–eugenol paste, or cold-curing acrylic resin. Each of these records is of only one positional relationship of the lower jaw to the upper jaw. Articulators may or may not have the capability of adjustment to all interocclusal records. It is at this point that differences in articulators become apparent when they are analyzed. Some are adjustable to centric relation records only, and others are adjustable to protrusive and centric relation records. Still others are adjustable to lateral relation records as well.

The mechanical features that determine whether an articulator can be adjusted to accommodate interocclusal records include (1) individually adjustable horizontal condylar guidances, (2) variable controls for the Bennett (direct lateral shift) movement, (3) variable intercondylar distance, (4) split-axis condylar guidance controls (to allow the Bennett movement in the instrument to be upward, downward, forward, or backward, as the articulator is moved into lateral positions), and (5) adjustable incisal guidance controls.

The recorded and adjusted relationships and positions of the casts on the articulators are accurate only at the positions at which the interocclusal records are made. All other relationships on the articulator are approximations.

Graphic record adjustment. Articulators designed for use with graphic records are generally more complicated than those used with interocclusal records. Since the graphic records consist of records of the extreme border positions of mandibular movements, the articulators must be capable of producing at least the equivalent of curved movements. The reason is that the border movements of the mandible are in curves.

These instruments and others similar to them are capable of reproducing, with reasonable accuracy, the border movements of the mandible, provided that the graphic records themselves are accurate. Accurate graphic records for this purpose are not too difficult to make, provided that the complicated kinematic face-bow and "jaw writing" apparatus is firmly attached to the jaws. This is a simple procedure if natural teeth exist in both jaws, but it becomes most difficult, and the records even unreliable, when patients are edentulous. This is especially true when the basal seats for the dentures are unfavorable.

Hinge axis location for adjusting articulators. All the instruments that can be adjusted to graphic records have one thing in common: the necessity for correct location of the opening axis of the mandible. A failure to correctly locate the "hinge axis" of the patient's mandible will make the correct adjustment of these instruments impossible.

One instrument, the Transograph, depends entirely on the accurate location of the hinge axis for its adjustment. It is adapted from a kinematic face-bow assembly, and the tests for accuracy are made with wax interocclusal records of centric position made in varying thickness. The Transograph provides no opportunity for adjustment to protrusive or lateral jaw relations.

SELECTION OF AN ARTICULATOR
FOR COMPLETE DENTURES

The large number of different designs of articulators available and the wide range of adjustment possibilities in these articulators can leave the dentist quite confused when one must be chosen. However, this need not be so. The choice of articulator must be made on the basis of what is expected of it. If occlusal contacts are to be perfected in centric occlusion only, a simple, sturdy, hinge type of articulator without provision for lateral or protrusive movements could be selected. This type of instrument has been called a one-dimensional instrument because only one interocclusal record is necessary for its adjustment and use.

If denture teeth are to have cross-arch and cross-tooth balanced occlusion, the minimum requirement is a semiadjustable articulator. This would be an instrument with individually adjustable condylar guidances in both the vertical and horizontal planes, such as the simple instruments in the Hanau University series, or the Whip Mix articulator.

If complete control of the occlusion is desired, a completely adjustable, three-dimensional articulator is of value. A three-dimensional articulator requires a centric relation record, a minimum of two lateral records, and some means for controlling the height and inclinations of the cusps. The records for their adjustment may be interocclusal records or three-dimensional graphic tracings made by a kinematic face-bow apparatus.

These more complicated articulators pose some problems for use in making complete dentures because of the resiliency of the soft tissues of the basal seat on which the recording bases must rest. Because the resiliency permits some movement of the bases in relation to the bone, the records made are not necessarily records of the true path of movement of the bone.

Therefore it becomes essential that the casts representing the patient's mandible and maxillae be oriented in the articulator similarly to the manner in which the jaws of the patient are oriented to one another and to the skull. To accomplish this orientation, certain measurements and records must be taken from the patient and transferred to the articulator to relate the patient to the articulator. Several articulators have been employed in the fabrication of complete dentures. We recognize that excellent results can be obtained with a wide variety of articulating instruments; however, we believe that extensive clinical experience and testing justify the recommendation of two articulators that are used extensively on the North American continent—the Hanau Model 130-28 and the Whip Mix articulators.

Relating the patient to the Hanau articulator

The Hanau articulator is a semiadjustable arcon type of instrument. It consists of an upper member containing the condylar guidance elements and a lower member to which the condylar spheres are attached. The upper and lower members are mechanically connected (Fig. 15-4).

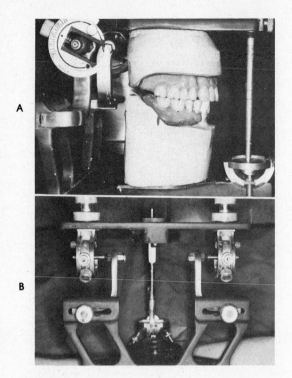

Fig. 15-4. Hanau Model 130-28 articulator. **A,** Side view. **B,** Rear view. Both views show that upper member of articulator carries "condylar housing" or simulated glenoid fossa. Mechanically connected lower member carries condylar spheres, which are contained in upper member's condylar housing.

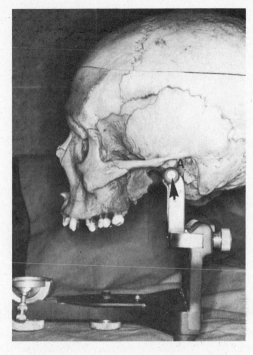

Fig. 15-5. Upper member of articulator has been replaced by a dry skull to simulate relationship of condylar housing, A, to condylar sphere *(arrow)*.

The Hanau articulator is classed as a modified two-dimensional instrument. The upper cast is oriented to the upper member (which represents the skull) by either a kinematic or arbitrary face-bow transfer record (see Fig. 15-5). The arbitrary face-bow is routinely used for complete dentures. The Hanau face-bow consists of a U-shaped frame or assembly that is large enough to extend from the region of the temporomandibular joints to a position 2 to 3 inches (5 to 7.5 cm) in front of the face and wide enough to avoid contact with the sides of the face. The parts that contact the skin over the temporomandibular joints are the condyle rods, and the part that attaches to the occlusion rims is the fork. The condyle rods are positioned on a line extending from the outer canthus of the eye to the top of the tragus of the ear and approximately 13 mm in front of the external auditory meatus (Fig. 15-6). This placement of the condyle rods will locate them within 2 mm of the true center of the opening axis of the jaws. The fork of the face-bow is attached to the maxillary occlusion rim so that the record is one of a simple measurement from the jaws to the approximate axis of the jaws (Fig. 15-7).

Theoretical evidence indicates that articulator adjustments for patients' varying intercondylar widths may be of significance in fixed prosthodontic procedures. This is probably not the

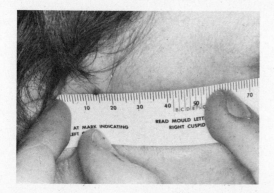

Fig. 15-6. Measurement of 13 mm on a line extending from top of tragus of ear to outer canthus of eye provides dentist with an arbitrary center for opening axis of mandible.

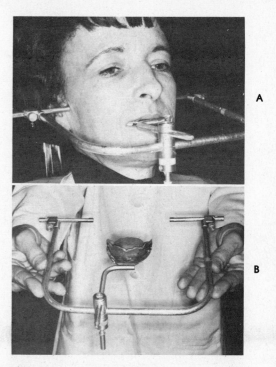

Fig. 15-7. A, Face-bow fork attached to maxillary occlusion rim and face-bow properly located on patient's face. **B,** Completed face-bow record.

case in the treatment of complete denture patients and is considered an elective procedure. The Hanau articulator is machined to accept different intercondylar distances and can be adjusted to each patient's intercondylar width (Fig. 15-8). In this manner, the location of the vertical axes of rotation of the patient's mandible can be approximated on either side of the articulator.

One orients the lower cast to the lower member of the articulator representing the mandible by relating the lower cast to the upper cast through an interocclusal centric relation record (Fig. 15-9).

The horizontal condylar guidances are adjusted by an interocclusal protrusive record. The lateral condylar guidances may be arbitrary or may be adjusted by right and left lateral interocclusal records. The lateral condylar guidances on this articulator do not make provisions for upward, downward, forward, or backward movement of the working condylar sphere.

The articulator is provided with an adjustable incisal guide table that is routinely used for removable prosthodontic restorations. The angulation of the lateral plates of the adjustable incisal guide table is calibrated in degrees, and the plates can be positioned at the desired lateral incisal guidance. The table is adjustable anteroposteriorly to provide the necessary guidance for protrusive movement.

The articulator has a straight incisal guide pin with a flat end, which permits movements on the adjustable incisal guide table. The incisal pin on the Hanau articulator is adjustable and allows for vertical changes without changes in position of the pin to the middle of the incisal guide table (Fig. 15-10).

Relating the patient to the Whip Mix articulator

The Whip Mix articulator is a semiadjustable arcon type of instrument, which consists of an upper member containing the condylar guidances and a lower member to which are attached the condylar spheres (Fig. 15-11). The upper and lower members are not mechanically con-

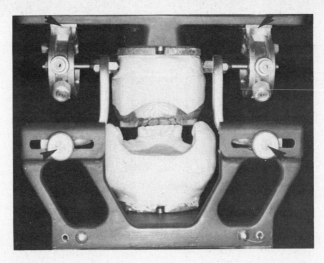

Fig. 15-8. Intercondylar width is adjustable *(arrows),* though this adjustment is rarely carried out in complete denture construction.

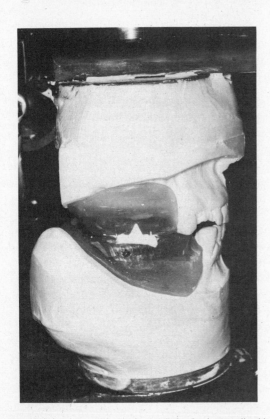

Fig. 15-9. Lower cast for an immediate denture patient is related on articulator by means of an interocclusal centric relation record. Maxillary cast is usually mounted first on articulator. In another technique both casts are mounted simultaneously.

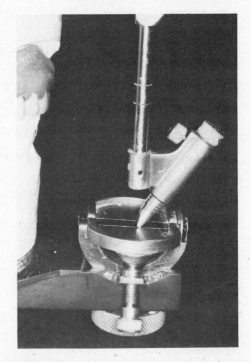

Fig. 15-10. Hanau incisal pin allows for vertical adjustments without moving away from middle of incisal guide table.

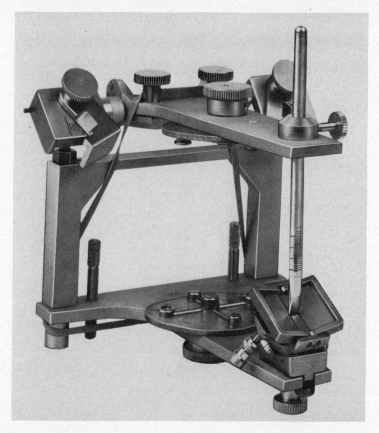

Fig. 15-11. Whip Mix articulator is a two-piece instrument designed on the arcon principle. (Courtesy Whip Mix Corp., Louisville, Ky.)

nected but can be held together when necessary by a rubber band.

The Whip Mix articulator is classed as a modified two-dimensional instrument. The upper cast is oriented to the upper member (which represents the skull) by either a kinematic or arbitrary face-bow transfer record. The arbitrary face-bow is routinely used for complete dentures. This arbitrary face-bow is positioned posteriorly by ear posts that fit into the external auditory meatus and anteriorly by a plastic nasion relator that fits into the concavity of the bridge of the nose. These three points establish an approximation of the axis-orbital plane on the patient so that this plane of reference can be transferred to the articulator.

The distance between the condylar spheres (intercondylar distance) is semiadjustable in a lateral direction and can be regulated for small (88 mm), medium (100 mm), and large (112 mm) intercondylar distances as determined by an indicator on the face-bow (Fig. 15-12, *A* and *B*). Metal shims permit the distance between the condylar guidance elements on the upper member to be adjusted in harmony with the intercondylar width of the condylar spheres on the lower member (Fig. 15-12, *C*). In this manner, the location of the vertical axes of rotation of the mandible can be approximated on the articulator.

One orients the lower cast to the lower member of the articulator representing the mandible

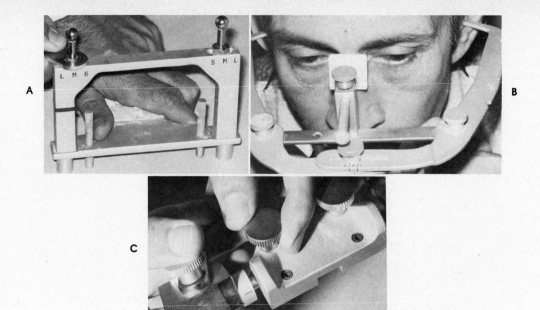

Fig. 15-12. A, Condylar spheres can be removed from frame of lower member of articulator and adjusted for varying intercondylar distances in accordance with needs of patient. Intercondylar disturbances are small, medium, and large, with a distance of 12 mm between each gradation. **B,** Face-bow is properly oriented to patient. Intercondylar width of individual patient is indicated by measuring gauge on anterior part of bow. Intercondylar distance for this patient is indicated as *M* (medium). **C,** One metal spacer is added on each side for a medium intercondyiar distance. This spacer will properly adjust condylar housing on upper member of articulator to fit condylar spheres when they are in medium position on lower member of articulator. Two metal spacers are required on both sides for a large intercondylar distance.

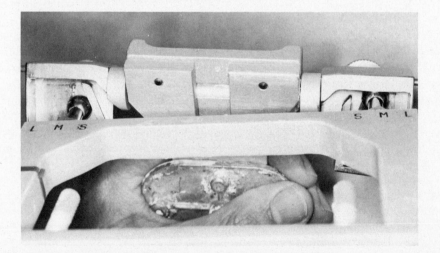

Fig. 15-13. Condylar housing and spheres of the Whip Mix Articulator, seen from below. Balancing condylar sphere on the left has been moved downward, forward, and inward as dictated by condylar guidances on left. Simultaneously, working condylar sphere on right has moved laterally (Bennett shift). Condylar housing will not permit full freedom of movement of working condylar sphere during this movement.

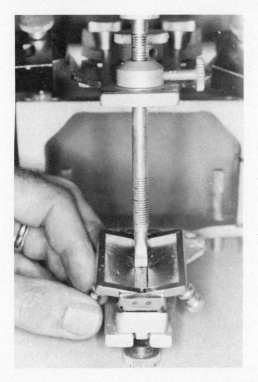

Fig. 15-14. Incisal guide table can be adjusted antero-posteriorly for protrusive movement, and lateral plates can be raised or lowered to be in harmony with lateral incisal guidance.

by relating the lower cast to the upper cast through an interocclusal centric relation record. The horizontal condylar guidances are adjusted by an interocclusal protrusive record, and the lateral condylar guidances are adjusted by right and left interocclusal lateral records. The lateral condylar guidances on the Whip Mix articulator do not make provisions for upward, downward, forward, or backward movement of the working-side condylar sphere (Fig. 15-13).

The articulator is provided with interchangeable fixed and adjustable incisal guide tables. The fixed table is constructed of plastic and can be individually modified by use of cold-curing acrylic resin. The adjustable incisal guide table is constructed of metal and is used for removable prosthodontic restorations. The lateral plates of the adjustable incisal guide table can be positioned at the desired lateral incisal guidance, and the angulation of the plates is calibrated in degrees. The entire table is adjustable antero-posteriorly to provide the necessary guidance for the protrusive movement (Fig. 15-14).

The articulator has a straight incisal guide pin. One end of the incisal guide pin is rounded to fit the concavity in the fixed incisal guide tables, and the other end is flat to permit movements on the adjustable incisal guide table. Since the incisal guide pin is straight, the vertical position of the pin in the upper member of the articulator changes the relation of the end of the incisal guide pin to the middle of the incisal guide table.

Orienting the upper cast on the Whip Mix articulator. The upper occlusion rim is placed in the patient's mouth. Preliminary adjustments are made so that the occlusal surface of the rim anteriorly is in the approximate position formerly occupied by the natural anterior teeth. The upper lip should be adequately supported, the incisal plane should parallel the interpupillary line, and the occlusal plane should roughly parallel a line from the ala of the nose to the tragus of the ear (Fig. 15-15). These modifications should be made quickly, since it is not necessary for the upper occlusion rim to be in its final form when it is used for orienting the upper cast on the articulator.

With the upper occlusion rim in the mouth, the face-bow fork is preliminarily positioned so that it is in line anteroposteriorly with the middle of the head, and a mark is made on the labial surface of the occlusion rim to indicate this position. Then the surface of the face-bow fork is heated, and it is attached to the occlusal surface of the upper rim with the mark on the labial surface being used as a guide to the proper position (Fig. 15-16).

The upper occlusion rim and the attached face-bow fork are placed in the patient's mouth. The patient is instructed to hold them in position with thumbs pressing against both sides of

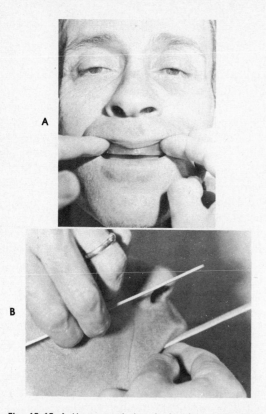

Fig. 15-15. A, Upper occlusion rim has been adjusted to represent approximate length of natural anterior teeth, with incisal plane parallel with interpupillary line. **B,** Occlusal plane of upper occlusion rim roughly parallels the ala-tragus line.

the bottom surface of the face-bow fork. The attachment mechanism for the face-bow is placed over the end of the face-bow fork, and the ear posts are guided into the external openings of the ears until they fit snugly. The anterior locking device on the face-bow is tightened to maintain this position, and a notation is made of the estimate of the cranial width as indicated by the marker on the front part of the face-bow.

The plastic nasion relator (nosepiece) is attached to the supporting crosspiece of the face-bow, and the face-bow is adjusted vertically so that the nosepiece fits into the concavity of the bridge of the nose (point nasion). The face-bow is securely locked to the fork in this position (Fig. 15-17). The nasion relator that determines the vertical position of the face-bow anteriorly forms a third point of reference and, together with the ear posts posteriorly, establishes the axis-orbital plane on the patient, which will be transferred to the articulator. The nasion relator has been designed so that when it is positioned at the nasion point, the face-bow will be located anteriorly in the approximate region of the infraorbital notch.

The ear posts are carefully disengaged from the ears, and the face-bow and attached upper occlusion rim are removed from the patient (Fig. 15-18, A). The condylar posts on the lower member of the articulator and condylar guid-

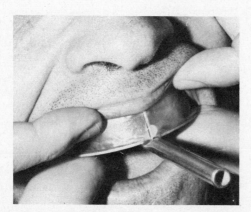

Fig. 15-16. Face-bow fork is attached to occlusal surface of upper occlusion rim.

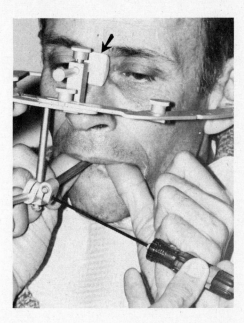

Fig. 15-17. Face-bow is properly oriented to patient's face with nasion relator *(arrow)* and is securely attached to face-bow fork. The patient is holding upper occlusion rim and attached face-bow fork securely in position on upper residual ridge during this procedure. Notice that face-bow is aligned at approximate level of infraorbital notch when positioned by plastic nasion relator.

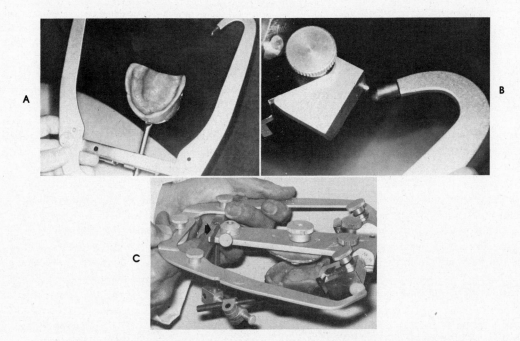

Fig. 15-18. A, Face-bow with attached fork and occlusion rim has been removed form patient. Notice that upper occlusion rim is lined with acrylic resin for accurate fit on cast and in mouth. **B,** Ear posts of the face-bow are attached to small metal rods extending from condylar housing. **C,** Forward end of upper member of articulator rests on anterior cross piece of face-bow *(arrow).*

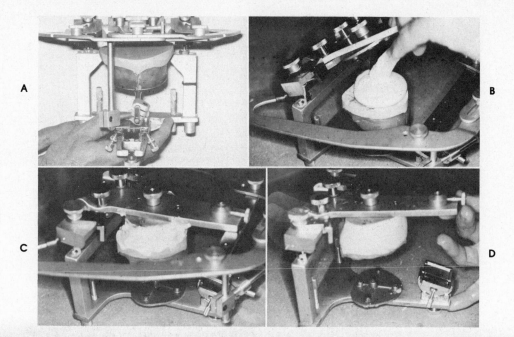

Fig. 15-19. A, Face-bow, occlusion rim, cast, and upper member of articulator are supported on lower member of articulator to facilitate mounting the upper cast. Lower member of articulator is used in this procedure for convenience only. **B,** With the upper member of articulator elevated, fast-setting plaster is distributed over top of upper cast. **C,** Upper member of articulator has been closed back into position on anterior part of face-bow. **D,** Mounting of upper cast on articulator is completed. Notice neat appearance of plaster that attaches upper cast to the mounting ring.

ance mechanisms on the upper member of the articulator are adjusted to correspond with the cranial width as indicated previously by the face-bow.

The face-bow holding the upper occlusion rim is attached posteriorly to the upper member of the articulator when the holes are fitted in the ear posts of the face-bow over small metal rods that extend laterally from each condylar housing (Fig. 15-18, *B*). The metal rods are located approximately 6 mm posteriorly from the actual transverse axis of the articulator to compensate for the location of the ear posts in the external auditory meatus, which are roughly the same distance posteriorly from the mandibular transverse hinge axis of the patient. The forward end of the upper member of the articulator, with the

incisal guide pin removed, rests on the anterior part of the face-bow (Fig. 15-18, *C*). Since the anterior part of the face-bow was positioned at the approximate level of the infraorbital notch on the patient's face by the nasion relator, the upper cast will automatically be oriented on the articulator in the same relationship as the upper jaw of the patient was to the temporomandibular joints posteriorly and to the infraorbital notch anteriorly (axis-orbital plane).

The upper member of the articulator and attached face-bow, occlusion rim, and upper cast can be conveniently supported by the lower member of the articulator while the upper cast is attached to the upper member of the articulator with fast-setting artificial stone (Fig. 15-19). The upper cast is now oriented on the upper mem-

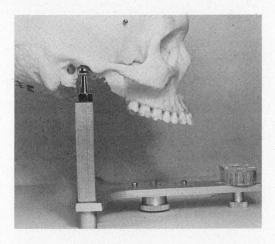

Fig. 15-20. A skull has been substituted for upper member of articulator to indicate manner in which relationship of upper cast to upper member of articulator simulates relationship of upper jaw to skull of patient. (From Hickey, J.C., Lundeen, H.C., and Bohannon, H.M.: J. Prosthet. Dent. **18:**425-437, 1967.)

ber of the articulator in a manner similar to that in which the upper jaw is oriented to the skull of the patient (Fig. 15-20).

Establishing the preliminary vertical relation of occlusion. The upper occlusion rim was preliminarily adjusted for facial support, vertical height, and the angulation of the incisal and occlusal plane. The face-bow was used to correctly orient the upper cast on the articulator. Refinements are now made in the form of the upper occlusion rim, with the fact kept in mind that the size and form of the rim represent the dental arch of the natural teeth plus the part of the residual ridge that has been lost by resorption. The length of the upper residual ridge in relation to the length of the upper lip can be helpful in developing the length of the occlusion rim anteriorly. If the upper lip is relatively long as compared to the length of the residual ridge, the level of the occlusion rim may be slightly above the vermillion border of the lip. If the upper lip is relatively short as compared to the length of the residual ridge, the occlusion rim may extend several millimeters below the border of the lip.

The height of the lower occlusion rim is preliminarily adjusted (with the upper rim out of the mouth) so that anteriorly it is at the level of the corner of the mouth and posteriorly at the level of the posterior one third of the retromolar pad. This height will approximate the level of the occlusal plane of the completed dentures. The lower rim is adjusted labially for proper support of the lower lip.

With both occlusion rims in the mouth, observations are made to determine what modifications may be needed to establish a preliminary vertical relation of occlusion. These observations include (1) a determination of the interocclusal distance, (2) measurements of the facial height at mandibular rest position when the occlusion rims are not in the mouth, as compared with measurements of the facial height at the vertical relation of occlusion established by the occlusion rims in the mouth, (3) the space between the rims during phonetic tests, and (4) the nature of the facial support of the patient. The occlusion rims are adjusted until an adequate interocclusal distance seems to have been established (Fig. 15-21).

Making the preliminary centric relation record. After the preliminary vertical relation between the jaws has been established with the occlusion rims, the preliminary centric relation record is made. Centric relation is *always* the horizontal relation used to orient the lower cast to the upper cast for edentulous patients.

With the occlusion rims in the mouth, sufficient trial closures in centric relation are practiced until both the dentist and patient become

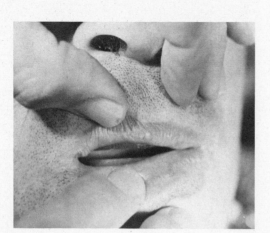

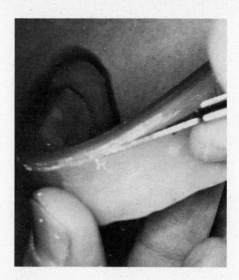

Fig. 15-21. Space between upper and lower occlusion rims indicates that an adequate interocclusal distance has been established when mandible is at the vertical relation of physiologic rest with maxillae.

Fig. 15-22. Lower occlusion rim is reduced to make space for recording medium so that centric relation record can be made as close to desired vertical relation as possible.

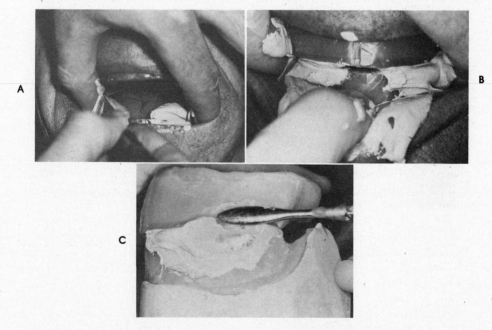

Fig. 15-23. A, With both occlusion rims in the mouth and supported, recording medium is added to occlusal surface of lower rim. **B,** Patient closes in centric relation as rehearsed previously. Closure is stopped at predetermined vertical relation, with no contact between opposing occlusion rims. **C,** Occlusion rims are placed on lower cast and securely sealed together before lower cast is mounted on articulator.

familiar with the position. The hand position used by the dentist and instructions to the patient are similar to those described previously.

When the patient can consistently follow the instructions, approximately 2 mm of wax are removed from the occlusal surface of the lower occlusion rim to provide space for the recording medium (Fig. 15-22). The centric relation record must always be made at or as close to the desired vertical relation as possible without contact of the opposing occlusion rims. The dentist observes the relationship of the occlusion rims when the mandible is in centric relation and stops the closure at the desired vertical relation

of occlusion during additional trial closures of the jaws. A space of approximately 2 mm should exist between the rims at the preliminary vertical relation of occlusion. Two V-shaped cross grooves are made in the occlusal surfaces of both occlusion rims in the molar region on both sides. These serve as keys for the recording material should the interocclusal record and rims come apart.

The recording medium, a fast-setting plaster-like material (Impressotex), is placed on the occlusal surface of the lower occlusion rim on both sides in the molar-premolar region. Under the guidance of the dentist, the patient closes the jaws into the recording plaster with the man-

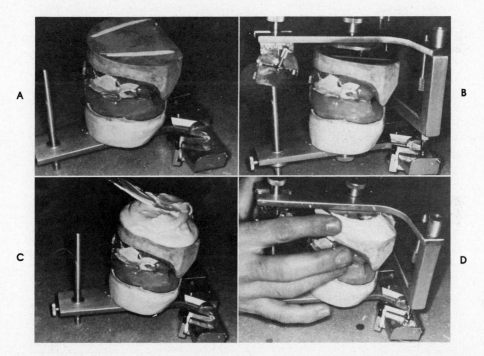

Fig. 15-24. A, Occlusion rims and lower cast are placed in position on upper cast, which is attached to upper member of articulator. **B,** Lower member of articulator is positioned on inverted upper member of articulator to make certain that there is adequate space between mounting ring on lower member of articulator and lower cast. **C,** With lower member of articulator removed, fast-setting plaster is distributed over surface of lower cast. **D,** Lower member of articulator is placed on upper member. Condylar spheres must fit snugly against posterior part of the condylar housings. Incisal guide table must be in contact with incisal guide pin. Lower cast is attached to lower member of articulator by fast-setting plaster.

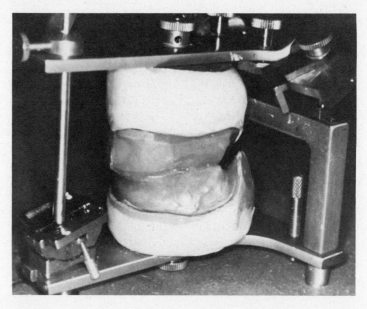

Fig. 15-25. Lower cast has been attached to lower member of articulator in proper relation to upper cast by means of interocclusal centric relation record. Notice neat appearance of mountings.

dible in centric relation. The same procedures are followed as were used in the trial closures. The closure is stopped when the occlusion rims reach the predetermined vertical relation (Fig. 15-23, *A* and *B*). It is essential that both rims be correctly positioned on the residual ridges while the record is being made.

After the recording medium has set, the patient opens the mouth carefully, and the occlusion rims and interocclusal record are removed (Fig. 15-23, *C*). They can often be removed as one unit. There must be no contact of the opposing occlusion rims posteriorly or through the plaster record. Such contacts would displace the tissues under the denture base, cause movement of the occlusion rims on the basal seat, or shift the mandible away from centric relation. If contact between the rims has occurred, a new interocclusal record must be made.

Some patients may have difficulty in maintaining the mandible in a fixed position while

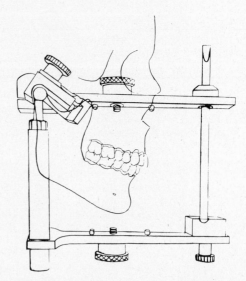

Fig. 15-26. Drawing of a skull has been superimposed on articulator to indicate how properly mounted casts are oriented to the articulator as jaws of patient are oriented to the skull. (From Hickey, J.C., Lundeen, H.C., and Bohannon, H.M.: J. Prosthet. Dent. **18**:425-437, 1967.)

the plaster interocclusal record sets. In these instances, wax instead of plaster is used as the recording medium.

Orienting the lower cast on the Whip Mix articulator. The lower cast is seated in position in the lower occlusion rim. The upper member of the articulator is inverted and placed on the laboratory bench with the incisal guide pin centered vertically so that it will contact the middle of the incisal guide table. The lateral condylar guidances are set at zero, and the horizontal condylar guidances at 35 degrees to support the condylar spheres. The upper occlusion rim with the lower rim and lower cast attached is properly positioned on the upper cast (Fig 15-24, *A* and *B*). Fast-setting artificial stone is distributed over the bottom surface of the lower cast and the mounting ring of the lower member of the articulator (Fig. 15-24, *C*).

The condylar spheres of the lower member of the articulator are placed in the condylar housing of the upper member, and the front part of the lower member is rotated downward until the incisal guide table contacts the incisal guide pin (Fig. 15-24, *D*). The condylar spheres must be in contact with the posterior part of the condylar housings. Additional artificial stone is added around the cast. A weight placed on the lower member of the articulator will tend to counteract the expansion of the artificial stone as it sets. The mounting must be neat (Fig. 15-25). Both casts are now oriented on the articulator in a similar manner to that in which both jaws are oriented to the skull of the patient (Fig. 15-26).

16

Selecting artificial teeth for edentulous patients

The selection of artificial teeth for edentulous patients requires a knowledge and understanding of a number of physical and biologic factors that are directly related to each patient. The dentist must perform this phase of prosthodontic care for edentulous patients, since he is the only person who can accumulate, correlate, and evaluate the biomechanical information so that the selection of artificial teeth will meet the individual esthetic and functional needs of the patient.

The selection of artificial teeth is a relatively simple, non–time-consuming procedure, but it requires development of experience and confidence. The dentist has many guides available to help him in selecting both anterior and posterior artificial teeth. However, any choice of artificial teeth must be considered as a preliminary selection until the teeth are arranged on the trial denture bases and can be critically viewed in the patient's mouth. Only then can the final selection be made.

ANTERIOR TOOTH SELECTION

The selection of anterior teeth for edentulous patients when all records of form, color, and size have been lost is a clinical procedure. The best way to determine the color, form, and size of the teeth is by trial in the patient's mouth.

The selection of the best possible teeth for each patient will have much to do with the eventual success or failure of complete denture service. Anterior teeth that are not in harmony with the patient's facial color, form, and size will cause problems in denture construction and in the reaction of the patient to the completed dentures. It is in this phase of denture service that the opportunity exists for an expression of the artistic ability of the dentist.

Much of the effectiveness of tooth selection depends on the ability of dentists to interpret what they see. The selection of teeth is not a mechanical exercise. Formulas, average values, and measurements can serve as a starting point but cannot take the place of good artistic judgment. Careful observation of the faces and teeth of people with natural teeth will develop a sense of dentofacial harmony that is the objective of tooth selection and esthetics. There must be harmony of color, form, size, and arrangement of teeth if dentures are to defy detection.

Preextraction guides

Preextraction guides include diagnostic casts, photographs, radiographs, observation of the teeth of close relatives, and extracted teeth.

Diagnostic casts of the natural teeth are the most reliable guides in both selecting and arranging anterior teeth (Fig. 16-1, *A*). In most instances, artificial teeth that are similar in appearance to the patient's natural teeth are desirable. The size and form of the anterior teeth can be determined on the diagnostic cast, and comparable artificial teeth are selected.

Frequently, patients can supply photographs that show the natural anterior teeth or at least the incisal edges of some teeth (Fig. 16-1, *B*). Photographs can provide information about the width of the teeth and possibly the outline form, which would be more accurate than other selection systems. In addition, an algebraic proportion may be established from the photograph. The unknown factor is the width or length of the natural central incisor. The known factors are the interpupillary distance of the patient, the interpupillary distance on the photograph, and the width or length of the central incisor in the photograph.

Intraoral radiographs made before the natural teeth were lost can supply information about the size and form of the teeth to be replaced and can sometimes be obtained from the patient's previous dentist. However, radiographic images are always slightly enlarged and may be distorted because of the divergence of the x rays. Patients are grateful for the extra effort of the dentist in this important aspect of their appearance.

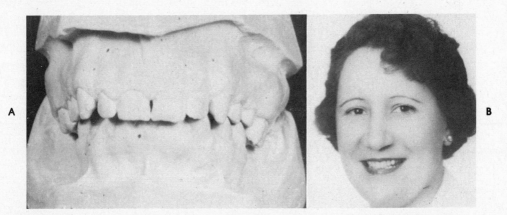

Fig. 16-1, A, Diagnostic casts provide best method of selecting artificial teeth that are similar in form and shape to natural teeth. **B,** Outline form and relative size of artificial teeth can be obtained from a photograph of patient that shows the natural teeth.

Sometimes patients keep extracted anterior teeth or dental casts given them by a previous dentist. The extracted teeth will provide excellent information as to the size and form for the artificial teeth but cannot be used in selecting color.

Size of anterior teeth

The size of the teeth should be in proportion to the size of the face and head (Fig. 16-2). Generally, larger persons have large teeth. However, there are variations in which a large person may have small teeth and spaces between the teeth or a small person may have unduly large teeth and much irregularity in their alignment. Tactful questions asked of the patient and photographs can reveal this information.

Women's teeth are often smaller than men's. This is especially true of the lateral incisors, which normally should be more delicate in women than in men. A distinct difference between the size of the central and lateral incisors is desirable, particularly in women.

The growth of alveolar bone requires the presence and eruption of teeth. Thus the size of the casts have a relationship to the size of the anterior teeth. However, when attempts are made to determine the size of artificial teeth by measurement of edentulous casts, the results will be incorrect. The teeth will be too small because of resorption of the residual ridges. If the width of the anterior teeth is to be determined by measurements, the occlusion rims should be contoured for esthetics, and the measurement made around the curve of the labial surface of the occlusion rim. The approximate location of the distal surfaces of the upper canines can be indicated by marks made on the upper rim at the corners of the mouth (Fig. 16-3, A and B). Then the distance between the marks is measured around the labial surface of the occlusion rim (Fig. 16-3, C), and anterior teeth of this width are arranged as indicated by the occlusion rim.

Other methods for selecting size of anterior teeth. An estimation of the position of the apex of the upper natural canine can be found by extension of parallel lines from the lateral surfaces of the alae of the nose onto the labial surface of the upper occlusion rim (Fig. 16-4), but this is not sufficiently reliable for use as the means for the final selection. Measurements on the occlusion rim will provide an indication of the width of the upper anterior teeth.

Anthropometric measurements can be helpful in the selection of artificial teeth. Studies of 555 skulls indicate that the greatest bizygomatic width divided by 16 gives an approximation of the width of the upper central incisor (Fig. 16-5), and that dividing by 3.3 provides an estimation of the overall width of the upper six anterior teeth. A face-bow may be used to determine the

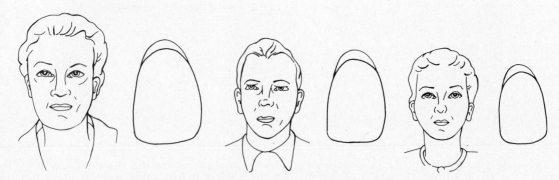

Fig. 16-2. Shapes of artificial teeth chosen to be in harmony with size of patient's face.

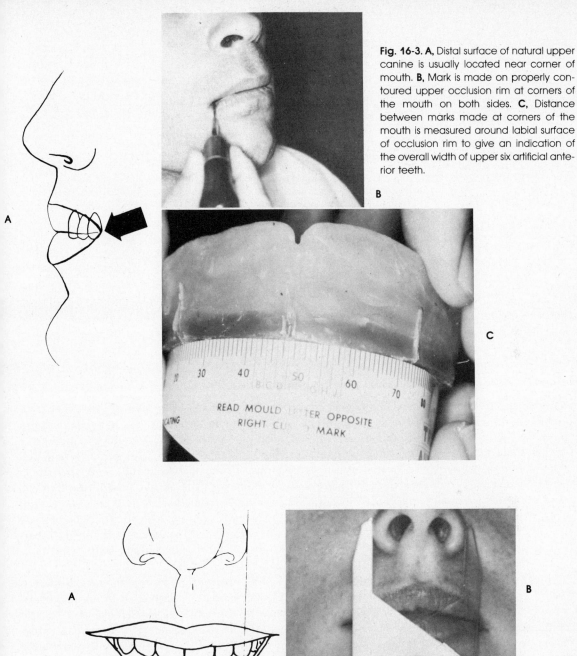

Fig. 16-3. A, Distal surface of natural upper canine is usually located near corner of mouth. **B,** Mark is made on properly contoured upper occlusion rim at corners of the mouth on both sides. **C,** Distance between marks made at corners of the mouth is measured around labial surface of occlusion rim to give an indication of the overall width of upper six artificial anterior teeth.

READ MOULD LETTER OPPOSITE
RIGHT CUSPID MARK

Fig. 16-4. A, Vertical line extending along lateral surface of the ala of the nose often may pass through middle of natural upper canine. **B,** Plastic measuring caliper is available that provides a measurement of the interalar width and suggests possible molds of artificial anterior teeth that are in harmony with this width.

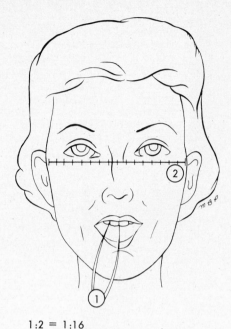

Fig. 16-5. Measurements on skulls indicate that width of natural central incisor, 1, is approximately 1/16 of the bizygomatic width, 2.

1:2 = 1:16

bizygomatic width. The ratio of the cranial circumference to the width of the upper anterior teeth has been shown to be 10 to 1 in over 90% of 509 subjects studied. As a general guide, upper anterior teeth whose overall width as listed on tooth-selection charts is less than 48 mm are relatively small teeth. Those listed as over 52 mm are relatively large teeth.

Form of anterior teeth

The forms of artificial anterior teeth should harmonize with the shape of the patient's face (Fig. 16-6). The outline form is considered from a front view of the patient and the labial surface of the upper central incisor. The outline form of faces can be grouped into three basic classes: square, tapering, and ovoid. These classes are further subdivided on the basis of a combination of the characteristics of the three classes. Other variations arise in the proportions of the length and width of the faces.

The same types of variations in the forms of teeth have been provided by the manufacturers

of artificial teeth. The dentist's problem is to select a tooth form that is in harmony with the form of the face of each individual patient. For this he should study faces of people and the forms of their natural teeth. Teeth that are in harmony with the outline form of the face will look good; teeth that are not in harmony with the face will not look so good. This kind of study will help dentists recognize harmony or disharmony of form when they work with their patients.

When the outline form of the patient's face is distinctly square, tapered, or ovoid, it is a mistake to use tooth forms that are also square, tapered, or ovoid. The use of extreme examples of teeth in each class with extreme examples of faces in the same class will emphasize a characteristic that may not be complimentary to the patient.

The teeth selected must be "nice-looking" in themselves. Some molds of teeth have pleasing forms; yet others look quite mechanical. The nice-looking teeth are much more easily

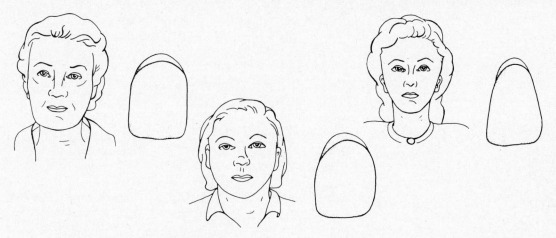

Fig. 16-6. Form of artificial teeth chosen to be in harmony with outline form of the patient's face.

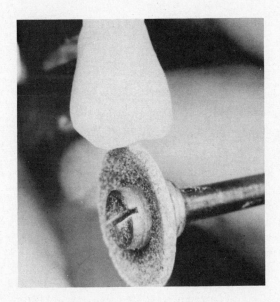

Fig. 16-7. Outline form of an upper canine is modified to make it more natural in appearance and acceptable for individual patient.

arranged into a pleasing coposition than teeth that have no esthetic value as individual teeth. The shape of the labial surface is probably more important than the outline form, which can be changed when the incisal edges of the teeth (Fig. 16-7) are ground. This grinding should be done on almost all anterior teeth according to the age of the patient.

The labial face of the tooth viewed from the

mesial aspect should show a contour similar to that of the face viewed in profile (Fig. 16-8, *A*). The three general types of profiles are convex, straight, and concave. The labial face of the tooth viewed from the incisal edge should show a type of convexity or flatness similar to that shown by the face viewed from under the chin or from the top of the head (Fig. 16-8, *B*).

The form of labial surfaces of anterior teeth

A   B

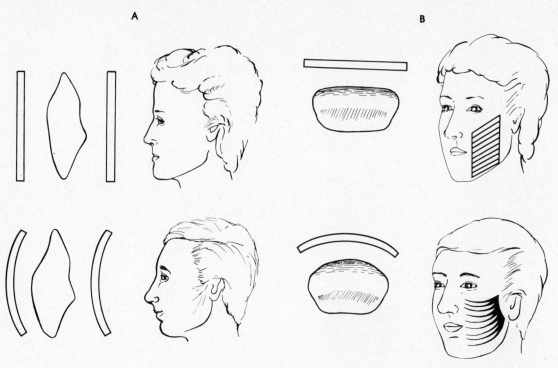

Fig. 16-8. A, Labial surfaces of artificial teeth chosen to be in harmony with profile of face. **B,** Labial surfaces of artificial teeth as viewed from incisal edge should be in harmony with convexity or flatness of face.

should follow nature. The profession must depend on the manufacturer for these forms. Curved, convex surfaces refract and reflect light and appear smaller than flat surfaces. The eye can measure a straight surface, whereas an optical illusion will be produced by a rounded surface. Tooth forms look more artificial when nature's curvatures are missing.

Curvatures of anterior teeth can be seen when observed from the mesial, distal, incisal, and labial surfaces. Other curvatures may be reverse curvatures in the form of minute irregularities. A study of natural tooth surfaces under a little magnification reveals no smooth, glassy surfaces. These minute irregularities should be reproduced in the artificial teeth to give a natural effect.

The contact areas or surfaces in the anterior teeth should show wear as occurs in natural teeth through life. Broadened contact areas look more natural because the long contact surfaces give a truer appearance of age.

Thicker teeth, labiolingually, can be rotated and spaced to give the three-dimensional depth so necessary for esthetics. Therefore thick teeth should be given the preference in selection.

Dentogenic concept in selecting artificial teeth

Tooth selection using the concepts of "dentogenics" is based on the age, sex, and personality of the patient. It seems reasonable that a large, rugged man would tend to have teeth of a size and form different from those of a delicate-appearing woman. The squareness of tooth form tends to portray masculinity, whereas more rounded incisal and proximal contours connote femininity (Fig. 16-9). Lateral incisors that are smaller than the central incisors tend to make the arrangement of the teeth appear more feminine than central and lateral incisors that are

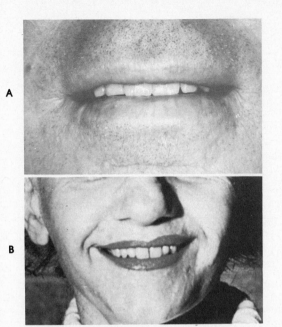

Fig. 16-9. Artificial teeth that are appropriate for this man, **A,** and for this woman, **B,** because of relative size, outline form, contour, and arrangement of teeth. Appearance of teeth for the woman, **B,** would be inappropriate for the man, **A.**

more nearly the same size. Dentogenic concepts provide useful information, which is used along with other methods of selecting artificial teeth.

Selection of artificial teeth under any concept is the responsibility of the dentist. A work authorization order that merely indicates the age, sex, and personality of the patient does not fulfill professional requirements.

Color of teeth

A knowledge of the physics, physiology, and psychology of color is of value in the selection of the color of teeth.

The colors recognized by the human eye are the effect of certain wavelengths of light on the retina. The colors of faces and teeth therefore come from the effects of reflected light on the rods and cones of the retina of the eyes. Although the human eyes can identify the various colors of the spectrum from red to violet, the

color of most concern to dentists is the yellow band in the spectrum. The reason is that the colors of teeth and faces are primarily yellows.

Color has four qualities: hue, saturation (chroma), brilliance (value), and translucency. All these are involved in the selection of teeth.

Hue is the specific color produced by a specific wavelength of light acting on the retina. It is the color itself, such as bluish, greenish, or reddish yellow.

The hue of the teeth must be in harmony with the color (hue) of the patient's face. If the two colors are in harmony, the effect will be pleasant as are two harmonious notes on a piano. If the color of the teeth and the color of the face are not in harmony, attention will be called to the teeth, just as a discord between two notes on a piano would be noticed whereas hundreds of harmonious notes would blend pleasantly together (Fig. 16-10). Disharmony of light waves or sound waves will attract attention. Disharmony of the hue of the teeth with the basic hue of the face will make dentures look artificial.

Saturation (chroma) is the amount of color per unit of area of an object. For example, some teeth appear more yellow than others. The hue could be the same, that is, the yellow in both teeth could be the same yellow, but there is more of it in some teeth than others.

Brilliance (value) refers to the lightness or darkness of an object. Variations in brilliance are produced by the dilution of the color (the hue) by white or black. When the yellow in teeth is diluted with white, the result is a light tooth; when the yellow is diluted with black, the result is a dark tooth. The relative amount of white or black in the teeth determines their lightness or darkness.

People with fair complexions generally have teeth with less color, and the colors are less saturated; thus the teeth are lighter and are in harmony with the colors of the face. People with dark complexions generally have darker teeth that are in harmony with the coloring of the face. However, the lightness or darkness (brilliance) of the face (the frame for the teeth in the mouth) can alter the apparent brilliance of the teeth.

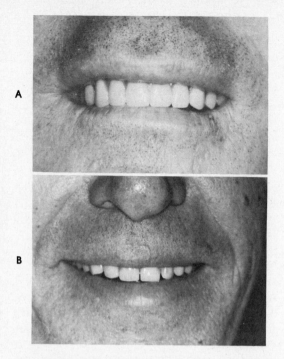

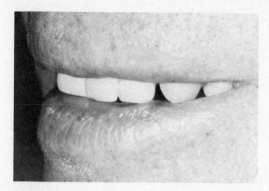

Fig. 16-11. Since this patient has a dark complexion, artificial teeth appear light, even though their color is comparatively very dark.

Fig. 16-10. A, Artificial teeth that are out of harmony with face in color, size, and shape. **B,** Size and color of artificial teeth blend with size and color of patient's face.

Light teeth in the mouth of a patient with a very light complexion may appear dark. Likewise dark teeth in the mouth of a patient with a very dark complexion may appear to be lighter than they are (Fig. 16-11).

Translucency is the property of an object that permits the passage of light through it but cannot give any distinguishable image. The light rays are so broken up and diffuse that the light cannot pass directly through the object as it would if the object were transparent. Translucency of artificial teeth has the effect of mixing the various colors (hues) of the porcelain in the teeth with the changing colors within the oral cavity. This results in teeth that look alive because of the changes in the light and color reflected from the teeth and passing through the teeth with different light sources. The apparent color of teeth is different when the lighting of

the interior of the oral cavity is changed. When the mouth is nearly closed, the teeth will appear darker than when it is open wide, with the interior of the oral cavity well lighted. Also, when light is reflected through the teeth from the oral cavity, the teeth will appear to be lighter and more pink than in other light situations. The pink color of the interior of the mouth shows through the translucent porcelain as it does through the enamel of natural teeth. For this reason, tooth manufacturers are striving to place translucent porcelain in the same places in artificial teeth as nature has placed enamel in natural teeth.

The basic color of Caucasian faces is yellow. Blue is the complementary color of yellow. So, if the dentist stares at a blue card or cloth for 30 seconds before observing the color of teeth and faces, he can make a more accurate observation of the yellow color. The problem is to distinguish between the various gradations of yellow, from reddish yellow to greenish yellow. The preparation of the retina of the eye to be more sensitive to yellow will simplify color selection.

A general classification of skin pigmentation is sallow, ruddy, olive, and swarthy. In hair colors there are black, brown, red, and blond. In eyes there are blue, gray, brown, and black. There are so many combinations of all of these factors that it would be impractical to manufacture enough shades to match them all. The color of the hair has been used by some dentists as a guide. This is unreliable and can be inaccurate because the color of hair changes more rapidly than the color of the teeth. Persons can change the color of their hair from week to week. The color of the eyes has been suggested as a guide to the color of the teeth. This is not sound, since the size of the iris of the eyes is so small in comparison with the area of the total face and the eyes are not close to the teeth.

The color of the face is the basic guide to the color of the teeth. It is the frame into which the picture (the teeth) must fit. The hue of the teeth must be in harmony with the colors in the patient's face in the same way as two musical notes must be in harmony to be pleasing to the ear. Saturation of color in the teeth must correspond to saturation of color in the patient's face. Brilliance of the teeth must correspond to the lightness or darkness of the patient's face. Teeth that are either too light or too dark will be conspicuous, and denture teeth should not be conspicuous. Translucency, which is a characteristic of enamel, makes possible some variation in the effect of the color with different lip and mouth positions. This variation is essential to the illusion of naturalness.

Age and tooth color. The colors of natural teeth change with age. They get progressively darker. In youth, the pulp chambers are large, and the red color of the pulp affects the total color of the tooth. Later, the pulp chamber becomes smaller as a result of the deposition of secondary dentin in it. This makes the tooth more opaque and reduces the effect of the color of the pulp. As wear occurs on the teeth as a result of toothbrushing and polishing, the surface of the tooth becomes more smooth and reflects more light. As abrasion occurs on the incisal edges of teeth, the enamel is lost, and with it the translucency of the incisal edges. Also, the dentin becomes exposed and picks up stains from the oral fluids, foods, medicines,

tobacco, etc. As a result, the teeth become darker and generally somewhat brownish. This is particularly apparent on the incisal edges of the lower anterior teeth.

The general rule is that darker teeth are more appropriate in older patients' mouths and lighter teeth are more harmonious in young patients' mouths. A record made of the color of a patient's teeth at 20 years of age will not be appropriate to use for the same patient at 60 years of age. The tooth color must be in harmony with the facial coloring at the time the dentures are made.

Some patients save their extracted teeth and suggest that the dentist match their color. A color selection made in this manner will always be incorrect. The color of teeth changes instantly when they are removed from the mouth because of the loss of the color from the pulpal tissue. The color blanches out further as the teeth dry out. Extracted teeth are valuable for the selection of the size and forms of teeth but not for color.

Selecting the color of artificial teeth. Observations of the shade-guide teeth should be made in three positions: (1) outside the mouth along the side of the nose, (2) under the lips with only the incisal edge exposed, and (3) under the lips with only the cervical end covered and the mouth open (Fig. 16-12). The first step will establish the basic hue, brilliance, and saturation; the second will reveal the effect of the color of the teeth when the patient's mouth is relaxed; the third will simulate exposure of the teeth as in a smile.

Basic considerations are harmony of the color of the tooth with the color of the patient's face and inconspicuousness of the teeth. The color selected should be so inconspicuous that it will not attract attention to the teeth. The color of the teeth should be observed on a bright day when possible, with the patient located close to natural light. The teeth should also be observed in artificial light, since denture patients are often seen in this environment.

The "squint test" may be helpful in evaluating colors of teeth with the complexion of the face.

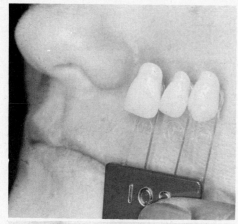

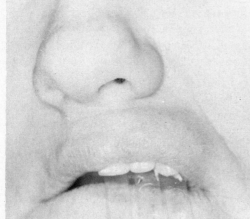

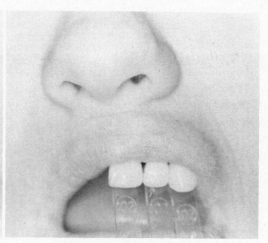

Fig. 16-12. Testing tooth color with shade-guide teeth. **A,** Color is matched with that of skin of cheek. **B,** Color is observed under upper lip with incisal edges exposed. **C,** Color is observed with labial surfaces uncovered and mouth open to observe effect on color when light is reflected through teeth from inside of mouth.

With the eyelids partially closed to reduce light, the dentist compares prospective colors of artificial teeth held along the face of the patient. The color that fades from view first is the one that is least conspicuous in comparison with the color of the face.

Preliminary try-in of selected teeth

Molds of anterior teeth that appear to be desirable can be easily appraised when they are arranged on the upper occlusion rim or on a tooth selector (Fig. 16-13). Anterior teeth must be selected with sufficient width to fill the available space adequately in the mouth and provide for placement or irregularities in individual tooth position. The final decision regarding the selection of anterior teeth is made by observations of the trial (wax) dentures in the patient's mouth. The most common error in the selection of artificial anterior teeth is to select teeth that are too small in size and too light in color (Fig. 16-14).

POSTERIOR TOOTH SELECTION

The posterior teeth should be selected for color, buccolingual width, total mesiodistal width, length, and type according to cuspal inclination and material. They should also be in accord with the size and contour of the mandibular residual ridge.

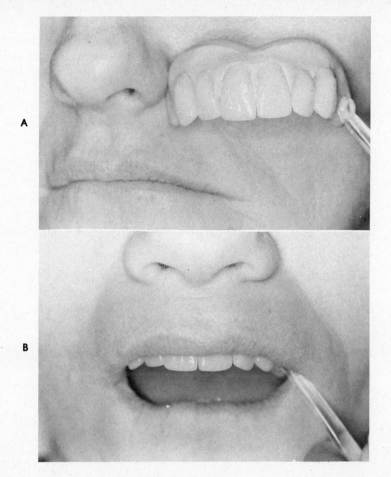

Fig. 16-13. Preliminary selection of artificial anterior teeth is arranged on a tooth selector, **A,** for quick observation in the patient's mouth, **B.**

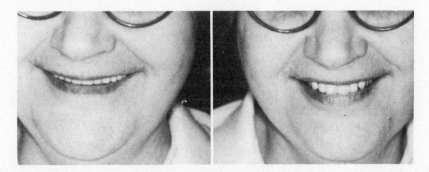

Fig. 16-14. *Left,* Artificial teeth that are too small and too light in color. The seemingly endless row of teeth, together with improper support of lips, creates what has been called the "denture look." *Right,* Artificial teeth that are of proper size and in correct position to support lips. The upper six anterior teeth fill available space, whereas in picture on left, eight to ten teeth appear to occupy the same space.

All posterior teeth are not exact reproductions of natural teeth, which is as it should be. A complete denture has an anchorage and support different from those of natural teeth, and therefore the occlusal surfaces of artificial teeth should be modified. Masticating efficiency is only one consideration in the selection of posterior tooth forms, since comfort, esthetics, and preservation of the underlying bony and soft tissue structures are also important factors.

Posterior denture teeth are generally classified into two types: anatomic teeth and nonanatomic teeth. Strictly speaking, all denture teeth are designed geometrically, but the term *ana-tomic* is used for those artificial posterior teeth that more nearly resemble the teeth of a dentition. Manufactured artificial tooth forms can only be a start in developing an occlusion. The dentist then modifies the forms of the occlusal surfaces and arranges the teeth to fit the plan of occlusion.

Buccolingual width of posterior teeth

The buccolingual width of artificial teeth should be greatly reduced from the width of natural teeth they replace. Artificial posterior teeth that are narrow in a buccolingual direction enhance the development of the correct form of

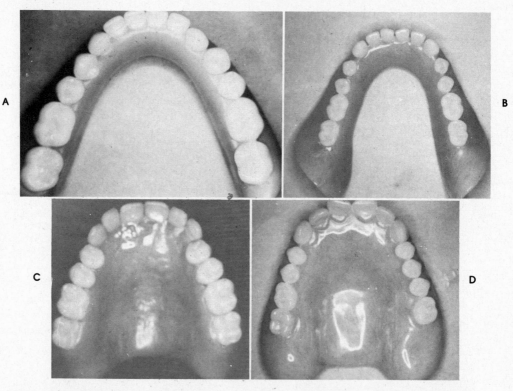

Fig. 16-15. A, Posterior teeth that are too wide in relation to size of denture base. **B,** Posterior teeth of proper size in relation to denture base. Notice that buccal and lingual flanges slope away from occlusal surfaces of posterior teeth. This form allows cheeks and tongue to help maintain lower denture in position on residual ridge. **C,** Upper posterior teeth are too large in relation to denture base. **D,** Upper posterior teeth of proper size in relation to denture base. Notice slope of upper buccal flanges in relation to occlusal surfaces of posterior teeth. Forces created on denture bases by cheeks will help maintain upper denture in position.

the polished surfaces of the denture by allowing the buccal and lingual denture flanges to slope away from the occlusal surfaces. This occlusal form permits forces from the cheeks and tongue to help maintain the dentures in position on their residual ridges (Fig. 16-15). Narrow occlusal surfaces with proper escapeways for food also reduce the amount of stress applied on food during mastication to the supporting tissues of the basal seat. On the other hand, the posterior teeth should have sufficient width to act as a table upon which to hold food during its trituration.

Mesiodistal lengths of posterior teeth

The length of the mandibular residual ridge from the distal surface of the canine to the beginning of the retromolar pad is usually available for artificial posterior teeth. Artificial posterior teeth are made available by the manufacturer with varying overall mesiodistal widths (Fig. 16-16, A).

After the six anterior mandibular teeth have been placed in their final position, a point is marked on the crest of the mandibular ridge at the anterior border of the retromolar pad. This is the maximum extent posteriorly of any artificial teeth on the mandibular ridge. However, if the residual ridge anterior to this point slopes upward, smaller teeth or fewer teeth must be used to avoid having teeth over a pronounced incline at the distal end of the ridge. A smaller number of smaller teeth will often prevent the lower denture from sliding forward when pressure is applied on the molar teeth.

A ruler can be used to measure from the distal surface of the mandibular canine to the point that has been marked at the end of the available space (Fig. 16-16, B). The total mesiodistal width in millimeters of the four posterior teeth is often used as a mold number. For example, mold 32L of the Dentists' Supply Company signifies that the four posterior teeth have a total mesiodistal dimension of 32 mm and a long occlusal cervical length.

The posterior teeth should not extend too close to the posterior border of the maxillary

denture because of the danger of cheekbiting. However, if the posterior teeth do not extend far enough posteriorly, the forces of mastication would place a heavier load on the anterior part of the residual ridges. When the mandibular ridge slopes up sharply at its distal end, the posterior teeth must not be placed on this slope (Fig. 16-16, C). To do so would cause the lower denture to slide forward when forces are applied to the posterior teeth over the slope.

Posterior teeth are not arranged over the retromolar pad. Because the histologic structure of the pad is too soft and too easily displaced, it would allow the denture to tip during mastication. For this reason, only three posterior teeth are used on each side of the denture for many patients (Fig. 16-16, D).

Vertical length of buccal surfaces of posterior teeth

It is best to select posterior teeth corresponding to the interarch space and to the length of the anterior teeth (Fig. 16-17, A). Artificial posterior teeth are made available by the manufacturer in varying occlusocervical lengths (Fig. 16-17, B). The length of the maxillary first premolars should be comparable to that of the maxillary canines to have the proper esthetic effect (Fig. 16-17, C). If this is not done, the denture base material appears unnatural back of the canines. If the ridge laps are fairly thin and long, the posterior teeth can be readily positioned over full ridges without sacrificing leverage or esthetics. The form of the dental arch should copy, as nearly as possible, the arch form of the natural teeth they replace.

Type of posterior teeth according to materials

Most artificial posterior teeth are made of air-fired or vacuum-fired porcelain, acrylic resin, or a combination of acrylic resin and metal occlusal surfaces (Fig. 16-18).

Acrylic resin posterior teeth wear away faster than porcelain teeth and stain easily for some patients. Therefore porcelain artificial posterior teeth are used except for selected patients.

Acrylic resin posterior teeth are used when

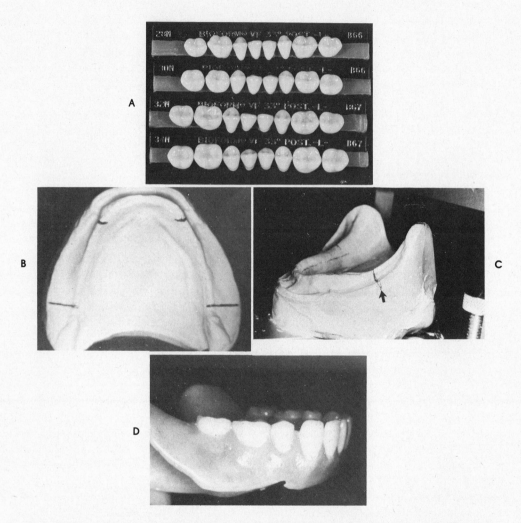

Fig. 16-16. A, Artificial posterior teeth are manufactured with varying mesiodistal widths. The four posterior teeth in mold 28M have a total mesiodistal width of 28 mm, whereas the four posterior teeth in mold 34M have a total mesiodistal width of 34 mm. **B,** Marks on cast indicate available space for artificial posterior teeth. **C,** Mark on cast *(arrow)* indicates to dentist or dental laboratory technician the distal extent of posterior teeth. **D,** Three posterior teeth are used on either side of lower denture because they adequately fill space available between distal surface of lower canine and retromolar pad or the beginning of a steep incline at distal end of mandibular ridge.

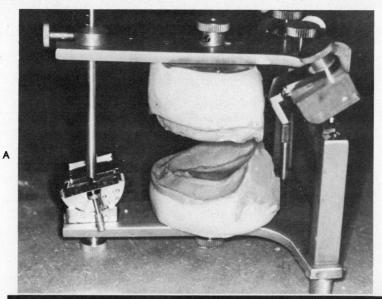

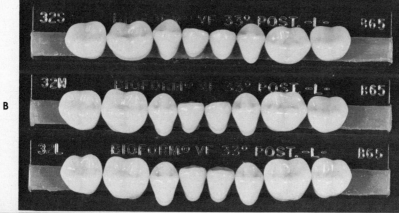

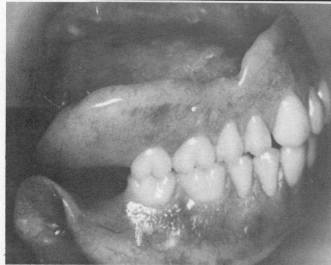

Fig. 16-17. A, Available interarch space between residual ridges is guide for length of posterior teeth, which in this situation will permit use of long posterior teeth. **B,** Artificial teeth are manufactured with varying occlusocervical lengths—32S, short; 32M, medium; and 32L, long. **C,** Length of posterior teeth is in harmony with that of canines. This is an important factor in esthetics when the patient is seen from the side.

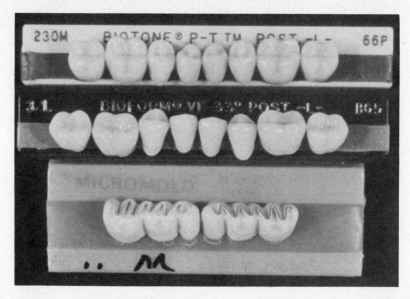

Fig. 16-18. Materials for posterior teeth. *Top,* Acrylic resin. *Middle,* Vacuum-fired porcelain. *Bottom,* Artificial posterior teeth in block form and made of acrylic resin with cobalt-chromium-steel metal inserts.

they oppose natural teeth or teeth whose occlusal surfaces have been restored with gold. This procedure reduces the possibility of the artificial teeth causing unnecessary abrasion and destruction of the natural or metallic occlusal surfaces of the opposing teeth. Gold occlusal surfaces can be developed for the artificial teeth and used in a similar manner (Fig. 16-19).

Acrylic resin artificial posterior teeth are also desirable when the tooth must be excessively reduced in length because of a small interarch distance. The chemical combination between acrylic resin teeth and the denture base prevents them from breaking away from the denture base. In addition, the plastic tooth is indicated when a tooth must be shaped to fit small spaces for esthetic purposes or be placed in contact with retainers for removable partial dentures.

Acrylic resin posterior teeth must not be used with porcelain anterior teeth on complete dentures. The resin posterior teeth will wear more rapidly than the porcelain anterior teeth and

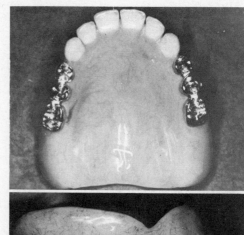

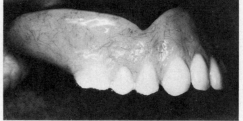

Fig. 16-19. A, Occlusal surfaces of posterior teeth have been cast in gold. **B,** Gold occlusal surfaces are barely visible when denture is viewed from the side.

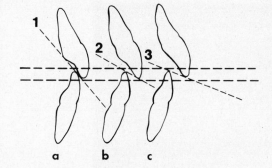

Fig. 16-20. a, No horizontal overlap with the resultant angle, *1.* **b,** Same vertical overlap but greater horizontal overlap with less incisal angle inclination, *2.* **c,** Same vertical overlap with still greater horizontal overlap and still less resultant incisal guide angle, *3.*

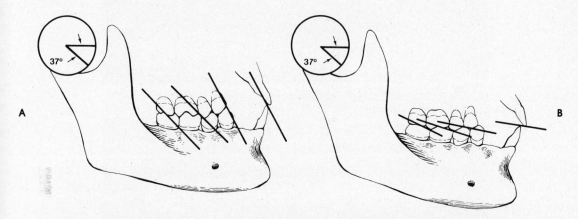

Fig. 16-21. Two figures with same condylar inclination but with different incisal guide inclinations. **A,** Steep vertical overlap with resultant steeper cusp inclines. **B,** Less steep incisal angle and resultant flatter cusp inclinations.

eventually create excessive and destructive occlusal forces in the anterior part of the mouth. The basal seat in this part of the mouth is usually least able to withstand any increased stresses.

Types of posterior teeth according to cusp inclines

The cuspal inclines for posterior teeth depend on the plan of occlusion selected by the dentist. For example, if a steep vertical overlap and low posterior tooth inclines are used, a spaced horizontal overlap of the anterior teeth must be used. If a flat or nearly horizontal incisal guidance angle is chosen, shallow posterior tooth

inclines should be selected, particularly if the condylar guidance also is shallow. In edentulous patients the incisal guidance angle is determined by the dentist; therefore the posterior tooth inclines are decided on when the horizontal overlap of the anterior teeth is set (Figs. 16-20 and 16-21). As has been mentioned, the try-in of the 12 anterior teeth aids in the selection of size and the final determination of the posterior cusp inclines. The influence of cusp inclines on denture stability is discussed in Chapter 21.

Posterior artificial teeth are manufactured with cusp inclines that vary from relatively steep to flat planes. The commonly used posterior

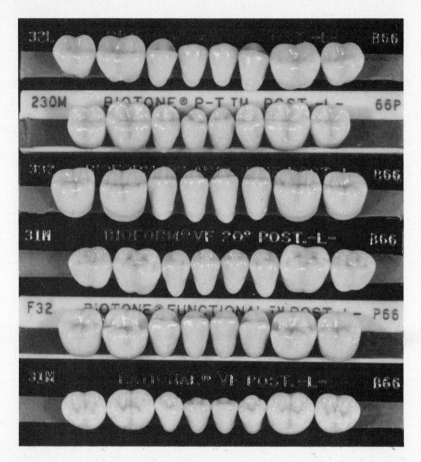

Fig. 16-22. Cuspal inclines of molds for posterior teeth. 32L (top), 33 degrees; 230M, 30 degrees; 33L, 30 degrees; 31M, 20 degrees; F-32, 10 degrees; 31M (bottom), 0 degrees.

teeth are those with cuspal inclinations of 33, 20, or 0 degrees (Fig. 16-22). The cuspal inclination is measured as the angle formed by the incline of the mesiobuccal cusp of the lower first molar with the horizontal plane.

The 33-degree posterior teeth offer the maximum opportunity for a fully balanced occlusion. However, the final effective height of the cusp for a given patient depends on the way in which the teeth are inclined (tipped) and the interrelation of the other factors of occlusion, that is, the incisal guidance, the condylar guidance, the height of the occlusal plane, and the compensating curve. Maintaining a shallow incisal guid-

ance compatible with esthetics allows a balanced occlusion to be developed with as little cusp height on the posterior teeth as possible, thus reducing lateral forces on the residual ridges. Research has indicated that anatomic teeth cause no more changes of supporting tissues or patient discomfort than other forms of posterior teeth.

The 20-degree posterior tooth is semianatomic in form and wider buccolingually than the corresponding 33-degree tooth. The 20-degree tooth provides less cusp height with which to develop balancing contacts in eccentric jaw positions that the 33-degree tooth does.

Nonanatomic teeth are advisable when only a centric relation record is transferred from the patient to the articulator and no effort is directed to establish a cross-arch balanced occlusion. Nonanatomic teeth are also effective when it is difficult or impossible to precisely record centric jaw relation from the patient or there are abnormal jaw relationships. However, it is a fallacy to believe that because posterior teeth contact evenly when the mandible is in centric relation, they will also contact evenly in eccentric mandibular positions unless specifically arranged to do so.

17

Preliminary arrangement
of artificial teeth

Once the casts have been tentatively mounted on the articulator, teeth are set in the occlusion rims so that more accurate observations can be made than was possible with the occlusion rims alone. The vertical jaw relations, established by adjustment of the occlusion rims, and the horizontal jaw relation (centric relation), established by a preliminary interocclusal record of centric relation, are likely to be incorrect. These records must therefore be recognized as tentative and subject to correction when new information is available.

The profile contours of the occlusion rims may also be incorrect and are subject to change when teeth and wax, instead of wax alone, control the contours of the lips. The carving of the labial surfaces of the occlusion rims must therefore be considered as tentative. The establishment of anterior tooth positions on the trial dentures is the dentist's responsibility and should preferably be carried out by the dentist or else be prescribed specifically to the dental technician.

Most dentists, however, prefer to carve the wax occlusion rims as accurately as they can for determining the desired amount of lip support and to have their assistant or technician make the preliminary arrangement of teeth as guided by these wax contours. Subsequently, these dentists make corrections in the tooth positions and even in the positions of the arches of anterior teeth when the wax trial dentures are observed in the mouth at the try-in appointment.

Other dentists will set the anterior teeth in the wax trial dentures themselves and thus reduce the time required for resetting the anterior teeth at the time of the try-in of the wax dentures. These dentists use the information they gained when the preliminary jaw relation records were made and other guides that might not be available to dental auxiliaries to assist them in the preliminary arrangement of teeth.

GUIDES FOR THE PRELIMINARY ARRANGEMENT OF ANTERIOR TEETH

The carved occlusion rims should provide reliable guides for placement of the anterior teeth in the wax occlusion rims. They indicate the likely anteroposterior and vertical positions of the incisor teeth on the basis of support they supply to the lips and mandible.

The length of time each jaw has been edentulous is in direct proportion to the amount of resorption that can be *expected*. The amount of resorption, in turn, can indicate the distance the teeth should be set from the residual ridge. If the patient's teeth have been out only 3 weeks, for example, the artificial teeth should be placed with the ridge lap of the tooth against the cast. But even this is not always correct. It may be that the patient lost the teeth as a result of severe periodontal disease that had destroyed much bone *before* the teeth were removed. Also, the patient may have lost some of the bone from the anterior part of the jaws through surgery at the time the teeth were removed. The dentist can learn about these possibilities while making the diagnosis and use the information when setting the central incisors in wax.

If the patient was edentulous for a long time or had natural teeth opposing a complete denture, much bone could have been lost from the residual ridge. In this situation, the artificial teeth should *not* be placed against the ridge. As a general rule, the longer the natural teeth have been out, the farther the artificial teeth should be from the residual ridge. This rule also applies when teeth are removed from the same mouth at different times. The shrinkage in this situation will be greater from one jaw than from the other one. The teeth should be placed closer to the residual ridge when there is less shrinkage and farther from the residual ridge when there has been more resorption. The objective is to place the occlusal plane of the teeth in the same position it occupied when the natural teeth were in place.

Relationship to the incisive papilla

The incisive papilla is a guide to anterior tooth position because it has a constant relationship to the natural central incisors. It is found in the lingual embrasure between these incisors. Naturally then, the incisive papilla is a guide to the position of the midline of the upper dental arch or, more specifically, to the position of the central incisors in the dental arch. The mesial surfaces of the central incisors of many people are not exactly in the center of their faces or mouths. When information on the position of the central incisors is available, the positions of the artificial teeth can be made more like those of the natural teeth and the teeth will look more natural. So, at least until the teeth are seen in the mouth, a line marking the center of the incisive papilla on the cast is extended forward onto the labial surface of the cast and then cut into the labial surface of the wax occlusion rim (Fig. 17-1). The central incisors are set on either side of this line. Their positions are quite similar to the positions of the natural teeth insofar as right and left orientation is concerned.

The incisive papilla is a guide also to the anteroposterior position of the teeth. The labial surfaces of the central incisors are usually 8 to 10 mm in front of the incisive papilla. This distance, for obvious reasons, will vary with the size of the teeth and the labiolingual thickness of the alveolar process carrying the natural teeth, so that it is not an absolute relationship. Furthermore, as severe resorption of the residual ridge in a vertical direction occurs, the incisive

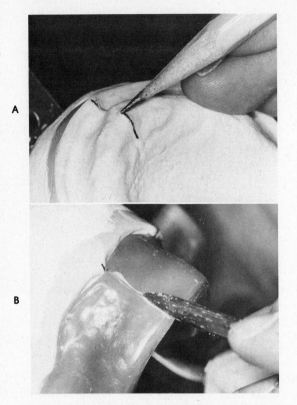

Fig. 17-1. Incisive papilla is used to locate midline of dental arch. **A,** Mark is made on cast through the center of the incisive papilla. **B,** Mark is transferred to occlusion rim as a guide to placement of the maxillary incisors.

papilla may move distally. Thus the distance from the incisive papilla to the labial surface of the teeth may become greater when much bone is lost from the maxillary residual ridge in a vertical direction.

Resorption of bone from the labial surface of the maxillary arch or surgical reduction of the labial plate of bone from the maxillae will cause the incisive papilla to *appear* to move forward. Obviously, this cannot happen, so an incisive papilla found on the labial-occlusal surface of a cast indicates that the anterior teeth must be set in front of the residual ridge by a distance that would correspond to the amount of change in the bone.

Relationship to the reflection

Another guide to the position of the two central incisors is the relationship of the labial surfaces of teeth to the reflection of soft tissues under the lip or recorded in the impression and cast. Notice in Fig. 17-2 that the labial surfaces and incisal edges of the teeth are anterior to the tissues at the reflection where the denture borders would be placed.

There is an obtuse angle between the labial surface of the root of a central incisor and the labial surface of the clinical crown of the tooth. This fact must be kept in mind when the artificial incisor is placed in the wax denture base, that is, the occlusion rim. The roots of the natural teeth extend into the alveolar process, with a relatively thin layer of bone over the labial surface of the root of the central incisor (Fig. 17-2). This relationship means that the labial surface of the residual ridge can be used as a guide to determining the proper inclination of the anterior teeth. *The accuracy of this guide decreases as the resorption of the residual ridge progresses,* but nevertheless the imaginary root of the artificial tooth must extend into the residual ridge, with allowance being made for the loss of bone structure, size, and shape. Clinical judgment is essential in the evaluation and application of these guides.

Factors governing the anteroposterior position of the dental arch

The anteroposterior position of the dental arch should be governed chiefly by consideration of the orbicularis oris and its attaching muscles and by the tone of the skin of the lips. Superficially, this means position and expression of the lips. The orbicularis oris affects and is affected by the following seven muscles: the quadratus labii superioris, caninus, zygomaticus, quadratus labii inferioris, risorius, triangularis, and buccinator. These muscles control expression and reflect the personality and appearance of every person wearing complete dentures. Dropping the orbicularis oris backward throws this entire group of muscles closer

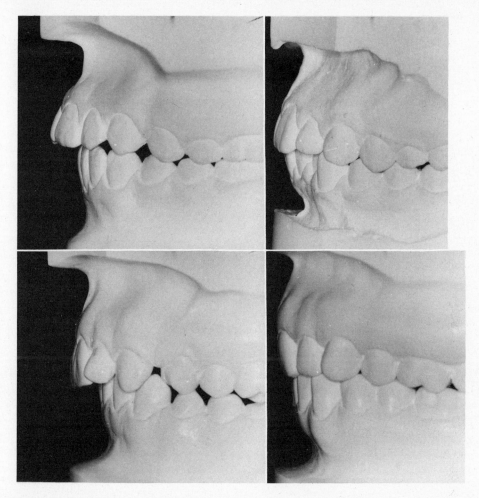

Fig. 17-2. Profile views showing relation of line of labial surface of central incisor to line of inclination of residual ridge.

to their origin and slackens them so that they cannot be effective when stimulated to contraction. The tone and action of these muscles depend on the anteroposterior support provided by the teeth and the denture base material.

Setting of teeth over the maxillary anterior ridge is often carried to an extreme, which undermines the esthetic result. The greatest harm is done in setting the maxillary anterior teeth back to the ridge or under the ridge, regardless of the amount of resorption that has taken place. A study of the anterior alveolar pro-

cess discloses the fact that the process is at an angle to the labial face of the maxillary incisors. In other words, its direction is upward and backward (Fig. 17-2). Therefore the crest of the ridge is considerably more to the posterior in a resorbed ridge than it is in a recent extraction. If the rule of setting teeth over the ridge is followed after the residual ridge has resorbed, prematurely aged appearance is the result (Fig. 17-3).

In Figs. 17-4 to 17-7 this cast was sawed in two along the median suture for a study of the rela-

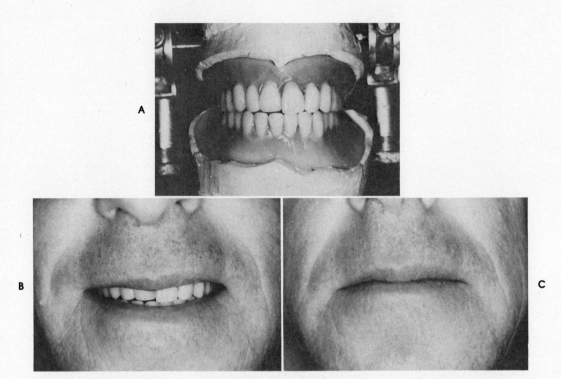

Fig. 17-3. A, Teeth are set on ridge, on the patient's right, and in a position that simulates their former natural position on the patient's left. **B** and **C** contrast this arrangement in patient's mouth. Left side of patient's mouth is esthetically more pleasing as a result. It must be emphasized that such a tooth arrangement is not always feasible or desirable, since it also depends on patient preference and circumoral changes.

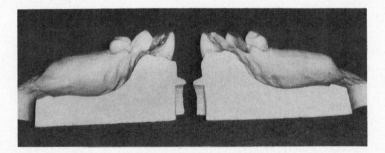

Fig. 17-4. Cast sawed in half showing relative positions of teeth.

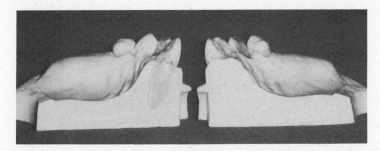

Fig. 17-5. Simulated inclination of central incisor root is drawn on cast.

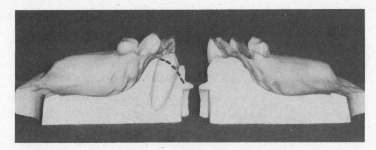

Fig. 17-6. Central incisor is removed from cast, and anticipated bony reduction is marked.

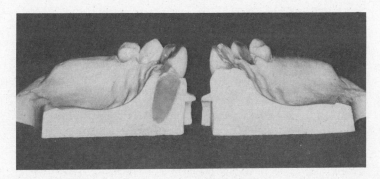

Fig. 17-7. An artificial tooth is waxed into place, replacing central incisor and restoring both tooth position and gingival tissue contour.

tive position of an artificial tooth to a resorbing ridge. One side of the cast was left intact to determine the former natural relation of the teeth to the maxilla. The central incisor was removed from the other side of the cast to show the evolution of an edentulous ridge, with the artificial tooth placed in relation to the ridge and to its former position as shown by the untouched half of the cast. This depicts how far upward and backward the tooth would have been placed had it been set to follow the edentulous ridge. If all the artificial teeth had been placed to follow this ridge, the orbicularis oris and its attaching muscles would have lost their correct anotomic relationship, and an aged, expressionless appearance would have resulted.

SETTING THE MAXILLARY ANTERIOR TEETH IN WAX FOR THE TRY-IN

The technique for setting anterior teeth in the wax occlusion rims is at the same time simple and exacting. If the occlusion rims have been accurately carved to support the lips and the maxillomandibular jaw relation, the occlusion rims are the guide to the anteroposterior position in the dental arch. If they were not accurately carved, the dentist must make observations of the alterations in labial surface contour that would be necessary when the teeth are set up. For example, if the lip needs more support when the occlusion rims are in the mouth, the incisors should be set in front of the labial surface of the wax rim. If the lips are too full at that time, more of the labial surface of the occlusion rims should be cut away before the teeth are set.

If the carving of the occlusion rims has been accurately done, cut away a small section of wax where a central incisor is to be placed. Then heat the wax where the occlusion rim has been cut away until the wax pools (becomes molten) in that place. This will provide a "socket" for the artificial tooth. Heat the cervical end of the tooth in a Bunsen burner and place it in the molten wax. The heated tooth will reheat the wax and allow it to be moved into the desired position with its mesial surface on the midline and the incisal edge just overlapping the occlusal surface of the lower occlusion rim. This process is repeated for setting the adjacent central incisor. (See Fig. 17-8.)

Then set the remaining upper anterior teeth in the wax, alternating their placement on the two sides of the dental arch. Care should be exercised to follow the arch form indicated by preextraction casts or photographs if they are available. If these records are not available, use the residual ridge as a reference, keeping in

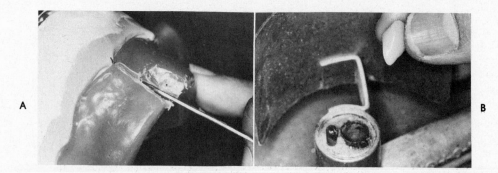

Fig. 17-8. A to G, Setting maxillary anterior teeth. **A,** Wax is pooled with a hot spatula to form a socket for central incisor. **B,** Cervical end of tooth is heated in Bunsen flame. (This is done only with porcelain teeth, since it would destroy plastic teeth.)   *Continued.*

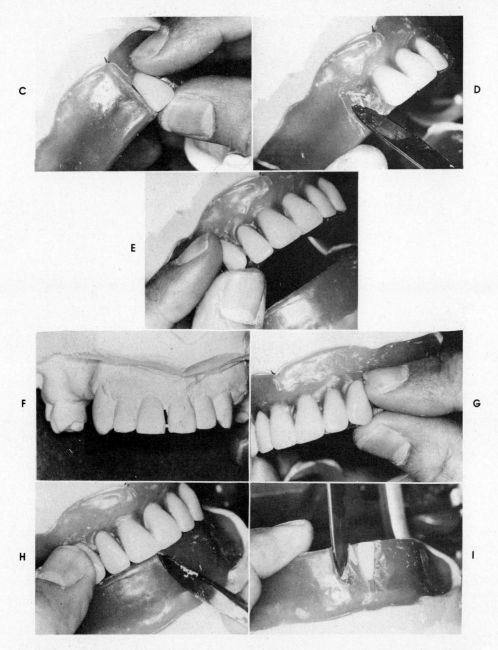

Fig. 17-8, cont'd. C, Heated end of tooth is placed in molten wax socket and moved to desired position. Heated tooth keeps wax soft enough that length, inclination, rotation can be adjusted as indicated by preextraction records. **D,** Socket is prepared for a lateral incisor. **E,** Position of the canine is adjusted to that of canine on diagnostic cast, **F. G,** Position of left canine is adjusted in wax. **H** and **I,** Setting mandibular anterior teeth. **H,** Midline for mandibular dental arch is marked to correspond with midline of maxillary dental arch. **I,** Mandibular incisors are set in the same manner as maxillary incisors.

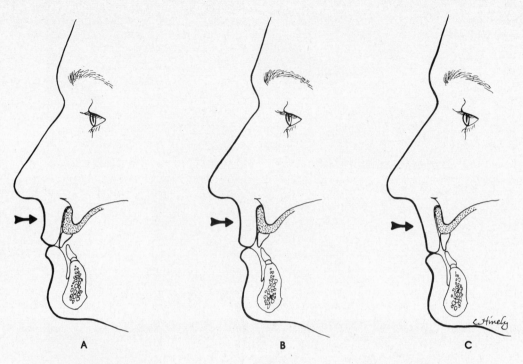

Fig. 17-9. Schematic drawings showing facial distortion because of incorrect positions of maxillary teeth. **A,** Favorable tooth and denture border position. **B,** Less favorable. **C,** Esthetically unfavorable restoration.

mind the history of the residual ridge—whether the teeth have been out a long time or bone has been lost from it by pathosis or by surgery. Always, the imaginary roots of the artificial teeth must extend into the residual alveolar ridge (before resorption), even though patients may wish it to be different. When the occlusion rim is removed from the cast, the dentist should observe the long axes of the teeth and visualize them as extending into the residual ridge. Be sure that the imaginary roots do not interfere with each other. One can best observed this by removing the occlusion rim from the cast and looking over the labial flange of the occlusion rim to visualize the imaginary roots extending into the alveolar groove of the trial denture base.

Importance of proper anteroposterior position of anterior teeth

In Fig. 17-9 is a series of drawings that show the importance of the teeth and the labial flange of the denture base to position and form of the lips. In Fig. 17-9, *A*, is shown the inclination that will maintain lip fullness and length in its natural form. To prevent the upper lip from thinning, lengthening, and losing the vermilion line contour, the incisors must be placed out to their former positions in order that the lip action will remain the same. In Fig. 17-9, *B*, are shown the incisors set with reduced vertical overlap, with resultant turning in and lengthening of the lip. In Fig. 17-9, *C*, are shown the incisor and border inclination in a still more lingual position that causes a thin, long, straight, and expressionless lip. This is attributable to the incline caused when the upper tooth is set back to contact the mandibular incisor.

Anterior artificial teeth should almost invariably be placed in exactly the same positions as those previously occupied by the natural teeth, and the labial surface of the denture base material should duplicate as nearly as possible the contour and position of the mucous membrane covering the alveolar ridge. To change either of these factors will change the support for the lips and the tone and action of the muscles involved in appearance and facial expression. Any attempt to reduce the horizontal overlap of the anterior teeth will alter the support of the lips. This may actually be indicated in some situations, for example, patients with maxillary protrusion (see Figs. 25-6 and 25-7), but it must be emphasized that such liberties are taken only in unusual and exceptional situations.

When the horizontal overlap of natural teeth is reduced to develop contacts in centric occlusion, unfavorable occlusal forces are applied on the anterior part of the residual ridges. The dangers from this source far exceed the possible dangers of unfavorable leverage that might be produced when the teeth are set where the natural teeth were. It is not necessary for the anterior teeth to contact in centric occlusion unless they did so as natural teeth. Even then, it is best that they be set just out of contact.

The relation of the maxillary and mandibular anterior ridges has an influence on the anteroposterior position of both the maxillary and the mandibular anterior teeth. A common error is to attempt to establish a standard vertical overlap and horizontal overlap without regard to the ridge relation. This is incorrect; the anteroposterior position of the teeth should vary with the anteroposterior relation of the residual ridges.

If the mandibular ridge should be forward of the maxillary ridge, as in prognathic patients, the upper anterior teeth should never be set labial to the mandibular teeth. They can be set end to end, with the incisal edges cut at an angle

that would have a seating action on the maxillary denture. When the prognathism is extreme, it is not possible to have tooth contact in the incisor region because the maxillary incisors would have to be placed too far anteriorly and too much leverage would result. Also, the tooth position would put the upper lip under too much tension.

Extremely high ridges may seem to create a problem unless one realizes that natural teeth once came out of these ridges. Insufficient space between the residual ridges is an indication that either the artificial teeth are longer than the natural teeth or the vertical dimension of the face is too short. However, if only parts of the ridges are too close together, the cause may be an excess of fibrous tissue on the ridge. This occurs most frequently in the upper tuberosity region, and surgical removal of excess fibrous tissue is indicated.

SETTING THE MANDIBULAR ANTERIOR TEETH IN WAX FOR THE TRY-IN

The lower anterior teeth are set in the lower occlusion rim so that the mesial surfaces of the two central incisors are in the same sagittal plane as the mesial surfaces of the upper central incisors. The same basic principles are involved in the arrangement of these teeth as apply to the arrangement of the upper anterior teeth. The roots of the mandibular incisors came out of the mandibular alveolar process. Therefore the imaginary roots of the mandibular anterior teeth must be positioned so that they would extend into the residual alveolar ridge if the roots were real. This will often place the mandibular teeth labial to the residual ridge. The reason for this is the fact that the mandibular natural teeth are most frequently labial to the apices of their roots. Observe the labial profile of the teeth in the diagnostic cast in Fig. 17-10.

Observations of the incisal edge, imaginary tooth apex, and the mandibular residual ridge are easily made by removal of the mandibular occlusion rim from its cast and sighting over the

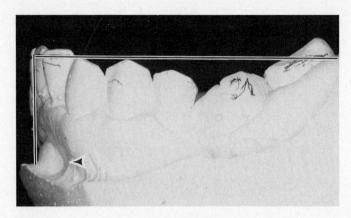

Fig. 17-10. Apices of imaginary roots of lower anterior teeth *(arrow)* are lingual to incisal edges and labial surfaces of crowns of teeth. When residual alveolar ridge resorbs, artificial teeth must be placed labial (anterior) to ridge if lip is to be properly supported.

labial surface of the labial flange from the basal surface of the occlusion rim toward the incisal edges. If the teeth are not properly inclined labiolingually, it will be apparent that the imaginary tooth roots could not be extending into the residual ridge.

Any difference in the arch form of the teeth and the arch form of the residual ridge can be easily detected by this same observation. It is important to recognize that the natural teeth erupted out of the alveolar process and that the artificial teeth must be placed so that their imaginary roots also could have erupted from the alveolar process when allowance is made for bone lost through disease, surgery, accident, or resorption.

The height to which the lower anterior teeth are set is tentatively determined by the height to which the mandibular occlusion rim had been built. Normally, this will allow for a slight vertical overlap of the upper anterior teeth over them. Before the first try-in, this overlap will be about 1.5 mm. Of course, this is subject to change after the trial dentures are seen in the mouth.

Horizontal overlap

The horizontal overlap of the maxillary over the mandibular teeth will be fairly uniform from one side of the dental arch to the other. The amount of projection of upper teeth over the lower teeth in the horizontal plane will vary with the amount of difference in the sizes of the two jaws. If the upper jaw is much larger than the lower one, the upper and the lower teeth should be placed where the natural teeth were, without attempting to make them be in contact in the centric jaw position. The upper teeth should be related to the upper jaw and the lower teeth to the lower jaw, regardless of their relationships to each other. To change from this basic position invites problems and either supports part of the face too much or another part of it not enough.

Remember that this first tooth setup is only tentative and that changes in the vertical or horizontal jaw relations will indicate the need for changes in the tooth positions. If the teeth are correctly set labiolingually in relation to their respective residual ridges, the subsequent changes will be only in their relative height and in the irregularities to be developed in their arrangement to make them appear more natural.

PRELIMINARY ARRANGEMENT OF POSTERIOR TEETH

The preliminary arrangement of the posterior teeth involves the application of principles sim-

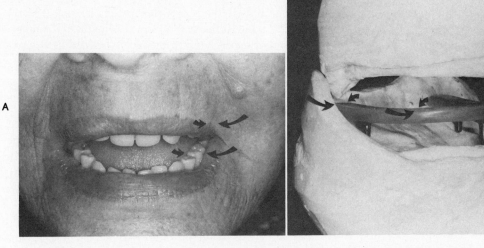

Fig. 17-11. The two sets of arrows in both **A** and **B** suggest relative orientation of occlusal plane's anterior (corner of mouth) and posterior (two thirds of the way up the retromolar pad) landmarks.

ilar to those followed in the tentative arrangement of the anterior teeth. The artificial posterior teeth should be placed as nearly as possible where the natural teeth were. This, in fact, is easier said than done, since there are not so many guides or indicators to posterior tooth position as there are to anterior tooth position. Therefore the final position of the occlusal plane, the final arch form, and even the final length (posterior extent) of the occlusal plane cannot be determined until the jaw relations are tested and found to be correct.

The tests are essential, and the posterior teeth must be arranged in such a way that the tests can be made. This means that the height and orientation of the occlusal plane are nearly correct, the opposing teeth have specific and precise relationships to each other, and the arch form of the lower dental arch must be nearly correct.

Orientation of the occlusal plane

Orientation of the anterior end of the occlusal plane is determined by esthetics. The vertical level at which the incisal edges of the anterior teeth are set is the level of the anterior end of the occlusal plane. If these teeth are set in the same positions that the natural teeth occupied, the front end of the occlusal plane will be correctly located.

The posterior end of the occlusal plane should be located so that (if it were extended) it would be level with the junction between the middle and the distal third of the retromolar pad. Stated another way, the distal end of the occlusal plane should be at a level two thirds the way up the retromolar pad as simulated in Fig. 17-11.

If it is assumed that the anterior teeth are correctly placed for esthetics, location of the posterior end of the occlusal plane in the same relation to the retromolar pads will place the occlusal plane at the level that is familiar to the tongue. If the occlusal plane is located at a higher or lower level to gain leverage advantage, the dentures will interfere with normal tongue action. This will be more dangerous to the stability of the dentures than unfavorable leverage.

The height of the occlusal plane in the anterior region of the arch in dentures is influenced by the length of the lips, ridge fullness, ridge height, amount of maxillomandibular space, and the incisal guide angle. The ridge height may be excessive in the mandibular anterior region and low in the maxillary anterior region, or vice versa, or both the anterior and posterior ridges may be high or low. These factors may influence the location of the occlusal plane for some patients, but the ideal is to locate the plane in the same position as it was when natural teeth were present. The maxillomandibular space and the ridge height and fullness in the posterior regions often influence the positioning of the occlusal plane even though they should not. Often the occlusal plane is marked out on the wax rims to follow an arbitrary line on the face. This line is usually taken from the ala of the nose to the tragus of the ear. However, it is not an accurate guide, since it varies just as much as the shapes of ridges vary.

The inclination of the plane as a whole is an important factor in stability or instability of dentures. If the plane is too low in the anterior region or too high in the posterior region, the maxillary denture will tend to slide forward under pressure. If the reverse is true (the plane too low in the posterior region and too high in the anterior region), the incline plane action under biting force will tend to cause the mandibular denture to slide forward. Ideally, the occlusal plane should parallel both residual ridges.

The vertical orientation and inclination of the occlusal plane is not a simple matter of dividing the maxillomandibular denture space equally. The division of this space is governed by the relative amount of bone lost from the two ridges. If more bone has been lost from the maxillae than from the mandible, the occlusal plane must be closer to the mandible than to the maxillae. If more bone has been lost from the mandible than from the maxillary jaw, the occlusal plane must be closer to the maxillae than to the mandible. The level of the occlusal plane must be placed as nearly as possible to the position of the occlusal plane of the natural teeth. It should *not* be placed at a level that would favor the weaker of

the two ridges (basal seats). The most reliable guides are the height of the corners of the mouth and the height of the retromolar pads. At this point in the procedure, the height of the anterior teeth is tentative and will be modified as indicated by observations made at the try-in.

Tentative buccolingual position of posterior teeth

The buccolingual position of the posterior teeth and the posterior arch form are determined anteriorly by the positions (or arch form) of the anterior teeth and posteriorly by the shape of the basal seat provided by the mandible. The curvature of arch of the anterior tooth arrangement starts from the front teeth in a pleasing curvature toward the posterior teeth. The posterior teeth must continue this curvature in such a way that the posterior teeth are properly related to the bone that supports them and to the soft tissues that contact their buccal and lingual surfaces. In the final tooth arrangement, the posterior part of the arch form will be determined to a great extent by the "neutral zone" between the cheeks and the tongue. This is the space developed by the removal of the posterior teeth and the loss of bone from the residual ridges. The pressure of the cheeks and tongue against the buccal and lingual surfaces of the erupting natural teeth were strong enough to influence their alignment in the dental arch. These same forces are applied against dentures (Figs. 17-12 and 17-13). Therefore the final arrangement of the arch form of the posterior teeth must be developed with respect for these external forces.

Leverage and posterior tooth positions. Posterior teeth would have their most favorable leverage if they were set close to the residual ridge and lingual to it. This is not practical because of the disturbing influence it would have on other relationships such as the vertical dimension of occlusion, face height, esthetics, and the space allotted to the tongue (Figs. 17-14 and 17-15).

Posterior teeth placed buccal to the ridge can cause a denture to tip when pressure is applied

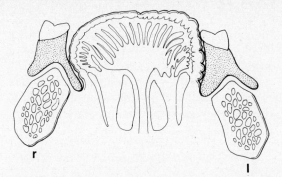

Fig. 17-12. Schematic drawing showing mandibular teeth too far to buccal side of ridge on right side and too far to lingual side of ridge on left side.

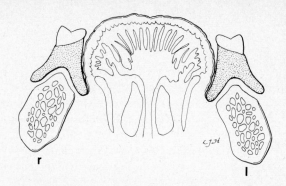

Fig. 17-13. Positions of mandibular teeth corrected from position shown in Fig. 17-12.

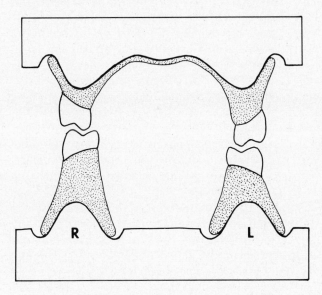

Fig. 17-14. *Right side,* Incorrect division of interridge space; *left side,* interridge space properly divided.

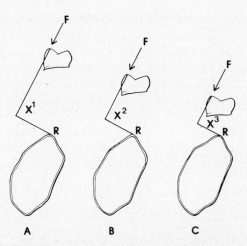

Fig. 17-15. Amount of leverage that is exerted on occlusal plane in relation to distance it is above the ridge. **A** to **C,** Occlusal plane at varying heights. Amount of leverage, X^1, X^2, X^3, may be established by the following formula: torque equals force *F,* times the distance of the line of application of the force to the fulcrum point, *R.*

on the tooth in that bad leverage position. The effect of such bad leverage is magnified as the occlusal plane is located further away from the ridge (the basal seat) (Fig. 17-15). The solution to the problem is to recognize the location of the occlusal surfaces of the natural teeth and to place the artificial teeth as nearly as possible in that position. However, this is not easily done when the upper jaw is wider or narrower than the lower jaw. These situations require special handling of the occlusal surfaces of the posterior teeth in their final arrangement into balanced occlusion.

Tentative arch form of posterior teeth

The basic principle for the buccolingual position of the arch form of the posterior teeth is that the arch of teeth should conform to the shape of the residual ridge. In other words, the teeth should be in a position to have erupted from the residual ridge. The basic rule, then, is that a perpendicular erected from the buccal side of the crest of the ridge should bisect the buccal cusp of the lower first molar. This principle and rule apply regardless of the differences in the widths of the upper or lower jaws. Therefore the arch form and buccolingual posterior tooth positions are keyed to the mandibular basal seat regardless of alterations that may be necessary if the upper jaw is wider or narrower than ideal. The form of each dental arch must be consistent and harmonious within itself and with its foundation. The tentative arrangement of the posterior teeth can respect these guides.

This thought regarding placement of the arch and occlusal plane can best be conveyed by thinking of each arch as a piece of wire or strip of carding wax that can be placed up or down or backward or forward and that can be bent wider or narrower.

Figs. 17-16 to 17-20 are a series of illustrations of the mandibular arch form, from a superior aspect, that show some errors in the mandibular arch position and form and a final favorable arch position and form. This series emphasizes the treatment of an arch as a unit before treatment of individual teeth in the final arrangement. Such an order of procedure saves time and more readily aids in obtaining the desired result.

Generally, the posterior teeth will fall between two lines extending posteriorly from the distal surface of the canines to the buccal and lingual margins of the retromolar pad.

SETTING THE POSTERIOR TEETH FOR THE TRY-IN

Posterior teeth are set up in tight centric occlusion. The mandibular teeth are set in the wax occlusion rim over the residual ridge in their ideal buccolingual position, and the maxillary teeth are set in a tight centric occlusion with them regardless of their buccolingual positions. The objective here is to have the intercuspation of the posterior teeth so precise that any deviation of this occlusion in the mouth will be easily detected. Thirty-degree teeth are probably more effective for checking the accuracy of jaw relations than 20-degree or 0-degree teeth. The incline planes of the 30-degree cusp teeth magnify horizontal errors in occlusion and make them easy to detect. The incline plane contacts between the teeth will reveal errors in centric occlusion in the mouth as the dentist instructs the patient to pull the jaw back and "close just until any tooth touches, then to close tight." Any touch of the teeth and slide from that contact can be felt in the fingers of the dentist making the observation. The touch and slide represent an easily detected error.

Guidelines for centric occlusion

There are three specifications for teeth in centric occlusion: (1) the upper teeth overlap the lower teeth, (2) the long axis of each upper tooth is distal to the long axis of the corresponding lower tooth, and (3) each tooth is opposed by two teeth, except for the lower central incisor and the upper last molar. These are the specifications for tooth arrangement in testing the accuracy of centric relation records and mounting of casts. The teeth must be set in these relationships for the dentist to be able to make the necessary tests and observations.

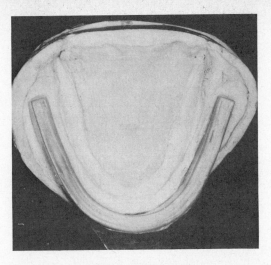

Fig. 17-16. Arch too wide.

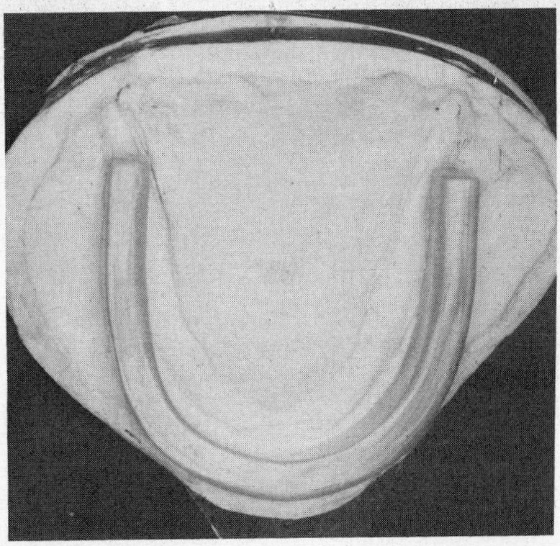

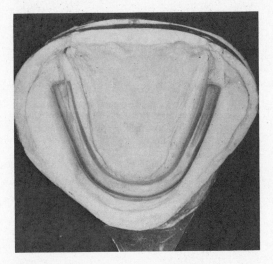

Fig. 17-17. Arch too wide in premolar region and too narrow in molar region.

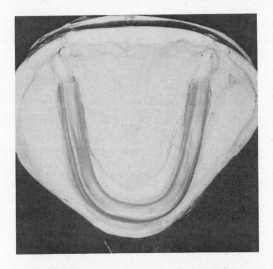

Fig. 17-18. Arch too narrow in molar region.

Fig. 17-19. Arch too far to lingual surface in anterior region.

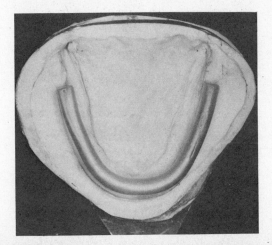

Fig. 17-20. Favorable arch form. Posterior part of it follows curvature of residual ridge.

There are two basic approaches to the arrangement of posterior teeth in centric occlusion. Both procedures are in current use. One involves setting the maxillary teeth first in relation to a line drawn over the crest of the mandibular ridge and then setting the mandibular teeth to the maxillary teeth. The other procedure involves setting each mandibular tooth or all the teeth before the corresponding maxillary tooth or teeth are set. This method permits the mandibular teeth to be set more accurately in relationship to the residual ridge than the first method does. Most residual ridges are curved laterally between the position of the canine and the retromolar pad. The teeth should be set to follow this curve to provide the maximum tongue space and balance the pressure of the tongue with the pressure of the cheek. If the posterior part of the dental arch was curved when the natural teeth were present, this same relationship should be established if the support of the cheeks is to be restored.

Procedure for setting posterior teeth into centric occlusion only

Arranging posterior teeth for a try-in is illustrated in Fig. 17-21. An alternative method of setting up nonanatomic posterior teeth is described in Chapter 21 and Figs. 21-44 and 21-45. *The latter method is very easy to carry out, since the features of their occlusal surfaces permits complete anteroposterior and buccolingual freedom of placement.*

Following is a description of the techniques for setting up cusp teeth:

Reduce the height of the posterior segments of the occlusion rim on one side, keeping the full height of the occlusion rims on the other side. This will make space for the teeth on one side and maintain the vertical dimension of the occlusion rims on the other side.

Pool enough wax distal to the maxillary canine to make a socket for the maxillary first premolar.

Heat the cervical end of the premolar and place it in the pooled wax so that its long axis is parallel with the buccal surface of the canine.

Place the second maxillary premolar in the wax with a similar alignment and length.

Pool the wax in the mandibular occlusion rim directly under the adjacent proximal surfaces of the upper premolars.

Heat the cervical end of the lower second premolar and place it in the pooled wax in such a way that it is too long. Then close the articulator to allow the upper teeth to force the lower tooth

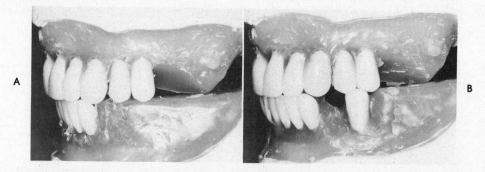

Fig. 17-21. Steps in arranging posterior teeth for try-in. **A,** Maxillary first and second premolars are set in alignment with maxillary canine to continue arch form established by anterior teeth. Premolar buccal surfaces parallel buccal surface of canine. Cervical end of each tooth is heated before it is set in its wax socket. **B,** Mandibular second premolar is set too high in pooled wax, and articulator is closed to push it down to its correct position. Heated cervical end of tooth keeps wax soft enough that tooth can be rotated or inclined as necessary. *Continued.*

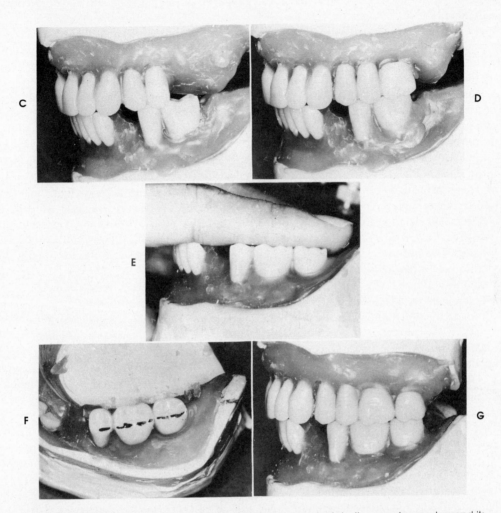

Fig. 17-21, cont'd. C, Mandibular first molar is set so that it contacts both second premolars and its buccal cusps would be bisected by a perpendicular erected on buccal side of crest of residual ridge. **D,** Maxillary first molar is set in pooled wax socket so that it is slightly too long. Then articulator is closed to force it into soft wax socket. An index finger can be used to assist tooth into its correct intercuspation and inclination by pressing against cervical end of tooth while the articulator is being closed. **E,** Mandibular second molar is set in a similar manner as mandibular first molar **(C).** The finger acts as a template to make certain that all the mandibular cusps are harmoniously related to each other and that the occlusal plane aims at a level near top of retromolar pad. **F,** Alignment of lower buccal cusps corresponds with curvature of arch form of residual ridge. **G,** Maxillary second molar is set too long in its wax socket and held at cervical end with index finger while articulator is closed. This procedure automatically intercuspates all the posterior teeth into tight centric occlusion.

into the soft wax. Hold a finger against the cervical end of the lower tooth to hold it and automatically keep the lingual cusp in contact with the upper two teeth.

Pool the wax distal to the lower second premolar for the first molar tooth. Heat the cervical end of this tooth and push it into the molten wax. Align it buccolingually in relation to the ridge crest as previously determined. Align the buccal and lingual cusps with those of the second premolar. Push it down into the wax so that its occlusal surface is aiming at a point near the top of the retromolar pad. Then close the articulator. This will bring the mesial inclines of the molar into contact with the distal inclines of the second premolar. The tooth contact should not disturb the position of the molar. If it does, push the molar further into the wax.

Pool the wax for placing the upper first molar and heat the cervical end of the tooth as was done for the others. Place the heated cervical end of the tooth in the molten wax, then holding the cervical end of the tooth in, close the articulator to seat the occlusal surfaces together.

Pool the wax for placing the lower second molar. Heat the cervical end of the tooth and push it into the molten wax in the desired buccolingual relationship with the cusps aligned with the cusps on the first molar and the occlusal surface aiming toward the point near the top of the retromolar pad. The index finger placed on top of the occlusal surfaces of the mandibular teeth at this time will reveal disharmonies in the height of the cusps and their alignment. Make the necessary adjustments.

Pool the wax in the position of the upper second molar and heat and place this tooth in position in the soft wax, but a millimeter or so too long. Then close the articulator while holding a finger against the cervical end of the upper tooth. This will occlude the teeth and position the molar in proper centric occlusion with the lower tooth.

Use a hot spatula to seal the wax around the cervical ends of all of the teeth.

Repeat the procedure on the opposite side.

Then after the wax is cooled, carve any excess wax from around the teeth and smooth the wax for try-in in the mouth.

The occlusion will be balanced only for centric occlusion for the try-in. The posterior teeth will have to be reset to develop balanced occlusions in the other jaw positions after verification of the jaw relations and final arrangement of the anterior teeth for esthetics.

Setting posterior teeth is essentially a mechanical problem, and their anteroposterior position depends on the proper anteroposterior setting of the anterior teeth. A change or shift in the position of the anterior teeth for esthetics would necessitate rearranging all the teeth. After the anterior setup has been accepted as final, the final anteroposterior position of the posterior teeth can be more readily determined.

After the positon of the anterior teeth has been determined in the mouth, it is possible to have an exact guide for the size of the posterior teeth. It may be necessary to change the size of the posterior teeth at this time. This distance between the distal surface of the mandibular canine and the mesial end of the retromolar pad is measured to determine the total anteroposterior space that may be covered by the teeth. The occlusocervical length of the posterior teeth is determined by the height and fullness of the ridges. The maxillae do not afford landmarks by which to measure, whereas the mandible rises with an upward curvature that prevents the setting of teeth too far posteriorly. The anterior teeth are in their final arrangement, and they establish the anterior limit of the posterior occlusion (Fig. 17-22). The distal limit of the extent of the posterior teeth is determined by the incline of the lower residual ridge. This may be as far forward as the normal position of the first molar tooth in some mouths. If a tooth is placed on this incline, the denture will tend to slide forward if any pressure is applied on the tooth. It may be necessary to omit an upper and lower premolar or molar from the dentures to avoid placing teeth on this incline. The bucco-

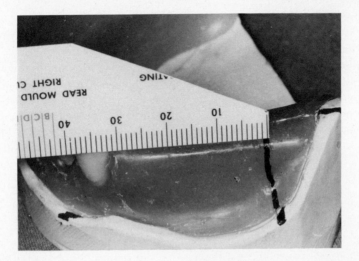

Fig. 17-22. Measurement for selection of size of posterior teeth. *Vertical line,* Anterior edge of retromolar pad. Posterior teeth should not be placed over retromolar pad or on upward incline of the lower residual ridge.

lingual width of the posterior teeth should be narrower than the width of the natural teeth to reduce biting pressure and to increase tongue space. Remember that many tongues become abnormally wide because of reorganization of their intrinsic musculature when posterior teeth are lost and not replaced. The decreased buccolingual diameter of the teeth also contributes to a more favorable slope of the lingual surface of the lingual flange.

GENERAL CONSIDERATIONS

The ideal position of artificial teeth is precisely the same as that of the natural teeth they replace. When this objective is achieved, the soft tissues of the face will be supported the same as they were when the natural teeth were present. The pressures of the soft tissues against the artificial teeth will be exerted as were exerted by these same tissues against the natural teeth when they were erupting into the mouth. These pressures were effective in aligning the natural teeth into the dental arch, and they can be effective in maintaining dentures in place. This is provided, of course, that the artificial teeth are aligned in dental arches that are in the

same positions as the dental arches of the natural teeth were. Tench has stated the situation graphically. He compared the cavity produced in a patient's mouth by the removal of the teeth and the subsequent shrinkage of the residual ridges with a cavity in a tooth. The space is available: it must be filled but not overfilled. The artificial teeth and the denture base material of the dentures should fill the usable space without interfering with the action of oral or facial structures.

The anterior teeth play an important part in three basic oral functions. These functions are esthetics, incision, and phonetics.

To fulfill their function in esthetics, artificial teeth must be of the same size and shape as natural teeth and occupy the same basic positions as natural teeth. Preextraction diagnostic casts and photographs can provide invaluable guides for the placement of these teeth if they are available. If not available, the judgment and knowledge of the dentist concerning dental and oral anatomy must serve as the guides. The dentist's judgment is based on knowledge of the changes that occur in the residual ridges after the teeth are lost and of the tone of the skin around the mouth as compared with that in other parts of the face.

The function of incision involves certain mechanical considerations that must be coordinated with occlusion of the posterior teeth. These are discussed in Chapter 21.

The functon of phonetics is closely associated with the tooth position for esthetics. In fact, phonetics can serve as a guide to esthetics and to the establishment of the vertical relation of the jaws.

Esthetics and leverage

Frequently, esthetics and leverage go hand in hand. For example, an arch that is too broad in the premolar region will cause the patient to have the appearance of too many teeth, and likewise this buccal position of the premolars will have improper tipping leverage. If the anterior teeth are set parallel to each other in every inclination and rotation, with perfect regularity and symmetry, they will have a bad esthetic effect. Nature has many apparent irregularities of anterior teeth, but they usually are not without a pattern that is more or less pleasing for an individual person. Irregularities can be used to great advantage in making dentures appear natural. To be effective, these irregularities must be correlated with the arch form and facial contour.

The details must be worked out by the dentist at the try-in. The irregularities must be of a type that could appear in nature and must not be irregular in an unnatural way. For example, if two teeth are to be inclined or overlapped, their positions should be such that their roots (if they had roots) would not interfere with each other or with the teeth adjacent to them. It is still not possible to have two things occupy the same space at the same time, even if they are imaginary roots.

Common errors

Some of the common errors in arrangement of teeth include (1) setting mandibular anterior teeth too far forward in order to meet maxillary teeth, (2) failure to make the canines the turning point of the arch, (3) setting mandibular first premolars to the buccal side of the canines, (4) setting maxillary posterior teeth over the ridge and then occluding the mandibular posterior teeth, bringing them too far to the lingual area in the second molar region and causing tongue interference and mandibular denture displacement, (5) failure to establish the occlusal plane at the proper level and inclination, (6) establishing the occlusal plane by an arbitrary line on the face, and (7) lack of rotation of the anterior teeth to give a narrower effect.

18

Perfection and verification of jaw relation records

The vertical and centric relations of edentulous jaws are tentatively established with the occlusion rims as described in Chapter 15. After the preliminary arrangement of the artificial teeth on the occlusion rims, it is essential that the accuracy of the jaw relation records made with the occlusion rims be tested, perfected if incorrect, and then verified to be correct. The dentist must assume that the preliminary jaw relation records were incorrect until they can be proved correct. This mental attitude of the dentist—attempting to prove that the jaw relation records are wrong—is essential in perfecting and verifying jaw relation records.

Patients should be advised to leave existing dentures out of the mouth for a minimum of 24 hours before the jaw relation records are perfected and verified at the time of the try-in appointment. Thus the soft tissues of the basal seat will be rested and in the same form as they were when the final impressions were made. If this procedure is not followed, the distorted condition of the soft tissue can prevent the registration of accurate interocclusal records.

The importance of perfection and verification of jaw relation records cannot be overstressed. The appearance and comfort of the patient, occlusion of the teeth, and the health of the supporting tissues are all directly related to the accuracy of the jaw relation records.

VERIFYING THE VERTICAL RELATION

The mandibular trial denture is placed in position in the mouth, and then the maxillary trial denture is inserted. The patient is instructed to close lightly so that the maxillary labial frenum can be checked to see that it is absolutely free. This is necessary before the relation of the lip to the teeth can be observed. If the border causes binding of the frenum, the labial notch should be deepened.

Next, a tentative observation of the centric occlusion is made. The balls of the index finger and thumb of the same hand are placed between the teeth, and the patient is directed to "pull your lower jaw back and close until you feel a back tooth touch." At the first contact, direct the patient to open and to repeat this closure, "only this time stop the instant you feel a tooth touch, then close tight." The procedure will reveal errors in centric relation by the touch and slide of teeth on each other. The errors in centric relation may interfere with tests for vertical relations.

Occlusal vertical dimension and vertical relation of the jaws must now be given careful consideration because the final positions of the anterior and posterior teeth depend to a great degree on the amount of interarch distance available. Unfortunately, there is no precise scientific method of determining the correct occlusal vertical dimension. The acceptability of vertical dimension of the dentures depends on the experience and judgment of the dentist. However, the factors that govern the dentist's final determination of this relation are in general based on the careful consideration of the following:

1. Preextraction records
2. Amount of interocclusal distance to which the patient was accustomed, either before the loss of natural teeth or with old dentures
3. Phonetics and esthetics
4. Amount of interocclusal distance between the occlusal surfaces of the teeth when the mandible is in its rest position

5. Study of facial dimensions and facial expression
6. Lip length in relation to teeth
7. Interarch distance and parallelism of the ridges as may be observed from the mounted casts
8. Condition and amount of shrinkage of the ridges

A combination of these factors and considerations may be used to aid in determining an acceptable vertical relation. An elaboration on the various theories is given in Chapter 12.

It is obvious that verification of vertical maxillomandibular relations is a challenge and that it requires considerable judgment of many factors by the dentist.

VERIFYING OR CHECKING CENTRIC RELATION

After the vertical relation has been determined, the centric relation is verified. Centric relation can be verified by intraoral observation of intercuspation of the teeth or by extraoral methods on the articulator.

Intraoral intercuspation of teeth to check centric relation

The test for accuracy of the preliminary centric relation record involves the observation of the intercuspation of the teeth in the mouth when the mandible is pulled back by the patient as far as it will go and closure is stopped at the first contact of the teeth. This observation is made by feel as well as by sight. The thumb and forefinger of the same hand are used to make the observation. The palm of the hand is turned toward the patient's face so that it covers the patient's eyes and the little finger is up. The ball of the index finger and the ball of the thumb are placed between the upper and lower teeth. The stability of the mandibular trial denture is maintained by both the left hand and the presence of the right thumbnail on the incisal edges or, if feasible, on the labiocervical aspect of the incisors and denture flange (Fig. 18-1). The right thumb acts as an anterior stop to control jaw closing (e.g., to prevent the patient slipping past

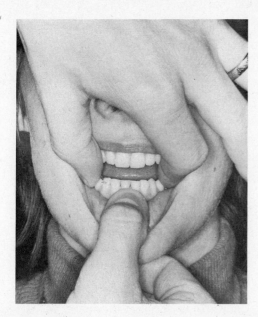

Fig. 18-1. Hand and finger positions used to check accuracy of centric relation records.

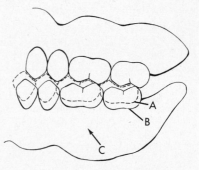

Fig. 18-2. An error in centric occlusion that is a result of an error in centric relation mounting will produce contact of inclined planes of cusps, *B*. Further closure will allow teeth to slide into centric occlusion, *A*. Path of closure is an arc, *C*, about posterior terminal hinge axis.

an initial premature occlusal contact into maximum tooth contact). The patient is instructed to pull the lower jaw back as far as it will go and to close just until the back teeth barely touch. Then the patient is told to close tightly. Any error in centric relation will be apparent when the teeth slide over each other, especially if anatomic teeth are used (Fig. 18-2). A second closure made with the same instructions and a stop of the closure at first contact will permit visual observation of the error.

An error in the mounting will cause some teeth to be out of contact when the first tooth contact is made. If the patient stops the closure at the instant the first teeth touch, the error will be indicated by the space between the lower tooth or teeth and the teeth it was intended to touch. The amount of error observed in this manner will be magnified by the effect of the inclined plane contacts. All the teeth that occluded uniformly on the articulator must have equally uniform contacts in the mouth, or the touch and slide observation will prove the mounting to be incorrect.

Once it is determined that the mounting is incorrect, a preliminary observation of esthetics is made. If the anterior teeth are not placed so as to support the lip properly, their positions are corrected. Then vertical overlap of the anterior teeth is carefully noted. This is important because the amount of vertical overlap of the anterior teeth will be the guide to the amount of closure permitted when the next interocclusal record is made.

Intraoral interocclusal records. The posterior teeth are removed from the lower occlusion rim, and both occlusion rims are placed in the mouth. Impression plaster, or an interocclusal registration paste, is mixed, and with the hands in the same position as for testing the previous record, the selected recording medium is placed on both sides of the lower occlusion rim in the molar and premolar regions. This may be done with a narrow plaster or cement spatula. Then the patient is instructed to pull the lower jaw back and close slowly until requested to stop and hold that position. The closure is stopped when the anterior teeth have the same vertical overlap as they had before the posterior teeth were removed. Thus the vertical relation of the two jaws will not be changed. When the plaster or registration paste is set, the new record is removed, toegether with the two occlusion

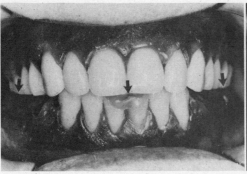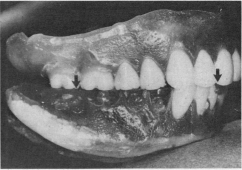

Fig. 18-3. Modified beeswax interocclusal record of centric relation is made to correct error in preliminary mounting of casts. Lower posterior teeth are removed to avoid any contact between upper and lower trial dentures. Vertical overlap of anterior teeth is guide to vertical relation at which centric relation is recorded. Beeswax tripod of stops identified by arrows.

rims, and the lower cast is remounted on the articulator. In an alternate technique an abbreviated beeswax occlusion rim is used to replace the removed posterior teeth (The rim may replace all the posterior teeth, or else a "tripod" of beeswax stops can be used; see Fig. 18-3). The patient is guided into the most retruded mandibular position at the selected vertical dimension when the upper posterior teeth will indent the softened opposing wax rims. The lower cast is remounted on the articulator, and the lower posterior teeth are reset into centric occlusion.

The occlusion rims, with the teeth in good tight centric occlusion, are returned to the mouth, and the same tests are made as before. If the teeth occlude perfectly and uniformly when the lower jaw is drawn back by the patient as far as it will go, the centric relation mounting may be assumed to be correct. There should be uniform simultaneous contact on both sides of the mouth, in the front and back, and without any detectable touch and slide of the teeth.

It is essential with this procedure that the dentist *try* to find an error in the previous record. He must assume that the record he has made is incorrect unless he cannot detect any touch and slide of the teeth. The entire procedure must be repeated until there is no doubt about the correctness of the relationship of the casts.

Extraoral method to check centric relation

Centric relation can be checked or verified by an extraoral method in which the observations are made on the articulator rather than in the mouth. This technique is an easy, hence attractive, one, but its use depends on one or two liberties being taken. The technique involves a centric relation registration in a soft wax placed between the opposing teeth. The teeth do not contact through the wax; hence the centric relation record is made at a slightly increased vertical dimension. While clinical experience endorses this technique, a purist could argue that such a verification record is only likely to work correctly if a kinematic hinge axis, rather than an arbitrary face-bow recording, was used originally. Since conclusive research to support such an argument is absent and since extensive clinical application of the technique has led to predictable and reproducible results, it deserves description.

Either wax, plaster, or a bite registration paste may be used as the recording medium in this technique. A piece of baseplate wax shaped like the dental arch, approximately one to two layers in thickness, is placed over the occlusal surfaces of the mandibular teeth, except that less wax should be used over the anterior teeth. This amount of thickness is chosen to eliminate the danger of making contact with the opposing

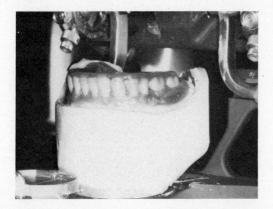

Fig. 18-4. Centric relation baseplate wax luted in the interproximal spaces.

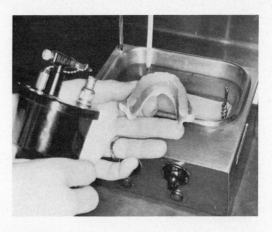

Fig. 18-5. Preliminary softening of wax by means of a hand alcohol torch.

teeth when biting pressure is first exerted and also to prevent a chilled layer of wax next to the teeth from interfering with equalized pressure. The maxillary teeth should not touch the wax on the mandibular anterior teeth. Contacts on wax on the anterior teeth tend to cause patients to protrude the lower jaw. The wax is luted into the interproximal spaces of the anterior and posterior teeth on the labial, buccal, and lingual sides. Before the wax is luted in position, the teeth and wax should be dried so that the luted wax will adhere firmly to the teeth and wax rim (Fig. 18-4). The surface of these layers of wax is first heated with an alcohol torch (Fig. 18-5). The flaming is done by going from side to side, allowing sufficient time for the heat to penetrate to the full depth of the wax. If this is not done, cold spots will be encountered, with resultant unequal pressure on the tissues. To further ensure a uniform depth of softened wax for making the record, the occlusal portion is dipped in water of 135° F (57° C) for a few seconds, and the depth of heat penetration is tested with an instrument. The wax should be softened throughout; if it is not, the dipping should be repeated (Fig. 18-6).

If stretching of the lips in placement of the mandibular trial base does not dislodge the maxillary trial base, the maxillary trial base is inserted first, and then the mandibular trial den-

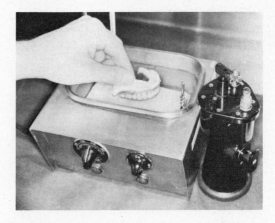

Fig. 18-6. Surface of baseplate wax given a final softening in water of 135° F (57° C).

ture is seated in position. Using the same hand position as described previously, the dentist instructs the patient to pull the lower jaw back and close the back teeth until requested to stop. This occlusal pressure should not be great enough to force the maxillary teeth through the wax to contact with any point of the opposing teeth. If patients do not respond to one method of retruding the mandible, they may respond to another. The various methods that may be employed have already been discussed. A minimum amount of occlusal pressure should be exerted on the wax by the patient. The patient

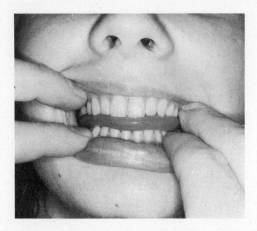

Fig. 18-7. Patient closing in most retruded position to determine accuracy of present mounting. Notice modified hand position and exaggerated bulk of wax used for photographic purposes.

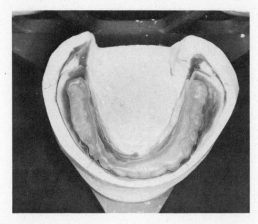

Fig. 18-8. Resultant indentations in wax for centric relation recheck. Notice that no tooth contact is made by opposing teeth.

maintains occlusal contact with the wax while it is chilling (Fig. 18-7). Chilling of the wax may be hastened by squirting a small amount of cold water into the mouth onto the wax, or a cotton roll dipped in ice water may be placed against the wax to aid in the chilling instead of the syringe being used. Both trial bases are removed from the mouth and chilled. The occlusal wax indentations and the opposing teeth are dried, and the indentations are examined carefully (Fig. 18-8).

The dentist may prefer to vary the technique just described by placing a double layer of soft wax (e.g., beeswax) over the posterior teeth only. Some clinicians maintain that this technique enables them to achieve better control of the patient's mandible (Fig. 18-9).

The wax record should show that there are indentations of all the opposing posterior teeth in the wax. No opposing maxillary tooth should penetrate the wax to strike the occlusal surface of any mandibular tooth. No imprints of maxillary anterior teeth should be seen in the wax. If this were to occur, it would be likely to result in deflective occlusal contact, with its resultant evils—shifting of the bases or a change in the

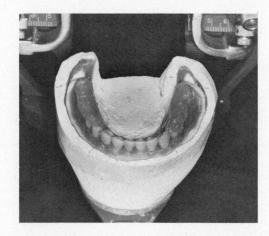

Fig. 18-9. Identical technique to that described in previous figure, except that anterior teeth are not covered with wax.

maxillomandibular relation, both horizontally and vertically. This first record is made to level the wax to the occlusal surfaces of the teeth so that the excess can be trimmed to give an even depth of wax throughout. This surface is again dipped in hot water of 135° F, and a new centric relation record is made in the mouth. The objective is to obtain shallow indentations made by all

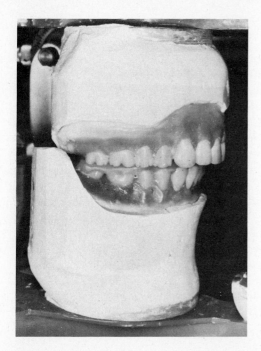

Fig. 18-10. Testing wax centric relation record to determine whether record from mouth coincides with centric relation record on articulator.

the teeth in the arch. Care must be taken that the patient does not close far enough to make any contact between the teeth. After the wax has been chilled, the trial dentures are placed on their casts, and the articulator is closed in centric relation into these indentations to see if the opposing teeth fit into the indentations in every way, that is, anteroposteriorly, laterally, and vertically (Fig. 18-10). It is surprising to what degree of exactness these teeth do fit into the indentations if the original centric interocclusal record and the check are both correct.

If the opposing teeth do not fit exactly into the indentations in the new record, it means that the original mounting was incorrect or that the patient gave an incorrect relation when making this interocclusal record. Therefore the surface of the wax record is again flamed, dipped into hot water, and reinserted into the mouth; and another attempt is made to get the mandible into its most retruded position while the patient closes into the wax. Again this record is tested on the articulator. If the relation on the articu-

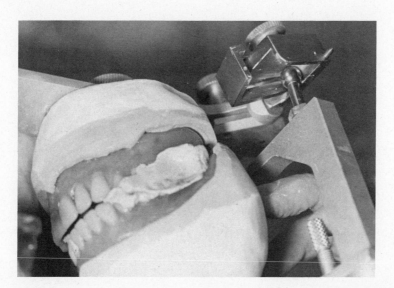

Fig. 18-11. Plaster interocclusal centric relation record is used to test accuracy of preliminary centric relation mounting on articulator. Location of condylar sphere in contact with posterior, lateral, and superior elements of condylar housing indicates that preliminary record and test record are clinically identical. Thus casts on articulator are assumed to be mounted in centric relation.

lator and the new record coincide, the mounting is considered correct. If the mounting does not check, the procedure in the mouth is repeated and tested on the articulator again. If the mounting does not check at this time, the mandibular cast should be separated from the mounting ring, and the cast should be remounted by means of the last interocclusal wax record. The new mounting is again checked in the same manner to prove or disprove its correctness.

It should be noted that intraoral records of maxillomandibular relations made in wax require more closing pressure by the patient than records made in soft plaster require. Consequently, the contacts of teeth will be more nearly uniform when heavy pressure is exerted, whereas records made in soft plaster will be more uniform at first tooth contact. Uniformity of contact at the first contact without pressure is less damaging to the tissues of the basal seat because the dentures do not have to displace any tissue for the teeth to meet evenly. When the denture bases must displace basal seat tissues to establish uniformity of tooth contact, the tissues subjected to this displacement are subject to trauma. Ultimately this leads to soreness or to loss of bone from the residual ridges.

When the initial registration (preliminary centric relation record) was made in plaster or a bite registration paste, the same recording medium should be used to verify the accuracy of the mounting on the articulator. Likewise, if wax was used, it should be the verifying medium. However, it is easier to distort wax when the record is removed from the mouth and tested on the articulator (Fig. 18-11).

19

Creating facial and functional harmony with anterior teeth

The anatomic structures that collectively form the face normally develop concurrently and are interdependent during function throughout life. Disruptive events in this homeostatic complex can range from relatively minor changes such as a deflective occlusal contact to major alterations in bodily form such as removal of the natural teeth, which drastically affects the form and function of the remaining living parts.

In this context of homeostasis, creating facial and functional harmony with anterior teeth becomes a biologic challenge of utmost significance. Not only must the teeth be the proper form, size, and color to harmonize with the face, but they must also become a functioning component in a living environment that depends on their proper position for its normal physiologic activity. This proper position allows patients to preserve their facial identity as it existed when natural teeth were present. The ability of patients to maintain their normal facial expression will likely be the most important psychologic factor in acceptance of the dentures.

ANATOMY OF NATURAL APPEARANCE AND FACIAL EXPRESSION

The dentist who is treating a patient with complete dentures has more to do with the beauty of the face than any other person. The appearance of the entire lower half of the face depends on the denture. It is usually not diffi-

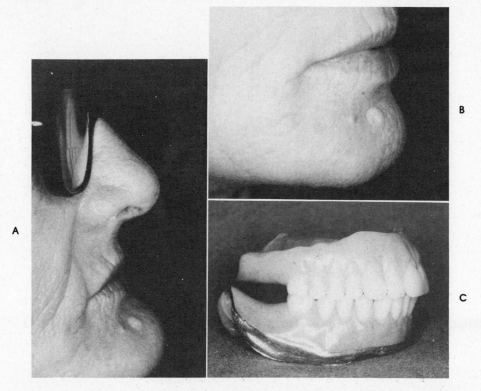

Fig. 19-1. A, Lower part of face lacks proper contour because of inadequate support for orbicularis oris muscle and muscles related to it. **B,** Facial contours have been properly restored. The tremendous improvement in appearance of patient is directly related to position of artificial teeth and form of supporting base material of the complete dentures, **C.**

cult on casual meeting to detect the person who is wearing poorly constructed dentures (Fig. 19-1). The characteristic thin, drooping upper lip that appears lengthened and has a reduced vermilion border is typical of malpositioned anterior teeth and probably a reduced vertical relation of occlusion. Tense, wrinkled lips often reveal the patient's efforts to hold the denture in place. The drooping corners of the mouth tell the story of the misshapen and misplaced dental arch form of anterior teeth, the thin denture borders, and often the reduced occlusal vertical dimension. The appearance of premature aging may not be caused by age itself but by the lack of support for the lips and cheeks because of the loss of teeth or their improper replacement. The

apparent extra fullness of the lower lip may be the result of too broad a mandibular dental arch or the elimination or reduction of the mentolabial sulcus. This may indicate that the lower anterior teeth have been placed too far lingually or that the labial flange of the lower denture base is overextended or too thick.

Normal facial landmarks

One must study normal facial landmarks before attempting to achieve the goal of natural and pleasing facial expression with complete dentures. The facial landmarks of the lower third of the face have a direct relationship to the presence of the natural teeth (Fig. 19-2). The contours of the lips depend on their intrinsic

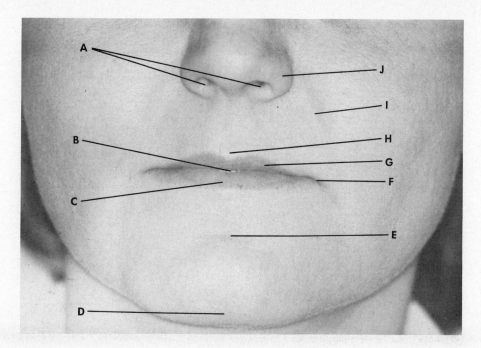

Fig. 19-2. Facial landmarks. *A*, Nares; *B*, rima oris; *C*, lower lip; *D*, mentum; *E*, mentolabial sulcus; *F*, angulus oris; *G*, upper lip; *H*, philtrum; *I*, nasolabial sulcus; *J*, ala nasi.

structure and the support for them provided by the teeth and the soft tissues or denture bases behind them. When the natural teeth are lost, these landmarks and surrounding facial tissues become distorted. To reestablish normal appearance and function, artificial teeth must be replaced in the same position as the natural teeth that were lost.

The lips vary in length, thickness, shape, and mobility in different patients. Such variance accounts for the degree of visibility of the upper and lower anterior teeth during speech and other facial expressions. When the mandible is in the resting position, the lips usually contact each other and turn slightly outward, exposing the vermilion border. The vertical groove in the middle of the upper lip is called the philtrum, and the horizontal groove midway between the vermilion border and the inferior border of the chin in the lower lip is called the mentolabial sulcus, or groove. Incorrect positioning of the

anterior teeth or supporting base material of complete dentures will alter the normal appearance of the vermilion border, the philtrum, and the mentolabial sulcus in edentulous patients.

The nasolabial sulcus, or groove, is a depression in the skin on either side of the face, which runs angularly outward from the ala of the nose to approximately just outside the level of the rima oris (Fig. 19-2). The zygomatic muscle has its origin on the zygomatic bone and angles downward and forward to be inserted at the corner of the mouth into the orbicularis oris muscle. The actions of the zygomatic muscle in elevating the corner of the mouth in smiling or laughing produce the nasolabial sulcus (Fig. 19-3). Many older patients want to have the nasolabial sulcus obliterated because the sulcus becomes a wrinkle as the skin loses its resilience. Removal of the fold has been attempted by thickening the denture base under the nasolabial fold, but the extra bulk in this location

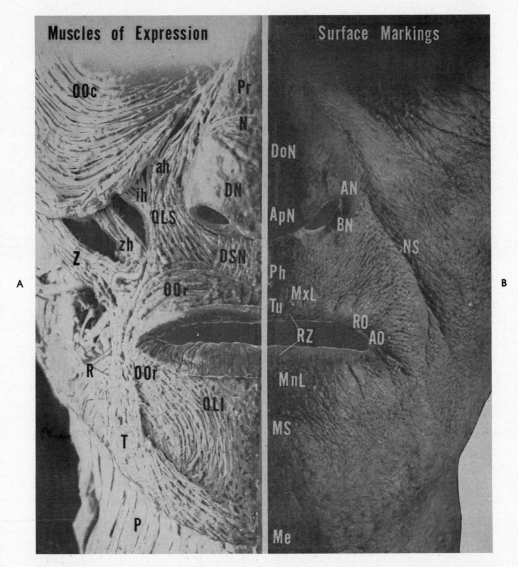

Fig. 19-3. Frontal view of the polyfunctional pyramid. **A,** Underlying superficial musculature. *OOc,* Orbicularis oculi; *Pr,* procerus; *N,* nasalis; *QLS,* quadratus labii superioris; *ah,* angular head; *ih,* infraorbital head; *zh,* zygomatic head; *DN,* dilator naris; *DSN,* depressor septi nasi; *Z,* zygomaticus; *R,* risorius; *OOr,* orbicularis oris; *T,* triangularis; *QLI,* quadratus labii inferioris; *P,* platysma. **B,** Surface anatomy. *DoN,* Dorsum nasi; *AN,* ala nasi; *ApN,* apex nasi; *BN,* basis nasi; *NS,* nasolabial sulcus; *Ph,* philtrum; *MxL,* maxillary lip; *Tu,* tubercle; *RO,* rima oris; *AO,* angulus oris; *RZ,* red zone or vermilion border; *MnL,* mandibular lip; *MS,* mentolabial sulcus; *Me,* mentum. (From Martone, A.L., and Edwards, L.F.: J. Prosthet. Dent. **11:**1010, 1961.)

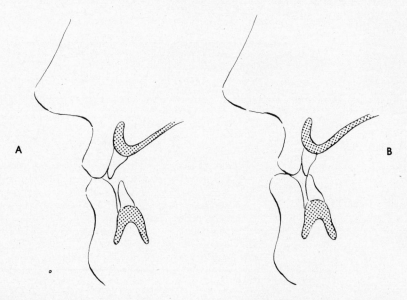

Fig. 19-4. A, Reproduction of patient's former horizontal overlap with proper facial contour. **B,** Horizontal overlap changed so that maxillary anterior teeth contact mandibular teeth with resultant damage to upper lip.

causes a very unnatural appearance. The sulcus is normal and should not be eliminated. The proper treatment is to bring the entire upper dental arch forward to its original position when the natural teeth were present and to maintain the original arch form of the natural teeth and their supporting structures. Thus the prominence of the nasolabial sulcus will be restored to its original contour.

In many patients the corners of the lip line (rima oris) will be as high as the center portion, but the lip line will not necessarily be straight all the way across.

The upper lip rests on the labial surfaces of the upper anterior teeth, and the lower lip rests on the labial surfaces of the lower anterior teeth and the incisal edges of the upper teeth. For this reason, the edge of the lower lip should extend outward and upward from the mentolabial sulcus. A reproduction of the horizontal overlap of the natural anterior teeth in the denture is essential to maintain proper contour of the lips (Fig. 19-4).

A study of the inclination of the osseous structure supporting the lower anterior teeth indicates that, in most patients, the clinical crowns of the lower teeth are labial to the bone that supports them. Likewise, a study of the inclination of osseous structure and the inclination of maxillary anterior teeth reveals that the upper lip functions on an incline (see Fig. 19-5). The neglect of these factors in the replacement of the natural teeth often causes the lip to be ill-formed and in time will cause vertical lines to form in the lip.

Maintaining facial support and neuromuscular balance

The orbicularis oris and its attaching muscles are important in denture construction inasmuch as the various contributing muscles have bony origins and their insertions are into the modiolus and orbicularis oris at the corner of the mouth (Fig. 19-6, A). Thus the functioning length of all these muscles depends on the function of the orbicularis oris muscle. The muscles that merge

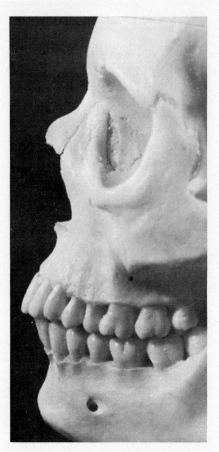

Fig. 19-5. Incisal edges and labial surfaces of lower anterior teeth are labial to bone supporting them. Inclination of labial plate of bone and labial surfaces of upper anterior teeth causes upper lip to function on an incline. It is easy to observe lack of support of lip that would result when artificial anterior teeth are positioned over crest of residual ridges. Resorption of the alveolar process in the mandibular anterior region after removal of the anterior teeth would move the residual bony ridge lingually at first and then labially as resorption continued.

into the orbicularis oris are the zygomatic, the quadratus labii superior, the caninus (levator anguli oris), the mentalis, the quadratus labii inferior, the triangularis (depressor anguli oris), the buccinator, and the risorius.

The orbicularis oris is the muscle of the lips. It is a sphincterlike muscle that is attached to the maxillae along the median line under the nose by means of a band of fibrous connective tissue known as the maxillary labial frenum and to the mandible on the median line by means of the mandibular labial frenum.

The buccinator muscle is a broad band of muscle forming the entire side wall of the cheek from the corner of the mouth and passing along the outer surface of the maxillae and mandible until it reaches the ramus, where it passes to the lingual surface to join the superior constrictor of the pharynx at the pterygomandibular raphe (Fig. 19-6, *B*). The two buccinator muscles and the orbicularis oris form a functional unit that depends on the position of the dental arches and the labial contours of the mucosa or the denture base for effective action.

With the loss of the teeth, the function of the orbicularis oris, buccinator, and attaching muscles are impaired. Since these muscles of expression are no longer supported at their physiologic length, contraction of the unsupported muscle fibers will not produce normal facial expression because the lips and face will not move naturally or may not move at all. The contraction simply takes up the droop in the muscle fiber itself. However, when this muscle

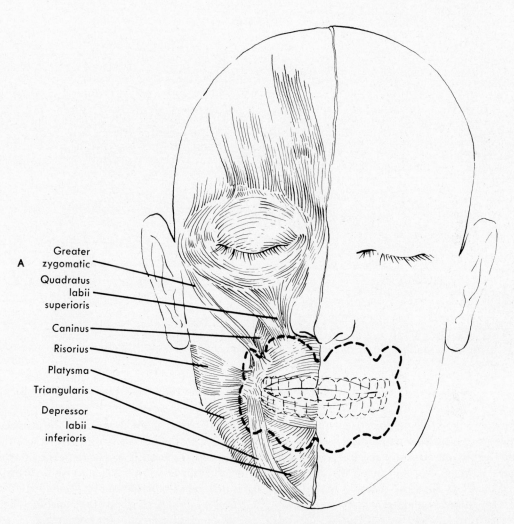

Greater
zygomatic

A

Quadratus
labii
superioris

Caninus

Risorius

Platysma

Triangularis

Depressor
labii
inferioris

Fig. 19-6. Muscles that maintain facial support. When artificial teeth and denture base material restore lips to their proper contour, the facial muscles will be at correct physiologic length and their contraction will cause normal facial expression of patient. **A,** Facial muscles as indicated.

Continued.

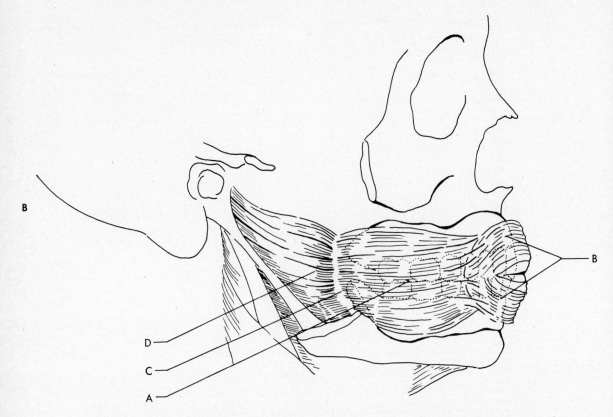

Fig. 19-6 cont'd. B, Functional unit of buccinator muscles, *A,* and orbicularis oris muscle, *B,* depends on position of upper denture for proper action. *C,* Pterygomandibular raphe. *D,* Superior constrictor muscle.

complex is correctly supported by complete dentures, impulses coming to the muscles from the central nervous system cause a shortening of the muscle fibers that will move the face in a normal manner. Thus the memory patterns of facial expression developed within the neuromuscular system when the patient had natural teeth will be continued or reinforced so that the patient's original appearance can be maintained (Fig. 19-7).

Three factors affect the face in the repositioning of the orbicularis oris with complete dentures: (1) the thickness of the labial flanges of both dentures, (2) the anteroposterior position of the anterior teeth, and (3) the amount of sep-

aration between the mandible and the maxillae (Fig. 19-8). If the jaws are closed too far and the dental arch is located too far posteriorly, the upward and backward positioning of the orbicularis oris muscle complex moves the insertion of all these muscles closer to their origins. This condition causes the muscles to sag when at rest and to be less effective when they contract. Such positions automatically drop the corners of the mouth, with the resultant senile edentulous expression, and may result in atrophy of the muscle fibers.

The proper width of the maxillary denture borders plays a great part in supporting the muscles and lengthening the distance that these

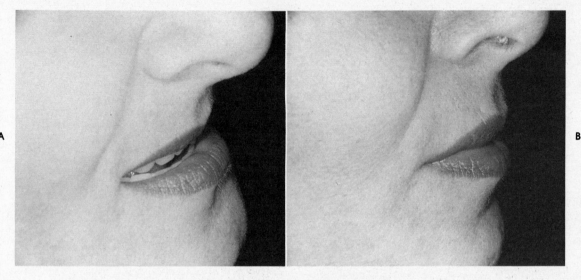

Fig. 19-7. A, Lips are improperly contoured and are not moving naturally during speech. The lack of facial expression results from inadequate support of the lips by the anterior teeth, improper thickness of the labial flanges, and an inadequate vertical relation of occlusion. **B,** Lips are restored to proper contour with new dentures.

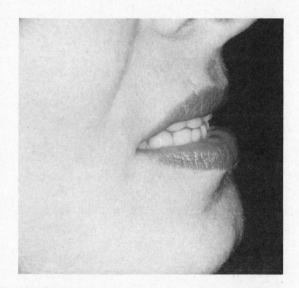

Fig. 19-8. Note activity of lips during speech when they are properly supported by new dentures. Compare with lack of activity in same patient in Fig. 19-7, A.

muscles must extend to reach their insertion. If the mouth has been edentulous a long time with considerable resorption of the residual ridges, the borders need to be thick to restore the position of these muscles (Fig. 19-9).

The advisability of repositioning protruding or slightly protruding anterior teeth to reduce their horizontal overlap and improve the appearance of patients is a serious mistake (Fig. 19-10). The muscles, teeth, and all associated structures grew simultaneously, and therefore the physiologic length of the muscles has been determined. In fact, the muscles of the face, cheeks, tongue, and lips helped to align the natural teeth in the dental arches. To move teeth back in dentures is to entail a loss of facial expression that may be more damaging to the appearance of the patient than the slightly protruding teeth. Individual pronounced irregularities may be improved, provided that the position of the dental arch in its support of the orbic-

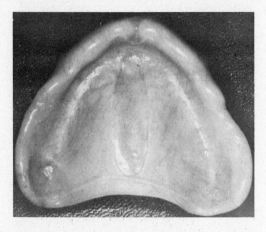

Fig. 19-9. Labial flange is thick at the borders. This thickness of the labial flange is in harmony with available space in patient's mouth because of resorption of upper residual ridge and is needed for proper support of upper lip.

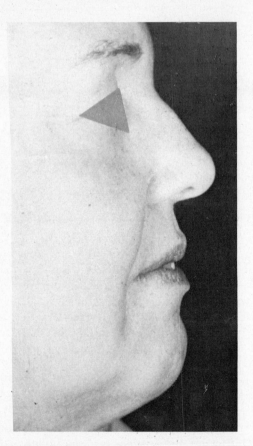

Fig. 19-10. Natural anterior teeth provide support for orbicularis oris muscle. The artificial anterior teeth must be in this same anteroposterior position to maintain proper length of muscle fibers.

ularis oris and its attaching muscles is not perceptibly altered.

Thus normal facial expression and proper tone of the skin of the face depend on the position and function of facial muscles. These muscles can function physiologically only when the dentist has positioned and shaped the dental arches correctly and has given the mandible a favorable vertical position. In addition, the dentures themselves must be pleasing and natural in appearance in the patient's mouth, a condition that is dependent on arrangement of the artificial teeth in a plan that simulates nature. This, then, is the challenge of creating facial and functional harmony with anterior teeth.

BASIC GUIDES TO DEVELOP FACIAL AND FUNCTIONAL HARMONY

After an acceptable vertical relation of occlusion has been determined and the horizontal relation of the casts on the articulator has been verified for centric relation, the appearance of the patient is studied, and modifications are made in the arrangement of the teeth to obtain a harmonious effect with the patient's face. The guides that are considered in developing facial and functional harmony include (1) evaluation of the preliminary selection of the artificial teeth, (2) the horizontal orientation of the anterior teeth, (3) the vertical orientation of the anterior

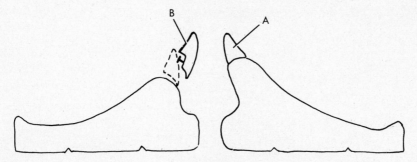

Fig. 19-11. *Right,* Cast representing original position of natural central incisor, *A. Left,* Cast showing artificial tooth, *B,* in correct position to restore the physiologic length of muscles for proper function. Tooth *(dotted line)* is incorrectly positioned when set to follow residual ridge.

teeth, (4) phonetics in orientation of anterior teeth, (5) the inclination of the anterior teeth, (6) harmony in the general composition of the anterior teeth, (7) refinement of individual tooth positions, (8) the concept of harmony with sex, personality, and age of the patient, and (9) correlation of esthetics and incisal guidance. Although these factors will be discussed individually for simplicity, they are interrelated in the actual clinical situation.

Evaluating the preliminary selection of artificial teeth

The preliminary selection of teeth must be critically evaluated for size, form, and color. The six upper anterior teeth, when properly supporting the upper lip, should be of sufficient overall width to extend in the dental arch to approximately the position of the corners of the mouth and still allow for individual irregularities of rotation, overlapping, and spacing. The canines should extend distally so that they can be the turning point in the dental arch. The form of the teeth should be harmonious with the face but not necessarily identical with the outline form of the face. The color of the teeth should blend with the face so that the teeth do not become the main focal point of the face. The anterior teeth are the principal ones to be considered in esthetics, though the posterior teeth,

involving height of plane and width of arch, play their part also. The dentist must make changes in the selection of teeth at this time if such changes will improve the appearance of the dentures.

Guides to horizontal orientation of the anterior teeth

The position and expression of the lips and the lower part of the face are the best guides for determining the proper anteroposterior orientation of anterior teeth. The other guides or measurements are secondary and must be ultimately related to the appearance of the patient.

The greatest harm done in esthetics is setting the maxillary anterior teeth back to or under the ridge, regardless of the amount of resorption that has taken place. A study of the anterior alveolar process discloses that its direction is upward and backward from the labial surface of the maxillary incisors (Fig. 19-5). Therefore, the crest of the upper ridge is considerably more posterior in a resorbed ridge than it was when the teeth were recently removed (Fig. 19-11).

Insufficient support of the lips resulting from anterior teeth that are located too far posteriorly is characterized by a drooping or turning down of the corners of the mouth, a reduction in the visible part of the vermilion border, a drooping and deepening of the nasolabial grooves, small

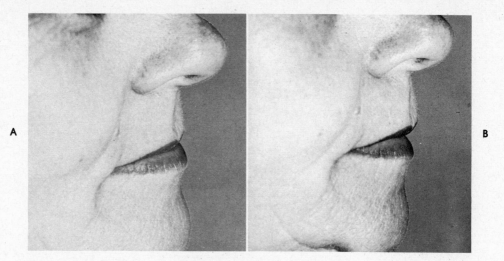

Fig. 19-12. A, Artificial anterior teeth are positioned too far posteriorly. Notice lack of tone in skin of upper lip. **B,** Artificial anterior teeth are positioned properly in an anteroposterior direction. Notice improved tone in skin of upper lip.

vertical lines or wrinkles above the vermilion borders of the lip, a deepening of the sulci, and a reduction in the prominence of the philtrum (Fig. 19-7, A).

A striking difference occurs when the anterior teeth are in the proper position (Fig. 19-12). The vermilion borders of the lip become visible, the corners of the mouth assume a normal contour, many of the small vertical lines above the vermilion border of the upper lip can be reduced or eliminated, and the tone of the skin surrounding the dentures will be similar in texture to that of the skin in other parts of the face that are not affected by position of the teeth. Although the nasolabial groove will still be present, the drooping appearance can often be considerably reduced. Nasolabial grooves should not be eliminated, and the dentist must be careful about what is told the patient in this regard. However, patients should be informed about the other improvements that can be made by the dentures which will produce a more youthful appearance.

Excessive lip support resulting from anterior teeth that are located too far anteriorly is characterized by a stretched, tight appearance of the lips, a tendency for the lips to dislodge the dentures during function, an elimination of the normal contours of the lips, and distortion of the philtrum and sulci (Fig. 19-13). A photograph of the patient with natural teeth can be most helpful in the placing of artificial teeth. The teeth can be arranged so that the appearance and contours of the lips and lower part of the face resemble that seen in the picture.

The relation of the maxillary and mandibular anterior ridge to each other has an influence on the anteroposterior position of both the maxillary and the mandibular anterior teeth. A common error is an attempt to establish a standard vertical and horizontal overlap without regard to the ridge relation. This procedure is incorrect because the anteroposterior position of the teeth must correspond to the positions of the ridges. If the mandibular ridge is forward of the maxillary ridge, as in prognathic patients, the upper anterior teeth should not be placed labial to the mandibular teeth. The anterior teeth can be set end to end, with the incisal edges at an angle that produces a seating action on the maxillary denture (Fig. 19-14).

A study of the position of natural teeth on

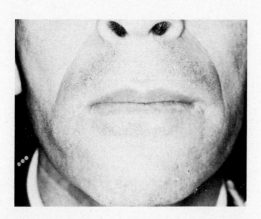

Fig. 19-13. Stretched appearance of lips and philtrum indicates that artificial anterior teeth are positioned too far anteriorly.

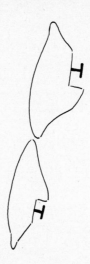

Fig. 19-14. Diagram showing correct inclination of teeth and incisal edges in moderate prognathic relations.

diagnostic casts can provide information that can be transferred to arrangement of artificial anterior teeth. As mentioned previously, the upper lip functions on an incline produced by the labial plate of the alveolar process and the crowns of the upper anterior teeth. The position of the natural anterior teeth makes their labial surfaces at least as far forward as the labialmost part of the reflection (Fig. 19-15, *A*). This information can be transferred to the position of the artificial anterior teeth on the trial denture base. Such a guide is also helpful in contouring of occlusion rims (Fig. 19-15, *B*) and in development of the preliminary arrangement of anterior teeth.

Observations of the position of the anterior teeth when the trial denture base is out of the mouth can be of assistance. The labial surfaces of many natural upper central incisors are approximately 8 to 10 mm in front of the middle of the incisive papilla. Measurements made with a Boley gage from the middle of the incisive fossa on the trial denture base to the labial surfaces of the artificial central incisors will reveal the relationship of these teeth to the incisive papilla (Fig. 19-16, *A*).

When the trial denture bases are viewed from

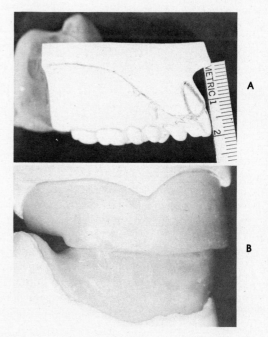

Fig. 19-15. A, Relation of labial surface of natural central incisor to reflection in this sectioned cast. **B,** Inclination of labial surfaces of wax occlusion rims should simulate that of natural situation seen in **A.** When occlusion rims slope lingually toward occlusal surface in anterior region, they will rarely, if ever, provide proper support for patient's lips.

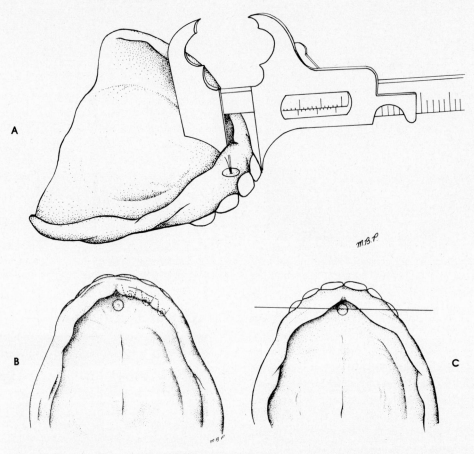

Fig. 19-16. Indications of correct anteroposterior position of artificial anterior teeth. **A,** By measurement from middle of incisive fossa on trial denture base to labial surface of central incisors. **B,** By visualization of imaginary roots of artificial anterior teeth. Imaginary roots will appear to be further in front of residual ridge when a great amount of resorption has occurred. **C,** By determining relationship of a transverse line extending between middle of upper canines to incisive fossa.

the basal surface, the labial surfaces of the anterior teeth should be apparent, and a visualization of their imaginary roots can be helpful. If the imaginary roots appear to be on the labial side of the residual ridge (making allowance for the bone loss from that part of the ridge), the anterior teeth will be very near to their correct labiolingual positions. If the imaginary roots appear to extend into the crest of the residual ridge, the artificial teeth are positioned too far posteriorly on the trial denture base (Fig. 19-16, B). The location of the incisive fossa in relation to the crest of the ridge gives an indication of the amount of resorption of the upper residual ridge. The greater the amount of resorption, the farther in front of the crest of the ridge the imaginary roots should appear.

An imaginary transverse line extended between the upper canines, as viewed from the basal surface of the upper trial denture base, should cross close to the middle of the incisive fossa when anterior teeth of the proper size are

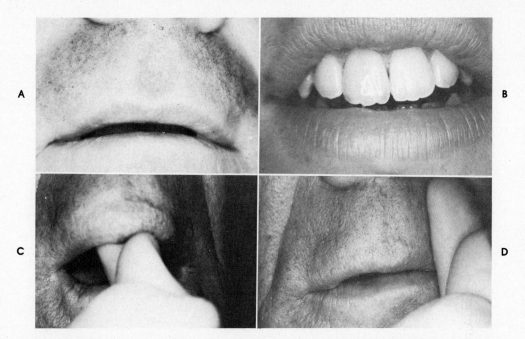

Fig. 19-17. A, Long upper lip obscures natural upper anterior teeth from view even during most speech. **B,** Relatively short upper lip exposes almost all the full crowns of upper central and lateral incisors. **C,** Upper lip is allowed to drape over index finger, which has been placed on incisive papilla. Thumb is in contact with vermilion border of upper lip. **D,** Amount of index finger that has been covered by upper lip is an indication of relative length of upper lip in relation to upper residual ridge.

located correctly in the anteroposterior position (Fig. 19-16, *C*). When the line falls anterior to the incisve fossa, the overall width of the anterior teeth may be too small, or the teeth may be positioned too far forward. When the line falls posterior to the incisive papilla, the overall width of the anterior teeth may be too large, or the teeth may be positioned too far back.

The use of phonetics in determining the horizontal orientation of the anterior teeth is discussed in a separate section of this chapter.

Guides to vertical orientation of the anterior teeth

The amount of the upper anterior teeth that will be seen during speech and facial expression depends on the length and movement of the upper lip in relation to the vertical length of the

dental arch. If the upper lip is relatively long, the natural teeth may not be visible when the lip is relaxed or even during speech (Fig. 19-17, *A*). In this situation, however, some teeth may be exposed when the person smiles. In other patients with relatively short upper lips, the full crown may be visible below the upper lip (Fig. 19-17, *B*). In some of these patients, a large amount of the mucous membrane (denture base) in addition to the teeth may be exposed when they smile.

In addition, the movement of the lips during function varies considerably among patients. Thus, when artificial teeth are placed in the same position as the natural teeth, the amount of the upper teeth that will be visible varies for each patient.

During a normal smile, the incisal and middle

third of maxillary anterior teeth are visible in almost all patients, and the cervical third in approximately half the patients. The incisal third of mandibular anterior teeth will be visible in most patients. Mandibular anterior teeth are seen to a greater extent than maxillary anterior teeth in about half the patients during speaking. In addition, mandibular anterior teeth increase in visibility in persons 40 years of age and older and are seen to a greater extent in men than in women.

A simple test can be used to estimate the length of the upper lip in relation to the residual ridges. The index finger is placed on the incisive papilla with the relaxed upper lip extending down over the finger (Fig. 19-17, *C*). The amount of the finger that is covered by the upper lip gives an indication of the length of the lip in relation to the residual ridge and the extent to which it will cover the upper anterior teeth (Fig. 19-17, *D*). An estimation of the amount of resorption of the residual ridge must be included in the mental calculation. Knowledge of the length of time the natural teeth have been out will help in making this estimate.

The lower lip is a better guide for the vertical orientation of the anterior teeth than the upper lip. In most patients, the incisal edges of the natural lower canines and the cusp tips of the lower first premolars are located at the level of the lower lip at the corner of the mouth when the mouth is slightly open (Fig. 19-18, *A*). Should the artificial lower anterior teeth be located above or below this level, then the vertical positioning of the teeth is probably incorrect (Fig. 19-18, *B*). In addition to any changes in the position of the lower teeth, the position of the upper teeth and the vertical relation of occlusion must also be considered because these factors are all closely interrelated. When the lower teeth are above the lip at the corner of the mouth, any one or a combination of the following conditions may exist: (1) the plane of occlusion may be too high, (2) the vertical overlap of the anterior teeth may be excessive, or (3) the vertical space between the jaws may be excessive. When the lower teeth are below the lip at the corner of the mouth, the opposite situations must be considered. The use of other observations and guides will help in deciding what corrections should be made.

Observations of the size of the trial denture bases can give clues to the vertical orientation of the anterior teeth. In most patients, the lower and upper natural teeth occupy approximately the same amount of the interarch space. Should the dimensions of the lower trial denture from the border of the base to the incisal edges of the teeth appear to be significantly different from the same measurement on the upper trial denture, then the plane of occlusion may need to be raised or lowered to make the trial dentures more similar in height (Fig. 19-19). These measurements are made from incisal edges to the denture borders. The vertical space between the jaws (vertical relation of occlusion) must also be considered because of its close interrelationship with the plane of occlusion. If there has been much more shrinkage from one jaw than from the other, the amounts of base material between the incisal end of the teeth and the basal surface of the denture will be quite different, even though the overall dimensions are similar.

A study of the location of the artificial anterior teeth and their imaginary roots in relation to the residual ridges on the trial denture bases can be of assistance in determining the position of the teeth. The artificial anterior teeth should be located vertically in the same positions as those previously occupied by the natural teeth. When it appears as though there is not sufficient interarch space to accommodate the upper and lower anterior teeth without significantly reducing their size by grinding, it is well to remember that at one time there was space for the natural teeth with an adequate interocclusal distance in the patient's mouth. Insufficient space between the residual ridges is an indication that either the artificial teeth are longer than the natural teeth or the vertical dimension of the face is too short.

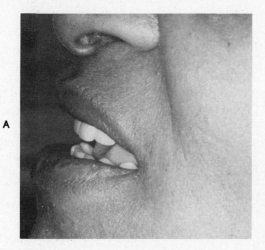

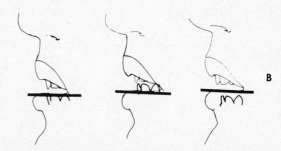

Fig. 19-18. A, Incisal edge of natural lower canine is located at level of lower lip at the corner of the mouth. **B,** Drawings showing artificial teeth in relation to lower lip. *Left,* Artificial teeth at the proper height; *middle,* lower artificial teeth are too high; *right,* artificial teeth are too low.

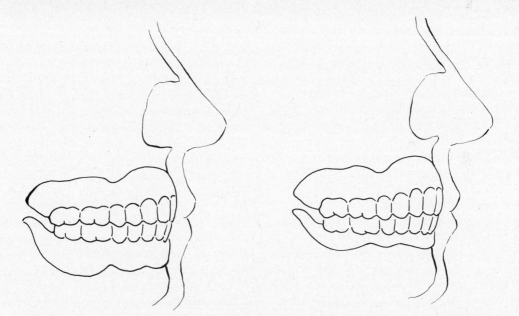

Fig. 19-19. *Left,* Upper and lower dentures appear to be approximately similar in height. *Right,* Upper denture is considerably larger in height than lower denture. Often this discrepancy in size between dentures indicates an incorrect vertical position of the artificial teeth.

Phonetics in orientation of anterior teeth

Phonetics, the production of speech sounds, can be used as a guide to the positions of teeth. To do this, however, it is necessary to know how the various speech sounds are made. Anterior tooth position is critical in the production of some sounds and not at all important in others.

As teeth are arranged for esthetics, it is not the speech sound itself that is critical. Instead it is the relationships of the tongue, teeth, denture base, and lips to each other. The sounds made by patients at the time of the try-in can never be as accurate as when hard denture base resin has been substituted for the trial bases and the patient has become accustomed to the dentures.

All speech sounds are made by controlled air. The source of the air is the lungs, and the amount and flow of the air is variable. The controls are the various articulations or "valves" made in the pharynx and the oral and nasal cavities. The structures involved in each valve constitute the basis for one classification of speech sounds. The valves used for modifying the flow of air to produce speech sounds include (1) the labial sounds, (2) the labiodental sounds, (3) the dental and alveolar (anterior) sounds, (4) the palatal sounds, and (5) the velar (posterior) sounds. The first four of these groups of sounds can be affected by the position of the teeth.

A voice sound is one that is initiated in the vocal cords, such as vowels a, e, i, o, and u and the voiced consonants b, d, g, j, v, m, n, l, and r. The voice sounds may or may not be a part of the sounds produced by the action of the valves. This makes possible the production of at least two speech sounds at each of the valves. Some voice sounds, too, may be made without involving the use of the air valves. These are modified when one changes the resonance of the oral and nasal cavities. Changes in resonance can change the sounds produced by some of the air valves.

Labial sounds. The labial sounds b, p, and m are made at the lips. In b and p air pressure is built up behind the lips and released with or without a voice sound. Insufficient support of the lips by the teeth and denture base can cause these sounds to be defective. Therefore the anteroposterior position of the anterior teeth and thickness of the labial flanges of dentures can affect the sounds b and p.

Labiodental sounds. The labiodental sounds f and v are made between the upper incisors and the labiolingual center to the posterior one third of the lower lip. If the upper anterior teeth are too short (set too high up), the v sound will be more like an f sound. If they are too long (set too far down), the f sound will be more like a v sound (Fig. 19-20, A). However, the most important information to be sought while the patient makes these sounds is the relationship of the incisal edges to the lower lip.

The dentist should stand alongside the patient and look down at the lower lip and the upper anterior teeth. If the upper teeth touch the labial side of the lower lip while these sounds are made, the upper teeth are too far forward, or the lower anterior teeth are placed too far back in the mouth (Fig. 19-20, B). In this situation, the relationship of the inside of the lower lip to the labial surface of the teeth should be observed while the patient is speaking. If the lower lip drops away from the lower teeth during speech, the lower anterior teeth are most likely too far back in the mouth (Fig. 19-21, A). If, on the other hand, imprints of the labial surfaces of the lower anterior teeth are made in the mucous membrane of the lower lip or if the lower lip tends to raise the lower denture, the lower teeth are probably too far forward, and this means that the upper teeth also may be too far forward (Fig. 19-21, B).

If the upper anterior teeth are set too far back in the mouth, they will contact the lingual side of the lower lip when the f and v sounds are made. This may occur also if the lower anterior teeth are too far forward in relation to the lower residual ridge. The observation made from the side and slightly above the patient will provide the necessary information for determining which changes should be made (see Fig. 19-20, B).

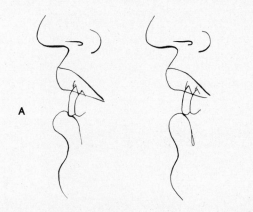

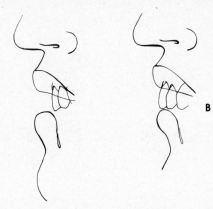

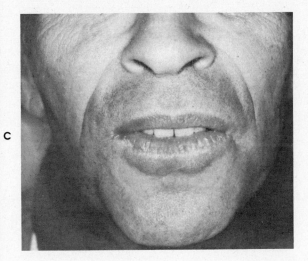

Fig. 19-20. Diagrams showing effects of tooth positioning on the sounds *f* and *v*. **A,** Upper artificial anterior teeth are too long, so that during the pronunciation of *f*, they contact the lower lip in a position similar to that producing the *v* sound. Hence the two may sound alike. **B,** Effects of anteroposterior position. *Left,* Teeth have been properly positioned. Notice that incisal edges contact posterior third of lower lip. *Middle,* Teeth have been positioned too far posteriorly. *Right,* Teeth have been positioned too far anteriorly. **C,** Incisal edges of central incisors contact the lower lip properly as the patient says, "fifty-five."

Fig. 19-21. Diagrammatic representations of effects of incorrect positioning of lower artificial anterior teeth. **A,** Teeth have been positioned too far posteriorly, so that a space develops between the lip and the teeth during pronunciation of words containing labiodental sounds. Arrow indicates that dentist observes this relationship by looking down at lower lip and anterior teeth. **B,** Lower artificial anterior teeth have been positioned too far anteriorly, so that the lower lip crowds into lower anterior teeth or may tend to raise the lower denture off the lower residual ridge during pronunciation of words containing labiodental sounds. The arrow indicates that dentist observes this relationship by looking down at the lower lip and anterior teeth.

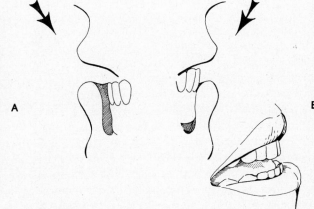

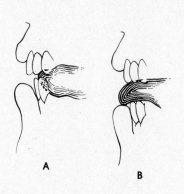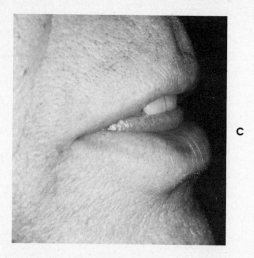

Fig. 19-22. Effects of vertical position of artificial anterior teeth on pronunciation of *th*. **A,** Tongue is prevented from extending properly between teeth. **B,** Tongue is extended between artificial anterior teeth when they are properly positioned. **C,** Note proper position of the tongue when this patient wearing complete dentures pronounced the word *thick.*

Dental and alveolar sounds. Dental sounds, such as *th* in *this*, are made with the tip of the tongue extending slightly between the upper and lower anterior teeth. This sound is actually closer to the alveolus (teeth ridge) than to the tip of the teeth. Careful observation of the amount of the tongue that can be seen with the words *this, that, these,* and *those* can provide information about the labiolingual position of the anterior teeth (Fig. 19-22). If about ⅛ inch (3 mm) of the tip of the tongue is not visible, the anterior teeth are probably too far forward (except in patients who had a Class II malocclusion), or there may be an excessive vertical overlap that does not allow sufficient space for the tongue to protrude between the anterior teeth. If more than ¼ inch (6 mm) of the tongue extends out between the teeth when such *th* sounds are made, the teeth are probably set too far lingually.

Other alveolar sounds, such as *t, d, n, s,* and *z,* are made with the valve being formed by the contact of the tip of the tongue with the anteriormost part of the palate called the alveolus or the lingual side of the anterior teeth. If the teeth are set too far lingually, the *t* in *tend* will sound

more like a *d*. If the anterior teeth are set too far anteriorly, the *d* sound will be more like a *t* sound. The palate of a denture base that is too thick in the area of the rugae could have the same effect.

The sibilants *s, z, sh, zh, ch,* and *j* (with *ch* and *j* being affricatives) are alveolar sounds because the tongue and alveolus form the controlling valve. The important observation to be made when these sounds are produced is the relationship of the anterior teeth to each other. The upper and lower incisors should approach each other end to end, but they should not touch. A phrase such as "I went to church to see the judge" will cause the patient to use these critical sounds. The relative position of the incisal edges when these sounds are made will provide a check on the total length of the upper and lower teeth (including their vertical overlap) (Figs. 19-23 and 19-24, *B*). More important, a failure of the incisal edges to approach each other exactly end to end will indicate a possible error in the amount of horizontal overlap of the anterior teeth (Fig. 19-24). This test will reveal the error, but it will not indicate whether it is

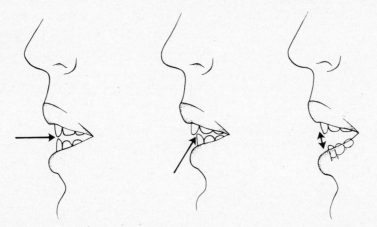

Fig. 19-23. Diagrams of vertical length of artificial anterior teeth during pronunciation of sibilants. *Left,* Proper vertical length. *Middle,* Anterior teeth are too long (excessive vertical overlap). *Right,* Anterior teeth are too short (inadequate vertical overlap).

the upper teeth or the lower teeth that are not in the correct labiolingual position.

The *s* sounds can be considered dental and alveolar speech sounds because they are produced equally well with two different tongue positions, but there can be some variation even behind the alveolus. Most people make the *s* sound with the tip of the tongue against the alveolus in the area of the rugae with a small space for the escape of air between the tongue and the alveolus. The size and shape of this small space will determine the quality of the sound. If the opening is too small, a whistle will result. If the space is too broad and thin, the *s* sound will be developed as an *sh* sound somewhat like a lisp. The frequent cause of undesired whistles with dentures is a posterior dental arch form that is too narrow.

A cramped tongue space, especially in the premolar region, forces the dorsal surface of the tongue to form too small an opening for the escape of air. The procedure for correction is to thicken the center of the palate so that the tongue does not have to extend up so far into the narrow palatal vault. This allows the escapeway for air to be broad and thin. A lisp with dentures can be corrected when the procedure is reversed and a narrow concentrated airway is provided for the *s* sound.

About one third of the people make the *s* sound with the tip of the tongue contacting the lingual side of the anterior part of the lower denture and arching itself up against the palate to form the desired shape and size of airway. The principles involved in such a palatal valve are identical to those involved in the other tongue position. However, the lower denture can cause trouble. If the lower anterior teeth are too far back, the tongue will be forced to arch itself up to a higher position, so that the airway would be too small and a whistle could result. If the lingual flange of the lower denture is too thick in the anterior region, the result will be a faulty *s* sound. It can be corrected when the artificial teeth are placed in the same position that the natural teeth occupied and the lingual flange of the lower dentures is shaped so that it does not encroach upon the space needed by the tongue.

Palatal and velar sounds. The truly palatal sounds, such as those in *year, she, vision,* and *onion,* present less of a problem for dentures. The velar sounds such as *k, g,* and *ng* have no effect on dentures.

Patient adaptation in phonetics. It is obvious that denture bases and the positions of teeth can affect the production of speech sounds, but fortunately people can learn to adapt their speaking

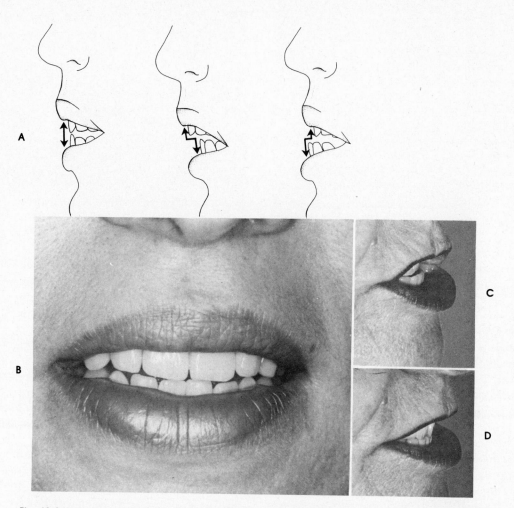

Fig. 19-24. Amount of horizontal overlap during pronunciation of sibilants. **A,** Proper amount of horizontal overlap *(left);* excessive horizontal overlap *(middle),* indicating that the upper teeth may be too far forward or the lower teeth too far back; insufficient horizontal overlap *(right),* indicating that the upper teeth may be too far back or the lower teeth are too far forward. **B,** Incisal edges of lower anterior teeth approach those of upper anterior teeth in an end-to-end relationship, indicating proper anteroposterior placement of teeth during pronunciation of sibilants. **C,** Lower anterior teeth have moved forward of the upper anterior teeth, indicating insufficient horizontal overlap. The lack of tone in the skin of upper lip and the small vertical lines above vermilion border indicate that upper anterior teeth do not properly support upper lip. **D,** Notice difference in appearance of upper lip and relationship of upper and lower anterior teeth during pronunciation of sibilants when teeth are in proper location.

habits to correct errors that may be caused by faulty tooth placement in dentures. For this reason, the sound of speech sounds is not a safe guide to tooth positions. The safe guide is the careful observation of the relationships of the lips and tongue to the teeth and the denture bases when certain sounds are made.

When these observations are made, the patient should be encouraged to speak normally without attempting to overcome any speech difficulty. When patients are aware of the dentist's real objective, they find it difficult to move the mouth normally. Dentists should watch the lips and tongue and pay minimal attention to the sounds of speech in order to get the most information about tooth position from phonetics.

Fortunately the relation of teeth and denture base surfaces and the retention of dentures to the production of sounds can be variable and yet not cause serious speech interferences. This variability is tolerated because the power of adaptability in phonetics is unusual. If it were not for this fact, it is doubtful if any patients wearing complete dentures would ever be able to articulate and enunciate properly. On the other hand, the more nearly duplicated the former conditions are in regard to the structures of the oral cavity, the better the speech of the denture patient will be. Functional contouring of the polished surface of the palate of the maxillary denture with mouth temperature wax is an example of simulating previous conditions that can improve the speech of the patient.

Inclination of anterior teeth

In some patients the upper anterior teeth are inclined labially in relation to the frontal plane when the head is erect (Frankfort plane parallel with the floor), whereas in other patients they are inclined more lingually (Fig. 19-25, A). Diagnostic casts, photographs, and what the patient remembers about the "slant of the upper front teeth" can help solve the problem concerning the inclination of the natural teeth.

A study of teeth in human skulls indicates that the roots of the anterior teeth are parallel to and

very close to the labial surface of the bone. Usually there is an obtuse angle between the bone and the labial surface of the teeth. In some skulls, the labial surface of the teeth is parallel to the bone, but also labialward to it. When the labial surface of the teeth is curved from cervical to incisal edge, the cervical one third of the tooth may appear to be continuous with the inclination of the labial plate of bone (Fig. 19-25, B). Diagnostic casts support this premise. When the natural teeth are removed with no unnecessary surgery, the original inclination of the labial plate of bone is preserved and will remain until considerable resorption has occurred, thus providing a guide to the inclination of the anterior teeth (Fig. 19-25, C). The inclination of the labial surface of the residual ridges as seen in edentulous casts can supply this information.

The profile form of the patient's face is often representative of the inclination of the anterior teeth that were found within the oral cavity. The lips supply the pressures from the outside that help determine the anteroposterior position and inclination of the anterior teeth. Thus it is logical to assume that the inclination of the anterior teeth parallels the profile line of the face (Fig. 19-26). Suggestions for individual tooth position to provide harmony between the inclination of the teeth and the profile line of the face is described later in this chapter (p. 403).

Harmony within the general composition of anterior teeth

A number of factors are interrelated in the general composition of the anterior teeth for a normal, pleasing appearance. Although these factors vary among patients, there is sufficient constancy to warrant individual attention. The topics that are discussed in providing harmony within the general composition of the anterior teeth include (1) harmony of arch form and form of the residual ridge, (2) harmony of long axes of the central incisors and the face, (3) harmony of the teeth with the smiling line of the lower lip, (4) harmony of opposing lines of labial and buccal surfaces, (5) harmony of teeth and profile

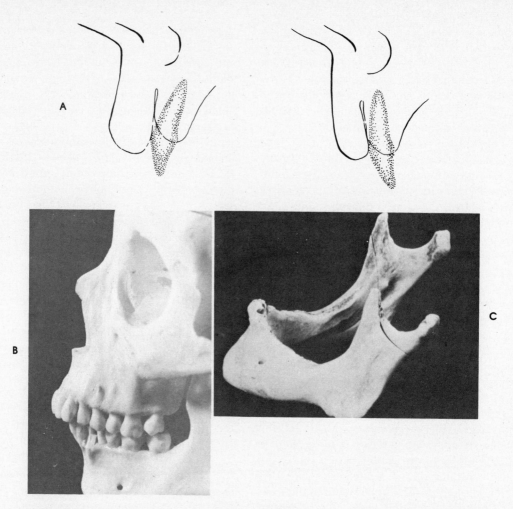

Fig. 19-25. Labial and lingual inclination of anterior teeth. **A,** Natural teeth have varying degrees of inclination. **B,** Notice inclination and position of the anterior teeth in relation to inclination of labial plate of bone. **C,** Inclination of this lower residual ridge provides information that lower anterior teeth, which it once supported, had a labial inclination.

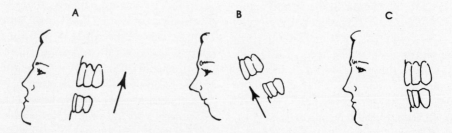

Fig. 19-26. Inclination of anterior teeth often parallels profile line of lower third of face.

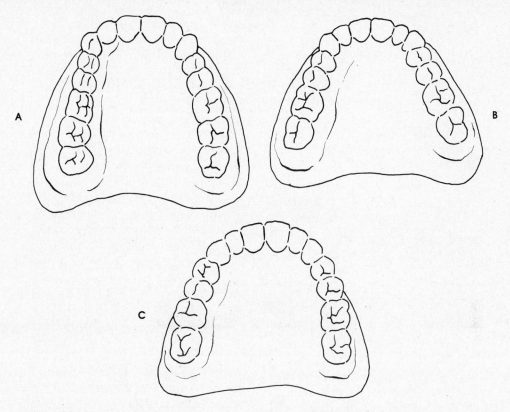

Fig. 19-27. Varying shapes of natural dental arches. **A,** Square arch; **B,** tapering arch; **C,** ovoid arch.

line, and (6) harmony of incisal wear and age.

Harmony of dental arch form and form of the residual ridge. The anterior arches may be classified in a general way as square, tapering, and ovoid, to follow the form of the dental arch when the teeth are present (Fig. 19-27). However, they cannot be closely classified as such because of the frequent intermingling of the characteristics of one form with another.

The central incisors in the square arch assume a position more nearly on a line with the canines than in any other setup. The four incisors have little rotation because these arches are wider than the tapering arch. This gives a broader effect to the teeth and should harmonize with a broad, square face (Fig. 19-28, *A*).

In the tapering arch, the central incisors are a greater distance forward from the canines than in any other arch. There is usually considerable rotating and lapping of the teeth in the tapering arch because there is less space in the arch. Therefore, crowding is the result. The rotated positions reduce the amount of tooth surface showing; therefore the teeth do not appear as wide as in other setups. This narrowed effect is usually in harmony with a narrower, tapering face (Fig. 19-28, *B*). In fact, the very narrowness of the tapered arch contributes to the narrowness and taper of the face. Natural teeth move in function, and this frictional movement wears the contact areas. Artificial teeth need to be ground on these corresponding contact areas to allow

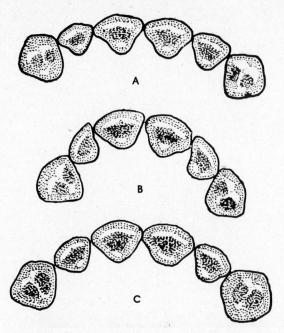

Fig. 19-28. A, Square anterior arch form; **B,** tapering anterior arch form; **C,** ovoid anterior arch form.

the necessary rotational positions and give the desired effect of a tapering setup.

The central incisors in the ovoid anterior arch are forward of the canines, in a position between that of the square and of the tapering arches. The teeth in this form of arch are seldom rotated. Therefore they show a greater amount of the labial surfaces than the tapering setup and, as a result, have a broader effect that should be in harmony with an ovoid face (Fig. 19-28, *C*).

The form of the palatal vault gives an indication of the original form of the dental arch before removal of the natural teeth and resorption of the residual ridge. A broad and shallow edentulous palatal vault indicates that the dental arch form originally may have been square; a high, V-shaped edentulous vault probably indicates a tapering dental arch; a rounded vault of average height may indicate an ovoid dental arch. Most patients exhibit some form of combination of these classifications.

The arch form of the artificial anterior teeth should be similar in shape to the arch form of the residual ridge, if one assumes there was no unnecessary surgery when the anterior teeth were removed (Fig. 19-29). This simple anatomic factor is often neglected and should be observed carefully. When the anterior teeth are arranged in an arch form that corresponds to the form of the residual ridge, often natural-appearing irregularities that may have been present in the patient's mouth will be reproduced.

Changing the shape and position of the artificial dental arch away from the form of the natural arch causes a loss in face form and expression that is highly unsatisfactory. A square arch form where the natural arch was more tapering will cause a stretching of the lips, with elimination of the natural philtrum. A tapering arch form of teeth where the natural dental arch was square will not adequately support the corners of the mouth for proper facial expressions.

The shape and position of the dental arch determines the size of the buccal corridor. The buccal corridor is the space between the buccal surfaces of the upper teeth and the corner of the mouth that is visible when the patient smiles. The space varies considerably among patients, and the size of the space is not critical. The presence of the buccal corridor helps eliminate an appearance of too many teeth in the front of the mouth. When the arch form of the posterior teeth is too wide or when the lips do not move to their full extent during smiling because of improper support, the size of the buccal corridor will be reduced or perhaps eliminated (Fig. 19-30).

Patients may request a change in the position or form of the dental arch. The dentist should not compromise with the patient on this point because the dentist will be blamed when unfavorable consequences result.

Harmony of the long axes of the central incisors and the face. One of the early observations that should be made in developing the arrangement of anterior teeth for the individual patient is the relationship of the long axes of the central inci-

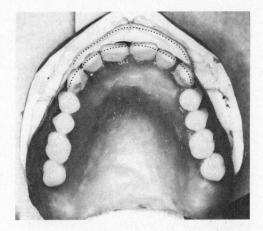

Fig. 19-29. Dotted lines indicate that arch form of artificial anterior teeth on trial denture base is basically similar to form of anterior part of residual ridge.

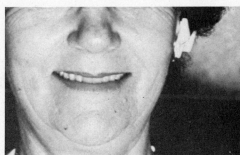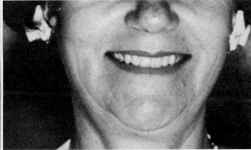

Fig. 19-30. *Left,* Buccal corridor is inadequate because of improper placement of upper teeth. *Right,* Anterior teeth are in proper position to support upper lip, and an adequate buccal corridor is present.

sors to the long axis of the patient's face. When the long axes of these teeth are not in harmony with the long axis of the face, the arrangement will not blend with the face, since the incisal plane of the anterior teeth will not be parallel with the interpupillary line (Fig. 19-31, *A*). This will cause an unpleasant disharmony of lines. It is a simple task to reset the central incisors to make their long axes harmonious with the long axis of the face (Fig. 19-31, *B*). If the central incisors must be divergent at their incisal edges, the midline of the dental arch should be at the center of the face. Then the lateral incisors and canines will almost automatically fall into their proper alignment, and the incisal plane will be in balance with the interpupillary line.

The long axes of the central incisors should be parallel with the long axis of the face, and the midline of the dental arch (the contact area between the central incisors) should be located near the middle of the face. This is determined when one drops an imaginary perpendicular line from the midpoint on the interpupillary line. The midline position of the natural central incisors can be estimated also by observation of the position of the incisive papilla on the cast and the corresponding fossa in the upper trial denture base, since the incisive papilla was located lingually and between the natural upper central incisors before their extraction.

The midline of the lower dental arch is between the central incisors and is usually

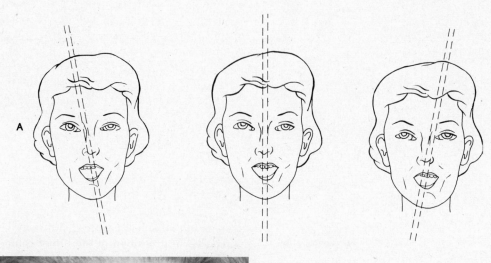

A

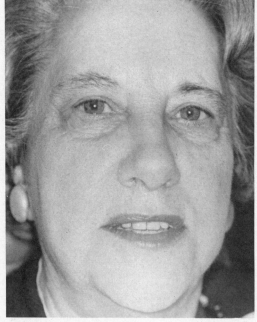

B

Fig. 19-31. Long axes of central incisors should be parallel with long axis of face. **A,** Middle drawing shows that such parallelism provides a necessary harmony of lines. Notice disharmony in drawings on the left and right. **B,** Long axes of artificial central incisors have been correctly aligned.

aligned with the midline of the upper central incisors. When the lower anterior teeth are correctly located anatomically in the lower dental arch, an imaginary line drawn anteroposteriorly through the middle of the lower denture should pass between the lower central incisors (Fig. 19-32). The maxillary and mandibular midlines fail to coincide in most adults with natural teeth.

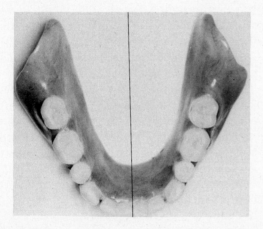

Fig. 19-32. Lower anterior teeth correctly positioned, as shown by imaginary line passing through middle of lower denture and between lower central incisors.

The application of these principles regarding the placement of central incisors and their inclinations may be modified to meet individual needs as indicated by preextraction records.

Harmony of the teeth with the smiling line of the lower lip. When a person smiles, the lower lip forms a pleasant curvature known as the smiling line. This can be used as a guide in arranging the upper anterior teeth.

When the line formed by the incisal edges of the upper anterior teeth follows the curved line of the lower lip during smiling, the two lines will be harmonious and will create a pleasing appearance. When the incisal edges of the upper anterior teeth form a curved line that is not in harmony with, or is opposite in contour to, the line formed by the lower lip during a smile, the contrast of the lines is disharmonious and will be displeasing in appearance (Fig. 19-33, *A*).

The vertical position of the upper canines is primarily responsible for the shape of the smiling line. When the canines are arranged so that their incisal edges are slightly shorter than the incisal edges of the lateral incisors, the smiling line will tend to parallel the lower lip when the patient smiles (Fig. 19-33, *B*). A reverse smiling line is one of the most frequent causes of artificial appearing dentures.

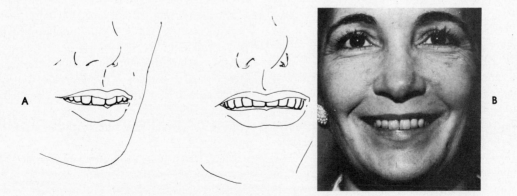

Fig. 19-33. Harmony of line formed by incisal edges of upper anterior teeth with line formed by curvature of lower lip. **A,** Lines are in harmony *(left)* and not in harmony *(right)*. Results are a pleasing and a displeasing appearance. **B,** Notice the harmony in this face.

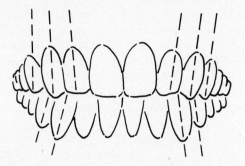

Fig. 19-34. Diagram showing balanced opposing lines. Dissimilarities in inclination, rotation, and position of teeth on either side of midline provide what is called asymmetrical symmetry, which is essential for natural-appearing teeth.

Harmony of opposing lines of labial and buccal surfaces. Setting teeth with their long axes parallel to each other is the thing that causes people to dread complete dentures because of their artificial appearance. Many patients are subconsciously irritated by this artificial appearance of dentures and find many other faults with them that they would otherwise overlook.

A well-balanced painting or drawing must have lines at opposing angles as well as some parallel lines. The same principle must apply to have a pleasing picture of the teeth. For example, if the teeth on both sides of the arch were inclined to be parallel to each other, they would make a most unsatisfactory-appearing denture. There should be asymmetrical symmetry in the arrangement of teeth (Fig. 19-34).

The labial and buccal lines must have opposing equivalent angles, or nearly so, to have a harmonious effect. For instance, if the maxillary right lateral incisor is set at an angle of 5 degrees to the perpendicular, the lateral incisor on the left side should be set at 5 degrees to the perpendicular in the opposite direction. The scheme of opposing angles should be carried to the maxillary canines and the mandibular opposing canines (Fig. 19-34). However, deviation in angulation can be arranged in different teeth on the two sides. Extra inclination of a lateral inci-

sor on one side can be balanced by inclination of the opposite canine; asymmetrical symmetry is the objective.

There should be harmony between the labial and buccal lines of the teeth and the lines of the face. Square and ovoid faces should have teeth that have lines that are more nearly perpendicular, whereas the teeth in tapering faces should have lines that are more divergent from the perpendicular.

An optical illusion can be created for patients who have a nasal deflection. Four of the maxillary teeth can be set at an opposite angle to the deviation making it less apparent.

Harmony of teeth and profile lines of the face. As a general rule, the labial surfaces of the maxillary central incisors are parallel to the profile line of the face. In prognathic patients with protruding mandibular incisors, the incisal edges of the maxillary teeth are out farther than the cervical ends of the teeth. In the opposite condition in which the mandibular incisors are retruded to some extent, the incisal edges of the maxillary teeth are inclined lingually more than the cervical ends of the teeth (Fig. 19-35).

When the maxillary central incisor is parallel with the profile line of the face, the lateral incisor should be set at an opposite angle to prevent parallelism from being predominant. For example, in patients with retrognathic jaw relations whose maxillary central incisors are out at the cervical ends, the lateral incisors could then be depressed at the cervical end to oppose the line that is made by the labial surfaces of the central incisors. For the prognathic patient, the incisal edges of the maxillary central incisors often are set labially. The maxillary lateral incisors could then be placed slightly out at the cervical ends to oppose the labial face line of the central incisors.

Most faces have a blending of two or three types of profiles. Arrangement of teeth for a harmonious appearance must be modified accordingly. The most predominating facial form can be helpful as a guide for positioning of the teeth.

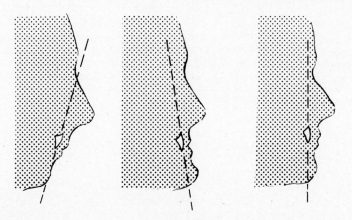

Fig. 19-35. Diagram showing labial face of central incisor parallel with profile line of face. Incisal third of tooth breaks lingually from profile line.

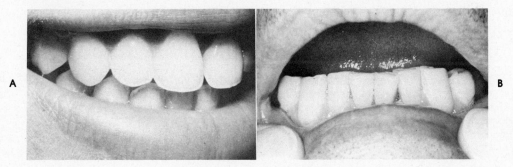

Fig. 19-36. Amount of wear on incisal edges of anterior teeth should be in harmony with patient's age. **A,** Lack of wear is compatible with youth. **B,** Extreme wear indicates a much older patient than the one seen in **A.**

Harmony of tooth wear and age. Incisal edges and proximal surfaces of anterior teeth wear concomitantly with age. This is another characteristic of natural teeth that must be incorporated in artificial teeth if they are to appear to be in harmony with the age of the patient. The incisal edges of denture teeth should *always* be ground to simulate the wear surfaces that would have developed at the age of the patient. Thus a young patient would likely exhibit a minimum amount of wear on the incisal edges of the teeth (Fig. 19-36, *A*), whereas an increased amount of incisal wear would be expected for an older patient (Fig. 19-36, *B*).

A sketch of the anticipated pattern of wear to be placed on the incisal edges of anterior teeth can be beneficial. The outline form of the artificial teeth is sketched on a piece of paper, and the anticipated changes that are to be created to simulate wear on the incisal edges are depicted on the drawing (Fig. 19-37). In general, more lingually placed upper teeth or parts of teeth will wear away more than more labially placed upper teeth. The greatest amount of wear on the

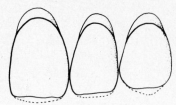

Fig. 19-37. Simple sketch made by dentist of the outline form of artificial teeth is helpful in planning incisal wear that will be incorporated for a particular patient. *Dotted line,* Original appearance of incisal edges of artificial teeth; *solid line,* incisal wear that is anticipated.

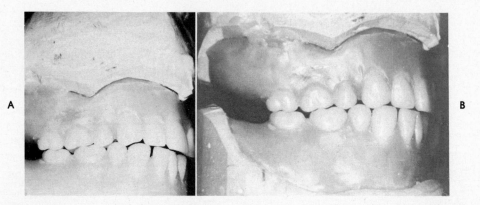

Fig. 19-38. A, Incisal wear on artificial anterior teeth. **B,** Pattern of incisal wear seen in **A** has been developed to improve appearance of denture and to assist in balancing the occlusion. Wear on upper canine has been placed at its proper location with lower canine in relation to balanced occlusion.

lower anterior teeth or parts of teeth will occur in the more anteriorly placed lower teeth. The simulation of wear on anterior teeth should be logically in harmony with the way it occurs when the upper and lower teeth pass over each other.

Developing incisal wear on artificial teeth during balancing and correcting the occlusion is a logical approach to this phase of esthetics. In this manner, the wear is placed on the teeth where it would have occurred during function and also where it assists in the mechanics of balancing the occlusion (Fig. 19-38).

The effect that the form of the tooth creates can be dramatically altered by reshaping of the tooth to simulate wear. The same mold of anterior teeth can be altered to help create a young, soft, feminine appearance for one patient or an older, vigorous, masculine appearance for another patient (Fig. 19-39, *A*).

Most patients who need dentures are at an age when the contact areas of their natural teeth have been worn, whether or not the teeth overlap each other. Therefore the artificial teeth should be altered so that they do not have the appearance of ball contact points with large interproximal spaces. If the teeth selected have contact points that resemble those of a young person's teeth, they should be ground to provide a more natural appearance (Fig. 19-39, *B*).

Refinements of individual tooth positions

One of the essential factors in satisfying patients with complete dentures is that the den-

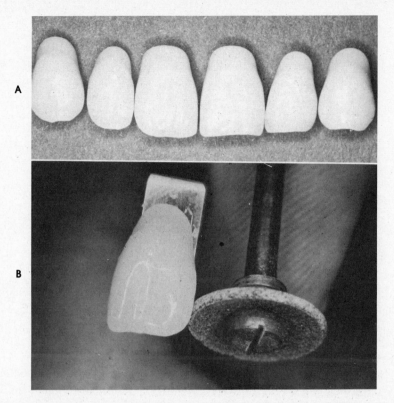

Fig. 19-39. A, The same mold of teeth has been modified so that the three teeth on the left depict youth and femininity, whereas the three on the right would be suitable for an older, masculine patient. **B,** Contact areas as well as incisal edges of artificial teeth must be modified to provide natural appearance.

tures be pleasing and natural in appearance. Dentures are not pleasing unless the teeth are arranged in a plan that nature developed. If patients have some anterior teeth remaining, diagnostic casts should be made as preextraction records to be used in selection and arrangement of the individual teeth. If dentists use preextraction records in construction of many dentures, they soon will learn nature's scheme in arranging teeth for those patients who have lost all teeth before a record was made. With patients for whom no preextraction records are available, dentists can select another cast of natural teeth and follow their arrangement as a guide.

Selection and placing of artificial teeth will not appear natural unless they are set with typical inclinations and rotations that the eye has been accustomed to seeing. These inclinations and rotations can cause the same teeth to appear as oversized or normal. For example, if the canine is rotated so that the eye can see only its mesial half, the tooth will look only approximately one half as large as if it were set so that the entire labial surface immediately meets the eye. Lateral and central incisors, especially in a tapering setup, do not show the entire labial surface when seen from directly in front of the patient. This reduction in the amount of surface that shows harmonizes with a tapering face.

A beginning point for studying the labiolin-

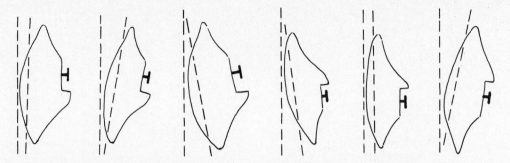

Fig. 19-40. Scheme showing normal labiolingual inclinations of the anterior teeth in relation to the perpendicular.

gual inclination of the maxillary anterior teeth in relation to the perpendicular is shown in Fig. 19-40. The labial surface of the maxillary incisors is parallel to the profile line of the face, which is almost perpendicular. The labial surface of the lateral incisors is in at the cervical end more than that of the adjacent teeth. The labial surface of the canines is out at the cervical end more than that of the other maxillary anterior teeth. The degree to which the cervical end of the canine extends outward usually is in harmony with the lateral lines of the face. The labial surface of the mandibular central incisor is in at the cervical end more than that of the lateral incisor or canine. The mandibular lateral incisor is out at the cervical end more than the central incisor, so that it is almost perpendicular. The mandibular canine is out at the cervical end at the same degree of angulation as the maxillary canine, except that it is at an opposite equivalent angle. The labiolingual inclinations of maxillary anterior teeth are intended to serve only as guidelines from which variations must be made if the individual patient's teeth are to appear natural.

A beginning point for studying the anterior teeth from the labial aspect in their mesiodistal inclination is shown in Fig. 19-41. The central incisor is almost perpendicular, whereas the lateral incisor is inclined distally at the cervical end more than any other anterior tooth. The canine is inclined toward the distal at the cervical end

more than the central incisor and less than the lateral incisor.

A beginning point for studying the rotational positions of the anterior teeth from an incisal aspect is shown in Fig. 19-42. The central incisor is slightly rotated from parallelism to a tangent of the line of arch contour. The lateral incisor is rotated to have its distal surface turned lingually at a considerable angle to a tangent of the line of the arch contour. The canine is rotated so that the distal half of the labial surface points in the direction of the posterior arch form. The mandibular incisors have a rotational position that generally is parallel to a tangent of the arch contour.

A beginning point for studying the superoinferior position of the six anterior teeth in relation to the incisal plane is shown in Fig. 19-43. The maxillary lateral incisor and canine are slightly above the level of the incisal plane.

All these positions of anterior teeth from the various aspects serve only as beginning points and must be varied into harmonious irregularities that are not foreign to any that nature has established. For example, a maxillary canine is seldom in at the cervical end and will appear completely artificial should this irregularity be attempted. The patient cannot point out the exact cause of the unnaturalness but will be aware that something is wrong. Although these are the beginning positions for studying teeth in

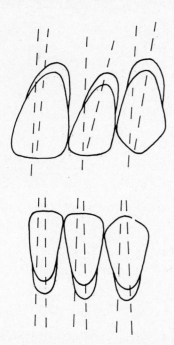

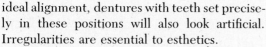

Fig. 19-41. Scheme showing mesiodistal inclination of anterior teeth in relation to the perpendicular.

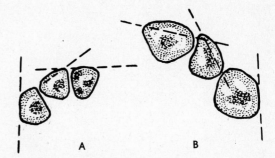

Fig. 19-42. Diagrams of incisal view of anterior teeth showing their angle of rotation. **A,** Mandibular. **B,** Maxillary.

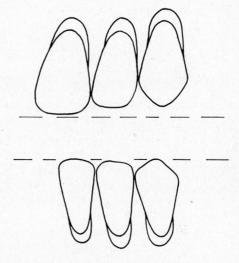

Fig. 19-43. Scheme of superoinferior positions of the anterior teeth in relation to incisal plane.

ideal alignment, dentures with teeth set precisely in these positions will also look artificial. Irregularities are essential to esthetics.

A number of irregularities are found so frequently that they appear natural when reproduced. In order to reduce the artificiality of dentures, it is well to make the teeth irregular. When this is done, the dentist must make a study of the common slight irregularities. Some of the slight irregularities of maxillary anterior teeth that may be used include (1) lapping the mesial surfaces of the maxillary lateral incisors slightly over the central incisors, (2) depressing the maxillary lateral incisor lingually so that the distal surface of the central incisor and the mesial surface of the canine are labial to the mesial and distal surfaces of the maxillary lateral incisor, (3) rotating the mesial incisal corner of the maxillary lateral incisor lingual to the distal surface of the central incisor, with the distal surface

of the lateral incisor flush with the mesial surface of the canine, and (4) placing the incisal edge of the lateral incisor much higher than the incisal edge of the central incisor and canine.

Irregularities of the central incisors may be developed by (1) overlapping of the labial incisal angle of one central incisor over the adjacent central incisor, (2) placement of one central incisor slightly lingual to the other central incisor without rotation, and (3) placement of one cen-

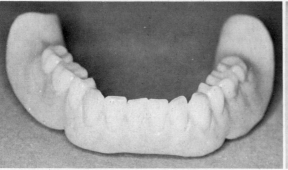
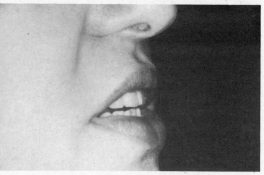

Fig. 19-44. A, Note mesial rotation of central incisors, rotation and position of lateral incisors, and mesial aspect of canines overlapping distal aspect of lateral incisors. **B,** Lower artificial anterior teeth appear natural in the patient's mouth.

tral incisor slightly labial to and slightly longer than the other central incisor.

The maxillary canine may be placed labially in the dental arch, giving this tooth considerable prominence. However, the canine must maintain a rotational position that does not expose the distal half of the labial surface to the eye when viewed from immediately in front. The canine must never be depressed at its cervical end. Rather, its labial surface should be more or less parallel to the side of the face when viewed from the front.

The mandibular anterior teeth can be made slightly irregular with much effectiveness if the irregularities are harmonious with nature's frequent irregularities. A setup that appears natural and decreases the artificial appearance is one in which both central incisors are forward and rotated mesially, one or both lateral incisors are lingual to the arch curve and slightly longer than the adjacent teeth, and the mesial surfaces of the canines overlap the distal surfaces of the lateral incisors (Fig. 19-44).

To overlap teeth in rotational positions and at the same time avoid excessive labiolingual irregularities, the lingual side of the proximal surface of the overlapping tooth must be ground. The overlapping contacts in natural teeth have been worn by the movement of the teeth on their con-

tact points in function. Therefore, to simulate worn natural overlapping, the more labially placed of two overlapped porcelain teeth must be ground on its lingual contact area.

Harmony of spaces and individual tooth position. The use of spaces between teeth can be effective to emphasize individual tooth positions and create a natural-appearing arrangement of teeth. A space is not usually desirable between the upper central incisors unless one existed between the natural teeth. Even then, if the space was large, a smaller space in the denture can create a similar effect and be more pleasing (Fig. 19-45, *A*). Spaces between central and lateral incisors, between lateral incisors and canines, and between canines and premolars are effective irregularities that are visible particularly when patients are seen from the side (Fig. 19-45, *B* and *C*). The location of spaces should be chosen carefully so as to maintain proper balance in the overall composition. Spaces must be designed so they can be self-cleansing.

Concept of harmony with sex, personality, and age of the patient

Frush and Fisher have stated that "creating the illusion of natural teeth in artificial dentures . . . is based on the elementary factors suggested by the sex, personality, and age of the

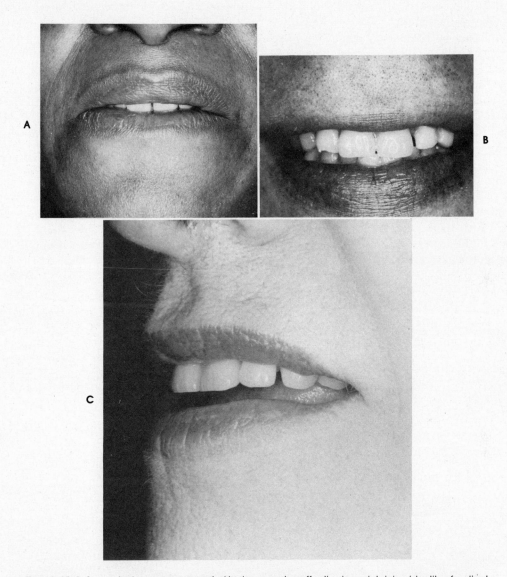

Fig. 19-45. A, Space between upper central incisors can be effective in maintaining identity of patient if such space was present between natural central incisors. **B,** Space between central and lateral incisors helps create a natural appearance in arrangement of artificial anterior teeth. **C,** Space between lateral incisor and canine provides a good esthetic effect when seen from the side. When seen from the front, the space is not noticeable (see Fig. 19-31, *B*).

patient. Femininity is characterized by curved surfaces, roundness, and softness in the form of the dentition, and a prominent smiling-line alignment of the anterior teeth. Masculinity is characterized by boldness, vigor, and square-ness in the dentition and a straightness of the incisal line of teeth. The personality spectrum is divided into delicate, medium, and vigorous, with connotations of personality variations with-in masculine or feminine classifications. It is related to the molds, colors, position of teeth, and form of the supporting matrix for the teeth. Age is depicted in dentures in various degrees by worn incisal edges, erosion, spaces between teeth and variations in the form of the matrix around the cervical end of the teeth.

Individual tooth form and position are also related to these concepts. The size and position of the central incisors dominate the arrangement of the six upper anterior teeth. Rotation of the distal surfaces anteriorly and placement of one central incisor bodily ahead of the other make the appearance of these teeth more vigorous (Fig. 19-46, A). Smaller lateral incisors with rounded incisal angles appear more feminine than larger ones (Fig. 19-46, B). Rotation of the lateral incisors will harden or soften the composition. Canines are positioned to complete the smiling line, rotated so that the mesial surfaces face anteriorly, abraded according to physiologic age, set with the cervical end out, and aligned with the long axis in a vertical direction when viewed from the side (Fig. 19-46, C).

The concept of the influence of sex, personality, and age provides additional information for developing harmony between the composition of tooth arrangement and the patient. Dentists must take full advantage of all concepts to create dentures that restore the natural appearance of their patients (Fig. 19-47).

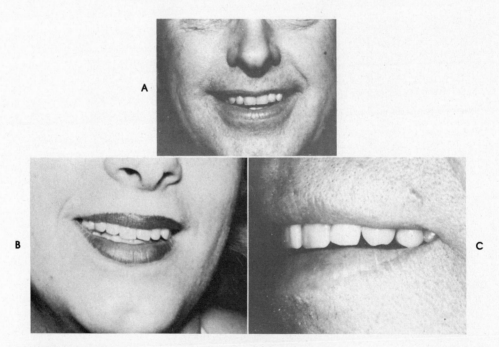

Fig. 19-46. A, Central incisors dominate appearance of the arrangement of artificial upper anterior teeth. **B,** Rounded incisal edges and relative size of upper lateral incisors provide a composition that is feminine in appearance. **C,** Notice location of upper left canine in relation to smiling line, wear on incisal edge, vertical long axis of tooth, and position of mesial surface.

Correlating esthetics and incisal guidance

The best plan of occlusion to enhance stability of complete dentures is one with a shallow incisal guidance inclination. The reduction in the vertical overlap of the anterior teeth may detract from the appearance of the dentures because it is likely to place the maxillary anterior teeth too high or the mandibular anterior teeth too low in the oral orifice. The simplest way to overcome this difficulty and still maintain a pleasing esthetic appearance would be to increase the horizontal overlap (Fig. 19-48). However, if this is done, the lip support or the occlusal vertical dimension would be changed. These procedures may not be feasible if the esthetics and mechanics are to be protected.

One can reduce the vertical overlap of the anterior teeth by increasing the interridge distance. However, this must not be done to the extent that it would encroach on the interocclusal distance. A compromise involves a slight shortening of the upper and lower canines while the full length of the incisors is maintained. In this situation, occlusal balance in the protrusive position might not be possible. However, balanced occlusion can be attained in the lateral

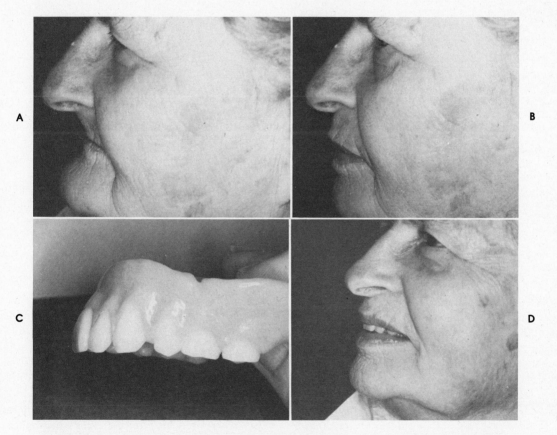

Fig. 19-47. A, Total lack of support of patient's face. Note prominence of chin. **B,** Lips have been restored to a natural position. Notice difference in appearance of chin and proper restoration of mentolabial sulcus. **C,** Upper anterior teeth on denture are arranged on an incline in relation to upper lip. Notice distance that anterior teeth are in front of residual alveolar ridge. **D,** Lips move naturally because the muscles that control facial expression have been restored to their proper physiologic length. Teeth appear natural because of their proper size, form, color, and arrangement.

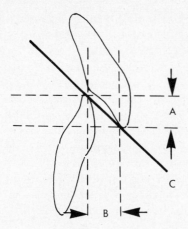

Fig. 19-48. Diagram of vertical and horizontal overlap. *A,* Vertical overlap; *B,* horizontal overlap; *C,* incisal guidance angle.

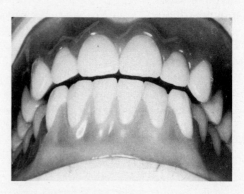

Fig. 19-49. Opposing anterior teeth should not contact when posterior teeth are in centric occlusion.

occlusions. Protrusive balance is less important than lateral balance because incision is performed consciously. The patient can control the amount and direction of force applied when he bites into food. On the other hand, chewing is carried out at a subconscious level. Patients do not think of the amount and direction of the force they apply. Consequently, they cannot protect themselves from forces that would dislodge their dentures. The angle of incisal guidance for lateral occlusion must be adjusted so that the posterior teeth can contact at the same time the upper and lower canines are end to end.

Even when the vertical overlap of the anterior teeth must be severe for proper esthetics, the opposing anterior teeth should not be in contact when the posterior teeth are in centric occlusion (Fig. 19-49). Such contact will eventually cause excess pressures from occlusion of the anterior teeth when the residual ridges resorb and the vertical relation of occlusion is decreased. Excessive force usually cannot be tolerated by the anterior part of the residual ridges and will likely cause increased resorption of bone and development of hyperplastic tissue in this region.

PATIENT ACCEPTANCE OF ARRANGEMENT OF ANTERIOR TEETH

Patients must be given the opportunity to observe and approve the final arrangement of the anterior teeth at the try-in appointment. The dentures should not be completed until approval is obtained. Even when patients indicate that they "do not care how their teeth look," they must be given full opportunity to inspect and approve the arrangement. These patients often become extremely concerned with their appearance when they begin to wear the dentures.

Patients should not be permitted to observe the trial dentures in the mouth until the dentist is satisfied with the composition as it is created. The premolars should be in the proper arch form, and the wax denture bases should be carved to approximate the final form. Initial reactions of patients can be long-lasting, and an unsatisfactory reaction to a partially completed arrangement of anterior teeth may cause continued problems even though the final appearance of the dentures is perfectly satisfactory.

Since the appearance of the dentures will be seen most often by other people during normal conversation, patients should first observe themselves in this situation. The patient is positioned 3 to 4 feet (1 to 1.3 m) in front of a large mirror with the trial dentures in the mouth and given the opportunity to observe the dentures during normal conversation and facial expression. If possible, another adult member of the family should also be asked to observe the patient during normal conversation. The reaction of the patient at this time can be critical to the eventual success of the dentures, so that this phase must not be done hurriedly or haphazardly.

The dentist should listen carefully to all comments that are made by the patient and never dismiss any of them as being silly or of no consequence. Some changes that the patient may suggest can be incorporated. However, other suggestions may not be advisable, and it will be necessary to explain to the patient that they are not anatomically feasible and would prevent the muscles in the cheeks and lips from properly moving the face. Many patients will be pleased with the appearance of the dentures and request few, if any, changes when the position of the artificial teeth approximates that of the natural teeth.

20

Completion of the try-in:
eccentric jaw relation records,
articulator and cast adjustment,
perfection of the posterior
palatal seal

When the final occlusion is developed and corrected on the articulator, it is essential that the movements of the articulator simulate mandibular positions or movements of the patient within the range of normal functional contacts of teeth. Thus the condylar elements of the articulator must be adjusted so that they approximate the condylar-guiding factors within the temporomandibular joints. These adjustments of the condylar elements of the articulator are made by means of interocclusal eccentric records.

PROTRUSIVE AND LATERAL RELATIONS

There seems to be confusion in the minds of many dentists as to what a protrusive registration is intended to attain. The idea that the angle and lines of the bony fossa completely govern the path of the condyle is erroneous. A study of the anatomy and function of the joint reveals the fact that the condylar path is governed partly in its shape and function by the meniscus. The meniscus is attached in part to the lateral pterygoid muscle and moves forward during opening and lateral mandibular movements. The path is controlled further by the shape of the fossa, the attachments of the ligaments, the biting load during movement (muscular influence), and the amount of protrusion. Variation in registrations can be caused by several factors. The registration may vary according to the biting pressure exerted after the mandible has been protruded. The condyle, not being locked on a path, is subject to change in its path with a variation of pressure. Undoubtedly, there is some leeway for adaptability to conform with the changing conditions of the teeth. Many parts of the body are phenomenal in their ability to adapt themselves to unusual conditions, and the temporomandibular joint is one of them. Not many complete dentures could be worn if this were not true. However, registration of normal comfortable movement of the condyle in its path, with subsequent harmonious centric and eccentric occlusion to conform with this, greatly augments lasting function of dentures. Therefore there seems little excuse for not registering this path, because it is not a difficult or time-consuming procedure in proportion to the results.

CONTROLLING FACTORS OF MOVEMENT

Edentulous patients bring only one controlling factor to the movement of the mandible, a fact that seems to be misunderstood generally. The misconception derives from the fact that many dentists think the condyle paths control the movement of the mandible entirely. In the laws of articulation, the incisal guidance provided by the anterior teeth is an important part of the control. This guidance is always decided by the dentist, whether consciously or not. With the Hanau and Whip Mix articulators, incisal guidance is controlled by the inclination of the incisal guidance mechanism, which is determined by the horizontal and vertical overlap of the anterior teeth. The incisal guidance is more influential in control of movement of the mandible than the condylar paths are because the condylar paths are farther away from the cusp inclines, which both the incisal angle and condyle angle influence.

ECCENTRIC RELATION RECORDS

The path of the condyle in protrusive and lateral movements is not on a straight line. The shape of the mandibular fossa is an ogee curve as viewed in the sagittal plane. This double curve will cause the apparent path of the condyle to be different with varying amounts of mandibular protrusion. The ideal amount of protrusion for making the record is the exact equivalent of the amount of protrusion necessary to bring the anterior teeth end to end. However, the mechanical limitations of most articulators require a protrusive movement of at least 6 mm so that the condylar guidance mechanisms can be adjusted.

Methods of registering the condyle path may be classified as intraoral and extraoral. Extraoral methods are generally exemplified by the Gysi and McCollum methods.

The intraoral methods may be listed as (1) plaster and Carborundum grind-in, (2) chew-in by teeth opposing wax, (3) chew-in modified by a central-bearing point, (4) Needles styli cutting a compound rim, (5) Needles method modified by a Messerman tracer, (6) protrusive registration in softened compound, (7) protrusive registration by plaster, and (8) protrusive registration in softened wax.

Lateral and protrusive condylar inclinations may be registered when straight protrusive movements are made. Many dentists consider these short-range lateral movements sufficiently indicative for practical purposes. However, for a complete registration, lateral records are necessary to indicate the limit of the range of movement, as shown by the Gothic arch (needle point) tracings.

Wax interocclusal records may be made on the occlusion rims before the teeth are set up or on the posterior teeth at the try-in appointment. Records made on occlusion rims must be considered tentative because the vertical and horizontal overlaps of the anterior teeth have not as yet been determined, and the exact amount of protrusion and the level at which the anterior teeth are to contact are still unknown. These preliminary records permit tentative adjustment of the condylar guidances on the articulator.

Plaster interocclusal records are made after

the anterior teeth have been arranged for esthetics and after both centric and vertical relation have been verified. If the horizontal overlap is sufficient to obtain enough protrusive movement of the lower jaw so that the articulator can be adjusted, this record will be adequate. It will be an accurate record of the relation of the jaws at their position during the function of incision. If the horizontal overlap of the incisors is too small to permit sufficient mandibular movement for adjustment of the condylar guidance, the patient must be instructed to protrude the jaw farther when the record is made. The minimum amount of protrusion for condylar guidance adjustment is 6 mm. This limitation is necessary because of mechanical deficiencies of most articulating instruments.

Lateral interocclusal records are made in a similar manner. The amount of lateral movement should be sufficient to place the upper buccal cusps over the lower buccal cusps.

Eccentric interocclusal records may be made with the guidance of extraoral tracings. While the tracing device is still attached to the occlusion rims, the amount of protrusive movement can be determined by observation of the distance between the apex of the tracing and the needle point. The amount and direction of the lateral movement can be determined by observation of the distance the needle point is from the apex of the tracing while the needle point is on one of the arcs of the tracing. When the needle point is 6 mm from the apex, the mandible in the first molar region will be approximately 3 mm lateral to its position in centric relation. The molar tooth will have moved laterally 3 mm. The reason for this is that the molar tooth is approximately midway between the tracing and the working-side condyle.

Protrusive interocclusal records for the Whip Mix articulator

After the try-in, the trial dentures are placed on the articulator. The lateral condylar guidances are set at 0 degrees so that the articulator will be moved in a straight protrusive direction. The horizontal condylar guidances are set at 25 degrees to give an indication of the space that will exist between the posterior teeth when the mandible is protruded.

The lower member of the articulator is moved forward approximately 6 mm with the teeth out of contact and then closed until the incisal edges of the lower anterior teeth reach the vertical level of the incisal edges of the upper anterior teeth. The 6 mm of forward movement that is necessary to permit proper adjustment of the horizontal condylar path of the articulator may bring the lower anterior teeth several millimeters in front of the upper anterior teeth.

The horizontal relation of the lower to the upper anterior teeth and the relationship of the midlines of the upper and lower anterior teeth are observed carefully, since they will be the guides to the dentist that the patient has closed in approximately the proper position when the protrusive record is made in the mouth (Fig. 20-1, *A*). Interfering opposing posterior teeth that contact before the lower anterior teeth reach the desired vertical relation should be removed from the wax occlusion rim.

When the dentist has become familiar with the relation of the lower to the upper anterior teeth in the protrusive position, the trial dentures are removed from the articulator and placed in the patient's mouth. The trial dentures are held in position by the dentist in the same way as for making the interocclusal centric relation record.

The patient is instructed to move his lower jaw straight forward and then to bite lightly on his front teeth. The dentist determines the amount and nature of the forward protrusion by his previous observation of the relationship of the anterior teeth on the articulator. The patient practices closing in the protrusive position under the guidance of the dentist until both become familiar with the procedure (Fig. 20-1, *B*).

A small amount of recording material that does not distort easily when set (impression plaster) is placed on the occlusal surfaces of the

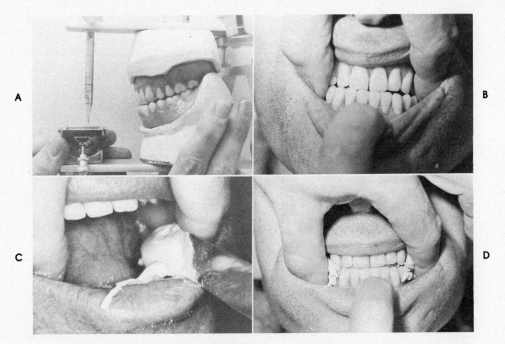

Fig. 20-1. A, Articulator (Whip Mix) is observed in protrusive position to determine amount of forward movement necessary to adjust condylar elements. This relationship will guide dentist when protrusive record is made in patient's mouth. **B,** Patient rehearses closing in protrusive position. Dentist observes anteroposterior relation of opposing anterior teeth and alignment of midlines between upper and lower central incisors as a guide to amount and direction of protrusive movement. Movement should be similar in nature to that observed previously on articulator. **C,** Fast-setting plaster is placed on occlusal surfaces of lower posterior teeth to serve as recording medium. **D,** Relationship of opposing teeth serves a guide for position of mandible when interocclusal protrusive record is made.

lower posterior teeth (Fig. 20-1, *C*). Then in a similar manner as in the practice sessions, the patient protrudes the mandible and closes into the recording material. The patient is instructed to stop the closure before the opposing teeth make contact and to hold the jaw lightly and steadily in the desired postion until the recording material sets (Fig. 20-1, *D*). The relationship of the lower anterior teeth to the upper anterior teeth in the patient's mouth should closely approximate the relationship observed on the articulator and during the rehearsal sessions.

The trial dentures and interocclusal record are removed from the mouth. The lateral condylar guidances on the upper member of the articulator are set at 20 degrees so that they will not

interfere if the mandible was not moved forward in straight protrusion, and the horizontal condylar guidances are set at 0 degrees. Then the trial dentures and interocclusal protrusive record are returned to the articulator (Fig. 20-2, *A*). The horizontal condylar housings are rotated individually until the guidance plates contact the condylar spheres (Fig. 20-2, *B* and *C*), and the angulation of the protrusive movement for both sides is recorded.

The advantages of the protrusive registration made in plaster, or recording material of similar consistency, are that the resistance to the biting force is minimal and uniform and that nothing guides the patient's mandible except the memory patterns of mandibular protrusion and the

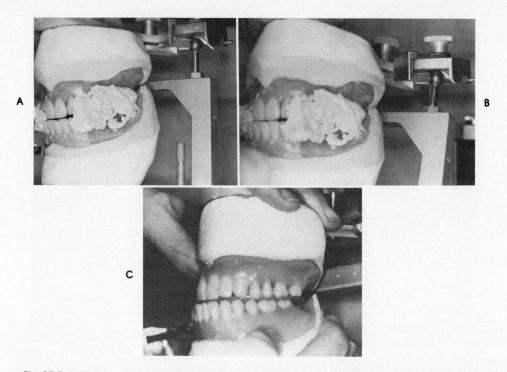

Fig. 20-2. A, Trial denture bases as positioned by interocclusal protrusive record are returned to Whip Mix articulator. Horizontal condylar guidance mechanism is not in contact with condylar sphere *(arrow).* **B,** Horizontal condylar mechanism has been rotated into contact with condylar sphere *(arrow),* thus establishing horizontal condylar guidance on articulator. **C,** Interocclusal protrusive record has been made with a wax interocclusal record. Articulator is adjusted in a similar manner to that in **B.**

instructions of the dentist. Also, the recording material will not be distorted during adjustment of the articulator.

Lateral interocclusal records for the Whip Mix articulator

The horizontal condylar guidances on the articulator are set at the angulation indicated by the protrusive interocclusal record, and the lateral condylar guidances are set at 20 degrees. With the trial dentures on the casts, the lower member of the articulator is moved in a lateral excursion with the teeth out of contact for a distance that will cause the balancing condylar sphere to move away from the centric position approximately 6 mm along the lateral condylar guidance. The articulator is closed in the lateral

position until the incisal edge of the lower left canine reaches the vertical level of the upper left canine. The amount of horizontal overlap between the canines in centric position will determine their relative relationship to one another in a 6 mm lateral excursion. The condylar sphere is moved approximately 6 mm to permit proper adjustment of the lateral condylar guidance on the articulator.

The relation of the lower canine and lower posterior teeth to the upper canine and upper posterior teeth is observed carefully with the articulator in the lateral position, since this will be the guide to the dentist that the patient has closed in approximately the proper position when the record is made in the mouth (Fig. 20-3, *A*). Interfering contacts of the poste-

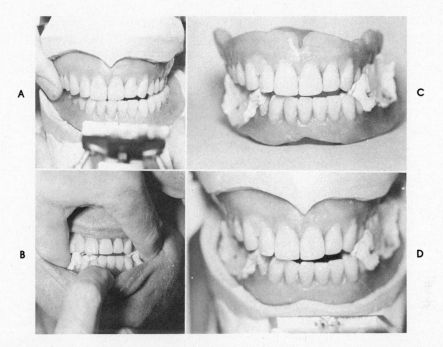

Fig. 20-3. A, Left lateral movement is made on articulator to determine relationship of opposing teeth. This relationship will guide dentist when lateral record is made in patient's mouth. **B,** After rehearsing procedure, a left lateral interocclusal record is made, using plaster as the recording medium. Relationship of opposing teeth in patient's mouth is similar to that observed on articulator. **C,** Trial dentures and interocclusal protrusive record have been removed from mouth, **D,** Trial dentures with interocclusal protrusive record have been returned to articulator.

rior teeth that occur before the canines reach the desired vertical relation should be eliminated by resetting or removal of the involved teeth.

When the dentist has become familiar with the relation of the lower teeth to the upper teeth in the lateral position, the trial dentures are removed from the articulator and placed in the patient's mouth. The trial dentures are held in position by the dentist in the same way as for making the interocclusal centric relation record.

The patient is instructed to move his lower jaw to the side and then close his teeth lightly together. If jaw exercises were prescribed at an earlier appointment, they should be of help at this time. The extent of the lateral movement is determined by the relationship of the lower teeth to the upper teeth as observed on the articulator. The patient practices the lateral movement under the guidance of the dentist until both become familiar with the procedure.

A small amount of recording material is placed on the occlusal surfaces of the lower posterior teeth of the trial dentures. A greater amount of the recording material must be placed on the balancing side than on the working side because the teeth on the balancing side will be farther out of contact than those on the working side during a lateral mandibular movement. Then, in a similar manner as in the practice sessions, the patient moves the mandible laterally and closes lightly into the recording material when instructed to do so by the dentist. The patient is instructed to stop the closure before the opposing teeth make contact and to hold the jaw lightly and steadily in that position until the plaster sets (Fig. 20-3, *B*). The relationship of the lower teeth to the upper teeth when the lateral record is made must closely approximate the relationship observed during the rehearsal sessions.

The trial dentures and lateral interocclusal record are removed from the mouth and returned to the articulator (Fig. 20-3, *C* and *D*). The lateral condylar guidance on the balancing side of the articulator is set at 45 degrees, and the horizontal condylar guidance is set at 0 degrees so that they will not interfere with the downward, forward, and inward position of the balancing condylar sphere, and the lateral codylar mechanism is rotated until it contacts the condylar sphere (Fig. 20-4). The angulations of both the horizontal and lateral condylar guidances are recorded for the lateral movement.

The same procedures are repeated to adjust the condylar mechanisms on the opposite side of the articulator. The patient moves the mandible in the oppoiste direction, a lateral interocclusal record is made, the record is transferred to the articulator with the trial dentures, the horizontal and lateral condylar guidances are adjusted, and the angulations are recorded.

Articulator adaptability to eccentric records

Mechanical limitations of the condylar guidances of the Whip Mix articulator can prevent the condylar spheres from assuming the same position as the condyles of the patient during certain mandibular movements. When this limitation exists, the condylar spheres will not fit the condylar housings properly when the teeth fit into the interocclusal record.

The horizontal condylar guidances of the Whip Mix articulator can be adjusted to record the position of the condylar spheres for an interocclusal protrusive record, since both condyles have moved downward and forward during this movement. However, for the interocclusal lateral record, the patient's balancing con-

dyle moves downward, forward, and inward while the working condyle rotates and moves laterally, usually with an upward or downward and a backward or forward component, depending on the anatomy of the temporomandibular joint. It is possible for the working condyle to move directly laterally in the horizontal plane with no upward or downward and backward or forward component during a lateral mandibular movement. However, it is unlikely that the anatomy of the temporomandibular joint would dictate this kind of movement. The condylar guidances of the Whip Mix articulator cannot be accurately adjusted to accommodate for the forward-backward and upward-downward movement of the working condyle during a lateral movement, since the articulator makes provision for only a direct lateral movement of the working condyle in the horizontal plane. For this reason, it is impossible to accurately adjust the condylar guidances of the Whip Mix articulator for many patients, using lateral interocclusal records. The approximation that can be recorded represents a limitation of this instrument.

The intercondylar width of the Whip Mix articulator is semiadjustable in increments of 12 mm. This feature, at least theoretically, permits the Whip Mix articulator to be adjusted with some lateral interocclusal records that the Hanau H-2 articulator could not accept.

Protrusive interocclusal records for the Hanau articulator

A roll of wax is placed over the occlusal surfaces of the mandibular teeth and is luted to the teeth and interproximal spaces. This wax is softened in hot water at 135° F (57° C) until the entire bulk is practically softened throughout. Both trial bases are placed in position on the casts, and the articulator is set ¼ inch (6 mm) in protrusion, with the condyle paths registering 25 degrees. At that position the upper member of the articulator is pressed into this warm wax to approximately one third of its depth. The mandibular trial denture is now removed from the

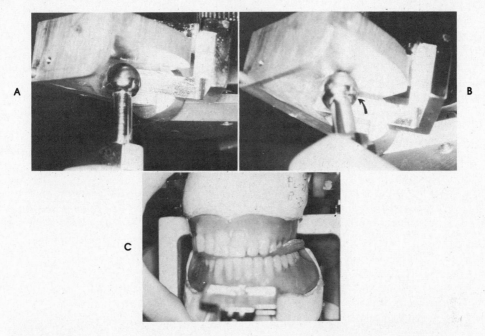

Fig. 20-4. A, Both horizontal and lateral condylar mechanisms are out of contact with condylar sphere as it is positioned in the housing by interocclusal lateral record. **B,** Horizontal condylar mechanism has been rotated into contact with condylar sphere to establish horizontal condylar guidance for left lateral mandibular movement. Lateral condylar guidance mechanism has been moved into contact with condylar sphere to establish lateral condylar guidance for lateral mandibular movement *(arrow).* **C,** Interocclusal left lateral record has been made, with wax as the recording medium. Articulator is adjusted as described in **B.**

cast, and the wax record is chilled thoroughly. Both the trial dentures are now placed in the patient's mouth, and the patient is taught how to protrude into these indentations. The patient is rehearsed in this protrusive action to prepare for making such a protrusive movement later when the wax is softened. The mandibular trial denture is now removed from the mouth, and the wax record is resoftened in hot water with care being taken not to destroy the indentations. The trial denture is now reinserted into the mouth, and the patient is told to feel carefully and move into these markings in the manner rehearsed previously. (The patient has been instructed not to exert occlusal pressure into these indentations until told to do so by the dentist.) The dentist observes carefully the position of the teeth in relation to the indentations, and when the teeth coincide with these markings, the patient is told to bite but is cautioned not to bite through the wax. The wax record is chilled in the mouth, removed, and examined to see that there is no contact between the teeth. The trial dentures are replaced on the articulator, and the articulator is protruded so that the maxillary teeth fit partially into the indentations. The locknuts for the condylar guidance slot adjustments are loosened. While pressure is exerted on the upper articulator member with one hand and the condylar guidance slot is worked back and forth with the other hand, a condylar path inclination is found that permits the teeth to stay in contact with the wax throughout. This adjustment is repeated for the opposite side. It is seen readily that too steep a path will prevent contact in the posterior part of the arch and that too horizontal a path will prevent contact in the anterior part of the arch. As was stated, one can arrive at a degree of incline of condylar path by having tooth contact with the wax throughout the arch. The condylar guidance slot is locked in the position thus obtained.

A protrusive record is first made on the articulator so that the correct amount of protrusive distance, which is also centered, will guide the patient's mandible to a desirable protrusive position. Unless the patient has a guide and is rehearsed, it is extremely difficult to keep the mandible from closing too far or not far enough in protrusive occlusion, or to the right or left in lateral occlusion, or in a combination of protrusive occlusion, or in a combination of protrusive and lateral. Such a record would give an unsatisfactory setting of the articulator. The record is made with a protrusive distance of ¼ inch (6 mm) because it is believed that with a shorter distance, the condyle would not move down its path a distance sufficient to be recorded on the instrument. A protrusive movement of more than ¼ inch is usually beyond the range of movement for the patient, and registration of a greater distance is not necessary.

An alternate procedure is one that involves the use of impression plaster for making the protrusive interocclusal record. After the try-in is complete, both trial dentures are placed in the mouth, and impression plaster is mixed to a heavy, creamy consistency. With the same hand position as used for making the plaster interocclusal record of centric relation, plaster is placed by means of a narrow plaster spatula on the occlusal surfaces of the mandibular premolars and molars on both sides. Then the patient is instructed to stick the chin out and bite on the front teeth. This will cause the patient to protrude the mandible to the place that the neuromuscular system had learned would bring the anterior teeth end to end. If the anterior teeth have been positioned where the natural teeth were, the mandibular incisiors will approach the maxillary incisors precisely in an end-to-end relation. (Obviously, if the anterior teeth have been set incorrectly, the jaw will be moved too far forward or not far enough.) The patient is directed to stop this closure *before* any tooth makes contact and to hold the jaw in that position until the plaster set. When the plaster has set, the trial dentures are removed, and the condylar guidance slots on the articulator are adjusted in the same manner as for the wax interocclusal record.

The advantages of the second method are that resistance to the biting force is minimal and uniform and that there is nothing to guide the patient's mandibular movement but the memory of the neuromuscular sense and the instructions of the dentist. Also, the plaster record will not be distorted by the procedures used to adjust the articulator.

PERFECTION OF THE POSTERIOR PALATAL SEAL

The posterior palatal seal is completed before the final arrangement of the posterior teeth because this final arrangement is a laboratory procedure and is done in the absence of the patient.

The posterior border of the denture is determined in the mouth, and its location is transferred onto the cast. A T burnisher or mouth mirror is pressed along the posterior angle of the tuberosity until it drops into the pterygomaxillary (hamular) notch (Fig. 20-5). The locations of the right and left pterygomaxillary notches are marked with an indelible pencil. On the median line of the anterior part of the soft palate are two indentations formed by the coalescence of ducts known as the foveae palatinae. The shape of these depressions varies from round or oval to oblong. The dentist can make them more readily discernible by having the patient hold the nose and attempt to blow into the nose. This causes the foveae palatinae and vibrating lie to be accentuated.

The vibrating line of the soft palate, which is a guide to the ideal posterior border of the denture, is usually located slightly anterior to the

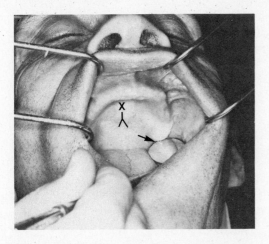

Fig. 20-5. Appearance of pterygomaxillary (hamular) notch *(arrow)* in the mouth is often deceiving. To be certain of its location, palpate it by means of a mouth mirror. *X,* Foveae palatinae.

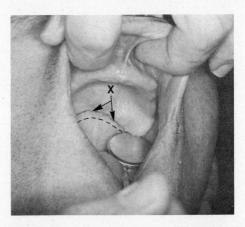

Fig. 20-6. Vibrating line has been traced on palatal tissues in indelible pencil. *X,* Vibrating line passes through hamular notch on both sides and slightly anterior to the foveae palatinae. Denture can end posterior to this line (dotted line indicates end of denture) because of gradual slope of palate.

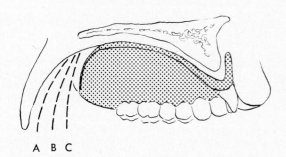

A B C

Fig. 20-7. Vibrating line and width of posterior palatal seal depend on soft palate form *A, B,* or *C. C* allows only a narrow posterior palatal seal; *A* allows widest posterior palatal seal.

foveae palatinae. However, the vibrating line may be on or slightly posterior to the foveae palatinae. The slight deviation from these markings is decided by the dentist. The dentist can decide by having the patient say *ah,* thus vibrating the soft palate. The dentist observes closely and marks the vibrating line with an indelible pencil (Figs. 20-6 and 20-7). The two pterygomaxillary notch markings are joined to the median line mark. The trial denture base is now inserted so that the indelible pencil line is transferred from the soft palate to the trial denture base, and the

excess baseplate is reduced to this line (Fig. 20-8). The trial denture base is placed on the cast, and a knife or pencil is used to mark a line, following the psoterior limits of the baseplate (Fig. 20-9). This line is marked laterally to a point 3 mm beyond the crest of the hamular notch.

The anterior line that indicates the location of the posterior palatal seal is drawn on the cast in front of the line that indicates the end of the denture (Fig. 20-10). The width of the posterior palatal seal itself is limited to a bead on the denture that is 1 to 1.5 mm high and 1.5 mm broad

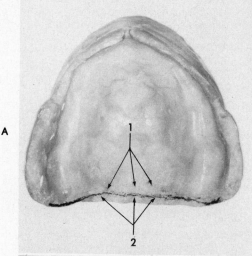

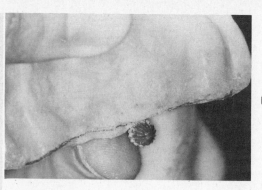

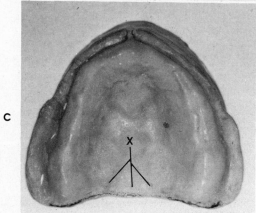

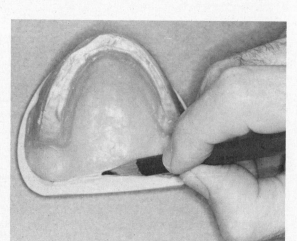

Fig. 20-8. A, Indelible pencil line across patient's palate (Fig. 20-6) has been transferred to denture base and can be seen rather indistinctly, *1,* anterior to solid line, *2,* that indicates end of denture. **B,** Trial denture base is shortened posteriorly to the indelible line with a vulcanite bur. **C,** Trial denture base posteriorly represents anticipated length of completed denture. *X,* Transfer of location of vibrating line from patient's mouth.

Fig. 20-9. Posterior extent of trial denture base is traced on cast.

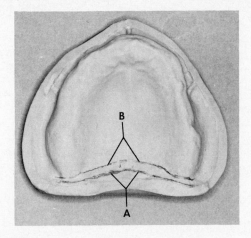

Fig. 20-10. Posterior line, *A,* indicates end of denture posteriorly across palate. Anterior line, *B,* indicates location of posterior palatal seal that will be carved into cast and transferred as a bead on the denture.

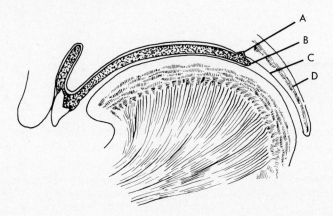

Fig. 20-11. Diagrammatic sagittal section of a denture in place in the mouth. *A,* Bead on denture is 1 mm high, 1 mm broad at its base, and 2 mm anterior to *B,* the end of the denture. *C,* Movable soft palate. *D,* Muscles of soft palate.

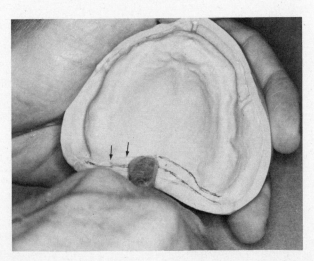

Fig. 20-12. A groove is carved on cast *(arrows)* with a large sharp scraper to form posterior palatal seal.

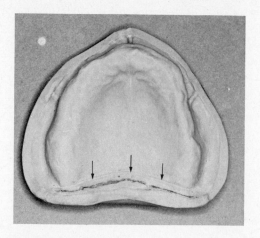

Fig. 20-13. Groove on cast *(arrows)* forms bead on finished denture (see Fig. 20-11).

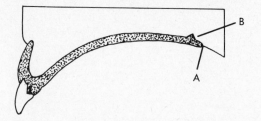

Fig. 20-14. Denture ends on the cast at *A*, and bead, *B*, is located 2 mm in front of vibrating line. Bead is extended laterally through center of hamular notches.

at its base (Fig. 20-11). A greater width creates an area of tissue placement that will have a tendency to push the denture downward gradually and to defeat the purpose of the posterior palatal seal. In other words, the posterior palatal seal should not be made too wide. Placement of tissue is made so that when the dentures move in function, as they always do, the placed tissue will move with the dentures and not break the seal.

A groove 1 to 1.5 mm deep is carved into the cast at the location of the bead. A large sharp scraper is used to carve this V-shaped groove through the hamular notches and across the palate of the cast (Figs. 20-12 and 20-13). The groove will form a bead on the denture that will provide the posterior palatal seal (Fig. 20-14). The bead will be 1 to 1.5 mm high, 1.5 mm wide at its base, and sharp at its apex. The depth of the groove in the cast is determined by the thickness of the soft tissue against which it will be placed, and the depth of the groove will determine the height of the bead.

The narrow and sharp bead will sink easily into the soft tissue to provide a seal against air being forced under the denture. If the bead has been made too high, the sharpness will make this apparent within 24 hours of the insertion of the dentures, and it can be easily relieved. The narrowness of the bead makes the seal with minimal downward pressure on the denture.

21

Arrangement of posterior teeth for functional harmony

Arrangement of artificial posterior teeth for functional harmony depends on a thorough understanding of occlusion. Occlusion is any contact between the incising or masticating surfaces of the upper and lower teeth. There are many kinds of occlusion that are significant in complete denture prosthodontics. The specifications for each kind of occlusion are related to other conditions at the time the occlusal contact is made. For example, centric occlusion is the relation of opposing occlusal surfaces that provides the maximum planned contact or intercuspation, or both, and it should exist when the mandible is in centric relation to the maxillae. All other occlusions are eccentric occlusions. Prostrusive occlusion refers to the occlusion existing when the mandible is moved forward from centric occlusion. Lateral occlusion refers to the occlusion existing when the mandible is moved laterally. Balanced occlusion refers to occlusion with simultaneous contacts of the occlusal surfaces of all or some of the teeth on both sides of the arch, regardless of the mandibular position.

The side toward which the mandible is moved is called the working side for purpose of identification. For the same purpose, the side opposite the working side is called the nonworking balancing side.

The setting of teeth includes orientation of the plane, shaping and positioning of the arch, inclinations and rotations for esthetics, and the mechanics for obtaining proper tooth inclination for balanced occlusion. Occlusion is too often construed as the only important objective in the setting of teeth. Such is not the case because, for example, the posterior dental arch could be too wide and still be in perfect balance. Nevertheless, despite perfect balance, the wide arch would cause failure of the dentures because of excessive leverage. The occlusal plane can be balanced and yet be too high or too low, with a ruinous result. Occlusion has to do with cuspal and incisal inclinations and their relation to other inclinations and jaw movements.

IMPORTANCE OF OCCLUSION

Occlusion is probably the most important subject in all disciplines of dentistry. Consideration of occlusal stresses, both vertical and lateral, and their components in the making of single tooth restorations is of prime importance in the preservation of the tooth, the teeth, and the restoration. Care should be used when one is finishing restorations so as not to take a tooth out of harmony or to leave it underfilled or overfilled. On the other hand, the entire occlusion should be tested for possible disharmony, which could be improved with a knowledge of what would constitute proper harmony in centric and eccentric positions in that dental arch.

MAINTENANCE OF ARCHES

In fixed restorations that replace one or several teeth, it becomes extremely important to establish optimally distributed stresses to preserve the supporting structures around the abutment teeth, which now have an extra load to bear. The future of that entire arch depends on the harmonious relation of all the teeth in centric and eccentric positions. There are times when the recuperative powers of the supporting tissues are so good that the supporting structures may tolerate an inharmonious occlusion. However as age increases and resistance to disease is lessened, the supporting structures will usually break down if they are overloaded

because of improper distribution of stresses. Repeated fracture of facings is not usually the result of failure in mechanical attachment or strength but of excessive loading caused by disharmony of cuspal inclines.

MAINTENANCE OF OCCLUSAL HARMONY

A contributing factor in the breakdown of supporting structures is unbalanced centric and eccentric occlusion.

In most parts of the body nature heals, compensates, or both, any disease and injury. However, nature does not heal and take care of dental caries, nor is it capable of taking care of the ravages of malocclusion. Therefore it is as important to understand occlusion in all its phases to repair and restore dental function as it is to restore individual tooth breakdown by dental caries.

Orthodontically, any movement of a tooth or teeth, however slight, will cause a change in the relationship of the inclines of the moved teeth to the remainder of the arch. Therefore the moment they are not held by an appliance, inharmonious inclinations soon shift them out of their acquired positions. For that reason, harmony of inclines throughout the dental arch is of paramount importance.

Difference in artificial and natural occlusion of teeth

It must be understood, however, that occlusion that is acceptable for natural teeth may not be acceptable for complete dentures. For example, with complete dentures, protrusive and lateral contact is preferred, whereas in natural occlusion this exact type of occlusal relationship is seldom needed.

The dentist must test and correct occlusion of the entire mouth for harmony of centric and eccentric occlusion before and after the construction of a partial denture. The remaining teeth are loaded to their maximum, and therefore distribution of vertical and lateral stresses must be executed carefully if the restoration and remaining teeth are to function efficiently and to result in no destruction of supporting structures.

Reduced inclines in dentures

The difficulties and handicaps of reduced anchorage in complete dentures demand the utmost in occlusal harmony. The dentist has the power to establish all factors of occlusion except the condylar path. Therefore the dentist has the opportunity to establish a reduced amount of displacing cusp inclinations and still maintain a harmony between the factors that will not disturb the stability of the complete dentures.

Rationale for arranging posterior teeth in balanced occlusion

During mastication, the teeth make contact to a variable extent on both the chewing side and the nonchewing side. A combination of tissue resiliency and denture movement during function accounts for the high frequency of the nonchewing, or balancing, side contacts. Denture movements occur regardless of the type of posterior occlusal forms used. Sheppard (1964) suggested the expression "enter bolus, enter balance" to account for this observation. Balanced occlusion can even be of questionable significance during mastication if interferences are built into the occlusion because of inaccurate jaw relation records. Studies in dentulous patients indicate that interferences on the nonchewing side have a damaging potential (Schuyler, 1935; Ramfjord, 1961). Interceptive occlusal contacts on the nonchewing side interfere with the delicate integrated neuromuscular coordination used in chewing. Not only are these interferences confusing and distressing to the patient, but they also impair masticatory efficiency (Feldman, 1971).

In longitudinal studies, Bergman and associates (1964 and 1971) have shown that after 2-year and 1-year periods of wearing complete dentures, defective occlusion was observed in several of the patients' dentures. When these observations are seen in the context of Tallgren's review (1972), the changes in occlusion or articulation are understandable. Changes in occlusal balance occur, regardless of the type of posterior tooth form used (Zarb and associates, 1970).

Although proof is lacking to support the validity of bilateral balance, balanced occlusion is essential during those times of tooth contact during mandibular movements when no food is in the mouth. The horizontal movements generated on an articulator do not simulate functional jaw movements; they in fact simulate parafunctional jaw movements (Fig. 21-1, A to C), and artificial teeth are balanced to provide maximum denture stabilization during these anticipated mandibular activities. Such a balanced occlusion can usually be readily obtained with anatomic teeth. This objective can also be achieved with nonanatomic teeth by the use of a compensating curve, ramplike type of arrangement and probably with the flat plane type of tooth arrangement as well (Fig. 21-1, D to G). Several clinicians dismiss the flat plane type of arrangement as ensuring contact in centric relation only. The premise must be postulated, however, that during jaw movements the combination of the exerted muscle forces and the resiliency of the supporting mucosal tissues will actually allow for a bilateral contact or balanced occlusion to develop in many patients over a limited range of mandibular movement. The exact range of freedom of parafunctional tooth contacts has not been determined. It is tempting to presume that this area is within the range of bilateral nonanatomic tooth contacts as arranged and so readily achieved on a flat plane.

There is a dearth of evidence to support any specific method or philosophy of articulation as being the optimal one. On the other hand, numerous clinical observations have been made that successful denture wearing is probably more dependent on a good patient-dentist relationship, coupled with a careful clinical technique, than on any particular technique per se.

There exists a distinct cosmetic limitation to the use of cuspless teeth. The concept of a flat occlusal plane that allows for maximum horizon-

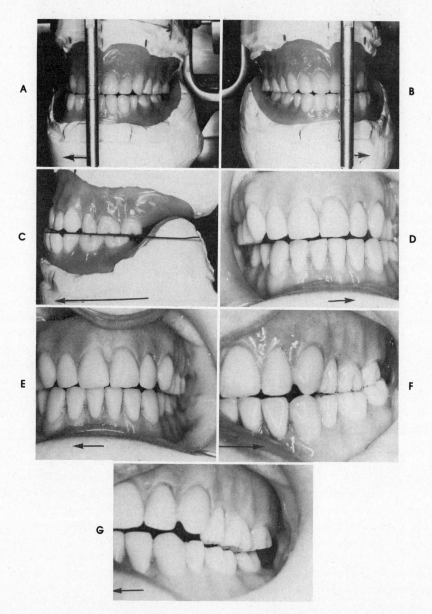

Fig. 21-1. A to **C,** Right, left, and protrusive mandibular excursions carried out on articulator to stimulate bruxing or parafunctional movements of the mandible. **D** and **E,** Intraoral views showing left and right excursions with posterior teeth set up on a flat plane. **F** and **G,** Left intraoral working and balancing contacts with posterior teeth set up so that the second molars serve as a ramp to maintain balancing contacts. These simulated movements are carried out in the mouth for parafunctional, rather than functional, purposes.

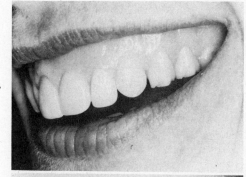

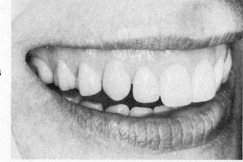

Fig. 21-2. Obviously unesthetic appearance of a nonana-tomic premolar, **A,** is remedied by recontouring of the mesial and distal marginal ridges, **B.**

tal mandibular movements is predicated on the use of a neutral or zero-degree incisal guidance. Most edentulous patients can be adequately treated by use of an incisal guidance with no vertical overlap of the anterior teeth. In most patients sufficient horizontal overlap of the incisors can be used to permit some jaw movement in a protrusive direction without seriously compromising the patient's esthetic appearance. However, when proper appearance of the patient requires a vertical overlap of the anterior teeth, cusp posterior teeth must be used (e.g., in a modified Angle Class II, division 2, type of anterior tooth arrangement). If an extra expenditure of time and effort should be required for using anatomic teeth in these situations, it is, of course, justified.

The actual morphologic shortcoming of a cuspless posterior tooth can frequently be com-pensated for by slight reshaping of the mesial and distal corners of the premolars with a sand-paper disk to develop the appearance of a cusp. A more pleasing esthetic result can then be obtained (Fig. 21-2).

TEMPOROMANDIBULAR JOINT DISTURBANCES

The temporomandibular joint probably influences the inclinations of teeth, and likewise the inclinations of teeth influence the joint. If the teeth and joint are in harmony as to their inclinations in centric occlusion and during eccentric movements, the joint can be expected to remain healthy. However, when the inclines of these factors are not in harmony because of loss and shifting of teeth, excessive wear of cusp inclines, or incorrectly constructed restorations such as inlays, crowns, fixed partial dentures, and removable partial and complete dentures, a pathologic condition may result. When these two factors are not in harmony, the joint may be the stronger of the two, in which case the teeth and supporting structures will be destroyed, or the reverse may be true, and the joint will bear the brunt of this malocclusion. This diseased condition of the joint may be manifest by clicking sounds, neuralgia, obscure headaches, pain and discomfort in the joint during mastication, a burning sensation of the tongue, and sometimes trismus of varying degrees. The presence of these symptoms must not be construed as the result of occlusal disharmony; yet this occlusal disharmony must always be investigated as a potential etiologic factor whenever these disturbances are present. The dental literature provides numerous examples of the correlation between occlusal disharmonies and temporomandibular joint dysfunction.

FACTORS OF CENTRIC OCCLUSION

Generally speaking, *occlude* in medical science means 'to close.' Therefore, the term *occlude* used in reference to the teeth should be taken to mean the position of the teeth in contact. Centric occlusion would mean, strictly speaking, that the teeth are in contact when the mandible is in centric relation to the head. However, centric occlusion is usually defined as that position of the maxillary and mandibular dental arches wherein the teeth are making maximum contact. (It must be remembered that centric occlusion is the normal termination of masticatory closure.) This definition then includes the position of the mandible when the teeth have been worn out of centric occlusion. For that reason, centric occlusion and centric relation with tooth contact may not coincide. Centric occlusion and centric relation in a child when the teeth are in contact under normal conditions are identical. As wear progresses and destruction takes place, the mandible gradually assumes a different position from centric relation. This is an extremely important factor in the registration of occlusal relations in complete denture construction of maxillary dentures, mandibular dentures, or both. This may readily be demonstrated by means of motion pictures showing the position of the mandible under heavy biting stress. In other words, a patient when chewing lightly may use habitual eccentric occlusion and relation. These may be protrusive or lateral or a combination of both relations, but when a resistant bolus of food is encountered, the mandible tends to work completely back to the retrusive position. For this reason, the relation of the patient's mandible to the maxillae should be recorded in the most retruded position in order to maintain maximum stability and efficiency.

UNDERSTANDING CENTRIC RELATION

Centric relation is defined as the most posterior relation of the mandible to the maxillae at the established vertical relation. This definition takes into consideration the three-dimensional nature of centric relation and the fact that the horizontal position of the *body* of the mandible changes with changes in its vertical relation, even though the condyles remain in their most posterior positions. It is more accurate than other definitions that are related to a technique used to locate or record it. For example, the definition that specifies centric relation as "the

most retruded position of the mandible from which lateral movements can be made at given degree of jaw separation" is based on the use of a Gothic arch (needle point) tracing technique for making the registration. This definition cannot be appropriately applied to some other methods for recording the centric relation. For example, interocclusal record techniques and hinge axis techniques for recording centric relation do not permit the use of any lateral movement when the centric relation record is made.

Vertical force applied while the centric relation record is made may be unevenly applied. This would cause more displacement on one side than the other, and the centric relation established from the uneven record would be incorrect, even though the bones of the jaws were in centric relation when the record was made. Also, the record can be incorrect, even when the mandible is in the position of centric relation, if the soft tissues of one part of the basal seat are thicker and therefore softer and more easily displaced than those of the other parts of the basal seat. In these situations the teeth of the dentures would touch first on the side where the greatest displacement had occurred, even though the bones of the mandible and the cranium were precisely in centric relation. The centric jaw relation must be recorded in such a way that the teeth will meet simultaneously at their first contact in centric occlusion.

Eccentric occlusion is defined as protrusive and right and left lateral contacts of the inclined planes of the teeth when the jaw is not moving.

Articulation can be defined as the relationships of the teeth during movements into and away from eccentric position while the teeth are in contact. It is occlusion in motion.

CRITICAL COMPONENTS IN THE ARRANGEMENTS OF POSTERIOR TEETH

The maxillary and mandibular natural teeth have a normal cuspal relation to each other that maintains their positional and functional relationship. In centric occlusion, this relation

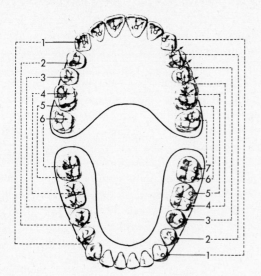

Fig. 21-3. Diagram with lines that connect from cusp, or point, on one denture to fossa on which it rests in centric relation on opposing denture. Three arrows indicate the directions in which this point or cusp travels in the working-side movement, the balancing-side movement, and the protrusive movement.

causes certain cusps to rest in opposing fossae. These cusps perform a definite function (Fig. 21-3). Nature maintains a certain harmony of inclines in eccentric positions. For instance, in left lateral movement wherein the left side becomes the working side and the right side the balancing side, the mandibular buccal cusps slide out between opposing maxillary buccal cusps to maintain contact. The maxillary lingual cusps on the left (working) side move between their opposing mandibular lingual cusps to maintain contact. The mandibular left anterior teeth slide out on the inclines of the maxillary left incisors to maintain contact. The lingual cusps of the maxillary teeth on the right (balancing) side slide on the inclines of the lingual surfaces of the buccal cusps of the mandibular teeth to maintain contact on this side. In such a left lateral movement, the lingual inclines of the maxillary buccal cusps and the buccal inclines of the mandibular lingual cusps on the left side and the lingual inclines on the left maxillary anterior teeth are in harmony with the lingual inclines of the mandibular buccal cusps on the right side. The inclination of the condylar path on the right side is also in harmony with these inclines in this movement. Other eccentric movements, if all conditions are normal, have comparable harmonies of cusp inclines in the various comparable positions.

Generally speaking, the same laws of occlusion apply in natural teeth as in complete dentures. However, the vertical overlap, and therefore the incisal guide angle, is already established in natural teeth, whereas the vertical overlap in complete dentures is partly in the hands of the dentist. It can be made at the sharp angle of 60 or more degrees or at the flatter angle of 5 or even 0 degrees, at the dentist's discretion, and still have harmonious occlusal balance. Nevertheless, not all inclines are desirable, even though they balance. The laws of occlusion can be made to apply, regardless of what the factors may be in natural or complete dentures. However, occlusal balance and harmony apply to and can be attained in all manner of combinations of controlling factors.

Two controlling end factors must be considered in complete denture occlusion: the condylar inclination and the incisal angle or incisal guide angle. In the edentulous patient only one factor, the condylar inclination, is determined by the patient. The dentist has no control over the condylar inclination that the patient possesses and cannot change or modify it to fit a theory. Any lack of harmony between tooth inclines and the condylar inclines could result in disturbances to the temporomandibular articulation and to lasting stability of the dentures. The other controlling end factor is established by the dentist in the choice of setting *but within the limits of esthetics*. It is understood that the more closely the incisal guide angle approaches zero degrees, the more stable the dentures will be because of the reduction of lateral inclines. However, there are limitations in this reduction that the dentist must consider, such as those of esthetics, ridge fullness, and ridge relation, any of which may change the incisal guide angle.

LAWS OF PROTRUSIVE OCCLUSION

The five principal factors in the laws of occlusion for protrusive movement, as stated by Hanau, are inclination of the condylar guidance, prominence of the compensating curve, inclination of the plane of orientation, inclination of the incisal guidance, and height of the cusps.

The order of the factors is revised, principally for clarity and convenience. A few words have been changed, such as *height* to *inclination*, because the inclination of the cusp is the more important factor to be considered in arrangement of the teeth.

The phrase *plane of orientation* has been changed to *orientation of the occlusal plane* because it describes more adequately the action that takes place. The word *orient* means 'to find the proper bearings or relations of.' Thus the term *orientation of the plane* is a factor to be determined, whereas the phrase *plane of orientation* implies that this factor already has been determined.

The five principal factors restated would be inclination of the condylar guidance, inclination of the incisal guidance, orientation of the occlusal plane, inclination of the cusps, and prominence of the compensating curve.

The first and second factors (inclination of condylar guidance and inclination of the incisal

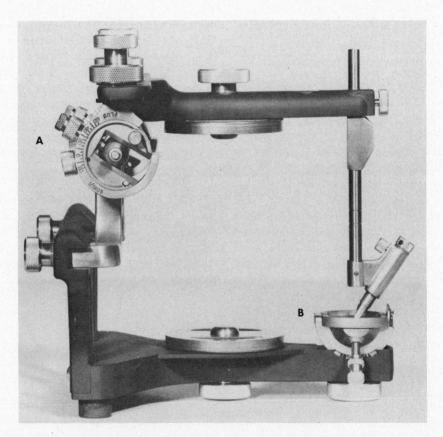

Fig. 21-4. A, Condylar inclination and, **B,** incisal guide incline are the controlling end factors and are determined before the three other factors are established by the dentist.

guidance) control the movements of the articulator, whereas the other three (orientation of the plane, inclination of the cusps, and prominence of the compensating curve) may be changed by the dentist to attain harmony among these five factors (Fig. 21-4).

Fig. 21-5 represents the first factor of occlusion, condylar inclination, which is the only factor given by the patient. This factor is obtained by means of protrusive registration.

As shown in Fig. 21-6, the condylar factor has been transferred to the condylar guidance setting on the articulator. Fig. 21-7 shows the incisal guide angle (the second factor of occlusion) as set by the dentist to determine the second controlling path of the articulator. This setting of the incisal guide angle is influenced by the amount of vertical and horizontal overlap that the dentist selects, which is really a cosmetic decision.

As has been stated, the two end factors are the condylar guidance and the incisal guidance. The condylar guidance is fixed by the patient, and the incisal guidance is governed mostly by the dentist's choice of the desired inclination. This inclination may be changed by the amount of vertical overlap and horizontal overlap. The greater the horizontal overlap, the more it reduces the angle of inclination, the vertical overlap remaining the same; of course, it goes without saying that the less the vertical overlap, the less the angle of inclination will be.

The mandible is guided into entirely different positions by changing the incisal inclination. The posterior teeth are closer to the action of the incisal inclination than they are to the condylar inclination (Fig. 21-8). Therefore greater influence is exercised on the teeth by the incisal inclination than by the condylar guidance.

In Fig. 21-9 are shown mandibles with different vertical overlaps. The mandible shown in A has a very shallow vertical overlap, with a resultant lowered cusp inclination, whereas the mandible shown in B has a steep vertical overlap and a consequent steep cusp inclination. In these drawings is shown how the cusp inclination is

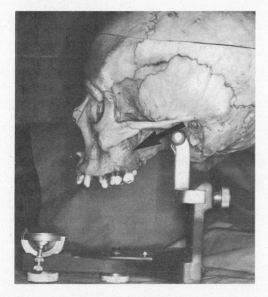

Fig. 21-5. Arrow simulates the condyle path inclination, which is the only control over jaw movement that an edentulous patient has.

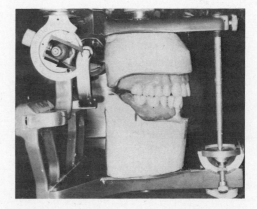

Fig. 21-6. Articulator mounting with the condyle path inclination shown in Fig. 21-5 transferred to the articulator condyle path on the instrument.

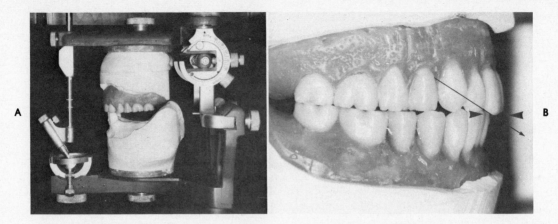

Fig. 21-7. Incisal guide angle, which is controlled by the dentist, is established on the articulator. **A,** A flat incisal guide table and, **B,** one of approximately 15 degrees (in this case shown at the incisor level). This angle was based on the dentist's choice of incisor teeth setup or overlap as dictated by cosmetic judgment.

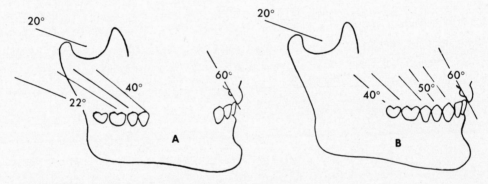

Fig. 21-8. A, Resultant cusp angulation if, hypothetically, the teeth were to be moved closer to the condyle influence. **B,** Same condyle and incisal inclinations, with the resultant cusp angulation when the teeth are moved forward closer to the incisal guide influence.

automatically determined from a rotational center that has been determined by lines drawn at right angles to the two determining end factors, the incisal and condylar guidance surfaces.

All actions in protrusive movement of the articulator are on arcs from a center that has been determined by the intersection of lines drawn at right angles to the guiding surfaces. These actions are controlled by the condylar guidance surface and the incisal guidance sur-

face. The steep vertical overlap places the rotational center below and posterior to the mandible, whereas the shallow vertical overlap places it above the mandible (Fig. 21-9). These are theoretical factors that help give a better understanding of articulator and jaw movements. However, in reality these movements need not be worked out in the construction of a denture because the articulator automatically establishes them.

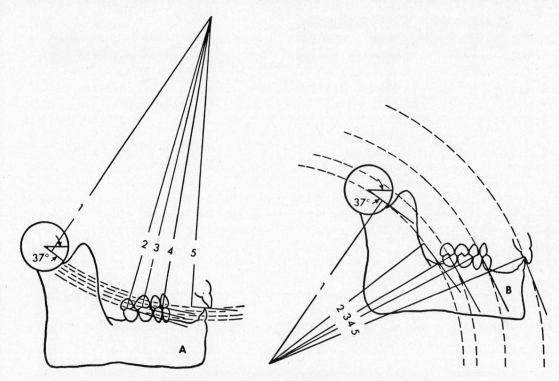

Fig. 21-9. A, Rotational center as a result of a shallow vertical overlap. **B,** Rotational center below the mandible as a result of a steep vertical overlap. Occlusion developed as in **B** would tend to push the upper denture forward more than occlusion with the rotational center above the level of the occlusal plane.

It must be reemphasized that the two end factors, condylar surface and incisal surface, establish and determine movement. The other three factors (orientation of the plane, inclination of the cusps, and prominence of the compensating curve) may be changed so that they will move on concentric curves, as represented in Fig. 21-9, lines 2 to 4. Notice that one can change the tooth inclines by inclining the occlusal plane up or down at the back, tipping the long axes of the teeth, or grinding the cusp inclinations. Notice further that teeth can be set on varying levels and still be in harmony of movement with the articulator. However, to locate an occlusal plane high or low to favor the weaker of the two ridges can cause both esthetic and mechanical trouble. If the soft tissues surrounding the dentures are

to function as they did for natural teeth, the occlusal plane should be oriented exactly as it was when the natural teeth were present. Thus the orientation of the occlusal plane becomes the third fixed factor of occlusion. By positioning the anterior teeth correctly for esthetic appearance and locating the posterior end of the occlusal plane approximately level two thirds of the way up the retromolar pad, the dentist fixes the orientation of the occlusal plane. Any necessary alterations for balancing the occlusion must therefore be made on other factors affecting the occlusion, that is, cuspal inclination or prominence of the compensating curve.

The inclination of the cusps of the teeth is the fourth factor of occlusion. The cuspal inclination of a tooth refers to the angle between the total occlusal surface of the tooth and the inclination of the cusp in relation to that surface. For example, the designation 33-degree tooth indicates that the mesial slopes of the cusps make a 33-degree angle with a plane touching the tips of all of the cusps of the tooth. In other words, if the long axis of the tooth is perfectly vertical, the plane of reference (the horizontal plane) would be at right angles to the vertical axis of the tooth. The mesial inclines would have a 33-degree angle to this horizontal plane.

The cusp inclination designated by the manufacturer, however, is not necessarily the effective inclination when the tooth is arranged in occlusion on the articulator. The basic inclination of the cusps is made steeper when the distal end of the lower tooth is set higher than the mesial end. The cuspal inclination can be reduced when the distal end of the lower tooth is set lower than the mesial end. Similar adjustments can be made in the inclinations of the buccal and lingual cusps when the buccolingual long axes of the teeth are tipped. Thus tipping the teeth can produce a compensating curve and make the effective height of the cusps greater or less. By this means, even zero-degree teeth can be arranged to present inclined planes to their opposing teeth.

The fifth factor of occlusion is the prominence of the compensating curve. The factor of the compensating curve is valuable because it allows the dentist to alter cusp height without changing the form of the manufactured teeth. Thus the dentist can make the cusps longer or shorter (steeper or flatter) simply by inclining the long axes of the teeth to conform to the end guidelines.

If the teeth themselves do not have cusps, the compensating curve can be used to produce the equivalent of cusps. The mesial inclines of the lower teeth can be thought of as actual segments of a compensating curve that is cut into pieces, with the pieces arranged in a more or less straight line. If each of these pieces were arranged to line up with all the others, the result would be a compensating curve with a single continuous surface. Such a surface can be used with zero-degree teeth.

It must be understood that the factors of occlusion are described separately for clarity but that they are adjusted simultaneously in the setting of the teeth to obtain harmony and balance with the movement of the articulator.

LAWS OF LATERAL OCCLUSION

The principal factors for lateral occlusion are similar to the ones given for protrusive occlusion. The two end factors controlling protrusive occlusion are condylar guidance inclines and incisal guide inclines. The two end factors controlling lateral movement are the condylar guidance incline on the balancing side and the lingual inclines of the upper buccal cusps and the buccal inclines of the lower lingual cusps on the working side. These inclines must be in harmony with the path of the lower canine to meet the upper canine end to end.

It is understood that there is more than one center of rotation in the movements of the jaw. In fact, the rotational centers are infinite in number. If the mandible rotates laterally with one condyle in a fixed position, it can generally be classified as having two rotational centers. However, the mandible can start in a protrusive position and then shift to lateral or to any intermediate position. Nevertheless, the movements of the mandible are controlled by both tooth and condyle factors and can be grouped into two general groups of rotational centers. When we stop at any given eccentric position, we can draw lines at right angles to the cusps upon which the mandible has stopped and determine the rotational center for that position. For instance, the mandible shown in Fig. 21-10 has moved to the left, and the mandibular teeth have stopped at a certain point on the opposing cusp incline on the left side. A line drawn at right angles to the buccal incline of the mandibular lingual cusp on the working side and another line at right angles to the lingual surface of the mandibular buccal cusp on the balancing side meet at *B*. All inclines involved in this left lateral

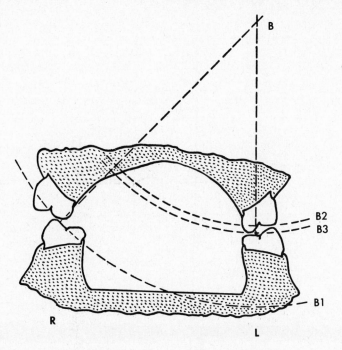

Fig. 21-10. Establishment of the center of rotation in a lateral movement by lines drawn at right angles to cusp inclines. *B1, B2,* and *B3* are concentric circles from the center *B.*

position must be on the curves of arcs drawn from this rotational center. The rotational center shifts according to the direction in which the mandible (or mandibular member of the articulator) moves from centric position. This rotational center is established by lines drawn at right angles to the working-side inclines, the balancing-side inclines, and the balancing-side condyle. These parallel arcs of concentric circles at varying distances from the center are all in harmony when in movement.

The rotational center may slide laterally while the mandible is in lateral occlusion. This lateral movement or shift of the mandible is the result of the movement of the condyles along the lateral inclines of the mandibular fossae. This translatory movement is known as the Bennett movement. According to the findings of Gysi, 15 degrees is the average Bennett movement. (It is well to remember that a rotational center can shift laterally and still form an arc from the shifting rotational center.)

Fig. 21-11 is a schematic drawing showing the effect of incisal and condylar inclination on posterior tooth cusp inclination on both the working and the balancing sides. Notice the difference in working-side and balancing-side inclines. In the example cited, this difference is attributable to the fact that the condyle on the working side neither rises nor falls but merely rotates (except for Bennett movement). For this reason, the working-side inclines are not so steep as the balancing-side inclines. Notice how the angle of inclination on the working side is less in the posterior area and greater toward the incisal area and how the degree of inclination changes with the distance away from the condyle and toward the incisal area and how the degree of inclination changes with the distance away from the condyle and toward the incisal area. If the

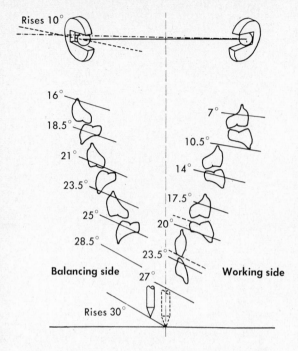

Fig. 21-11. Influence of incisal guidance and condylar inclines on the working and balancing sides. Condylar guidance, 10 degrees; incisal guidance, 30 degrees.

degree of inclination of the incisal guidance were zero, all the working-side inclines would be zero. Since in this instance the incisal guidance is 30 degrees, we start with a smaller degree of angulation in the posterior region and gradually increase toward 30 degrees as the incisal area is approached.

The balancing-side inclines are steeper than the working-side inclines because there are two factors of angulation: the incisal, 30 degrees, and the condylar, 10 degrees. The dentist controls the setting of the incisal inclination, and the patient registers the condylar inclination; then the articulator automatically controls the inclinations of the teeth in all positions after the dentist has moved the teeth so that they are in contact in all movements, that is, have obtained harmony and occlusal balance.

In the discussion of occlusion it was pointed out that the edentulous patient provides the condyle inclination and nothing regarding incisal inclination. It has been noted further that the condyle inclination is not the only influential factor; in fact, it is not so great a factor as the amount of vertical overlap or incisal guidance (the dentist's decision) is. With an edentulous patient there is no way of knowing what the incisal guidance factor was in the natural dentition or what it should be in the complete dentures. Therefore, of necessity the dentist must select the amount of vertical overlap or incisal inclination. A study of the geometric influences of inclines shows that reduction of cusp inclination is a great stabilizer for dentures. The obvious question that arises is with regard to the advisability of having flat occlusal surfaces throughout. This theoretically cannot be done and have bilateral balance, since the condyles do not presumably move horizontally. Therefore, again in theory, there must be some inclination of the occluding surfaces to harmonize with the downward movement of the mandible. Since the stability of dentures varies with cusp inclination, an inclination that is as flat as possible is selected for complete dentures. A brief study of the effect of vertical forces on varying degrees of inclination will emphasize the desirability of the greatest possible cusp reduction for stabilization. A study of Fig. 21-12 shows this graphically. In A it will be seen that the tooth and diagrammatic incline cause the buccal surface to shift. In B less shifting influence is shown. In C there is still less, and in D there is no shifting influence at all. These diagrams show readily that inclines disturb stability of dentures and should be reduced to a minimum. Occlusion is one of the retentive and stabilizing forces that impressions cannot overcome, no matter how great an amount of initial retention they may possess.

One related factor that may seem contradictory to the foregoing must be mentioned here. Reduction of cuspal inclines does not necessarily eliminate lateral forces on teeth and dentures. Mastication with cusp teeth is accomplished

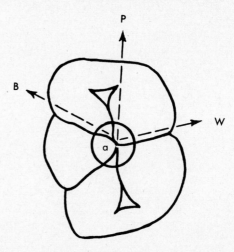

Fig. 21-13. Directional movement of maxillary cusp on posterior mandibular tooth. *a,* Maxillary cusp; *B,* direction of balancing movement; *W,* direction of working-side movement; *P,* direction of protrusive movement.

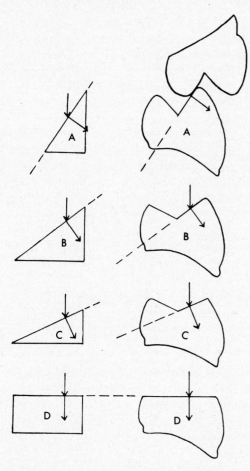

Fig. 21-12. Comparative study of the resultant forces of inclines.

with essentially vertical closing forces. The cusps cut, tear, and shear, as well as crush, food. Teeth with zero-degree cusps cannot shear food *unless* some horizontal movement is included in the chewing cycle. This horizontal movement induced by the muscles of mastication transmits horizontal forces to the supporting structures and may cause more denture movement than the cuspal inclines.

In Fig. 21-13 are shown the directional movements of the mandible as described by the cusps over their opposing surfaces. If one assumes that the circle, *a,* is an opposing maxillary cusp mov-

ing over the surfaces of a mandibular first molar, the anteroposterior arrow, *P,* shows the direction of contact between the cusp and the inclined plane in a straight protrusive movement. Arrow *B* indicates a lateral movement, which is diagonal in the balancing direction, and arrow *W* shows the movement of the cusp in the working direction. One must not take for granted that the mandible makes only these three grooved movements. It can make all movements that may be composites of *B* and *P* or *P* and *W*, which means that the mandible can move and occupy any part of the space between arrows *B* and *W*.

Well-formed, unworn, and healthy natural teeth in normal occlusion guide the mandible through these general directional movements. With the dental arch intact and with good supporting structures, the periodontium of such teeth will stand the shock of guiding the mandible. On the other hand, the support for denture bases is such a small fraction of the support for natural teeth (Chapter 1) that denture bases should have only a small fraction of the lateral and protrusive cusp inclines of natural teeth.

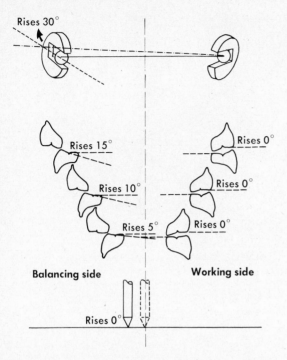

Fig. 21-14. Schematic drawing of cuspal inclinations with a steep condylar guidance and horizontal, or zero-degree, incisal guidance.

Such a realization almost implies an ideal of zero-degree guidance for both the incisal and condylar factors of occlusion. Hence the final argument between the two occlusal morphology schools (anatomic versus nonanatomic) hinges on the dentist's perception of the importance of a patient-determined versus a dentist-determined condylar guidance.

If the plan of occlusion is to have the least possible cuspal inclines, teeth should be selected and arranged according to this plan. Posterior teeth should have no more than a 5-degree angle in the premolars and should then become progressively steeper in the second molar region, depending of course on the condylar guidance. However, if the vertical overlap of the anterior teeth develops an incisal guidance steeper than 5 degrees, teeth with steeper cuspal inclinations must be used.

This plan of occlusion for complete dentures calls for the reduction of all inclines or cusps that interfere with the movement between incisal guidance and condylar guidance. Denture bases can ill afford cusps that travel in established grooves. This means that the incisal pin is not limited to the outside path of a Gothic arch, but can travel anywhere within this outside path. It should travel on any combination of protrusive and lateral movements without striking the slightest rise or unevenness. Occlusion should be smooth running.

In Fig. 21-14 is shown the scheme for selecting, setting, and grinding to fit a plan of horizontal incisal guidance and whatever condylar guidance the patient may have (30 degrees in the illustration). As will be seen, the working-side inclines on all the teeth are horizontal. These working-side inclines are determined by the horizontal movement of the working-side condyle, which merely rotates and does not rise or fall, and by the incisal guidance, which moves sideways but does not rise or fall. The balancing-side inclines start at zero degrees, or nearly so, in the premolar region and increase progressively as they approach the 30-degree balancing condyle inclination.

OCCLUSAL SCHEMES USED IN COMPLETE DENTURES FOR EDENTULOUS PATIENTS

The form of posterior teeth should be selected in the context of the dentist's broad objectives to fulfill the requirements of (1) esthetics, (2) harmonious function, and (3) maintenance of hard and soft tissues of the edentulous arches. Every dentist aims at fulfilling these objectives, regardless of the posterior tooth form selected. Posterior tooth forms have aroused a great deal of controversy among clinicians and researchers. Generally, most of the participants in the debate on the ideal posterior tooth form believe that the argument is settled and their opponents are wrong. Direct evidence is lacking to support any one concept.

There are several schools of thought on the choice of occlusal forms of posterior teeth for

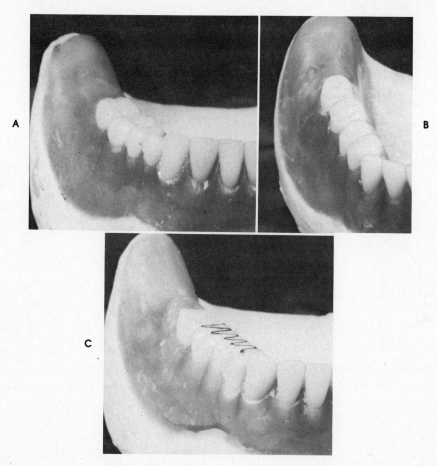

Fig. 21-15. Three of several occlusal schemes represent varying concepts in arrangement of posterior teeth. **A,** Anatomic occlusion using 33-degree posterior teeth set with a compensating curve. **B,** Occlusion using posterior teeth set with a buccolingual reverse curve on the premolars and first molars and with the second molars shaped and positioned to provide balancing contacts. **C,** Nonanatomic occlusion using zero-degree posterior teeth with embedded matallic "cutters" to enhance masticatory efficiency.

prosthetic restoration (Fig. 21-15), though only the two major ones are described here. These are the anatomic and nonanatomic techniques of posterior tooth morphology.

Anatomic teeth

The proponents of anatomic teeth insist that nature designed the tooth in a form best suited for the function of mastication. Cusp teeth have cutting blades so arranged that a part of the

nearly vertical closing force can shear food. Their contours can crush and triturate food when the proper forces are applied. Adequate sluiceways or escapes for food are present, which avoids the need for excessive pressures. The chewing efficiency of anatomic teeth for some foods is greater than that of the modified tooth forms. The cuspal inclinations facilitate the development of bilateral balance (contact) in the various eccentric occlusions. Cusps provide

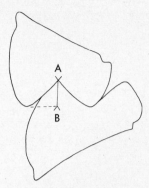

Fig. 21-16. Distance *A-B* represents the thickness of the occlusal pattern in eccentric occlusions.

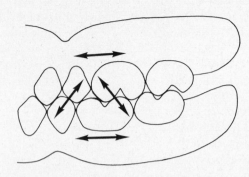

Fig. 21-17. Any possible tendency toward rotation produced by balancing tooth inclines is neutralized by the opposing inclines of cusps on the working side.

thickness of the occlusal pattern in eccentric occlusions, which is an aid in the development of balanced occlusion (Fig. 21-16).

Cusp teeth provide a resistance to denture rotation in relation to each other and to their bases, which is lacking in flat-cusp teeth (Fig. 21-17). The interdigitating cusps on the working side provide neutralizing incline plane contacts that tend to prevent rotation of the denture bases.

Nonanatomic teeth

Dentists who support the second school of thought, the concept of nonanatomic teeth, base their hypotheses on the following evidence (Feldmann, 1971).

Tooth contacts occur during mastication on the chewing and, even more frequently, on the nonchewing sides. These contacts may occur irrespective of the form or arrangement of artificial teeth used. Tooth contacts also occur during swallowing and sleep. Most tooth contacts tend to be fleeting in nature, with the possible exception of the prolonged contacts occurring during parafunctional movements. A good deal of evidence supports the conclusion that patients do most of their chewing in centric occlusion, indicating that this position is aimed for during jaw closure. Tooth contacts do not always occur in

the same horizontal position. Patient posture and denture base dislodgment, or movement, probably influence the location of these contacts. A cuspless occlusal scheme eliminates the possibility of deflective occlusal contacts when there is no food in the mouth.

The use of the patient's centric relation position does not imply that the patient is expected to masticate and swallow exclusively in that position. Many jaw closures also occur not only in proximity to but also anterior to the centric relation. This supports the concept that an area of freedom of tooth contact in the occlusion anterior and lateral to the centric relation should be provided for in any occlusal scheme. Such freedom is easily achieved by use of cuspless teeth.

The use of cuspless teeth involves the expenditure of less laboratory time and effort and can thus reduce the cost of treatment or save working hours for the dentist. The economic responsibility to the patient and the expense of the dentist's time are vitally connected with the phase of denture construction. This argument may be a significant one in the context of today's socioeconomic realities.

Advantages cited for nonanatomic teeth include (1) versatility of use, hence their employment in Class II and Class III jaw relationships; (2) permitting closure of the jaws over a broad contact area; (3) creating minimal horizontal pressures; (4) allowing for easier servicing of the complete dentures; and (5) allowing construction of dentures with a simple technique and articulator.

Those who prefer the nonanatomic occlusal forms claim that damage to the basal seat of the dentures is caused by the intercuspation of the cusp teeth as the vertical dimension of occlusion is lost through shrinkage of the ridges. The loss of the denture foundation permits the jaws to close beyond the level at which occlusal contact was made when the dentures were first inserted. Such action causes the body of the mandible (and the lower teeth) to move forward. Because of the forward movement of the body of the mandible, the mesial inclines of the cusps of the lower teeth make their first contacts against the distal inclines of the cusps of the upper teeth. Thus the teeth can no longer contact in centric occlusion though the mandible is in centric relation. Such a malrelation forces the upper denture forward and the lower denture backward.

On the other hand, nonanatomic teeth suffer from the following disadvantages: (1) their anatomic form is esthetically inferior to that of cusp teeth (Fig. 21-18); (2) some patients complain of their inability to penetrate food effectively, which renders the dentures mechanically inefficient; and (3) they probably require the application of force in a nearly horizontal direction of jaw movement to shear food, and this results in lateral forces against the residual ridges.

Several other schools of thought on posterior tooth form and arrangement are also in evidence, each receiving varying support from different teaching centers and practitioners. In the absence of conclusive research on this matter, it appears reasonable to suggest that any tooth form, properly used, can fulfill the dentist's and patient's objectives of a functional and esthetically pleasing result. Such a result should also be accompanied by a commitment to the objective of minimal supporting-tissue changes in a longi-

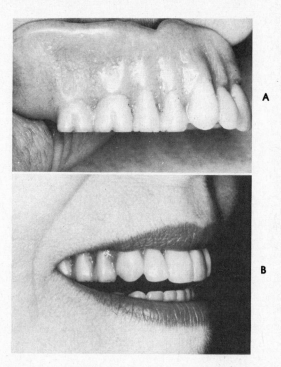

Fig. 21-18. A, Extraoral and, **B,** intraoral views of a nonanatomic posterior tooth arrangement, illustrating the poor cosmetic effect achieved. See Fig. 21-2 for a solution to this problem.

tudinal context. The latter objective is often described, though it is rarely encountered.

TECHNIQUES FOR ARRANGING CUSP TEETH IN BALANCED OCCLUSION
Technique setting each mandibular posterior tooth before corresponding maxillary tooth set

The anterior teeth are set first to their correct positions as indicated by esthetics. If the ridge relations are normal and the vertical and horizontal overlaps are approximately 1.5 mm each, the mandibular first premolar is set first. If the horizontal overlap is more than 1.5 mm, the maxillary first and second premolars are set first, and the first mandibular premolar is set after all the posterior teeth are set. In either situation, the primary consideration is that the first premolar follow the form of the residual ridge. Its buccal surface should be parallel to the buccal surface of the canine, and it should be set slightly farther buccally than the canine but *never* farther buccally than the buccal flange.

When the ideal situation is assumed, the mandibular first and second premolars are set to conform to the shape of the residual ridge. Then the maxillary first premolar is set into centric occlusion with the two lower premolars. If a space develops between the maxillary canine and premolar, the maxillary second premolar is set in alignment in the upper arch. Then the two mandibular premolars are removed, and the mandibular second premolar is set in centric occlusion with the maxillary premolars. The mandibular first premolar is fitted between the canine and premolar after the necessary amount is ground from its mesial surface. The first three premolars set are the key to the relative anteroposterior intercuspation of all the remaining posterior teeth.

Once the premolars are set and properly related to each other, positioning of all the remaining posterior teeth is quite simple. Each mandibular tooth is set before the corresponding upper tooth. It is positioned buccolingually so that a perpendicular erected to the buccal side of the crest of the residual ridge would bisect its buccal cusp. The vertical height of its occlusal surface is adjusted so that it is on a line from the mandibular canine to a level near the top of the retromolar pad. After it is set, the maxillary tooth is set to occlude with it. If the wax in the place the tooth is to be set is pooled with a hot spatula and the cervical end of the tooth is heated, the tooth can be set so that it is slightly too long. Then the articulator is closed so that the opposing teeth push the tooth up to the desired level. The index finger holds the cervical end of the tooth in place while the articulator is closed. This will develop the desired lingual cusp contact. The same procedure is used for setting all the remaining teeth.

A similar procedure can be used to set the teeth into balanced occlusion. The tooth is set into the wax so that it is too long; then the articulator is first closed in the lateral position, opened, and then closed in the centric position, opened, and then closed in the lateral position again. This procedure will cause the tooth to rotate on its long axis or tip. Thus the inclines of the cusps will guide the tooth into its proper position. The finger must keep the cervical end of the tooth from skidding laterally, and the articulator *must* be opened and closed into the desired position. The teeth *must not* slide on each other as the articulator is moved from one position to the other.

When the teeth are being set into balanced occlusion, the amount of lateral movement to be used is that necessary to bring the maxillary and mandibular canines into an end-to-end relation to each other.

No attempt is made to balance occlusion until the try-in is complete, esthetics are satisfactory, the centric relation record is correct, and the condylar guidance has been set. In centric occlusion, the cusps are resting in their opposing fossae, from which they were designed to balance (Figs. 21-19 and 21-20).

Final balancing of the teeth is attained when one changes three factors: the compensating curve, the orientation of the plane, and the inclination of the cusps after the two end factors, the incisal guidance and the condylar guidance, have been established.

Balancing of the teeth must not be allowed to change the contacting of the pin on the incisal guide table. To allow them to do so would be to change a controlling factor.

The articulator, when moving into lateral position, should show the cusps of the maxillary teeth traveling across the intercusp spaces and grooves of the mandibular teeth as points A of the maxillary teeth travel across points B of the mandibular teeth on the buccal inclines of the working side (Fig. 21-21).

On the lingual inclines of the working side, points A travel across points B on the mandibular teeth, as shown in Fig. 21-22. On the balanc-

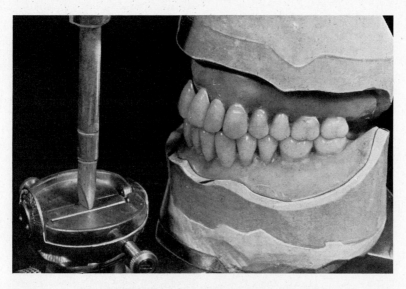

Fig. 21-19. Buccal view of teeth in centric occlusion.

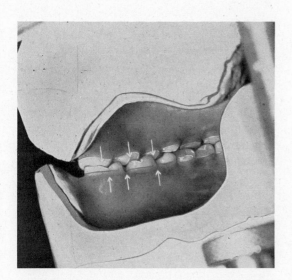

Fig. 21-20. Lingual view of teeth in centric occlusion.

ing side the lingual cusps of the maxillary teeth should be in contact with the buccal cusps of the mandibular teeth (Fig. 21-23).

Technique setting maxillary teeth first

The maxillary posterior teeth are set up, starting with the first premolar and continuing to the second molar, without placing the teeth in close proximal contact. This slight opening of the contact points allows the mandibular teeth to better assume their correct and important mesiodistal relation to the maxillary teeth. To place the maxillary teeth in their correct buccolingual position, a straightedge is placed over the crest of the mandibular ridge, as indicated by the markings on the artificial borders of the mandibular cast (Fig. 21-24). A line is scratched in the wax, with a straightedge as a guide (Fig. 21-25). The lingual cusps of the maxillary teeth are placed over this line (Fig. 21-26). The mandibular teeth then assume their buccolingual and mesiodistal position by intercuspating with the maxillary posterior teeth. Since intercuspation with an intercuspating tooth is very exacting, one can do it best by placing the mandibular first molar in position first. To place the first molar and still

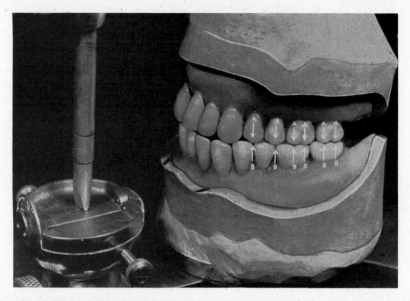

Fig. 21-21. Buccal view of teeth in left lateral position on the working side. Points *A* pass across points *B*.

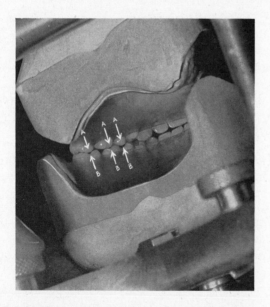

Fig. 21-22. Lingual view of the teeth in working position. Points *A* cross points *B*.

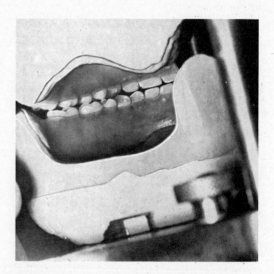

Fig. 21-23. Lingual view of the teeth in balancing position.

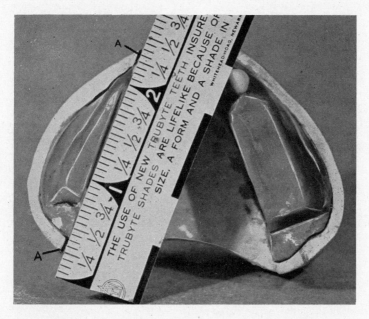

Fig. 21-24. Line to indicate crest of mandibular ridge between points *A*.

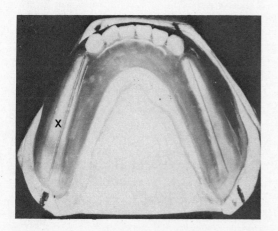

Fig. 21-25. Line, *X,* drawn between points on the artificial border of the cast. This line is only a guide. The teeth should be set on a curve conforming to shape of residual ridge.

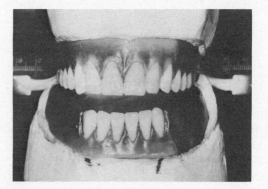

Fig. 21-26. Lingual cusps are placed directly over the lines on the mandibular occlusion rim. (See Fig. 21-25, *X.*)

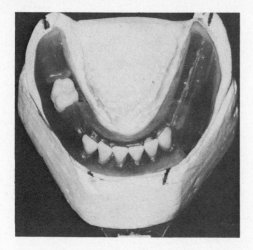

Fig. 21-27. First molar in place.

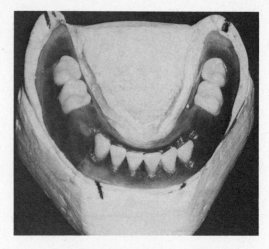

Fig. 21-28. Second molars in place.

preserve the location of the crest of the ridge on the remainder of the occlusion rim, a block of wax approximately the size of the tooth is removed (Fig. 21-27). By placing the mandibular first molar in position without adjoining teeth, the dentist can more easily determine its correct anteroposterior position. If the dentist were to start with the mandibular first premolar, the varying vertical overlap might crowd the tooth into difficult intercuspation with the maxillary teeth. This crowding would be carried into placement of all the mandibular posterior teeth. For that reason, placement of the mandibular first premolar is left to the last to take up all the variation in vertical and horizontal overlap of the anterior teeth. The first premolar is then ground to fit the remaining space.

The teeth are not arranged for balance at this time, since they are set only in their correct centric positions to the opposing teeth. Inclinations for balance are completed after the posterior teeth are all in position.

The second molar is now placed into position and has only one possible interference in assuming its correct anteroposterior position (Figs. 21-28 and 21-29).

The mandibular second premolar is next

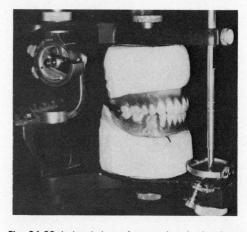

Fig. 21-29. Lateral view of second molar in place.

placed into position after another block of wax is cut away in this area (Fig. 21-30).

The mandibular first premolar is the last tooth to be placed and usually needs to be ground because vertical overlap for the patient is usually greater than the amount of vertical overlap with which the teeth were originally set up in creation of the master molds by the manufacturer (Fig. 21-31). Manufacturers could not make as many molds as there are varying ridge relations.

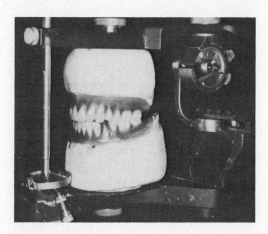

Fig. 21-30. Mandibular second premolar in place.

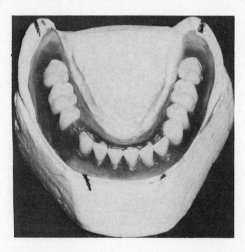

Fig. 21-31. Mandibular first premolar was too wide for space available.

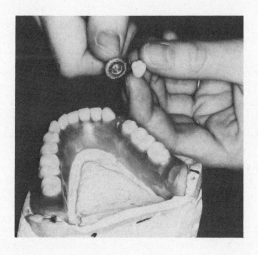

Fig. 21-32. Mandibular first premolar being ground to fit the remaining space.

For that reason, teeth must be ground and shaped to fit the space available (Fig. 21-32).

Another reason the mandibular first premolar is chosen as the last tooth in the arrangement is that it has only the buccal cusp in occlusion and does not affect esthetics as greatly by being reduced in size as would the maxillary first premolar, which shows more plainly as the lips move.

One of the common errors that cause anatom-ic teeth to be set inefficiently as to leverage and esthetics is the attempt to use a given mold of teeth without altering a single tooth. This usually crowds the mandibular anterior teeth too far forward, gives a wide effect in the premolar regions, and upsets the correct intercuspation and occlusion. The procedure in this discussion allows latitude in positioning the teeth by placing them in two sections: anterior teeth and posterior teeth. Then, in arranging the posterior

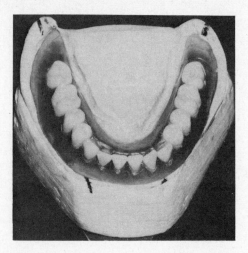

Fig. 21-33. Occlusal view with all mandibular teeth in place.

teeth, the mandibular first premolar is the only tooth that needs to be ground and adjusted to take up the ridge-relation variance. It is believed that this requires a minimum amount of effort for the achievement of acceptable leverage and esthetics (Fig. 21-33).

TECHNIQUES FOR ARRANGING CUSPLESS TEETH INTO OCCLUSION

Cuspless occlusal schemes may be designed with either a compensating curve or on a flat plane.

Cuspless teeth with a compensating curve

The arrangement of the posterior teeth is quite similar to that described in the segment on arranging anatomic teeth with a compensating curve. The teeth are set in the wax occlusion rim with use of the established contours of the occlusion rims and markings on the casts as guides. The teeth are arranged to contact maximally on a compensating curve and to harmonize with the controlling end factors (the right and left condylar inclinations and the incisal guidance). With cuspless teeth it is necessary to use a zero-degree incisal guidance to develop balancing contacts in the protrusive position (Fig. 21-34).

Practical experience indicates that it is not always possible to arrange nonanatomic teeth in balanced occlusion with a compensating curve alone. The difficulty lies in the absence of cusp height in the nonanatomic teeth. In these situations protrusive lateral balance can be attained on the articulator by use of a second molar ramp (Fig. 21-35, *A* and *B*). Even then, complete balance in all excursions is not feasible, and the dentist has to settle for a three-point balance effect (Fig. 21-35, *C*). If a vertical overlap of the anterior teeth is needed for esthetic reasons, a sufficient horizontal overlap must be introduced to prevent disocclusion of posterior teeth in a protrusive contact movement (Fig. 21-36).

It must be emphasized that using nonanatomic teeth with a compensating curve, with or without a balancing ramp, entails laboratory procedures that are not as timeconsuming as those employed in the use of posterior teeth with cusps.

Flat plane occlusion with cuspless teeth

The technique for arranging cuspless teeth on a flat plane is predicated on several premises that are distinct departures from what has been described in this chapter.

Complete denture–wearing patients should avoid incising with their anterior teeth. If they will recognize this limitation, no balancing contact will be necessary for protrusive occlusions. To assist patients in this effort, the anterior teeth are set with an incisal guidance as close to zero degrees as possible. Most patients can tolerate such as incisal guidance without a serious esthetic compromise. Occasionally, however, the patient's or dentist's desire to achieve an optimal cosmetic result necessitates a vertical overlap of the anterior teeth. This can generally be accommodated by the use of a sufficient horizontal overlap to allow a range of uniform posterior tooth contact anterior to the centric relation position (Fig. 21-36).

The condylar inclinations on the articulator are set at zero degrees while the cuspless teeth are arranged (Fig. 21-37, *A*). In this manner,

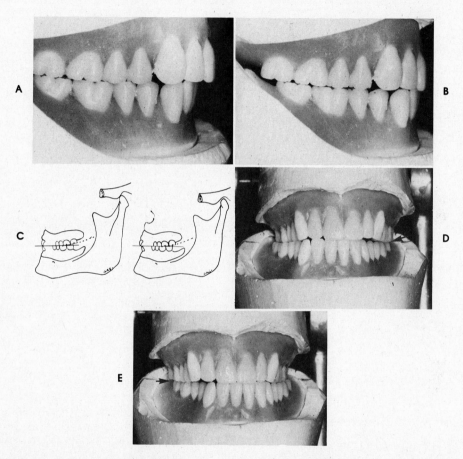

Fig. 21-34. Cuspless teeth are arranged on articulator to contact maximally on a compensating curve. **A,** In centric relation and, **B,** in a straight protrusive excursion. Both the incisal guide table on the articulator and the incisal guidance of the artificial teeth equal zero degrees. No vertical overlap of the anterior teeth is present, as represented diagrammatically in **C. D** and **E,** Right and left mandibular lateral protrusive excursions are simulated on the articulator. In both excursions, balancing-side contacts are evident *(arrows).*

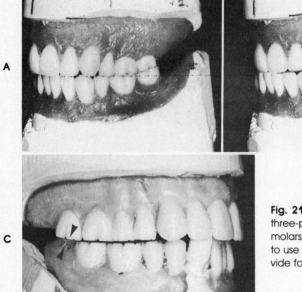

Fig. 21-35. Occasionally the dentist has to settle for a three-point balanced occlusion by setting the second molars on a ramp, **A** and **B**. If it is not technically feasible to use an artificial tooth, the wax can be carved to provide for a balancing side contact, **C**.

incising is avoided, and cusp projections above the occlusal plane are absent in the posterior segments. The Hanau or Whip Mix articulator is thereby reduced to a simple hinge articulator. With the mandibular occlusion rim on its cast in the articulator, the maxillary posterior teeth are set in the maxillary wax rim. The teeth are positioned to occlude with the flat surface of the mandibular occlusion rim and to approximate the position of the maxillary occlusion rim contour, which was previously determined. The markings established by the dentist on the maxillary cast are also used as guides in the arrangement of the teeth. The completed maxillary set-up will usually show the incisal edges of the anterior teeth, and the occlusal surfaces of all the posterior teeth to be flat against a flat plane (Fig. 21-37, *B* and *C*). Occasionally the maxillary anterior teeth are placed slightly lower in relation to the posterior occlusal plane, which results in improved cosmetic appearance. In this situation, the horizontal overlap should be adequate to allow a gliding range of posterior teeth without "tripping" the dentures.

The mandibular teeth are next arranged to maximally contact the upper teeth (Fig. 21-38). Each tooth in turn is placed in a soft wax socket made in the occlusion rim, which has been heated with a spatula, and the articulator is closed while the tooth is oriented bucolingually to conform to the contoured lower occlusion rim, to the markings on the cast, and to the maxillary teeth. The anteroposterior relation of the upper and lower teeth to each other is not critical because of the absence of cusps that would require intercuspation. Any combination of premolars or molars can be used to fill the available space. The posterior limit of the extent of these teeth is the point at which the mandibular ridge begins to curve upward (Fig. 21-39). Sometimes the large size of a patient's mouth or the patient's preoccupation with the number of

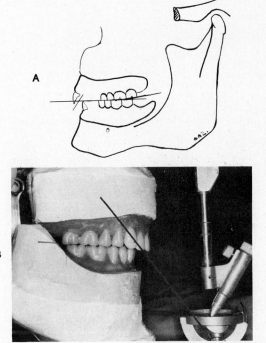

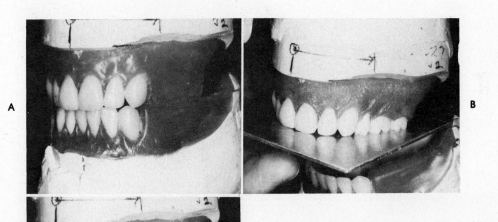

Fig. 21-36. Sufficient horizontal overlap is present in the anterior teeth to compensate for the required vertical overlap introduced for cosmetic reasons. **A,** Diagrammatic and, **B,** articulated denture setup.

Fig. 21-37. A, Anterior teeth are positioned with a zero-degree incisal guidance. **B** and **C,** Maxillary setup is completed so that incisal edges of anterior teeth and occlusal surfaces of all posterior teeth are flat against a flat plane.

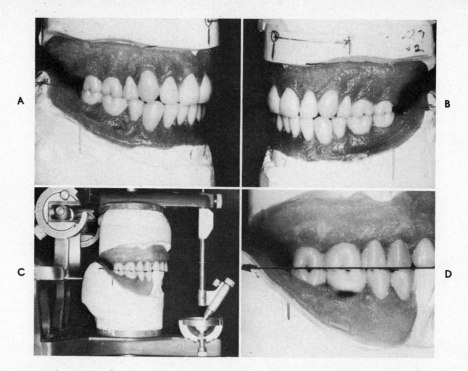

Fig. 21-38. A and **B,** Mandibular posterior teeth are arranged to maximally contact the maxillary teeth. **C,** In this case the condylar guidance and the incisal guide table on the articulator are set at zero degrees. **D,** Completed posterior tooth arrangement conforms to a flat plane.

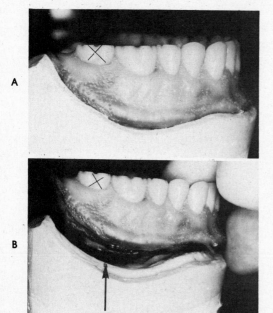

Fig. 21-39. A, Dentist should avoid setting up the last artificial mandibular tooth on slope of ridge. **B,** Cast should be marked at point where mandibular ridge begins to curve upward.

teeth present on the denture necessitate placing second or even third molars on this slope. In such situations, these teeth must not make contact with their antagonist or antagonists. In the horizontal plane, the maxillary teeth usually overlap the mandibular ones. Flat-cusp teeth are readily arranged to accommodate a unilateral or a bilateral crossbite situation.

REFERENCES

Bergman, B., Carlsson, G.E., and Ericson, S.: Effect of differences in habitual use of complete dentures on underlying tissues, Scand. J. Dent. Res. **79**:449-460, 1971.

Bergman, B., Carlsson, G.E., and Hedegård, B.: A longitudinal two-year study of a number of full denture cases, Acta Odontol. Scand. **22**:3-26, 1964.

Feldmann, E.E.: Tooth contacts in denture occlusion—centric occlusion only, Dent. Clin. North Am. **15**:875-887, 1971.

Ramfjord, S.P.: Dysfunctional temporomandibular joint and muscle pain, J. Prosthet. Dent. **11**:353-374, 1961.

Schuyler, C.H.: Fundamental principles in the correction of occlusal disharmony, natural and artificial, J. Am. Dent. Assoc. **22**:1193-1202, 1935.

Sheppard, I.M.: Incisive and related movements of the mandible, J. Prosthet. Dent. **14**:898-906, 1964.

Tallgren, A.: The continuing reduction of the residual alveolar ridges in complete denture wearers: a mixed-longitudinal study covering 25 years, J. Prosthet. Dent. **27**:120-132, 1972.

Zarb, G.A., Lewis, D.W., and Scrivener, E.W.: A clinical study of the effects of complete dentures on the oral tissues, Program and Abstracts of IADR Forty-third General Meeting, New York, 1970, No. 413, p. 152.

22

Appearance and functional harmony of denture bases

Three principal factors are concerned in the functional harmony of denture bases. They are the basal or impression surface, the leverage position and occlusal surface of the teeth, and the shape or form of the polished surfaces of the dentures (Fig. 8-1).

An increase in size of the basal surface increases the amount of adhesion, the amount of border seal, and the amount of biting resistance. These factors are discussed in Chapters 7 and 9.

The most important of all factors are the occlusal surfaces. They are discussed in Chapter 21 and therefore are not considered here except with the other two factors.

The third factor, which is usually overlooked, is the shape of the polished surfaces. This shaping of the polished surfaces should be given careful consideration. The two end factors in determining inclination of the polished surface are the width of the border and the buccolingual position of the teeth. The middle factor is the fullness given to the wax to obtain convexity or concavity.

Figs. 8-1 and 8-2 show the inclined plane action of the muscles of the cheek and tongue in gripping a bolus of food. This action may be described by the illustration of a patient chewing a small pickled onion, with the tongue and cheek holding the onion in place over the occlusal surfaces of the teeth while closing pressure is exerted upon it. This force exerted in the direction of the occlusal plane by the tongue and cheek can act as either a placing or displacing agent, depending on the shape of the polished surface.

A further study of Figs. 8-1 and 8-2 shows the power of inclined plane forces on the shape given the polished surfaces as a mechanical aid or detriment in retention. For instance, when the lingual and buccal borders of a mandibular denture are being shaped, they can be made concave so that the tongue and cheek will grip and tend to seat the denture. In the opposite case where the lingual and buccal surfaces were made convex by waxing and a narrow impression base was used, the inclined plane forces resulting from pressures of the tongue and cheeks would tend to unseat the denture. The buccolingual position of the teeth is important because the farther toward the cheek the teeth are, the greater the unseating inclined plane action becomes. A buccal position of the teeth would necessitate shaping the surface of the denture base in such a manner that the muscle action of the cheeks would tend to unseat the mandibular denture.

The buccal surface of mandibular dentures in the first premolar region should be shaped carefully so as not to interfere with the action of the modiolus connecting the facial muscles with the orbicularis oris muscle. This connecting point of muscles will displace the mandibular denture if the polished surface incline is toward the cheek or if the arch in the premolar region is too wide. These factors in function and retention of dentures seem to be little understood.

WAXING

As has been stated, the form of the polished surfaces of a denture influences its retentive quality. In addition, it influences the esthetic values of the denture. The wax surfaces around the teeth are known as the art portion of the polished surface and should, for esthetic reasons, imitate the form of the tissues around the natural teeth. Any fancy or artificial festooning is distinctly out of place. A slight root projection to follow the individual tooth should be carried out. The upper part of the polished surface is known as the anatomic portion and should be formed in such a way as to lose none of the original border width of the impression. A slight surplus should be allowed for loss of base material during finishing.

The form of the denture bases between the teeth and the denture border should be shaped in such a manner as to aid retention by the mechanical directional forces of the muscles and tissues (Figs. 8-1 and 8-2). Generally speaking, fullness on the buccal and labial surfaces of the mandibular and maxillary dentures is desirable, and the opposite is true on the palatal surface of the maxillary denture to allow all the possible space for the tongue. The speech of the patient will be handicapped unless a contour comparable to that of the palate before the natural teeth were lost is developed. The thickness of the palatal part of the base will vary with the loss of bone from the residual alveolar ridge. The lingual flange of the mandibular denture should have the least possible amount of bulk except at the border, which should be quite thick. This thickness is under the narrower portion of the tongue, and it greatly enhances the seal by contacting the mucolingual fold.

An excess of baseplate wax is added onto the buccal and labial surfaces of the mandibular and maxillary trial dentures. The bulk of the wax is cut back to the outer border of the cast (Fig. 22-1), and then the small end of a knife is held at a 45-degree angle to the tooth surface to form the wax gingival margin (Fig. 22-2). The common tendency is to cut this line too straight across from interproximal to interproximal and not leave enough wax in the interproximal spaces (Fig. 22-3). It is well to leave a surplus of wax along the gingival line at this time and then retrim when a complete view of the entire waxing is possible. Triangular markings can be placed as a guide to the length and position of the root indications, as long as it is kept in mind

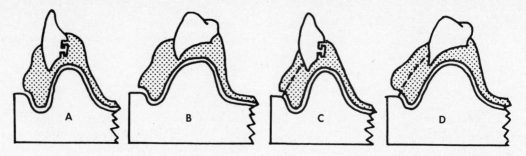

Fig. 22-1. Diagrams **A** and **B** show amount of wax added. **C** and **D** show line for reduction.

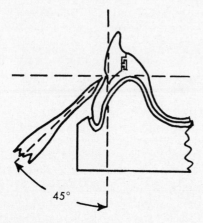

Fig. 22-2. Diagram illustrating angle at which knife is held in cutting gingival line.

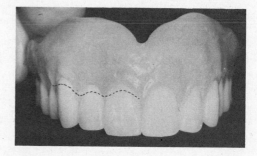

Fig. 22-3. Gingival line cut with the proper contour, and imperfectly cut *(dotted line).*

that the root of the maxillary canine is the longest, that of the lateral incisor the shortest, and that of the central incisor of a length between these two (Figs. 22-4 and 22-5). On the mandibular denture, the root of the canine is the longest, that of the central incisor the shortest, and that of the lateral incisor between these two. The wax is scraped out of the spaces between these triangular indications, after which the wax root indications will become manifest (Fig. 22-6). These sharp and rough root indications are now rounded with a large scraper and the spatula (Figs. 22-7 and 22-8). They should not be overemphasized.

The lingual surface of the mandibular denture may be made slightly concave without the concavity being extended under the lingual surface of the teeth. A projection of the tooth beyond the polished surface acts as an undercut into which the patient's tongue will slip, thereby causing the denture to be unseated (Fig. 22-9).

The palatal surface of the maxillary denture should be waxed to a neary uniform thickness of 2.5 mm. Thus, when the processed resin is smoothed and polished, the palate will be as thin as possible and yet be sufficiently thick to provide adequate strength. Lingual festooning

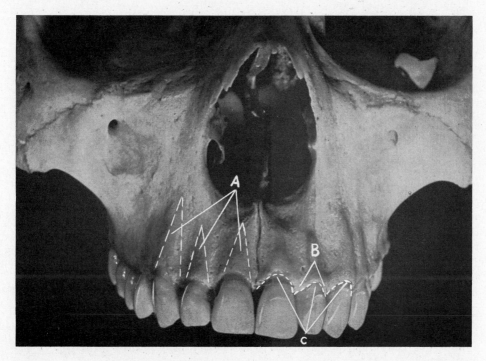

Fig. 22-4. *A,* Root indications viewed on skull; *B,* continuous gingival prominence; *C,* contour of gingival line.

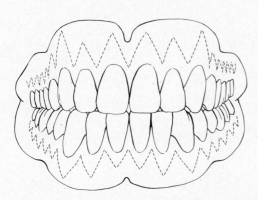

Fig. 22-5. Scheme showing location and various lengths of root indications to be made in wax.

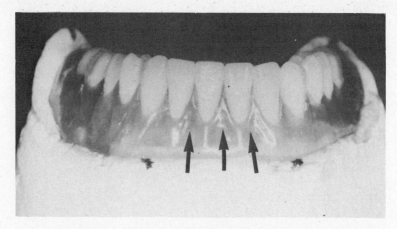

Fig. 22-6. Preliminary removal of wax between lines of root indications.

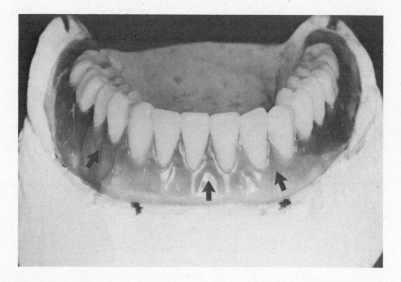

Fig. 22-7. Depressions between root indications smoothed with the wax spatula.

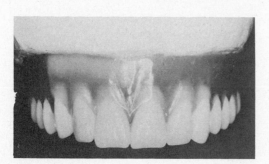

Fig. 22-8. Entire wax-up, with root indications given a final smoothing.

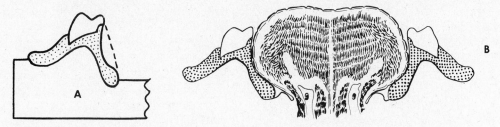

Fig. 22-9. A, Proper form of lingual polished surface contour. **B,** Relative position of tongue to lingual surface of denture base.

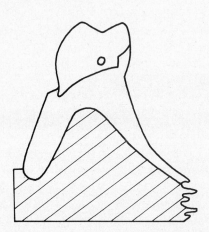

Fig. 22-10. Normal lingual contour of artificial posterior teeth is established during waxing procedure.

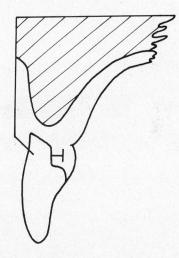

Fig. 22-11. Lingual contour of artificial upper central incisor has been reestablished in waxing procedure. This contour aids phonetics and provides a natural feel to the patient's tongue.

restores part of the lingual surface of the tooth that is not supplied in artificial teeth. Wax is added and carved on the lingual side of the artificial teeth to imitate the normal lingual contours of each tooth (Figs. 22-10 and 22-11).

MATERIALS USED FOR DENTURE BASES*
Acrylic resin

The material most often used in making denture bases is polymethyl methacrylate (PMMA)

*We wish to acknowledge the assistance of Dr. Carl W. Fairhurst, Regents Professor and Coordinator of Dental Physical Sciences, Medical College of Georgia School of Dentistry, Augusta, Georgia.

and is commonly called acrylic resin. PMMA is modified by the addition of cross-linking monomers that increase craze-resistance and rigidity. Pigment is added for color. PMMA is a solid polymer composed of long straight chains of molecular units of methyl methacrylate. Methyl methacrylate is a liquid monomer. Denture base resins are supplied as a liquid monomer and powder polymer. The liquid wets the powder and forms a binder when it hardens.

Two methods of polymerizing or hardening the resin are employed, heat cure and chemical cure. The heat cure is accomplished when the heat attacks the initiator (benzoyl peroxide) in the powder, which in turns acts on the methyl methacrylate to form a polymer. The chemical cure differs only in that an activator in the liquid attacks the initiator when the liquid and powder are in contact.

Metal denture bases

Metal denture bases may be made from a number of different materials such as gold, aluminum-manganese, platinum, Stellite (cobalt-chromium) alloys, and stainless steel (Fig. 22-12).

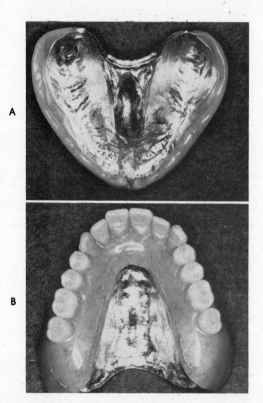

Fig. 22-12. Metal bases for complete dentures. **A,** Gold or Stellite alloy metal bases cover the palate and residual ridges, with the borders formed in acrylic resin. **B,** Notice distribution of metal and acrylic resin and also that lingual surfaces of artificial teeth have been restored with acrylic resin. The posterior palatal seal area need not be made out of metal. A "mesh" area here will provide excellent retention for an acrylic resin posterior palatal seal.

The *advantages* of metal denture bases are principally as follows:
1. Better thermal conductivity as compared to resins
2. Increase in tissue tolerance because of a less-irritating surface and increase in stimulation from heat and cold
3. Reduction of bulk across the palate, an important factor to the patient since more tongue space is created
4. Increased accuracy of fit of the denture base on the mucosa of the basal seat
5. Increased weight causing increased stability of lower dentures

Some *disadvantages* of metal bases are the following:
1. Greater initial cost and greater restorative cost
2. Difficulty and expense of rebasing and regrinding occlusion of metal dentures
3. Less margin of error permissible in the posterior palatal seal on a metal denture

FORMATION AND PREPARATION OF THE MOLD

After the trial dentures have been waxed, they are prepared for flasking. A Hanau ejector type of flask is used to facilitate removal of the trial denture after processing without danger of breaking the denture.

The trial denture is tested in the flask to determine its height in relation to the height of the bottom half of the flask (Fig. 22-13). The top half of the flask is placed in position to determine whether the teeth are too high in relation to the top of the flask. Approximately ⅛ to ¼ inch (3 to 6 mm) of space should be available between the teeth and the top of the flask. If the teeth are too high, the cast must be reduced in thickness. The artificial rim of the cast should be flush with the top of the bottom half of the flask to prevent possible breakage of the cast in later separation of the two halves of the flask (Fig. 22-14).

The distal ends of the lower cast may be high in relation to the remainder of the cast and extend close to the posterior edge of the flask. This condition causes the distal ends of the cast to be at an acute angle to the rim of the flask. Thus the distal ends are vulnerable to breakage, and careful consideration is demanded when this angle is reduced so that the top half of the flask will separate easily.

A mix of artificial stone is placed in the bottom half of the flask, and the cast, which has been

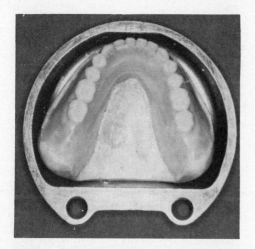

Fig. 22-13. Lower wax denture pattern and its cast in middle of bottom half of lower flask. (From Javid, N.S., and Boucher, C.O.: J. Prosthet. Dent. **29:**581-585, 1973.)

painted with separating medium (Fig. 22-15), is placed down into the stone until the artificial rim of the cast is nearly on a level with the top edge of the flask. The stone is leveled to a line between the edge of the cast and the rim of the flask.

After separating medium has been applied to the exposed stone in the flask, a core of artificial stone, 2 to 4 mm in thickness, is developed around the labial and buccal surfaces of both wax dentures, on the lingual surface of the lower wax denture, and the palatal surface of the upper wax denture. The top of the cores should be 2 to 3 mm below the occlusal plane of the teeth (Figs. 22-16 to 22-18). V-shaped grooves are placed in the cores so that they will separate with the top half of the flask.

Separating medium is applied on the exposed surfaces of the core, and the top half of the flask is placed in position. The two flask halves must meet exactly. Then a mix of artificial stone is poured up to the level of the incisal edges of the anterior teeth and the tips of the cusps of the posterior teeth (Fig. 22-19). The exposed stone is painted with separating medium, the flask is completely filled with artificial stone, and the lid of the flask is placed in position.

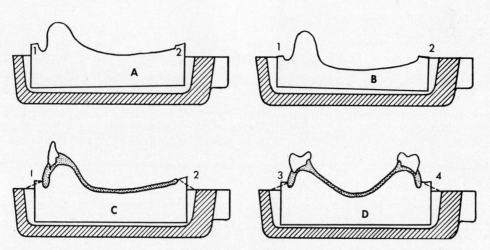

Fig. 22-14. Scheme illustrating first half of flasking of maxillary trial denture. **A,** Cast too high in flask in areas *1* and *2*. **B,** Areas *1* and *2* at a favorable level. **C,** Areas *1* and *2* should be beveled. **D,** Areas *3* and *4* to be beveled.

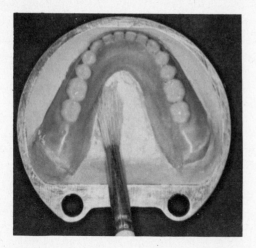

Fig. 22-15. Separating medium applied on the exposed stone of the land. (From Javid, N.S., and Boucher, C.O.: J. Prosthet. Dent. **29**:581-585, 1973.)

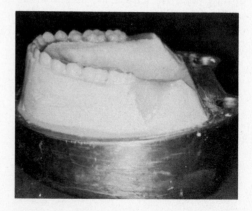

Fig. 22-16. Buccal and lingual cores around lower denture with V-shaped grooves (side view). (From Javid, N.S., and Boucher, C.O.: J. Prosthet. Dent. **29**:581-585, 1973.)

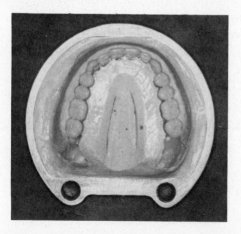

Fig. 22-17. Buccal and lingual cores around upper denture with V-shaped grooves (top side). (From Javid, N.S., and Boucher, C.O.: J. Prosthet. Dent. **29**:581-585, 1973.)

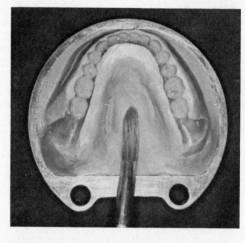

Fig. 22-18. Labial, buccal, and lingual cores coated with a separating medium. (From Javid, N.S., and Boucher, C.O.: J. Prosthet. Dent. **29**:581-585, 1973.)

The flask is placed in boiling water and allowed to remain from 4 to 6 minutes according to the size of the flask. The flask is removed from the water and opened from the side opposite the greatest undercut of the cast. After the flask is opened, the surplus wax is washed out with a stream of boiling water. When the water has been drained from the flask, the mold is washed again with boiling water containing a detergent, and then again with clean boiling water. Solvents such as chloroform are not used because of their effect on acrylic resin.

After the stone is dry, but still hot, the inside of the mold and the cast is painted with a tinfoil

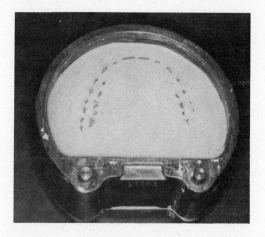

Fig. 22-19. After upper half of flask is put in place, a heavy mixture of dental stone is poured up to the level of the tips of the cusps. (From Javid, N.S., and Boucher, C.O.: J. Prosthet. Dent. **29:**581-585, 1973.)

substitute using a camel's hair brush (Fig. 22-20). The tinfoil substitute must not come in contact with the teeth or pool in the mold around the teeth. The tinfoil substitute is allowed to dry, and a second coat is painted on the inside of the mold. The flask is allowed to cool to room temperature.

PACKING THE MOLD

An acrylic resin dough is made by mixture of the powder (polymer) and liquid (monomer) in accordance with the manufacturer's directions. Monomer is a sensitizer that can cause an allergic contact eczematous reaction on the skin or mucous membrane. When the monomer is completely polymerized, it is no longer a sensitizer or elicitor of allergic reactions. When the mixture has reached a dough consistency, it is placed between two plastic sheets and formed into a roll about 1 inch (2.5 cm) in diameter. The roll is flattened so that it is about ¼ inch (6 mm) in thickness, and pieces are cut to approximate the length of the flanges and the size of the palate (Fig. 22-21, *A*). The pieces are positioned around the buccal, labial, and palatal surfaces of the upper mold (Fig. 22-21, *B* and *C*) and around the buccal, labial, and lingual surfaces of the lower mold (Fig. 22-22, *C*). The flask is closed in a press with a sheet of separating plastic between the two halves until they are almost in approximation (Fig. 22-21, *D*). Then the flask

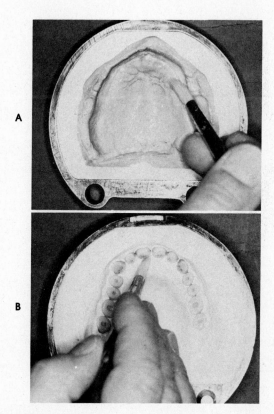

A

B

Fig. 22-20. A, Flask has been separated and the wax removed. Tissue surface of upper cast is painted with a tinfoil substitute. **B,** All wax has been removed and teeth are in their proper places in the mold. Stone is painted with a tinfoil substitute, which must be kept out of contact with teeth.

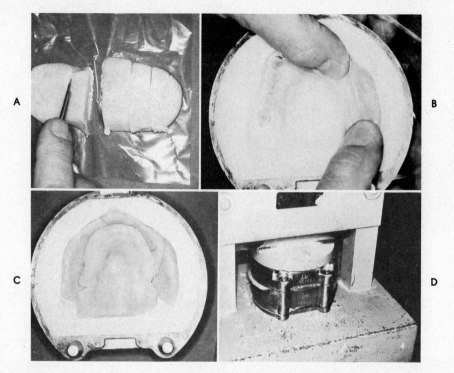

Fig. 22-21. A, Acrylic resin dough is formed into a cylindrical mass and cut into pieces of the approximate size of the mold. **B,** Section of the acrylic resin dough is placed in mold for upper denture. Dough is carried to place with cellophane to prevent contamination. **C,** Acrylic resin dough is distributed throughout upper mold. **D,** Flask is closed slowly in automatic press.

is opened, the excess flash resin is cut away precisely at the denture border, and additional resin is added at those places that are deficient (Fig. 22-22). This trial packing procedure is repeated until the mold is filled and no flash is formed. Then the flask is closed completely without the separating sheet. The slightest discrepancy in the closure of the two halves of the flask will cause an error in the occlusion.

The flask is transferred to a spring clamp. The spring clamp should be closed tightly, but the spring should not be fully compressed. This will allow the resin to expand upon processing and then finally to contract while still under pressure. After a wait of 30 to 60 minutes to allow the liquid to penetrate the powder thoroughly, the flask and clamp are placed in a curing unit. The denture is processed for 9 hours in water held at a constant temperature of 165° F (73.5° C), or another accepted processing procedure is used. Conventional acrylic resins are processed at temperatures from 135° to 180° F. No significant distortion takes place when the acrylic resin is processed at or below the manufacturer's recommended temperature. However, the level of monomer remaining in the cured acrylic resin clearly affects the degree of cytotoxicity of the denture base material. The flask is allowed to cool to room temperature.

PRESERVING THE ORIENTATION RELATIONS

Deflasking is completed, and the processed dentures are left on the casts. The casts and dentures are fitted back onto the mountings on the articulator, and the processing changes are observed. The processing changes are usually

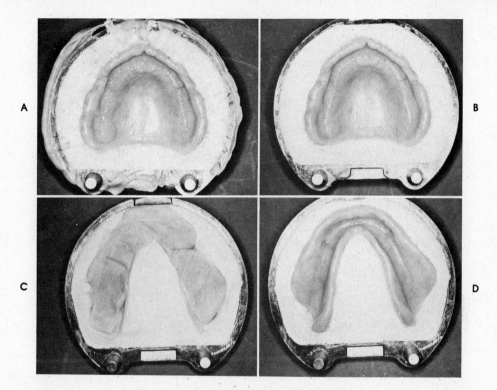

Fig. 22-22. A, Excess acrylic resin in mold has been forced between two halves of the flask during initial trial packing procedure. **B,** Excess acrylic resin in upper mold has been removed through a series of trial packing procedures. **C,** Acrylic resin dough is distributed throughout lower mold. **D,** Excess acrylic resin in lower mold has been removed through a series of trial packing procedures.

not corrected at this time, since new interocclusal records will be made from the patient.

The upper cast is attached to the upper mounting, and a record of its relationship to the articulator is made in plaster of paris on the remounting jig. Fast-setting plaster is spread on the jig, and the teeth of the upper denture are pressed into the plaster while the cast is in its keyed position in the mounting plaster on the upper member of the articulator. The plaster on the jig is allowed to set (Fig. 22-23).

SHAPING AND POLISHING THE CURED RESIN BASES

The dentures are removed from the artificial stone casts. The feather edges of the denture base material are removed with files, scrapers, and burs. Care must be used with rotating instruments because enough heat can be gener-

ated during grinding to cause distortion of the denture base. The feather edges around the gingival line of the teeth are cut down by means of burs and chisels to conform with the desired contour. Any difficulty encountered during polishing of the dentures is caused by the fact that they are not properly prepared for polishing. With burs, stones, chisels, and sharp scrapers, the surface is shaped until it presents a smooth, clean surface. No plaster and no deep scratches should remain after the preparation for polishing. It is impossible to retain the desired contour of the dentures if abrasives such as pumice are used for all the finishing.

A rag wheel and felt cone with pumice are used to finish the palatal portion of the upper denture. A single-row brush wheel and a rag wheel about ¼ inch (6 mm) in width are used

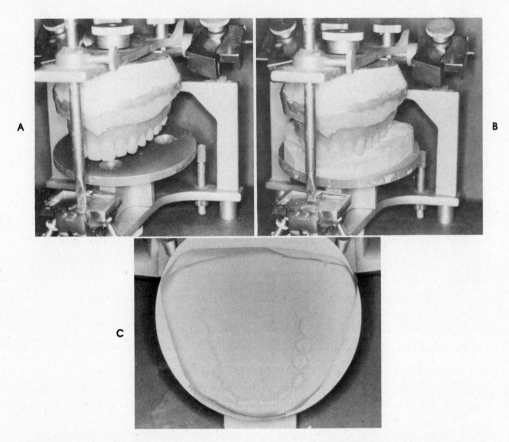

Fig. 22-23. A, Upper cast and processed upper denture are attached back onto mounting on articulator with sticky wax. Remounting jig is positioned on lower member of articulator. **B,** Upper denture is closed into plaster that has been placed on remounting jig so that occlusal surfaces of teeth will make an imprint in plaster. **C,** Plaster record of occlusal surfaces of teeth on upper denture will permit the denture, after deflasking, to be repositioned in proper relationship to upper member of articulator.

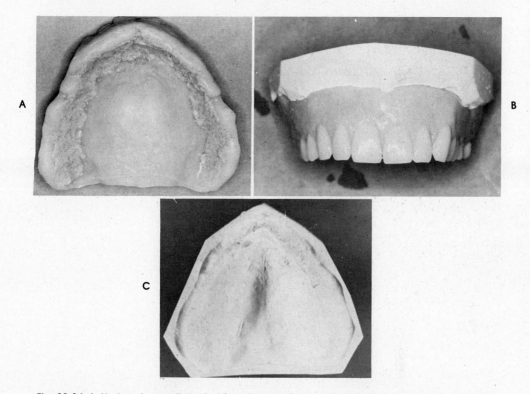

Fig. 22-24. A, Undercuts are eliminated from tissue surface of denture when they are filled with wet tissue paper. **B,** Upper remounting cast has been poured in upper denture. **C,** Upper denture has been removed from upper remounting cast. Denture must fit back on the cast easily and accurately.

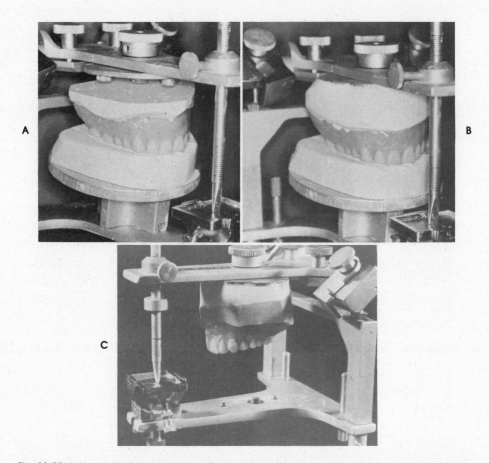

Fig. 22-25. A, Upper denture and remounting cast have been repositioned in imprints of the teeth in plaster index on remounting jig. **B,** Remounting cast has been attached to mounting ring on upper member of articulator by quick-setting plaster. **C,** Remounting jig and plaster index have been removed from lower member of articulator. Upper completed denture and remounting cast are located in same relation on articulator as established originally by face-bow record.

with pumice to smooth the labial and buccal surfaces of the denture without destroying the contour. A final high polish is given all the surfaces with a rag wheel and polishing material (tripoli, tin oxide and water, or Shure Shine).

CONSTRUCTION OF REMOUNTING CASTS

Remounting casts serve as an accurate, convenient, time-saving method of reorienting the completed dentures on the articulator for occlusal corrections. All undercuts on the tissue surface of the dentures are filled with wet tissue paper, Mortite (a caulking compound), or wet pumice (Fig. 22-24, *A*).

Remounting casts are poured into the denture using quick-setting plaster or artificial stone. After the plaster has set, the excess is trimmed down to the border (Fig. 22-24, *B*), and the dentures are removed from the remounting casts. The block-out material is then removed from the undercut areas, and the dentures are cleaned. The casts are examined to see that the grooves formed by the border of the dentures are not over 1 mm in depth. Excessive depth of the grooves jeopardizes exact placement of the dentures each time they are removed and placed back on the cast (Fig. 22-24, *C*).

With the remounting jig and index in position on the mandibular member of the articulator, the maxillary denture and remounting cast are placed into the plaster indentations. The maxillary remount cast is attached to the maxillary member of the articulator by means of quick-setting plaster (Fig. 22-25).

23

Completion of the rehabilitation of the patient

The moment new dentures are placed in a patient's mouth, all the procedures involved in denture construction are subject to review and reevaluation. The choice of procedures, the technical effectiveness of the procedures used, and the skill used in carrying out the procedures are exposed to three evaluations. These evaluations are made by the dentists who rendered the service, the patients who are to use the dentures, and the friends and associates of the patients.

DENTISTS' EVALUATIONS

Evaluations made by dentists should be the most critical, for they are the only ones who can know the possibilities and limitations in the treatment of their patients. In this moment of truth, dentists must know and recognize and admit (at least to themselves) any deficiencies in the prosthodontic service provided. If they are not completely honest with themselves at this point, if they are not informed about the type of observations that should be made, and if they are not extremely critical of the results of the treatment, they are not rendering a truly professional service. But, worse than that, the quality of the denture service to other patients will deteriorate. If, as a part of the treatment of edentulous patients, dentists make complete dentures that they consider to be perfect, their next dentures are likely to be not so good. In other words, if dentists cannot find anything at all that they would try to change in treating the same patient again with complete dentures, they are not so critical of their own efforts as they should be. The maintenance of quality of prosthodontic service depends on a constant vigilance and self-discipline. The forgetting curve takes its toll in technical skills and procedures just as it does in didactic knowledge. A critical evaluation by the dentist of every prosthodontic service rendered will tend toward a constant improvement of the service. This is an essential part of the care of denture patients after new dentures have been provided.

PATIENTS' EVALUATIONS

Patients' evaluations of their new dentures are made in two phases. The first is the reaction to the completed dentures the first time they are placed in the mouth. Two attitudes are possible: hopeful confidence or fear and apprehension. Patients' frame of mind at this time will depend largely on the dentist, but it may be affected by their previous experiences in denture wearing and by comments made by other people. If adequate diagnoses were made before any treatment was started, all misconceptions and inaccurate information will have been brought to light. At that time wise dentists will have allayed the patients' fears and corrected their misinformation, and instructions regarding the use of dentures will have been started. These dentists will have demonstrated to their patients that they are treating them properly and that they have used the utmost care in the technical procedures involved in building the dentures. Thoroughness in each step from diagnosis to insertion is apparent to patients—and this builds confidence. Patients sense carelessly or hastily carried out techniques, just as they recognize care used in making impressions and jaw relation records and in arranging the teeth for esthetics. A failure to spend adequate time at the try-in appointment leads to trouble on insertion of the dentures. If confidence cannot be earned and established *before* the day the den-

tures are placed in the mouth, the treatment after this time will be more complicated.

FRIENDS' EVALUATIONS

When patients leave the dental office with their new teeth, it is with mixed emotions. They want their friends to notice their improved appearance; they hope their friends and relatives will compliment them and confirm their judgment of the choice of the dentist they have made; and, of course, they still wonder how they will progress with eating and speaking. They need help. If people comment about about their new teeth, some patients may wonder if the teeth look natural, and if they do not comment about them, the patients may wonder if their friends are just being kind. In reality, if people comment about the teeth, it *may* be because the dentist failed to achieve a natural-appearing result.

The evaluations made by friends of patients are most likely to be inaccurate. Friends cannot know how the dentures feel; they cannot judge the efficiency of the dentures in eating and speaking; they cannot know the difficulties encountered by the dentist because of the poor foundation on which dentures may have been built. They cannot understand the possible lack of coordination of the patient or the ineptness of some patients in attempting to follow instructions or to use the dentures. The patients themselves may recognize these difficulties as partly their responsibility, but the comments of friends may cause them to blame the dentist for problems that may have been beyond the dentist's control. Such well-meaning friends may add to patients' difficulties because they have not been exposed to the information supplied to the patient by the dentist during the course of construction of the dentures. The only apparent way to guard against patients being misinformed by their friends is to take the lead and make certain that patients have been correctly informed. This process can be a continuing one and should start at the time the diagnosis is made.

TREATMENT AT THE TIME OF INSERTION OF DENTURES

The insertion of new dentures in a patient's mouth involves more than seating the dentures and telling the patient to call if there is any trouble. It is at this time that the dentist's evaluation is started. Also, there are certain technical procedures that must be carried out. The dentures, having been processed and polished, are not completed. The inaccuracies of the materials and methods used to get the dentures to this stage must be recognized and eliminated *before* the patient wears the dentures.

The inaccuracies may be the result of (1) technical errors or errors of judgment made by the dentist, (2) technical errors developed in the laboratory, or (3) inherent deficiencies of the materials used in the construction of the dentures. Regardless of the source of the inaccuracies, they should be corrected *before* the patient is permitted to use the dentures.

Before one places the dentures in the patient's mouth, the denture *flanges* should be examined to make certain that they are not too thick, and the denture *borders* should be examined to make certain that they are well rounded with no obvious overextension. If carefully border-molded impressions have been made, the flanges and borders should require no alteration at this time—provided, of course, that the laboratory operations have respected those borders. If a penciled outline on the cast has been used to indicate the extent of the flanges, more changes in border form will be necessary than when accurately border-molded impressions have been used. If the laboratory technician has disregarded the borders recorded by the impression on the cast or has disregarded the instructions relating to the flanges and borders, some alteration of the borders may be necessary at the time of insertion.

The dentist's objective, however, should be to make the impressions and casts so perfectly that there is no doubt in the mind of the technician about the form and extent of borders and flanges when the dentures are polished. If accurately

formed borders have been made on the impressions, the borders of the dentures should *not* be altered or polished until the dentures have been used for 24 hours. By avoiding any polishing of the borders, the dentist can easily detect any overextension at the first adjustment appointment. The impressions should be so accurate that the basal surface and the denture borders will not need any adjustment on the day the dentures are inserted.

Another observation should be made by the dentist immediately on the *first* insertion of the dentures. The occlusion should be checked the *very first time* the teeth are permitted to touch.

The patient should have been instructed to keep any previous dentures out of the mouth for 12 to 24 hours immediately before the insertion appointment. This is essential if the new dentures are to be seated on healthy, undistorted tissues. If the tissues have been distorted by the old dentures, the new ones cannot seat perfectly even if they fit perfectly. Improper seating of dentures at this time can cause the appearance of errors in occlusion or fit that would not exist if the tissues were undistorted. Unnecessary adjustments of any type to correct such apparent errors, if made at this time, can cause irreparable damage to the dentures. This caution is predicated on the requirements that the patient be without *any* teeth for 24 hours (or more if necessary) to get the tissues healthy before the final impressions were made and that no teeth be used by the patient until the jaw relation records were verified at the try-in.

Occlusion of all complete dentures should be perfected before the patient is allowed to wear them. This is true regardless of the technique or instruments used for making the impressions, making the jaw relation records, arranging the teeth into balanced occlusion, and processing the dentures. Construction of dentures for a patient involves many separate but related procedures. An error in any one of them could contribute to an error in the occlusion of the completed dentures.

ERRORS IN OCCLUSION

The errors in occlusion that may be observed on the first insertion of dentures can result from a number of things. These include a change in the state of the health of the temporomandibular joints, inaccurate maxillomandibular relation records made by the dentist, errors made in the transfer of the maxillomandibular relation records to the articulator, failure to seat the occlusion rims correctly on the casts, ill-fitting temporary bases, failure to use the face-bow and subsequently changing the vertical relation on the articulator, incorrect arrangement of the posterior teeth, failure to close the flasks completely, use of too much pressure in closing the flasks, or warpage of the dentures by overheating them in polishing operations. All these are possible errors of technique on the part of the dentist or laboratory technician.

Each of the procedures offers the possibility of an undetected error that might not be noted until the dentures are placed in the patient's mouth. Even then errors in occlusion may not be apparent unless other procedures are used to test for them. These errors in occlusion must be eliminated before the dentures are worn by the patient, or the soft tissues that are interposed between the bone and the dentures will be distorted in the attempt to eliminate the errrors.

Errors in occlusion of dentures may be the result of unavoidable changes in the denture base material itself (Fig. 23-1). Acrylic resins shrink when they change from a moldable to a solid form by polymerization. These resins have a high coefficient of thermal expansion, so that in cooling after polymerization is complete they shrink and this causes warpage. The greatest amount of denture deformation, or warpage, occurs when the dentures are removed from the casts. Further warpage may occur if too much heat is generated in polishing the dentures. Subsequently, the resin will absorb water in use, and this will expand the resin. All these processing changes are inevitable, though some of them can be minimized by careful and special techniques.

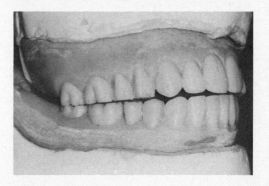

Fig. 23-1. Processed dentures are replaced on articulator while they are still on their casts. The changes that occurred in processing the acrylic resin bases caused errors in occlusion.

It is true that these changes are relatively small and that the soft-tissue covering of the maxillae and mandible will give, or be displaced, enough to allow dentures to be seated and tolerated by most patients. However, these discrepancies will alter the relationships of the teeth to each other. Such changes in occlusion should be eliminated before the dentures are worn by the patient.

Maxillomandibular relations are bone-to-bone relations, and as such they represent the relationships between solid objects, the maxillae and the mandible. These bones are covered by mucosa and submucosal tissues, which are resilient and displaceable. Because of this displaceability, some dentists have considered that the dentures settle into the tissues and that small errors in occlusion will correct themselves. If this is true, it is done at the expense of the health of soft tissues and eventually at the expense of bone, because bone is a more plastic tissue than mucosa. Bone, in time, will change to relieve soft tissues of excess pressure. Thus failure to correct occlusion before the patient wears the dentures can cause destruction of the residual alveolar ridges.

Part of the error in occlusion can be eliminated by replacement of the casts with the processed dentures still on them on their original mountings on the articulator and modification of the occlusal surfaces of the teeth by selective grinding (Fig. 23-1). This procedure can eliminate most of the errors that are a result of processing changes. However, it will not eliminate any errors produced by the impressions or jaw relation records, and it will not eliminate the errors that develop when the dentures are removed from the casts or when they are polished. Therefore new interocclusal records of centric and eccentric relations should be made at the time new dentures are first inserted in the patient's mouth.

Further errors in occlusion may develop after dentures have been worn by the patient. The resins of which the denture bases are made will absorb water. When this occurs, the bases expand and warp slightly. This change can alter the relationships of the inclined planes of the cusps of anatomic (cusped) teeth. When the residual ridges supporting the dentures are favorable, this altered relationship may not be noticeable to the patient. However, if one or both of the residual ridges are badly resorbed, the patient may experience soreness under the dentures as a result of malocclusion. In this situation, the dentures should be remounted on the articulator with new interocclusal records of centric and eccentric relations. Then the occlusion should be corrected by further selective grinding. The temptation to alter the denture bases should be resisted until it has been established that there is no error in occlusion.

Checking for errors in occlusion

The technique for checking to determine whether there are errors in occlusion is not difficult, but it does require willingness to see the error. Dentists must approach this observation with a negative attitude. They must *assume* that an error exists and should *try* to find it. If they simply tell the patient to bite up and then look at the teeth, the error in occlusion will not be detected. With these instructions, the patient will close the teeth together, and they will touch and slide into centic occlusion without this touch and slide being noticed by either the dentist or patient. The dentures may shift on the ridges or the mandible may move into an eccentric position without detection.

A method that is effective for detection of errors in occlusion involves a test in which the denture bases are kept firmly seated on their foundations and the dentist *feels* the touch and slide of teeth while the patient keeps the mandible back as far as it will go as the teeth are closed to occlusal contact. The *amount* of occlusal error and the *location* of the deflective occlusal contacts are not important in this test. The amount and location of the errors can be determined after the dentures have been remounted on the articulator. These usually minute errors cannot be located accurately enough in the mouth to be eliminated without remounting of the dentures on the articulator. If articulating paper is used in the mouth to locate the interceptive or deflective occlusal contacts, shifting of the denture bases or eccentric closures made by the patient or the presence of saliva will prevent the articulating paper marks from recording errors. Errors in occlusion are easily detected and corrected on the articulator.

Hand position for tests of occlusion. The left hand of a right-handed dentist is used to maintain the dentures in position and to *feel* the touch-and-slide error in the occlusion (the right hand of a left-handed dentist is used for this purpose). The hand is turned so that the little finger is up and the palm of the hand is toward the patient's face. The ball of the thumb and the ball of the index finger are placed between the upper and lower teeth. The fingernail of the other hand is placed on top of the incisal edges of the lower anterior teeth.

The patient is then instructed to pull the lower jaw back and *close slowly* until a *back tooth* touches. The words *close* and *back* are emphasized to cause the patient to retrude the mandible to the position of centric relation. When the first tooth contact is made, it will be felt by the thumb and forefinger that are against the teeth.

If there is an error, the finger and thumb will feel the slide that follows the first tooth contact. In the first attempt the patient will usually close too rapidly to stop when the first tooth contact is made. Therefore a second closure is directed in the same way except that the patient is told this time to *stop* just the instant that any tooth contact is felt. As the lower teeth approach the upper teeth, the fingernail is removed from the incisal edges of the lower anterior teeth, and the word *slowly* is repeated so that this movement will not be too fast for the observation to be felt by the fingers. When the first contact is made, the error in occlusion may be visible *if* the patient stops the closure *at the very first contact*. If the patient closes too tightly, centric occlusion may *appear* to be correct, even though it is not.

The word *bite* and *bite up* are studiously avoided because their use will tend to obscure errors in occlusion. The word *bite* implies the use of force, which is not desired in this operation. It also invites protrusion because protrusion of the mandible is necessary when a bite of something is to be taken. The word *close* should be used to eliminate the tendency toward protrusion of the mandible or the exertion of force at the time of this observation and test.

During this test, no pressure is exerted on the mandible in an attempt to retrude it. The patient should supply all the force to produce the desired motion and action of the mandible. If attempts to push the mandible back are made, the patient will tend to resist this force and push the mandible forward. The patient must pull his own mandible back.

The hand position described earlier is of the utmost importance. The balls of the finger and thumb, being partly between the occlusal surfaces of the teeth, provide slight resistance to the closure and keep the dentures seated on their respective basal seats. Their sensitivity makes it possible for the amount of resistance to be uniform on the two sides as they are slowly withdrawn from between the teeth. The palm of the hand prevents the patient from seeing the dentist's eyes and reacting to the expression on the dentist's face. The tone of the voice and the instructions to the patient should be such as to inspire confidence, cooperation, and relaxation. If the dentist is irritated—or lets the patient think so—the patient cannot follow the instructions. The palm of the hand shields the dentist's face from the patient.

A common error in this procedure is to approach the patient from the front with the index fingers of the two hands of either side of the dentures. The dentist-patient positional relationship invites errors in observation of occlusion. More pressure will be applied by the finger against the cheek on the side on which the dentist stands. This will cause the patient to move the mandible slightly in that direction. The finger and thumb of only one hand should be in the patient's mouth at the time the first tooth contact is made.

INTEROCCLUSAL RECORDS FOR REMOUNTING DENTURES

The dentures must be remounted on the articulator to do the selective grinding necessary for the perfection of the occlusion. Interocclusal records of centric relation and protrusive relation are necessary for this procedure.

The errors in occlusion should be eliminated on the articulator rather than in the mouth. If these corrections are attempted in the mouth, it is difficult to see the errors because the soft tissues will be distorted and obscure the errors and the articulating paper will not mark efficiently. On account of the resiliency of the soft tissues under the dentures, the denture bases will shift in relation to the underlying bone when there is an error in occlusion and the teeth are rubbed together. The articulating paper marks are likely to be incorrect, and most important, the control of jaw position depends entirely on the ability of the patient to place and move the jaw correctly. Much of the selective grinding done according to articulating paper marks made in the mouth actually increases the amount of error in the occlusion. When new interocclusal records are

made and the completed dentures are remounted on the articulator, the errors in occlusion are easily visible, easily located, and easily
corrected by selective grinding. Properly made
interocclusal records will not cause the denture
bases to slip or rotate in relation to their bony
foundations. And, on the articulator the dentures will be firm on their remount casts. The
points of contact and errors of occlusion can be
observed visually, with magnification if desired,
and articulating paper marks can be quite easily
made on the dry teeth.

There is another advantage to making these
corrections away from the patient. The interocclusal records, of course, are made in the
patient's mouth, and from the patient's standpoint this is just another step in the construction
of the dentures. On the other hand, if the grinding of occlusion is attempted in the presence of
the patient, the operation *appears* to the patient
to be one of correcting an error made by the
dentist. Thus there is a psychologic advantage in
doing the grinding in the laboratory.

Protrusive interocclusal record

The protrusive interocclusal record is made
first for convenience. The patient should be
instructed to keep the previous dentures, if any,
out of the mouth for 24 hours before insertion of
new dentures.

The new dentures are placed in the mouth,
and the patient is instructed to pull the mandible back, to close, and to hold a firm closing
pressure on them. A small amount of impression
plaster or bite registration paste is mixed, and
when it has reached the consistency of thick
cream, the left hand is placed in the position as
for checking occlusion. Then a narrow plaster
spatula is used to place equal amounts of plaster
on the occlusal surfaces of the premolar and
molar teeth on each side (Fig. 23-2). The patient
is directed to move the mandible forward and to
bite easily on the front teeth. The closure must
stop *before* the anterior teeth touch (Fig. 23-3).
After the plaster has set hard, the dentures are
removed from the mouth, and the protrusive

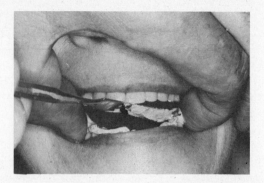

Fig. 23-2. Finger and thumb help to maintain dentures in
position while plaster or a bite registration paste is placed
on molar and premolar teeth with a narrow spatula.

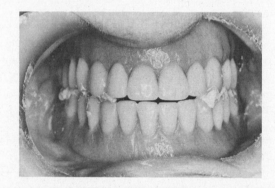

Fig. 23-3. Protrusive interocclusal record. Closure is
stopped before any teeth make contact.

interocclusal records are marked *LP* for the left-
side record and *RP* for the right-side record and
are laid aside.

Interocclusal record of centric relation

The dentures are cleaned and reinserted into
the mouth. The patient is instructed to pull the
mandible back and hold a firm closing pressure
on the dentures. Impression plaster or a bite
registration paste is mixed as for the protrusive
interocclusal record. The patient is directed to
open, and the left hand is placed so as to maintain the dentures in position and shield the eyes
of the patient so that verbal directions will be

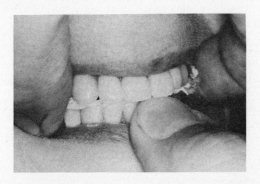

Fig. 23-4. Fingernail of index finger is on incisal edges of lower anterior teeth while patient pulls lower jaw back and closes into soft plaster on premolars and molars.

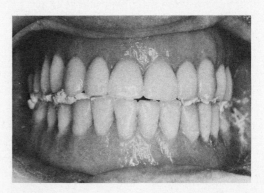

Fig. 23-5. Centric relation interocclusal record is made without any tooth contact.

followed. The hand is inverted so that the palm is facing toward the patient's face with the little finger up, and the ball of the finger and ball of the thumb are placed against the buccal surfaces of the teeth on both sides. Then the registration material is placed on the lower premolars and molars on both sides of the denture. With the material in position, the fingernail of the right index finger is placed on top of the lower incisor teeth, and the patient is instructed to pull the lower jaw back as far as it will go and *close* on the back teeth (Fig. 23-4). However, as the lower teeth approach the upper teeth, the right index finger is withdrawn so that only the finger and thumb of the left hand remain in the mouth. *The closure must be stopped before any teeth touch*. The patient is asked to hold that position, and as soon as the registration material has started to set, the left hand is removed. The patient should hold the teeth together until the material has set hard. In reality, the teeth never touch, but the patient cannot tell that they are not in contact (Fig. 23-5). When the material has set hard, the dentures are removed from the mouth. If the interocclusal record has been penetrated by any tooth, a new record must be made. Any contact of teeth or of the denture bases will produce an incorrect record.

Whenever a centric interocclusal record is made, the word bite *must* be studiously avoided. To be asked to bite invites the patient to protrude the mandible as for incision of food. Since there are no tracings or mechanical devices to show the relative horizontal position of the mandible to the maxillae, the choice of words in the instructions to the patient, the hand position, and the amount of closure permitted become extremely important factors for obtainment of an accurate record of centric relation.

REMOUNTING THE MANDIBULAR DENTURE

The maxillary denture will have been mounted on the articulator by means of the remount jig. This procedure will have preserved the face-bow orientation of the dentures.

The maxillary denture is seated in its remount cast, and the interocclusal record of centric relation places the mandibular denture in the desired relation to the upper denture (Fig. 23-6, A).

The undercuts in the mandibular denture are blocked out with disposable tissue or caulking compound. Then plaster or stone is built up on the mandibular member of the articulator to such a height that when the articulator is closed the plaster will engage the borders of the mandibular denture (Fig. 23-6, B to D).

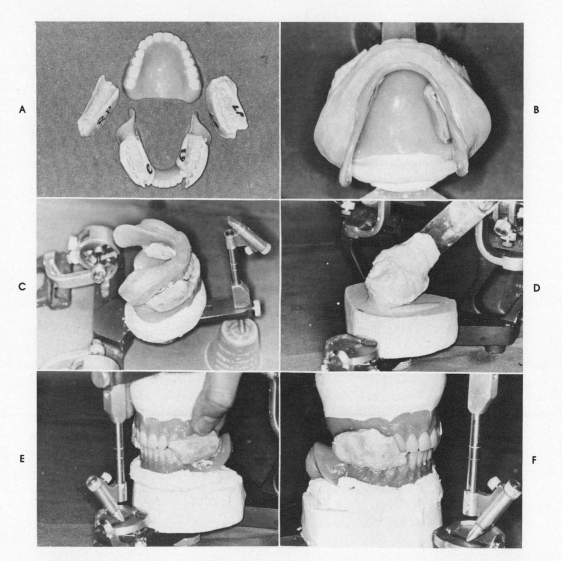

Fig. 23-6. A, Protrusive interocclusal records are made and laid aside. Then the interocclusal records of centric relation are made. **B,** Undercuts are blocked out of mandibular denture with caulking compound. Mandibular denture is seated on centric relation interocclusal record with maxillary denture. **C,** Assembled dentures are placed on mounting plaster on upper member of articulator. **D,** Impression plaster is placed on original mounting plaster on lower member of articulator. **E,** Mandibular denture is held in place in interocclusal record and lowered into soft plaster on lower member of articulator. **F,** Lower denture is attached to articulator in centric relation. If a remount cast had been made, it would have been placed on lower denture and attached to articulator with plaster.

ARTICULATOR ADJUSTMENT

After the mounting plaster has set, the protrusive interocclusal records are substituted for the centric interocclusal records, and the condylar guidances on the instrument are readjusted (Fig. 23-7). The horizontal condylar guidances are loosened, and the mechanism is rotated until both dentures are perfectly seated in the mounting plaster and in the protrusive interocclusal records. The horizontal condylar inclination on each side is recorded on the mounting plaster. These numbers are then used with the formula for setting the lateral condylar guidance. The horizontal condylar guidance, divided by 8, plus 12 equals the lateral condylar guidance, that is, $\frac{H}{8} + 12 = L$. The thumb nut above the condylar guidance mechanism is loosened, and the guidance mechanism is rotated around the vertical axis until the numbers correspond with the resultant of the formula. Then the thumb nut is tightened.

ELIMINATION OF OCCLUSAL ERRORS IN ANATOMIC TEETH

Final correction of any occlusal disharmony that may exist in dentures from any cause is made at this time by means of selective grinding. Selective grinding permits the desired factors of both tooth form and occlusion to be retained.

Articulating paper of minimum thickness is used to mark the actual contacts of the teeth. Thicker paper used to disclose interfering points in centric and eccentric occlusions gives deceptive results.

The articulating paper is interposed between the teeth, and markings are obtained by tapping the teeth together (Fig. 23-8). This can be done on both sides at the same time if two pieces of thin articulating paper are fastened together in front with a paper clip. After the first action on the articulating paper only the few high spots appear. These are removed after a test to determine whether to reduce the mandibular or the maxillary teeth at the points of contact (Fig. 23-

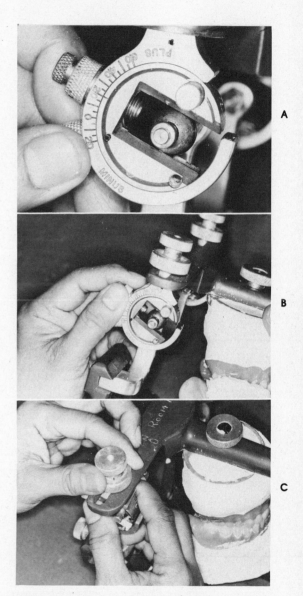

Fig. 23-7. A, Protrusive interocclusal records are in place, and horizontal condylar guidance is loosened and rotated to neutral position. **B,** Horizontal condylar guidance is adjusted so that both dentures stay seated on their plaster mountings and in the protrusive interocclusal records. **C,** Lateral condylar guidance is adjusted by rotation.

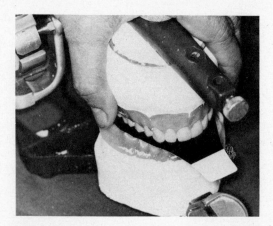

Fig. 23-8. Completed dentures mounted on articulator preparatory to the preliminary occlusal corrections. *A,* Articulating paper in place to mark occlusal contacts in centric relation.

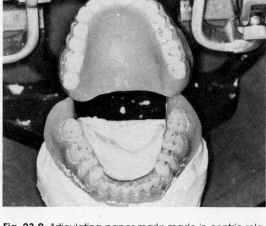

Fig. 23-9. Articulating paper marks made in centric relation show interceptive or deflective occlusal contacts in centric occlusion. Grinding is to be done only in fossae and not on cusps.

9). This grinding is done by means of mounted Chayes stones No. 16, 11, and 5. The marking process and the grinding procedure are repeated until practically all the teeth have contact in centric occlusion. During this centric grinding procedure, the incisal guide pin is relieved of contact on the incisal guidance table to allow for the slight reduction of the vertical dimension that must necessarily take place.

After the centric deflective occlusal contacts have been removed, the pin is placed in contact with the incisal guide table and is kept in contact through the remainder of the grinding procedure. Thin articulating paper is placed over the occlusal surfaces of the teeth on both sides, the articulator is moved into one of the lateral positions, and the contacts are marked on both sides for the same lateral movement (Fig. 23-10). A study of the markings shows contact of the maxillary and mandibular buccal and lingual cusps and the maxillary and mandibular incisors on the working side (Fig. 23-11). Marks are also shown on the lingual cusps of the maxillary teeth and on the buccal cusps of the mandibular teeth. If the pin rises away from the incisal guide table dur-

ing this lateral movement, the buccal cusps of the maxillary teeth and the lingual cusps of the mandibular teeth on the working side are reduced by means of a mounted stone. The balancing-side markings are reduced on the lingual side of the buccal cusps of the mandibular teeth to reduce balancing-side deflective occlusal contacts. The registration of these markings is continued with the same lateral movement, including the intermediate movements, and grinding of these high spots is continued until the pin stays in contact in all lateral and intermediate movements. This marking and grinding procedure is repeated for the right lateral movement (Figs. 23-12 and 23-13). Grinding to correct occlusion in lateral occlusions is limited to altering the lingual inclines of the upper buccal cusps and the buccal inclines of the lower lingual cusps on the working side and to altering the lingual inclines of the lower buccal cusps on the balancing side. After centric occlusion has been perfected, the lingual cusps of the upper teeth and the buccal cusps of the lower teeth must not be shortened.

If the grinding has been carried out in both

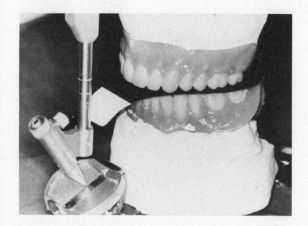

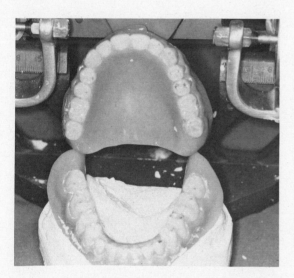

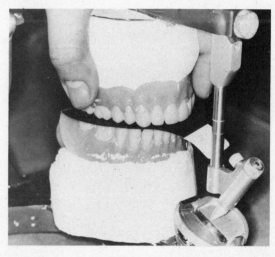

Fig. 23-10. Articulating paper is used to locate deflective occlusal contacts in left lateral occlusion. Notice position of incisal guide pin, which has resulted from movement of articulator into the left working position.

Fig. 23-11. Marks on buccal cusps of upper left posterior teeth and lingual cusps of lower left posterior teeth indicate contacts in the left lateral occlusion. These surfaces are ground to develop uniform contacts. The lingual cusps of upper teeth and the buccal cusps of lower teeth are not ground even though they have marks from the articulating paper.

Fig. 23-12. Articulator is moved between right lateral occlusion and centric occlusion, with articulating paper between teeth to locate deflective occlusal contacts in the lateral excursion. Notice position of incisal pin on incisal guidance table.

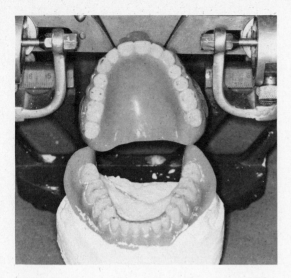

Fig. 23-13. Articulating paper markings in right lateral excursion. Marks on buccal cusps of upper right posterior teeth and lingual cusps of lower right posterior teeth indicate contacts in the right lateral occlusion. These surfaces are ground to develop uniform contacts. The lingual cusps of the upper teeth and the buccal cusps of the lower teeth are not ground even though they show marks from the articulating paper.

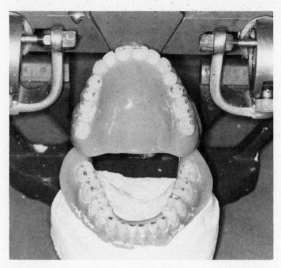

Fig. 23-14. Markings made by movements in all directions indicate uniform contacts.

right and left lateral and intermediate movements, the protrusive grinding will have been accomplished. Testing with articulating paper should show contact throughout the arches of the maxillary and mandibular dentures (Fig. 23-14). Inasmuch as denture teeth are fastened together as a unit, it is permissible to relieve the centric contact of the four incisors. This relief may be made at the time of setting the teeth, which will permit the use of a vertical overlap without increasing the incisal guide angle.

Carborundum paste for correcting occlusion

Carborundum paste should not be used to eliminate errors in occlusion of cusp teeth. If Carborundum paste is used to remove errors in centric and eccentric occlusions, occlusal vertical dimension will be reduced, and the area of contact of the tooth surfaces will be increased unnecessarily. The stresses of mastication will

be distributed improperly, and the loss of sharpness of the cusps will cause a decrease in the size and number of food exits. If it is used at all, smoothing of minute irregularities by the paste must be limited to one or two gliding movements of the articulator (Fig. 23-15).

Types of occlusal error in centric occlusion and their correction

Three types of occlusal error can exist in centric occlusion, and each can be corrected by specific grinding for that error.

1. Any pair of opposing teeth can be too long and hold other teeth out of contact. For correction of the error, the fossae of the teeth are deepened by grinding so that the teeth, in effect, telescope into each other (Fig. 23-16, A). The cusps are not shortened in this procedure.

2. The upper and lower teeth can be too nearly end to end. For correction of the error, grinding is done on the inclines of the cusps in such a way as to move the upper cusp inclines buccally and the lower cusp inclines lingually. In this process, the central fossae are made broader, the lingual cusp of the upper tooth is made more

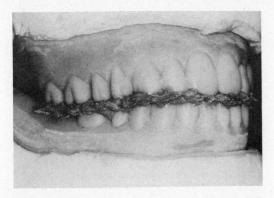

Fig. 23-15. Final smoothing can be done by abrasive paste, *A*, in one or two gliding movements of articulator.

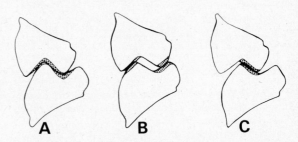

Fig. 23-16. Correction of errors in centric occlusion. Grind shaded areas if teeth are too long, **A**, if teeth are too nearly end to end, **B**, and there is too much horizontal overlap, **C**.

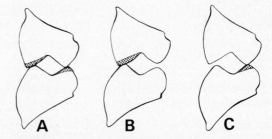

Fig. 23-17. Correction of errors on working side. The interfering cusps are shortened as indicated by shaded areas. **A**, Both buccal and lingual cusps are too long. **B**, Buccal cusps are too long. **C**, Lingual cusps are too long.

narrow when it is ground from the lingual side, and the buccal cusp of the lower tooth is made more narrow when it is ground from the buccal side (Fig. 23-16, *B*). The cusps are not shortened.

3. The upper teeth can be too far buccally in relation to the lower teeth. For correction of the error, the lingual cusp of the upper tooth is made more narrow by broadening of the central fossa, and the buccal cusp of the lower tooth is moved buccally by broadening of the central fossa (Fig. 23-16, *C*). In effect, the upper lingual cusp is moved lingually and the lower buccal cusp is moved buccally so that the teeth telescope into each other. The cusps are not shortened in this process.

Types of working-side occlusal errors and their correction

Six types of errors can exist in the occlusal contacts on the working side. Each of these will cause other teeth to be held out of contact in working occlusion, and each requires selective grinding of specific cusp inclines for its elimination.

1. Both the upper buccal cusp and the lower lingual cusp are too long. For correction of the error, the length of these cusps is reduced by grinding to change the incline extending from the central fossa to the cusp tip. The central fossa is not made deeper, but the upper buccal cusps and the lower lingual cusps are made shorter so that the other teeth will touch in that position (Fig. 23-17, *A*).

2. The buccal cusps make contact but the lingual cusps do not. For correction of the error, the buccal cusps of the upper teeth are ground from the central fossa to the cusp tip to shorten the cusp and change the lingual incline of the cusp so that it is less steep (Fig. 23-17, *B*).

3. The lingual cusps make contact but the buccal cusps do not. For correction of this error, one shortens the lower lingual cusps by chang-

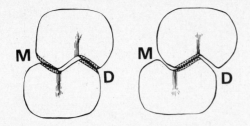

Fig. 23-18. To correct errors in mesiodistal relationship of teeth, grind where areas are shaded. *M,* Mesial surface; *D,* distal surface.

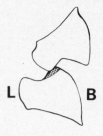

Fig. 23-19. To eliminate deflective occlusal contact on balancing side, grind lingual incline of lower buccal cusp. *L,* Lingual surface; *B,* buccal surface.

ing the buccal incline of the lower lingual incline so that it is not so steep. The upper lingual cusp is not shortened, and the central fossa is not made deeper (Fig. 23-17, *C*).

4. The upper buccal or lingual cusps are mesial to their intercusping positions. This error may occur along with any of the three errors just listed. For correction of this error, the grinding is done so that the mesial inclines of the upper buccal cusps are moved distally when the cusps are narrowed and the distal inclines of the lower cusps are ground to move them forward. The same cuspal inclination is maintained in this procedure (Fig. 23-18, *left*).

5. The upper buccal or lingual cusps are distal to their intercusping positions. This error may also occur along with buccolingual errors. For correction of the error, grinding is done from the distal side of the upper cusps and from the mesial side of the lower cusps (Fig. 23-18, *right*).

6. The teeth on the working side may not contact. The cause of this error is excessive contact on the balancing side.

Types of balancing-side errors and their correction

There are two types of balancing-side errors:

1. The balancing-side contact is so heavy that the working-side teeth are held out of contact. For correction of this error, paths are ground through the buccal cusps of the lower teeth to reduce the incline of the *part* of the cusp that is preventing the teeth on the working side from contacting (Fig. 23-19). As much as possible of each interfering cusp is preserved. No grinding is done from the lingual cusps that may be involved in this contact.

2. There is no balancing contact on the balancing side. To correct this error, it is necessary to shorten the buccal cusps of the upper teeth and the lingual cusps of the lower teeth on the *working* side. In this process, the lingual inclines of the buccal cusps of the upper teeth and the buccal inclines of the lingual cusps of the lower teeth are made less steep. No grinding is done in the central fossae (Fig. 23-17, *A*).

ELIMINATION OF OCCLUSAL ERRORS IN NONANATOMIC TEETH

Examination of the occlusion at the time of denture insertion often reveals one or more discrepancies. These discrepancies may be attributable to teeth coming out of alignment during the final stages of the laboratory procedure. An interocclusal centric relation record is made in a bite registration material with the opposing teeth just out of contact (Fig. 23-20). The dentures are mounted on the articulator, and the following procedures are undertaken:

1. Gross premature (interceptive occlusal) contacts in centric relation are removed by grinding, after being detected by the use of articulating paper between the teeth (Fig. 23-21). The same procedures are used to locate and

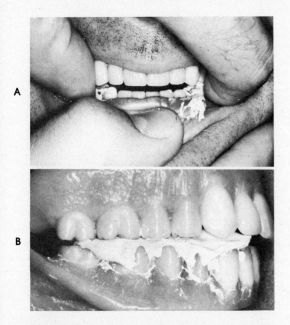

Fig. 23-20. A, Mandible is guided into centric relation position. **B,** Quick-setting plaster record is made with the teeth just out of contact.

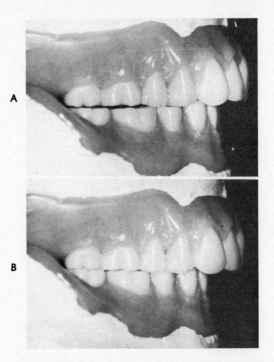

Fig. 23-21. Gross interceptive occlusal contact in premolar region, **A,** is removed so that maximal intercuspation occurs at centric relation position, which was transferred to the articulator, **B.**

remove all occlusal interferences in the lateral and protrusive occlusions. The grinding is done on the occlusal surfaces of teeth that appear to have been tipped or elongated in processing. In eccentric occlusion, no grinding is done on the distobuccal portion of the lower second molar. All balancing-side grinding is done on the lingual portion of the occlusal surface of the upper second molar.

2. Abrasive paste is placed on the teeth on the articulator. These teeth are milled with abrasive paste when the upper member of the articulator is moved in and out of protrusive and right and left lateral excursions. When the teeth slide smoothly through all excursions, the dentures are removed from the articulator and washed. Seldom is any correction necessary to attain a bilaterally balanced occlusion.

3. Spot grinding is done to correct the small discrepancies in centric relation that usually remain after the grinding with abrasive paste.

The dentist adjusts them after identifying the discrepancy with tabulator ribbon or articulating paper—using a light tapping motion with the articulator—and grinding the marks to ensure even occlusal contact in centric occlusion.

ADVANTAGES OF BALANCED OCCLUSION IN COMPLETE DENTURES

What is the advantage of balanced occlusion in dentures when a bolus of food on one side separates the teeth so that they could not possibly be in balancing contact on the opposite side? This question has aroused in the minds of many dentists the suspicion that balancing occlusion is a fetish of college professors and a few specialists. Many dentures are not balanced, since a large proportion of the profession is not thoroughly convinced of the value of balanced occlusion in relation to the effort involved in securing it. If a bolus of food were between the teeth on one side most of each of the 24 hours, there would not be much object in having an exact balanced occlusion. However, teeth make contact many thousands of times a day in both eccentric and centric positions, with no food in the mouth during nonfunctional mandibular movements. Even while chewing, the teeth cut through to contact every few fractions of a second. A balanced occlusion ensures even pressure in all parts of the arch, which maintains the stability of the dentures when the mandible is in centric and eccentric (parafunctional) positions.

ELIMINATION OF BASAL-SURFACE ERRORS

All surfaces of the completed dentures must be critically examined for small projections caused by imperceptible discrepancies in the cast or in the investing materials. A magnifying glass used in addition to a digital inspection of the denture bases can be effective in locating such irregularities. All denture borders and especially the frenal notches must also be examined carefully for sharp edges that will create considerable discomfort for the patient. Sharp borders, particularly in the frenal notches, must be carefully rounded before the initial placement of the dentures.

The removal of base material from the tissue surfaces of dentures to eliminate "pressure spots" that may be revealed by pressure-indicating paste or wax should be unnecessary. The fact that this procedure usually is carried out at the first appointment subsequent to the insertion of dentures indicates that many of these pressure spots may be the result of distortion of tissues by the occlusion.

However, pressure-indicator paste can be helpful when bilateral undercuts on the residual ridge interfere with initial placement of the dentures or when pressure spots were present in the final impression. The pressure-indicator paste is brushed on the tissue surface of the denture base in a thin layer so that the brush marks are visible and run in the same direction. In this

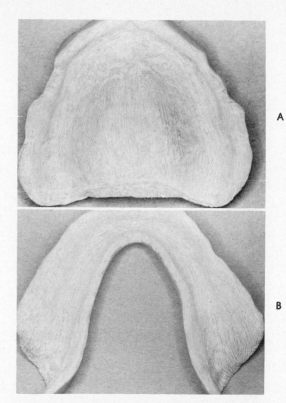

Fig. 23-22. A, Pressure-indicator paste is distributed in a thin, even layer across tissue surface of upper denture. **B,** Pressure-indicator paste is distributed in lower denture so that brush marks run in a similar direction. This method of distribution aids in determining interferences that may prevent proper placement of denture and detection of potentially harmful pressure spots.

manner, tissue interferences encountered during placement of the dentures or excessive pressure on the residual ridge can be more easily interpreted than without the paste (Fig. 23-22). Then the painted surface is sprayed with a silicone liquid.

The denture is carefully placed on the residual ridge and pressure is applied by the dentist on the occlusal surfaces of the teeth to determine the location of pressure spots in the denture base that displace soft tissue (Fig. 23-23). A repeated recording should be made for verification of pressure spots, and the denture base is carefully relieved (Fig. 23-24). When tissue

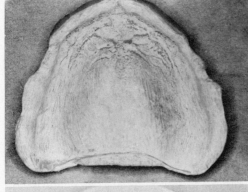

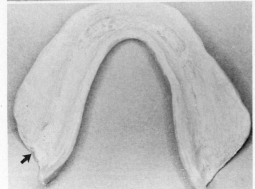

Fig. 23-23. A, Marks showing through pressure-indicator paste reveal location of pressure spots exerted by denture on residual ridge. The pressure spot in region of left hamular notch was also present in final impression. Notice that posterior palatal seal bead shows through pressure-indicator paste indicating that desired seal is being provided. **B,** Pressure areas showing through in alveolar groove anteriorly and retromolar fossa *(arrow)* should be relieved, since this is not primary stress-bearing area for lower denture. The exposed borders of lingual flange are not necessarily significant at time of initial placement of lower denture but may be of importance if correlated with unnecessary movement of denture or soreness in patient's mouth in alveololingual sulcus at a later date.

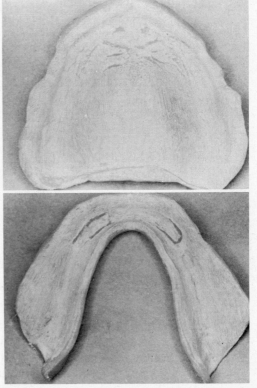

Fig. 23-24. Pressure spots seen in Fig. 23-23 have been carefully relieved with a No. 8 round bur. A minimum of denture base material is removed.

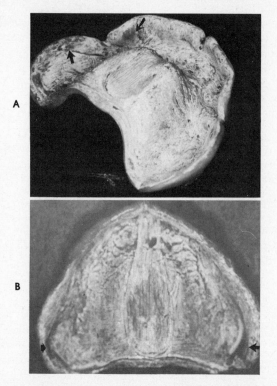

Fig. 23-25. A, Tissue interferences in placement of denture can be seen by pressure areas on flange just distal to canine fossa and just below border of buccal flange in molar region *(arrows)* in this immediate upper denture. **B,** Pressure areas just below border of buccal flanges in region of posterior part of maxillary tuberosities *(arrows)*.

interferences (undercuts) are present, the denture coated with pressure-indicator paste is seated on the residual ridge until resistance is met. The marks in the paste indicate where the denture base should be relieved to accommodate for the undercuts (Fig. 23-25). Pressure-indicator paste is *not* required for every new denture but only when there is a definite indication that it may be helpful.

SPECIAL INSTRUCTIONS TO THE PATIENT

Educating patients to the limitations of dentures as mechanical substitutes for living tissues must be a continuing process from the initial contact with the patient until adjustments are completed. However, certain difficulties that will be encountered with new dentures and information related to the care of dentures should be reinforced at the time of initial placement of the dentures. Forewarning patients makes them more tolerant of problems and less likely to incorrectly relate them to the fit of the dentures. Explanations provided after problems develop are often interpreted by patients as excuses made by the dentist for dentures that function less than satisfactorily.

Individuality of patients

Patients must be reminded that their physical, mental, and oral conditions are individual in nature. Thus they cannot compare their progress with new dentures with other persons' experiences. What is annoying and painful to some may be of secondary importance to others. Chewing and speech patterns with new dentures that are considered successful by some persons may be interpreted as totally unsuccessful in the minds of others. In addition, adaptability to new dentures is modified by age. Persons who make the adjustment to new dentures during middle age will probably experience considerably more difficulty with their replacement 15 years later, even though the new dentures may be technically superior to the original dentures.

Patients tend to forget the severity of problems with the passage of time. Many persons indicate that their dentures have always been comfortable, even though they may have had a difficult adjustment period. Such remarks can be discouraging to patients with new dentures unless they have been advised of this possibility.

Appearance with new dentures

Patients must understand that their appearance with new dentures will become more natural with time. Initially the dentures will feel strange and bulky in the mouth and will cause a feeling of fullness of the lips and cheeks. The lips will not adapt immediately to the fullness of the denture borders and may initially present a distorted appearance. Muscle tension may cause an awkward appearance that will improve after the patient becomes relaxed and more self-confident.

Patients should be instructed to refrain from exhibiting their dentures to curious friends until they are confident and competent to exhibit them at their best. When patients are not careful in following these instructions, they may likely become unfairly critical of the dentures and develop an attitude that will be difficult for the dentist to overcome. During the edentulous or partially edentulous period, gradual reduction of the interarch distance and collapsing of the lips will have occurred. These changes have usually been so gradual that the family and friends were not aware that they have occurred. Therefore a repositioning of the orbicularis oris muscle and a restoration of the former facial dimension and contour by the new dentures may seem like too great a change in the patient's appearance. This can be overcome only with the passing of time, and patients are advised to persevere during this period of readjustment.

Mastication with new dentures

Learning to chew satisfactorily with new dentures usually requires a period of at least 6 to 8 weeks. Patients will become discouraged unless they are aware that this learning period should be expected. New memory patterns often must be established for both the facial muscles and the muscles of mastication. Once the habit patterns become automatic in nature, the chewing process can take place without conscious effort. The muscles of the tongue, cheeks, and lips must be trained in the art of maintaining the dentures in position on the residual ridges during the masticatory process. Patients can be told that "these muscles must learn what they should and should not do."

Mastication is additionally impaired because of the excess flow of saliva for the first few days after placement of new dentures. However, in a relatively short period of time, the salivary glands accommodate to the presence of the dentures, and production of saliva returns to normal.

Patients should begin chewing relatively soft food that is cut into small pieces. If the chewing can be done on both sides of the mouth at the same time, the tendency of the dentures to tip will be reduced. Patients should be told that during this early period, mastication should be attempted on simple types of food such as crackers, soft toast, or chopped meat and that no attempt should be made to masticate resistant food. Also, during the learning period of mastication patients are advised to be away from critical observation of friends or members of the family, since the patients will be awkward in the beginning phases of chewing and susceptible to embarrassment and discouragement. Kindly but misplaced joking remarks and comments by members of the family may readily lead patients to a denture-conscious complex that will be reflected in the attitude toward the dentist and the dentures.

When biting with dentures, patients should be instructed to place the food between the teeth toward the corner of the mouth, rather than between the anterior teeth in the front of the mouth. Then, the food is pushed inward and upward to break it apart rather than downward and outward as would be done if natural teeth were present. Inward and upward forces tend to seat the dentures on the residual ridges rather than displace them.

Occasionally, edentulous patients have gone without dentures for long periods of time and have learned to crush food between the residual ridges or perhaps between the tongue and the hard palate. These persons usually experience increased difficulty in learning to masticate with new dentures, and the time period for adjustment will likely be extended.

Patients should be told that the position of the tongue plays an important role in the stability of the lower denture, particularly during mastication. Patients whose tongues normally rest in a retracted position in relation to the lower anterior teeth should attempt to learn to position the tongue farther forward so that it rests on the lingual surfaces of the lower anterior teeth. This position helps develop stability for the lower denture.

Speaking with new dentures

Fortunately, the problem of speaking with new dentures is not so difficult as might be expected. The adaptability of the tongue to compensate for changes is so great that most patients master speech with new dentures within a few weeks. If correct speech required exact replacement of tissues and teeth in relation to tongue movement, no patient could ever learn to talk with dentures. The necessity of additional bulk of material over the palate would cause a lasting impediment of speech. Even a 0.5 mm change at the linguogingival border of the anterior teeth would cause a speech defect, especially in the production of *s* sounds, if it were not for the extreme adaptability of the tongue to these changes. For that reason, tooth positions that restore appearance and masticatory function usually do not produce phonetic changes that are too great to be readily compensated. However, a study of tongue positions is valuable and gives an appreciation of the value of positioning the dentures in the relation formerly occupied by the natural teeth.

Speaking normally with dentures requires practice. Patients should be advised to read aloud and repeat words or phrases that are difficult to pronounce. Patients usually are much more conscious of small irregularities in their speech sounds than those to whom they are speaking.

Oral hygiene with dentures

Patients must be convinced of the importance of maintaining good oral hygiene for the health of the oral cavity. Plaque, stain, and calculus accrue on dentures and oral mucosa of edentulous patients in a similar fashion as in the mouths of dentulous patients. Dental plaque is an etiologic factor in denture stomatitis, inflammatory papillary hyperplasia, chronic candidiasis, and offensive odors, and it must be removed.

Patients should be told that their dentures must be thoroughly brushed at least twice daily and rinsed after meals whenever possible. The denture should be removed from the mouth and cleaned with a soft brush, using a dishwashing detergent or a toothpaste low in abrasives as the cleansing agent. Regular tooth paste contains an abrasive material that will wear away the surface of acrylic resin. The dentures should be brushed over a basin partially filled with water or covered with a wet washcloth to prevent breakage should they be dropped. Soaking dentures in a glass of water containing a mixture of one teaspoon of Calgon and one teaspoon of Clorox for 30 minutes once a week will remove most stains. Then the dentures must be rinsed thoroughly. Mersene (Colgate-Palmolive Co., New York, N.Y.) is effective in removing plaque from dentures.

The mucosal surfaces of the residual ridges and the dorsal surface of the tongue should also be brushed daily with a soft brush. This procedure provides stimulation for increased circulation and removes plaque and debris that could cause irritation of the mucous membrane or offensive odors.

Preserving residual ridges

The residual ridges were not intended to bear the stresses of mastication that are created by complete dentures. Therefore patients, especially when their general health is somewhat impaired, may expect some irritation and discomfort of the oral tissues. No two patients' mouths will react alike, since some tissues tolerate stress better than others. Therefore the expectancy in this regard cannot be predicted exactly. Patients must be made aware of these varying and unpredictable conditions.

If some irritation of the tissues is experienced, patients are advised to remove their dentures and rest the mouth for a time. More harm than good is done by telling patients that they must keep their dentures in the mouth constantly during this initial adjustment period, since they will become highly nervous and fatigued and be unnecessarily discouraged about their final successful wearing of the dentures. However, patients are requested to wear the dentures for several hours before an adjustment appointment so that the sore spots will be visible and accurate corrections to the dentures can be made. Patients must be cautioned concerning the critical nature of adjustments to the dentures. They must be convinced that the *dentist* is the only person qualified to undertake this most important aspect of the denture service. Obviously, patients should never attempt to adjust the dentures themselves.

Patients should be told that dentures must be left out of the mouth at night to provide needed rest from the stresses that they create on the residual ridges. Failure to allow the tissues of the basal seat to rest may be a contributing factor in development of serious oral lesions such as inflammatory papillary hyperplasia or may increase the opportunity for the growth of fungus infections such as candidiasis. When dentures are left out of the mouth, they should be placed in a container filled with water to prevent drying and possible dimensional changes of the denture base material.

Residual ridges can be ruined by use of denture adhesives and home-reliners, and patients should be cautioned about their use. When patients begin using these materials, they will soon feel insecure without them. Adhesives and especially home-reliners invariably modify the position of the denture on the residual ridge, which can result in a change in both the vertical and centric relations. The residual ridges can be irreparably damaged in a short period of time.

The special instructions must include directions for continued periodic oral examinations for edentulous patients. The tissues supporting dentures change with time, and the rate of change depends on both local and general factors. Good dentures eventually become ill-fitting dentures that can damage the mouth without the patient being aware that anything is wrong. Pathosis, which may or may not be associated with the dentures, can develop in the edentulous oral cavity. All edentulous patients should be examined by a dentist at least once a year and should be placed on a recall list for that purpose.

Educational material for patients

Since the education of patients is so critical to the success of new dentures, many dentists provide the patient with written instructions or other formal education material that has been developed. In studying the material, patients become aware that dentures are not permanent, that the mouth changes, and most importantly, that the proper care they provide for themselves may be the deciding factor in the success they will experience with dentures.

Denture patients need guidance after they have their new teeth. Much of this can be provided orally while the dentures are being constructed. But this is not enough. People remember less of what they hear than of what they see. For this reason, it is wise to provide denture patients with printed information about their new teeth, about the care of them, about cleaning them, about using them, and, not least important, about the periodic inspections that will be necessary later.

A number of books or pamphlets about the care and use of dentures are available. One or more of these should be given to each patient to read during the construction of the dentures. The information contained in them will help patients learn to use their new teeth and to recognize the fact that they need periodic professional dental supervision after they have dentures. These supplements to treatment are more important than some of us may recognize. After all, everyone knows how to make toast in an electric toaster, yet when you buy one, you get a set of directions for its use. If patients are to have adequate care after they get their new teeth, they should have some readily available source of information about them.

24

Maintaining the comfort and health of the oral cavity of rehabilitated edentulous patients

Treatment with complete dentures is not really successful unless patients wear them. Therefore complete denture service cannot be adequate unless patients are cared for after the dentures are placed in the mouth.

In many instances, the most crucial time in the success or failure of dentures is the adjustment period. The dentist is responsible for the care of the patient throughout this period, and it may require a number of appointments. It is important that the dentist and patient have a clear understanding as to the financial implications of the adjustment period. This relates to the philosophy of the dentist in patient management.

The complete cooperation of the patient during the adjustment period is essential. In educating patients, the dentist must explain to them the problems that they are likely to face during the adjustment phase and the procedures that both the patient and the dentist must follow to alleviate these problems.

TWENTY-FOUR HOUR ORAL EXAMINATION AND TREATMENT

An appointment for a 24-hour adjustment should be made routinely. Patients who do not have this attention have more trouble than those who are cared for within 24 hours of the insertion of the new dentures. This is the critical period in the denture-wearing experience of the patient. When the patient returns for the 24-hour adjustment, the dentist can ask, "How is the patient with the sore mouth?" This invites patients to describe their experiences and soreness, if any. The dentist must listen carefully to the patient and on the basis of these comments can learn approximately where to look for trouble. The statements may furnish valuable information about psychologic problems that may be developing.

Examination procedures

The occlusion should be observed before the dentures are removed from the mouth. To do this, the ball of the thumb and the ball of the index finger of the left hand are placed between the upper and lower teeth when the mouth is open. The palm of the hand is facing the patient, with the little finger up. The patient is directed to pull the lower jaw back and close on the back teeth. As this is done, the fingers are slowly withdrawn to the buccal sides of the teeth so that they can *feel* the teeth touch. If the teeth *touch and slide*, there is an error in centric occlusion. When such an error is detected, the dentures are placed on their remount casts on the articulator, and the occlusion is rechecked there. If the same error is found on the articulator, it is eliminated by selective grinding. If there is an error in the mouth and none is found on the articulator, new interocclusal records of the centric and protrusive relations must be made. The mandibular remount cast is removed from the articulator, and the lower denture is remounted before the occlusion is corrected.

After the occlusion has been tested, a thorough visual and digital examination of the oral cavity is performed to determine the location of sore spots. The examination begins with the mucosa of the upper buccal vestibule, proceeds, around through the labial vestibule and the buccal vestibule on the other side of the mouth, with careful observation of the frenums. The hamular notches and the hard and soft palates are examined for signs of abrasion. The area of

the coronoid process is palpated, and the patient is asked if any tenderness is felt in that region.

The lower dental arch and associated dental structures are systematically examined both visually and digitally. The tissues lining the vestibular spaces and the alveololingual sulcus, particularly the mylohyoid ridges and the retromylohyoid spaces, are observed carefully. The sides of the tongue and the mucosal lining of the cheeks must also be inspected.

Adjustments related to occlusion

A number of problems can result from errors in occlusion. Soreness may develop on the crest of the residual ridge from pressures created by heavy contacts of opposing teeth in the same region. Soreness may also be seen on the slopes of the residual ridge as a result of shifting of the denture bases from deflective occlusal contacts (Fig. 24-1). Before unnecessarily shortening or excessively relieving the denture base, one must observe the occlusion carefully in the mouth and on the articulator, giving particular attention to the possibility of heavy balancing contacts that will cause rotation of the denture bases. The correction is made on the articulator by development of a pathway on the lower tooth for the offending upper cusp. Such errors in occlusion are almost impossible to locate in the mouth because of movement of the denture bases on the supporting soft tissues.

Small lesions on the buccal mucosa of the cheek in line with the occlusal plane indicate that the patient is biting the cheeck during mastication. The lesion will be located on the mucosa adjacent to the offending teeth. This problem can usually be corrected by reduction of the buccal surface of the appropriate lower tooth to create additional horizontal overlap, thus providing an escapeway for the buccal mucosa.

Patients may complain, "My dentures are tight when I first put them in my mouth, but they seem to loosen after several hours." This symptom usually is an indication of errors in the occlusion and can often be corrected after new interocclusal records are made, the dentures are

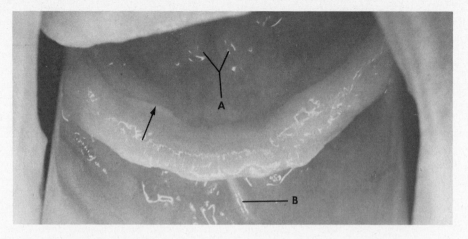

Fig. 24-1. Lesion *(arrow)* on mucosa of lingual slope of lower residual ridge is likely related to errors in occlusion that cause denture base to shift and thus impinge on mucosa. *A,* Sublingual caruncles; *B,* lower labial frenum.

remounted, and the occlusion is adjusted on the articulator. The dentures become loose because the deflective occlusal contacts cause a continual shifting of the bases on the basal seat. Although this problem may develop by the time of the 24-hour adjustment, it is more likely to be seen a little later on.

Adjustments related to the denture bases

A number of problems caused by new dentures are related to the denture bases themselves. Lesions of the mucosa in the reflections are most often caused by denture borders that are too sharp or denture flanges that are overextended. Sometimes, the labial notch of the denture may be sharp or insufficient in size, and the frenum becomes irritated. Usually the notch needs to be deepened slightly and also made rounded and smooth (Fig. 24-2). Widening of the notch may not be necessary and could result in a reduction in retention of the denture. The notch is deepened with a fissure bur. Then the denture base material is made round and smooth by the use of a sharp scraper and a Burlew disk, followed by pumice on the tip of a felt cone or a brush wheel.

Soreness created by extra length of the anterior part of the lingual flange should not be confused with soreness on the slopes of the ridge resulting from occlusion. An indelible pencil mark is placed either on the sore spot in the mouth or on the denture base and is transferred accordingly to accurately locate the correct site for reduction of the denture border (Fig. 24-3). The denture border is carefully shortened with a sharp scraper and carefully polished with pumice and a rag wheel.

Lesions in the region of the hamular notch must be considered carefully. If the irritated tissue is posterior to the notch, the denture base is too long and should be shortened. However, if the soreness is in the notch itself, the posterior palatal seal is likely creating too much pressure, and the inside of the tissue surface of the denture base should be relieved very cautiously. A mistake in judgment at this point might reduce or eliminate the seal of the upper denture. The notch should be carefully palpated to aid in making this diagnostic determination (Fig. 24-4).

Soreness may develop along the crest of the lower ridge when spiny projections of bone remain in this region (Fig. 24-5, *A*). Precautions

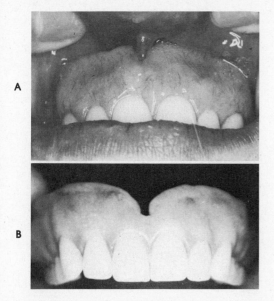

Fig. 24-2. A, Labial notch must accommodate action of labial frenum. **B,** Notch must be sufficiently deep with rounded, smooth borders.

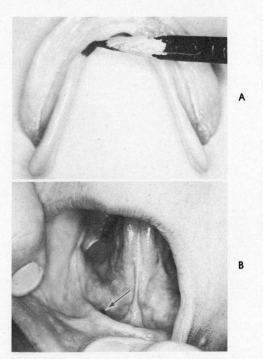

Fig. 24-3. A, Indelible mark is placed on border of lingual flange at site judged to correspond with sore spot in mouth. **B,** Mark is transferred to mucosa in the floor of the mouth *(arrow).* The relationship of the mark to the sore spot provides information as to necessary location for relief of border of lingual flange.

should be taken in the impression procedure but may not always be adequate. The denture base is coated with pressure-indicator paste, the denture is placed in the mouth, and pressure is directed on the occlusal surfaces of the teeth in a vertical direction (Fig. 24-5, *B*). The denture base is relieved in the locations as indicated, using a round bur.

Lesions of the mucosa lining the retromylohyoid fossa can be caused by excess pressure or length of the denture flange (Fig. 24-6, *A*). Often patients will complain of soreness when they swallow or state that "I feel like I have a sore throat." The denture base should be shortened, or the tissue surface should be relieved to reduce pressure, depending on the location of the lesion (Fig. 24-6, *B*). Complaints of soreness during swallowing are also frequently related to irritation in the region of the mylohyoid ridges.

Since additional stress is placed on the buccal shelf of the lower jaw during impression proce-

dures, differential diagnosis of soreness in this area may be necessary. If the irritation is related to the length of the buccal flange (Fig. 24-7, *A*), which can be determined when the denture border in the mouth is compared with the location of the lesion, then the length of the flange should be shortened. However, when the sore spot is on the mucosa overlying the buccal shelf, the denture base in that region is relieved. Pressure-indicator paste can be helpful in determining the location of this kind of lesion (Fig. 24-7, *B*). The denture base is relieved slightly with a sharp scraper, and in this instance the length of the flange is not reduced.

Excessive pressure from the lower buccal flange in the region of the mental foramen may

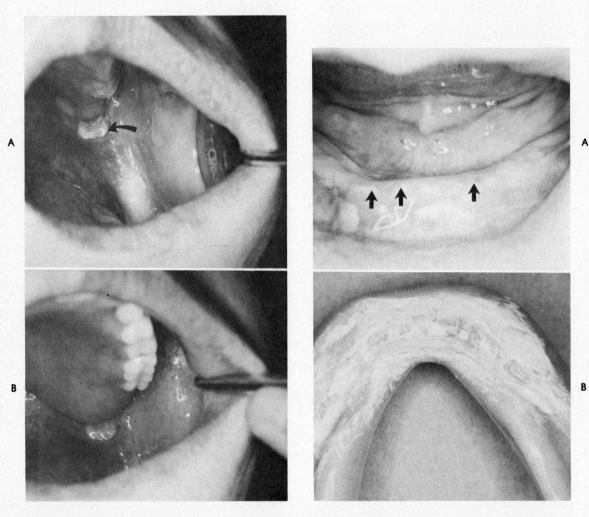

Fig. 24-4. A, Sore spot *(arrow)* is posterior to hamular notch, indicating that denture base is too long in this region. **B,** After adjustment of denture, notice that sore spot is visible posterior to border.

Fig. 24-5. A, Spiny projections of bone *(arrows)* underlie mucosa covering the crest of this lower residual ridge. **B,** Pressure spots in indicator paste denote location of necessary relief. The denture base will be adjusted with a No. 8 round bur.

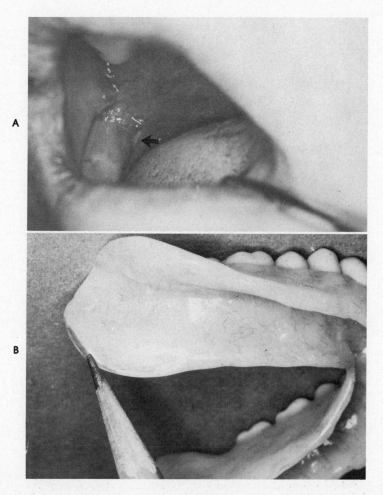

Fig. 24-6. A, Lesion on mucosa lining retromylohyoid fossa *(arrow)* is caused by excess length and pressure from denture base in this region. **B,** Pencil mark indicates site of correction for lesion seen in **A.**

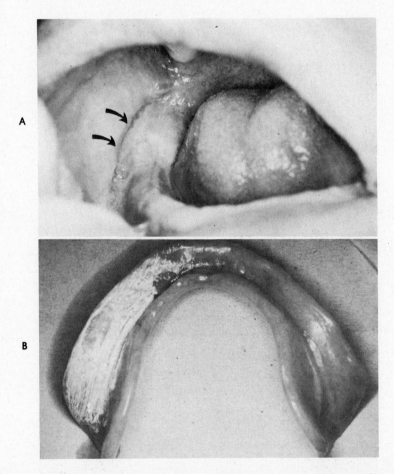

Fig. 24-7. A, Line of irritation *(arrows)* is caused by an overextension of buccal flange of lower denture. **B,** Pressure spot in indicator paste represents the part of the denture base that is placing excessive pressure on mucosa of buccal shelf (not related to **A**).

cause a tingling or a numbing sensation at the corner of the mouth or in the lower lip. This results from pressure on the mental nerve and occurs particularly when excess resorption has occurred, causing the mental foramen to be located near the crest of the lower residual ridge. A similar situation can occur in the upper jaw from pressure on the incisive papilla, which is transmitted to the nasopalatine nerve. The patient may complain of burning or numbness in the anterior part of the upper jaw. Relief may be required in the upper denture base in this region.

Patients may return for the initial adjustment appointment complaining that their dentures cause them to gag. The problem may actually be related to the dentures themselves, or there may be a psychologic component, or both. When the problem is denture related, usually it will be the upper denture although on occasion the lower denture or both dentures may be involved. Most often the gagging may relate to the posterior border of the upper denture. The border may be improperly extended, or the posterior border seal may be inadequate (Fig. 24-8). The gagging seems to be caused most often from a making and breaking of the posterior palatal seal as the tissue posterior to the vibrating line moves upward and downward during function. When the vibrating line has been properly located, it is not necessary and usually not desirable to extend the posterior border of the upper denture more than 2 mm past this point. If the posterior palatal seal is inadequate, modeling compound can be added to reshape this part of the upper denture and determine if this will help alleviate the situation. Then the modeling compound can be replaced with acrylic resin. Occlusion can also be a factor, since shifting of the denture bases may cause the making and breaking of the posterior palatal seal and result in gagging.

On occasion, patients will state that the upper denture comes loose when they open their mouth widely to bite into a sandwich or to yawn. Generally this complaint indicates that the dis-

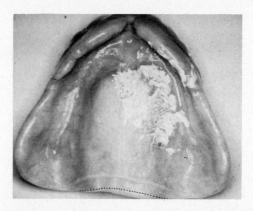

Fig. 24-8. Overextended posterior border of an upper denture. When posterior border was shortened to length as approximately indicated by the dotted line, denture no longer caused gagging when in the patient's mouth.

tobuccal flange of the upper denture is too thick and interferes with normal movements of the coronoid process (Fig. 24-9). The borders of the upper buccal flanges should properly fill the buccal vestibule. However, the distal corners of the denture base below the borders must be thin to allow the freedom necessary for movement of the coronoid process.

Again, in discussion with patients, they may indicate that the upper denture tends to loosen during smiling or other forms of facial expression. Excessive thickness or height of the flange of the upper denture in the region of the buccal notch or posterior to the buccal notch may cause this problem (Fig. 24-10). As the buccal frenum moves posteriorly during function, it encroaches on a border that is too thick and loosens the denture. Reduction of the width of the border posterior to the upper buccal notch will often help alleviate this problem.

Modifications of the denture base must be carefully made. To grind away parts of the base unnecessarily can cause further difficulty. The overextended parts of the denture base must be carefully reduced with a sharp scraper according to the amount of inflammation caused. Then the borders must be polished wherever they have

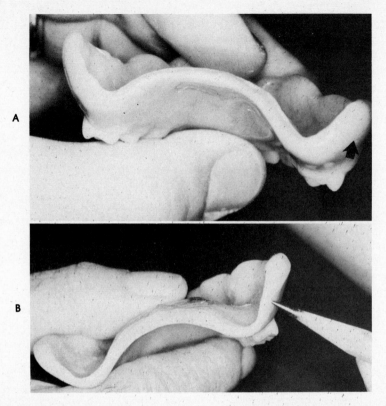

Fig. 24-9. A, Distobuccal flange of upper denture is too thick below border *(arrow).* **B,** Flange is proper thickness.

been modified. An unpolished border may lead to further inflammation, even though it is not overextended. If the border is polished by the dentist, any modification by the patient is apparent.

SUBSEQUENT ORAL EXAMINATIONS AND TREATMENTS

Dentures require inspection and may require further adjustment after they have been used by the patient. During the first 2 months, the acrylic resin base materials absorb water. This addition of water to the resin can change the size and shape of the dentures. Even though these changes are small, they may be sufficient to change the occlusion. Minute changes in occlusion can cause soreness by causing the dentures

to shift or slide in function. Soreness reported by patients in this situation is most likely to be on the lingual side of the mandibular ridge in the region of the canine and first premolar. The cause is most likely to be deflective occlusal contact between the last molar teeth diagonally across the mouth, and this incorrect contact will be on the balancing inclines of the lower second molar.

The occlusal error may be observed and corrected by placement of the dentures on their original remount casts on the articulator in most instances. However, if the bases have changed so that they do not fit the remount casts the way they did originally, it is necessary to make new remount casts and new interocclusal records. The remount jig record will permit the upper denture to be remounted without a new face-bow transfer record being made.

When the dentures do not fit the remount casts at this time, the patient should be required to keep the dentures out of the mouth for 24 hours before the new interocclusal records are made. This will permit the soft tissues of the basal seats to regain their healthy, undistorted forms.

After the new records are made, the occlusion is corrected by selective grinding by the same procedure as was used at the time of their insertion. It is interesting that the changes in occlusion are likely to be small, but the soreness they produce is very real and disturbing to the patient. Dentists should not succumb to the temptation to grind from the denture base without determining the real cause of the trouble.

Sometimes generalized irritation or soreness of the basal seat will develop (Fig. 24-11). Although this condition might be attributable to a number of factors such as an excessive vertical relation of occlusion, nutritional or hormonal problems, or unhygienic dentures, it may likely result from occlusion. As indicated previously, errors in occlusion should be suspected when a patient states that "My dentures are tight when I first put them in my mouth in the morning, but seem to loosen later in the day." A collection of calculus on the teeth on one side of the denture is also an indication of the need for correcting the occlusion.

Certain symptoms at an adjustment appointment may indicate insufficient interocclusal distance. The patient's comments may go something like this: "After I have worn my new dentures for several hours, the gums of both of my jaws get sore and the muscles in the bottom part of my face seem tired." On removal of the dentures, the mucosa of the basal seat may exhibit a generalized irritation. These symptoms indicate that when the patient's mandible is in the resting position, there is not sufficient space between the opposing teeth to allow the supporting structures of the residual ridge and the involved muscles to rest normally. If this is true,

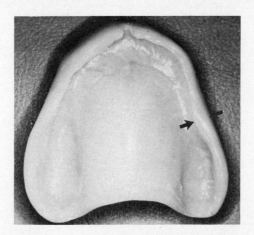

Fig. 24-10. Note excess thickness of right buccal border in region of buccal notch *(arrows)*. The buccal frenum moving posteriorly over this border during facial expression can loosen or unseat upper denture.

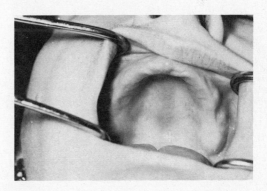

Fig. 24-11. Note generalized irritation and erythema of mucosa of basal seat of upper residual ridge. Occlusion is often primary contributing etiologic factor. The dentures should be remounted on articulator with new interocclusal records, and the occlusion adjusted.

there are several choices. Sometimes creation of a small amount of additional interocclusal distance will solve the problem, and the dentist can do this by returning the dentures to the articulator and reducing the vertical dimension of occlusion by grinding the artificial teeth. The amount of clearance between the anterior teeth and esthetics are the limiting factors in this procedure, and another 1 to 1.5 mm of interocclusal distance may be created in this manner. In other instances, it may be necessary to reset the artificial teeth of one or both dentures. The decision as to which teeth should be moved is based on the guides for establishing esthetics and the vertical dimensions of occlusion. Finally, in some instances, the dentures must be remade.

Periodic recall for oral examination

When patients are dismissed at the end of adjustment appointments, they are instructed to call for an appointment if they have any prob-lems. Some difficult patients should be scheduled for appointments periodically, perhaps at 3- to 4-month intervals. This procedure helps the patients' morale and also tends to eliminate their seeking adjustment appointments on a weekly basis or even more often.

Every denture patient should be placed on a recall program just as any other patient. The dentist should not hesitate to inform his patients that occlusal corrections, relining, new dentures, or other fairly involved procedures may be indicated as changes in the mouth continue to occur.

SECTION FOUR

Rehabilitating partially edentulous patients with special complete dentures

25

Tooth-supported complete dentures

Loss of teeth, especially mandibular teeth, will frequently lead to a rapid reduction in the height of the alveolar process (Tallgren, 1966, 1969; Carlsson and Persson, 1967) (Fig. 25-1, C). This morphologic change in the residual alveolar ridges is considered to be a major oral disease entity (Atwood, 1971), yet an effort to preserve the patient's oral health is limited by an incomplete understanding of the biomechanical and systemic factors influencing the reduction of residual ridges.

Dentists have long recognized the difference that the presence of teeth makes to alveolar ridge integrity (Fig. 25-1, A and B). It appears that the presence of a healthy periodontal membrane helps maintain alveolar ridge morphology.

In the past few years, several authors (Lord and Teel, 1969; Brewer and Fenton, 1973; Toolson and Smith, 1983) reported on favorable results obtained by constructing complete dentures over retained teeth or roots, or both, that may or may not be prepared. Much has been written about the benefits a patient obtains from such overdenture techniques. These benefits include better preservation of ridge height and improved denture stability. Longitudinal support has been lacking for the claim that the retention of tooth roots and their periodontal ligaments ensures better levels of alveolar bone. However, at least one pilot study by Crum and Rooney (1978) lends credence to the clinical observation that overdentures do contribute to alveolar bone maintenance.

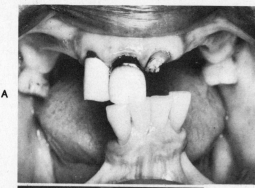

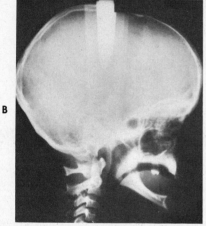

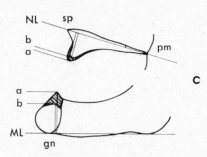

Fig. 25-1. A, Dramatic residual ridge reduction of mandibular edentulous segments is contrasted by integrity of alveolar ridge level where incisors are present. **B,** Virtual absence of alveolar bone is seen in mandible of a 13-year-old male patient whose dentition is congenitally absent. **C,** Measurements of alveolar resorption. The anterior height of upper and lower alveolar ridges at two stages of observation (*a* and *b*). The difference, *a − b*, represents reduction in height of alveolar ridges between stages of observation. *Shaded area,* Resorption. (**C** from Tallgren, A.: J. Prosthet. Dent. **27**:120-132, 1972.)

MUCOSAL COVERAGE OF ROOTS

Herd (1973) suggested that retained roots are accepted by the tissues and develop a nonfunctional type of periodontal membrane attached to a cellular cementum. His conclusions were based on a clinical, radiographic, and histologic study of 228 human retained root tips. In 1975, Guyer published a report in which he described selective retention of submucosally submerged vital roots to improve the contour of the edentulous ridge. Welker and associates (1978) replicated Guyer's technique on eight patients and observed them over a 5-year period. Their technique appeared successful insofar as it met patient satisfaction and dentist approval. This technique deserves further investigation but is not described in this chapter, since it is still at an early stage of development.

INDICATIONS AND CONTRAINDICATIONS

Over dentures, which may be of the partial or complete type, were initially prescribed for patients with congenital or acquired intraoral defects (Fig. 25-2). In recent years they have been prescribed for patients with badly worn down teeth (Fig. 25-3), for those patients with only a few remaining teeth (Fig. 25-4, *A* to *D*), or where aberration in jaw size or positions have developed (Fig. 25-4, *E* to *K*). The cosmetic and functional results obtained are excellent, and the retention of a few of a patient's teeth is frequently of immense psychologic value to the patient. The tooth-supported complete denture is a viable and simple alternative to the usual complete denture therapy. The application of this technique is virtually unlimited and depends on the dentist's judgment, skill, and

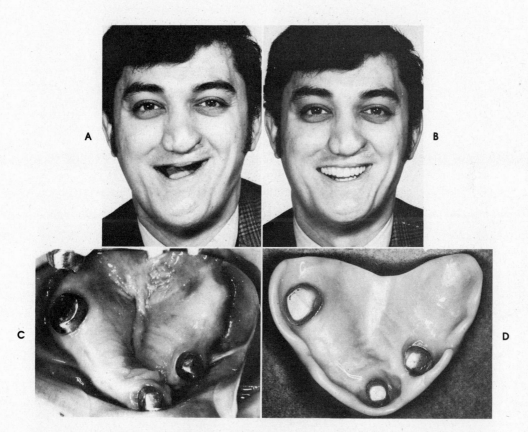

Fig. 25-2. A and **B,** Young adult whose congenital anomaly of a cleft lip and palate has been surgically repaired. **C,** Mirror reflection of maxillae, showing the remaining maxillary teeth prepared for gold copings, which in turn were related to fitted copings embedded in the maxillary denture, **D.**

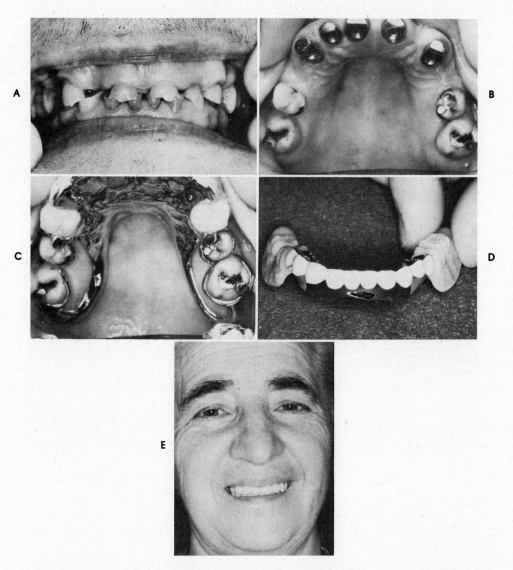

Fig. 25-3. A, Badly broken-down dentition in a 62-year-old female patient. **B** and **C,** Maxillary anterior teeth are restored with gold copings, and a maxillary cast removable partial denture is built over these copings. **D,** Mandibular dentition is restored with a part-overlay cast removable partial denture. **E,** Restored vertical dimension of occlusion improves cosmetic appearance of patient.

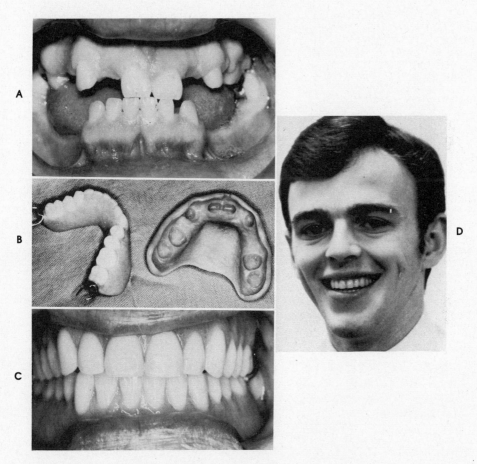

Fig. 25-4. A to **D,** Congenitally missing teeth have undermined both appearance and functional efficiency of this patient. Overlay dentures are used to create a normal appearance. **E, F, I,** and **J,** Pretreatment pictures of a patient whose complaint of mandibular dysfunction and poor cosmetics was attributable to a reduced vertical dimension of occlusion. **G, H,** and **K,** A maxillary overdenture resolved this patient's problem. (**A** and **D** courtesy Dr. A.H. Fenton, University of Toronto.)

Continued.

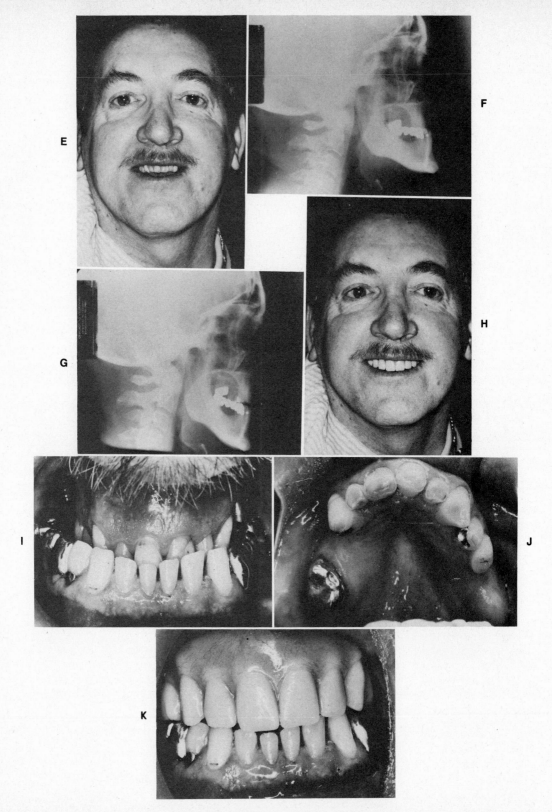

Fig. 25-4, cont'd. For legend see p. 513.

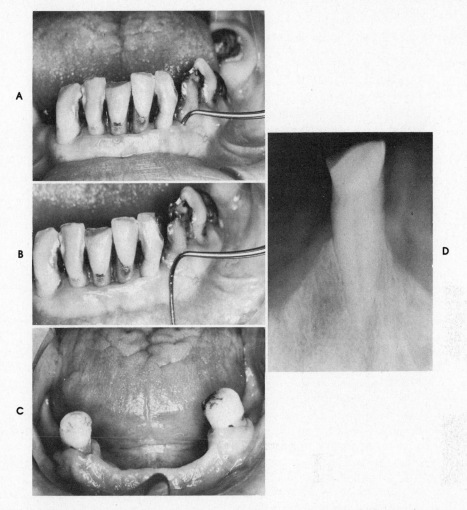

Fig. 25-5. A and **B,** Extensive bone loss negates use of these remaining teeth for abutment service. A healthy periodontium, seen clinically in **C** and radiographically in **D,** qualifies these teeth for selection as abutments.

versatility and, above all, the patient's motivation to maintain an impeccable oral environment. *Covering teeth and gingival tissues with overdentures is not conducive to maintaining a plaque-free environment*. Therefore it is not surprising that clinical experience with overdenture patients reveals a significant frequency of caries and gingival disease around the abutments. Caries may develop in a short period of time (Toolson and Smith, 1983), and some patients are more susceptible than others. This problem appears to be significantly reduced by the application of fluoride solutions to the prepared abutment teeth. A recent report by McDermott and Rosenberg (1983) underscores the value of using overdentures for the irradiated patient.

Contraindications are relatively few and are essentially related to an absence of patient motivation. Most patients who are candidates for their first complete dentures have at least one or two teeth that can be saved by periodontal treatment, an improvement in the crown/root ratio, and endodontic therapy.

SELECTION OF ABUTMENT TEETH

The critical factor in the selection of abutment teeth appears to be the status of the periodontium and the alveolar bone surrounding the teeth (Fig. 25-5). It is easy to argue that as many teeth as possible should be retained, but consideration should be given to the following factors:

1. Cost. A considerable expense may be incurred if several teeth are to be retained, treated endodontically, and covered with gold copings. Furthermore, isolated teeth seem to be preferable to several adjacent teeth (for example, in the anterior part of the mandible), since it can be argued that the latter may lead to a greater risk of gingival damage from interproximal increased plaque accumulation.

2. Preference for anterior over posterior teeth. The anterior alveolar ridge appears to be more vulnerable to reduction than the posterior alveolar ridges. Broken-down crowns on posterior teeth can also be restored with pin-amalgams or composites and used as removable partial denture abutments rather than overdentured ones without a cosmetic compromise (Zarb and associates, 1978).

3. The presence of teeth that are already endodontically treated. These teeth will lend themselves to the technique with minimal alterations.

4. Preference for mandibular over maxillary overdentures. However, maxillary overdentures are prescribed and maxillary anterior tooth roots are retained if the mandible has a large number of remaining teeth such that the occlusal support in the mandible is considerably greater than that in the maxillae.

PREPARATION OF ABUTMENT TEETH

Various methods and devices have been proposed (Dolder, 1961; Preiskel, 1968) for preparing abutment teeth for the overlay prosthesis. It is our impression that the essential feature in

this technique is not the type of attachment used but the following basic principles:

1. An abutment root or tooth should be chosen that is surrounded by healthy periodontal tissues (Fig. 25-6). The latter may already be present, or else is achieved by appropriate periodontal therapy.

2. Maximum reduction of the coronal position of the tooth should be accomplished. A better crown/root ratio is established, and minimal interference is encountered with the placement of artificial teeth.

3. The routine use of endodontically treated teeth helps achieve the second principle. However, some patients have advanced pulpal recession, usually combined with extensive tooth wear, which will allow for coronal reduction without the need for endodontic treatment (Fig. 25-7).

4. The need for a gold coping or a crown-and-sleeve-coping retainer as described by Yalisove (1966) depends on several factors. Frequently a devitalized, broken tooth can be restored with an alloy or a composite and rounded off and polished with fine sandpaper disks (Fig. 25-8). Occasionally a gold coping is necessary, and this may be prepared with or without a post or retentive pins, depending on the amount of tooth structure remaining above the gingival attachment. The gold coping (Fig. 25-9) does involve an additional expense, but some patients are uncomfortable with the sight of "unprotected" roots in their mouths. The patient's susceptibility to caries has to be considered, and when in doubt, it is better to use a gold coping on abutment teeth. Tooth preparation is similar to that for a complete gold crown, with a combination of shoulder and chamfered gingival margins as dictated by the amount of residual tooth structure. It must be emphasized that the main objective in using this technique is the preservation of alveolar bone and not the introduction of a technique for more retentive dentures. Consequently a simple, short, convex abutment preparation (with or without a casting) appears to be the ideal root surface preparation (Warren and Caputo, 1975).

5. The patient must be well motivated to maintain the hygienic phase of periodontal care. Regular follow-up visits are essential, and oral health maintenance measures are periodically reviewed and revised as necessary. Fluoride gel is prescribed for daily application to the inside of the overlay denture, which will bring the fluoride into intimate contact with natural tooth structure. Extensive experience with young, caries-susceptible cleft palate patients using the fluoride gel in this manner supports this directive. The fluoride is a 1% neutral pH sodium fluoride solution in liquid or gel form. It may cause irritation or a burning sensation in the tissues of some patients, and in these cases, the frequency of application is reduced from daily to two to three times per week.

6. The occasional need for removal of one or more abutment teeth used in this manner must be expected. The cause is usually a periodontal abscess, and removal of the affected tooth with appropriate filling in of the contacting site in the overlay denture can be carried out readily and inexpensively.

CLINICAL PROCEDURES

The clinical procedures will vary depending on whether a tooth-supported complete denture is being constructed or the procedure will be an immediate-insertion tooth-supported complete denture.

Tooth-supported complete denture

The important principles of complete denture construction must be respected before the mechanical ingenuities of particular types of

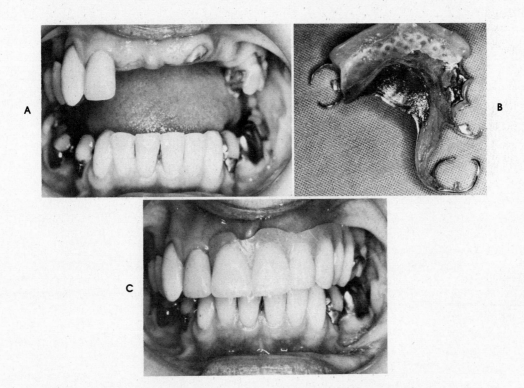

Fig. 25-6. A, Healthy root can be retained and covered by a removable prosthesis, **B** and **C.** This design will help maintain bone level in canine area as long as tissues surrounding residual root are maintained in a sanitative phase.

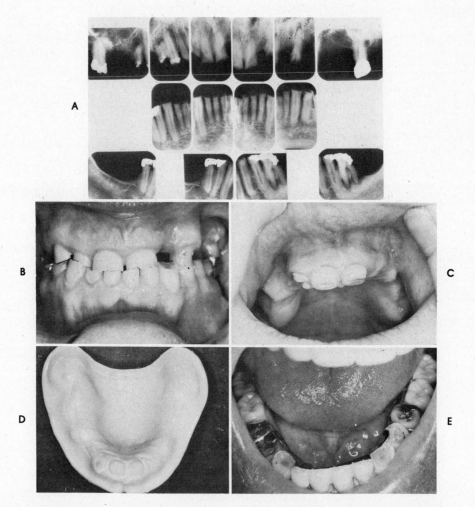

Fig. 25-7. Advanced pulpal recession, **A,** in this patient whose dentition showed considerable wear and neglect, **B.** Three maxillary anterior teeth were retained, **C,** and an overlay denture constructed, **D.** The badly worn anterior mandibular teeth were reduced, polished, and partially "restored" with a cast removable partial denture of the overlay type.

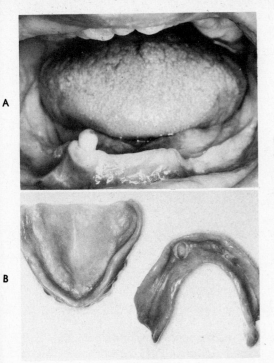

Fig. 25-8. A, Devitalized single tooth is restored with a composite restoration, and the crown/root ratio is improved by crown reduction and rounding off with sandpaper disks. B, Complete denture is constructed over this abutment tooth. (Courtesy Dr. A.H. Fenton, University of Toronto.)

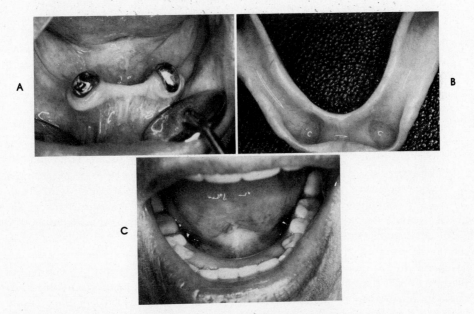

Fig. 25-9. A, Gold copings are used to protect and partially restore mandibular canines. B, Overdenture is hollowed out in these areas to conform to abutments' contours. C, Cosmetic merits of complete denture are in no way compromised.

attachments are considered (Preiskel, 1967). These principles are identical to those already described in previous chapters, and they should be meticulously followed and carried out. A well-executed complete denture technique does not need to rely on mechanical contraptions, frequently of a stress-breaking variety, to achieve the objectives embarked on in the treatment of complete denture patients.

One problem of tooth-supported complete denture service is the occasional tendency for some patients to demonstrate an untoward gingival response around the abutment teeth (Fig. 25-10). Following are factors that may cause gingival irritation:

1. Movement of the denture base (more apparent in mandibular dentures) with the development of a loading factor at the gingival margins
2. Poor oral hygiene and failure by the patient to observe the discipline of plaque removal and to pay sufficient attention to tissue rest and periodic recall assessments
3. Excess space in the prosthesis around the gingival margins surrounding the abutment teeth, which leads to the development of a "dead space" that is a potential source of inflammation

Clinical experience indicates that a slight space around the gingival margin is essential to avoid overloading this particularly vulnerable site. This observation applies to mandibular dentures, especially, since they appear to become unstabilized more easily than maxillary dentures. On the other hand, a dead space will frequently lead to a combined hypertrophic and hyperplastic response of the gingival margin, a reaction somewhat similar to that elicited by a relief chamber in a complete maxillary denture. Our experience has been that the hollowed-out area in the resin overlay denture should be lined with a treatment liner–tissue conditioner at the time of denture placement. The resiliency of such a material, combined with its need for frequent replacement, can create an optimal

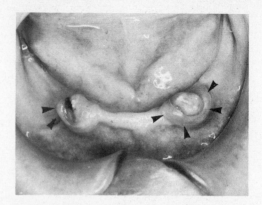

Fig. 25-10. Gingivitis *(arrows)* occurring around abutments of an overlay denture as a result of imperfect hygienic measures by patient.

arrangement for periodic recall appointments.

Immediate tooth-supported complete denture (Fig. 25-11)

The clinical procedures for immediate tooth-supported complete dentures are identical to those described in Chapter 26, except that the coronal reduction of the selected abutment teeth is carried out at the time of the extraction of the remaining teeth. The teeth to be retained are prepared on the master cast to approximate the shape of the eventual coping. The remaining teeth are trimmed away in the usual manner. Consequently, the processed immediate denture will demonstrate depressions on its impression surface that will conform to the surfaces of the teeth to be retained. The endodontic treatment is completed one or more appointments before the immediate denture insertion, or else just before the combined surgical-prosthetic appointment. Some dentists prefer the latter because removal of the tooth's crown facilitates the endodontic procedure. Immediate denture insertion and follow-up procedures are carried out in the usual manner. The need for refining the impression surface of the denture in the operated and coping sites by the addition of a treatment resin is essential because rapid tissue changes are to be anticipated. When healing has

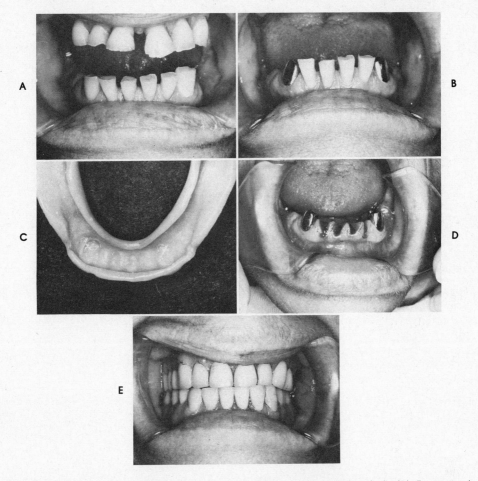

Fig. 25-11. A, Candidate for immediate dentures because of advanced periodontal disease and tooth mobility except for mandibular canines. The decision to retain the canines as abutments for a mandibular overdenture enables dentist, **B,** first to restore the canine; **C,** prepare the dentures; **D,** prepare the mouth surgically; and **E,** insert the immediate overlay denture. (Courtesy Dr. Francis Zarb, University of Toronto.)

taken place, any necessary copings are prepared, and the prosthesis is refitted.

LONGITUDINAL STUDIES

The well-deserved preoccupation on the dentist's part with retaining patients' teeth has led to a dramatic surge of interest in the overdenture concept. Several reports have been published and many anecdotal claims have been made, but there has been a lack of well-documented, long-term clinical follow-up of these patients. Current research (Toolson and Smith, 1983; Fenton and Hahn, 1978) endorses the claim that overdentures are a dramatically effective alternative to conventional complete denture therapy, and their use in routine practice is assured. But the very nature of overdenture design and its relationship to plaque must always be kept in mind if this excellent treatment modality is to fulfill its potential.

REFERENCES

Atwood, D.A.: Reduction of residual ridges: a major oral disease entity, J. Prosthet. Dent. **26:**266-279, 1971.

Brewer, A.A., and Fenton, A.H.: The overdenture, Dent. Clin. North Am. **17:**723-746, 1973.

Carlsson, G.E., and Persson, G.: Morphologic changes of the mandible after extraction and wearing of dentures; a longitudinal clinical and x-ray cephalometric study covering 5 years, Odontol. Revy **18:**27-54, 1967.

Crum, R.J., and Rooney, G.E., Jr.: Alveolar bone loss in overdentures: a 5-year study, J. Prosthet. Dent. **40:**610-613, 1978.

Dolder, E.J.: The bar joint mandibular denture, J. Prosthet. Dent. **11:**689-707, 1961.

Fenton, A.H., and Hahn, N.: Tissue response to overdenture therapy, J. Prosthet. Dent. **40:**492-498, 1978.

Guyer, S.E.: Selectively retained vital roots for partial support of overdenture, J. Prosthet. Dent. **33:**258, 1975.

Herd, J.R.: The retained tooth root, Aust. Dent. J. **18:**125-131, 1973.

McDermott, I.G., and Rosenberg, S.W.: Overdentures for the irradiated patient, J. Prosthet. Dent. **51:**314-317, 1984.

Preiskel, H.W.: Prefabricated attachments for complete overlay dentures, Br. Dent. J. **123:**161-167, 1967.

Preiskel, H.W.: An impression technique for complete overlay dentures, Br. Dent. J. **124:**9-13, 1968.

Tallgren, A.: The reduction in face height of edentulous and partially edentulous subjects during long-term denture wear; a longitudinal roentgenographic cephalometric study, Acta Odontol. Scand. **24:**195-239, 1966.

Tallgren, A.: The effect of denture wearing on facial morphology; a 7-year longitudinal study, Acta Odontol. Scand. **25:**563-592, 1969.

Toolson, L.B., and Smith, D.E.: A five-year longitudinal study of patients treated with overdentures, J. Prosthet. Dent. **49:**749-756, 1983.

Warren, A.B., and Caputo, A.A.: Load transfer to alveolar bone as influenced by abutment designs for tooth-supported dentures. J. Prosthet. Dent. **33:**137-148, 1975.

Welker, W.A., Jividen, G.J., and Kramer, D.C.: Preventive prosthodontics—mucosal coverage of roots, J. Prosthet. Dent. **40:**619-621, 1978.

Yalisove, I.L.: Crown and sleeve-coping retainers for removable partial prostheses, J. Prosthet. Dent. **16:**1069-1085, 1966.

Zarb, G.A., Bergman, B., Clayton, J.A., and MacKay, H.F.: Prosthodontic treatment for partially edentulous patients, St. Louis, 1978, The C.V. Mosby Co.

26

Immediate denture treatment for patients

Immediate dentures are dentures constructed before all the remaining teeth have been removed and inserted immediately after the removal of the remaining teeth. This method of treatment may be used with a single complete denture or with both maxillary and mandibular complete dentures. When both maxillary and mandibular immediate complete dentures are proposed, it is advisable to construct them simultaneously. This will ensure that cosmetic or occlusal irregularities in the remaining dentulous arch will not interfere with tooth positioning in the immediate prosthesis.

INDICATIONS FOR IMMEDIATE DENTURE SERVICE

The indication for immediate denture service is the dentulous or partially edentulous patient whose remaining natural teeth have to be extracted (Fig. 26-1). Dentists have used the treatment plan of rendering a patient edentulous, waiting several months for healing of the oral tissues, and subsequently constructing complete dentures. This view has been almost completely abandoned because of the following obvious advantages of immediate denture treatment:

1. The humiliating, edentulous period of healing is unnecessary. This is critical for all patients who cannot afford loss of social or business prestige.

2. There is usually less pain because the denture acts as a protecting splint over the operated

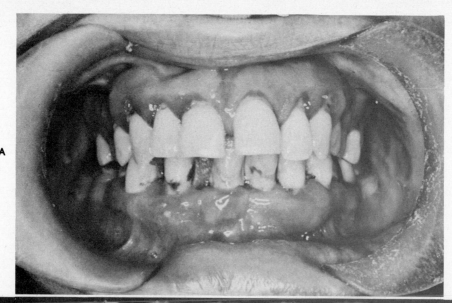

A

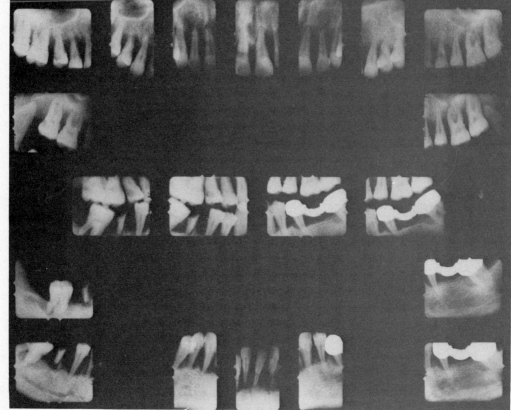

B

Fig. 26-1. A to **D,** An attractive cosmetic natural tooth arrangement is regrettably ruined by the appalling neglect in this mouth. Immediate dentures had to be prescribed.

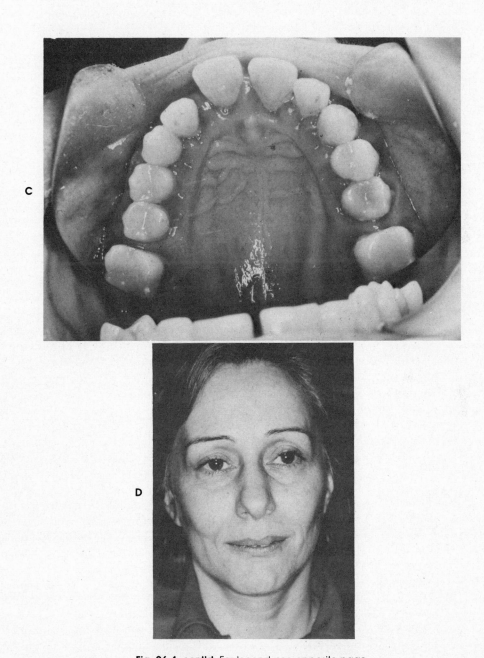

C

D

Fig. 26-1, cont'd. For legend, see opposite page.

sites. The discomfort and the inconvenience associated with learning to manipulate the dentures can be endured at the same time as the patient is recovering from the surgical operation.

3. The patient is spared the inconvenience and distress of several months of inability to masticate food and an inevitable major dietary modification.

4. Appearance is affected minimally, since cheek and lip support are maintained. The morphologic face height is also maintained (Carlsson and Persson, 1967), and the tongue does not spread out as a result of lack of contact with teeth.

5. It is easier for the dentist to place the teeth in their former identical positions, should this be desired. As a result, more faithful reproduction of individual variation of teeth, arch contours, and positions are possible. The dentist can use the remaining teeth as guides for orienting the anterior teeth in their vertical and anteroposterior positions and for duplicating the anterior dental arch width. In this manner, the positions of the anterior teeth can be accurately reestablished.

6. The availability of tissue conditioners and new border-molding materials provide the dentist with enormous scope for ensuring easy and correct modification of the immediate prosthesis. These materials can be applied both at the insertion stage and at the subsequent appointment stages, with a net effect of ensuring immediate and continuous excellence of prosthesis fit and comfort for the patient. *It is tempting to suggest that the advances in these dental materials have virtually eliminated all contraindications to the immediate denture service.*

Bone reduction

Bone often seems to resorb more rapidly without the stimulation supplied by the immediate denture base for functional rebuilding. Dentists have used this argument to justify immediate denture service as opposed to a period of time without teeth after their extraction and before the construction of complete dentures. The longitudinal studies of Carlsson and Persson (1967) and Carlsson and associates (1967) revealed that the choice between the two methods was not a critical factor when considered in the context of bone resorption. Their work indicated that bony reduction was related to denture-wearing habits and hence loading of the denture-bearing tissues and not to the timing of the prosthetic service. Their histologic examinations also failed to demonstrate differences between the two methods of treatment.

CONTRAINDICATIONS TO IMMEDIATE DENTURE SERVICE

There are a few minor disadvantages to the immediate denture service, since more "maintenance work" is required than with the conventional service. The maintenance effort is related to the need to maintain the fit of the dentures and the stability of the occlusion in the context of the ongoing changes in the recently surgically treated supporting tissues. Interim relines with tissue conditioners will therefore be needed. The number of these relines (one to three in the first year of immediate denture wear) will depend on the rapidity of alveolar bone resorption. However, it must be emphasized that these reline procedures are simple to carry out and not very time-consuming. The major changes in denture-supporting tissues take place within 8 to 12 months (Wictorin, 1969), and at this time a reline with a hard acrylic resin is usually carried out (see Chapter 28). Quite obviously the patient undergoing immediate denture treatment should be advised of these additional procedures. This will ensure complete understanding of the patients responsibilities for both regular appointment followup and the professional fees entailed.

DELAYED AND TRANSITIONAL DENTURES

Rarely, some dentists will elect to treat patients with poor oral health and systemic discease (usually renal or cardiac) with a delayed immediate denture insertion. In this approach the prepared dentures are inserted 1 to 2 weeks (or even longer) after the extractions. The objective here is to avoid the "make and break" contact of the denture with the surgically treated tissues, which may cause transient bacteremia during the early postoperative period. Some dentists will, on occasion, prescribe transitional dentures. These are interim immediate dentures usually fabricated by use of a modified and abbreviated form of the technique described in this chapter. The objective is to use these dentures until stability of the denture-supporting tissues is achieved and then to fabricate new dentures. Although this approach does have its merits, it is inevitably far more expensive and is not a better health service than the approach we are recommending.

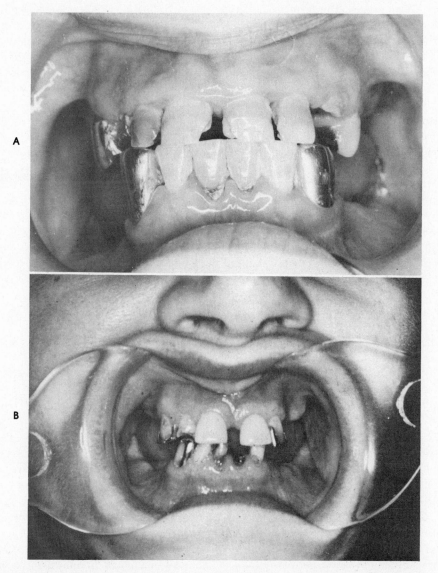

Fig. 26-2. Presence of centric stops in two patients prevents reduction of interarch distance and facilitates establishment of a vertical relation of occlusion for immediate denture construction.

PREIMPRESSION PROCEDURES

After the decision has been made to make immediate dentures, the optimal plan is to remove all posterior teeth except unilateral or, preferably, bilateral opposing premolars. Frequently, especially in Angle Class I patients, opposing incisors or canines are retained. These opposing teeth serve as centric stops (Fig. 26-2) to prevent reduction of the interarch distance during the healing period. The removal of the posterior teeth 4 to 6 weeks before impression making ensures the dentist greater ease for establishing the height and width of the posterior borders for the finished dentures.

It is possible to avoid a two-stage surgical procedure and to make impressions with the posterior teeth present (Fig. 26-3). However, the dentist's chances of making accurate impressions of the potential basal seat areas are then curtailed. This technique is usually reserved for patients whose oral health status is so depleted that total, as opposed to serial, extractions are mandatory.

A general scaling and curettage is usually indicated before the prosthetic appointments. A sanitative, or hygienic, phase of the oral tissues will reduce edema and facilitate the surgical procedure and postoperative healing. Frequently an occlusal adjustment of the remaining natural teeth is indicated. The very factors that indicate the need for tooth extraction (e.g., extensive caries, periodontal disease, extrusion, and drifting of teeth) are often associated with occlusal discrepancies that affect the registration of maxillomandibular relations. The establishment of a centric occlusion that coincides with centric relation will ensure that the patient's incorrect maxillomandibular relationship will not be carried over into the prosthetic occlusion.

The diagnostic or the final working casts will supply all the necessary information regarding the teeth, other than their shade and color. A record can be made of the anterior teeth to show all the individual characteristics that the dentist may elect to include in the tooth setup (Fig. 26-4).

CLINICAL PROCEDURES

With some modifications, the procedures used for making immediate dentures are similar to those described for making complete dentures for edentulous patients.

Preliminary impressions and diagnostic casts

The impressions are made in a stock perforated tray, which is adapted to the soft tissue forming the reflections by bending of the flanges and addition of utility wax on the borders (Fig. 26-5, A). The center of the palatal area in the maxillary tray is also covered with wax to effect a closer approximation of the tray to the palatal tissues (Fig. 26-5, B). The wax borders ensure proper extension of the impression along with adequate support for the alginate (irreversible hydrocolloid) impression material. Should the wax show through the first impression surface as a result of tissue contact, it will not harm the impression, since its softness does not cause undue pressure. The diagnostic casts prepared in this manner are usually quite adequate for the construction of custom trays. They are rarely accurate enough to be used as final working casts because the stock trays do not fit properly and tend to distort the border tissues. (See Fig. 26-6.)

Custom trays, final impressions, and casts

The fabrication of custom trays depends on the final impression technique to be used. We have employed two techniques with consistently excellent results. The first technique is shown in Fig. 26-7. Custom autopolymerizing (cold-curing) resin trays are made over a cast with a wax spacer. A tripod-stop effect is established on the incisal edges of the remaining teeth anteriorly and in the posterior palatal seal area and buccal shelf areas posteriorly. The tray is tried in the mouth to check its extension and adaptation. The tray is corrected, and its borders are molded as described in Chapter 8. The tray is prepared for the final irreversible hydrocolloid impression when several retentive perforations are made and an adhesive is applied to its tissue surface. If, on the other hand, a light-

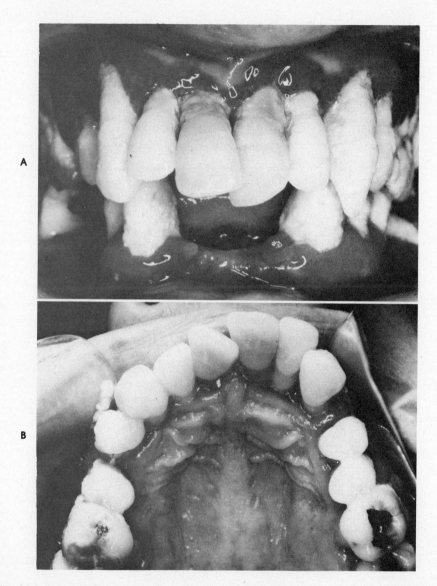

Fig. 26-3. A and **B,** Clinical and, **C** and **D,** radiographic pictures of patients with advanced peri-odontal disease who are candidates for the immediate denture service. In these situations, a two-stage surgical procedure is impractical and should be avoided. Quite obviously the resultant natural tooth arrangement in **A, B, E,** and **F** should *not* be duplicated.

Continued.

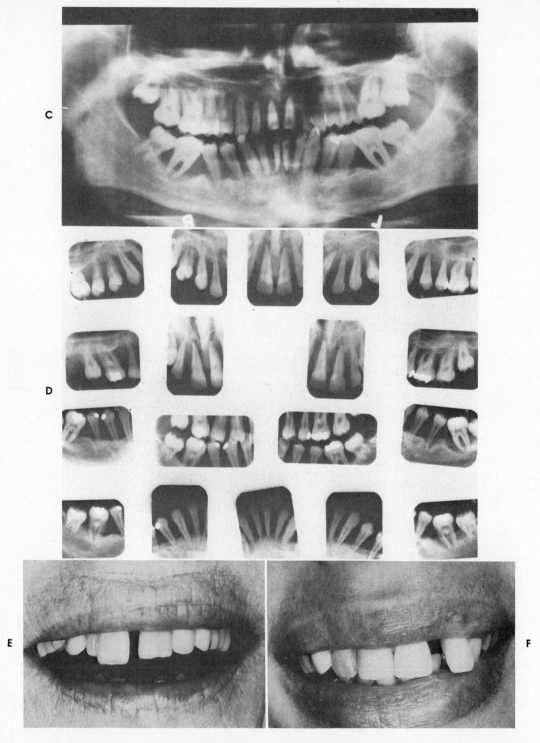

Fig. 26-3, cont'd. For legend see p. 529.

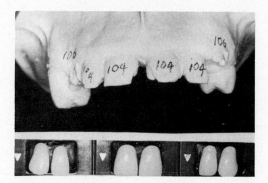

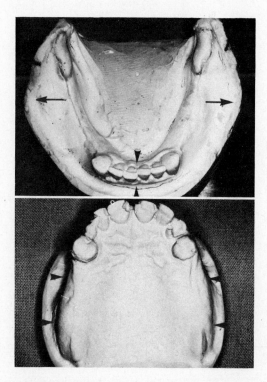

Fig. 26-4. Noting the shade characteristics on the diagnostic cast is a useful aid for the dentist in shade selection.

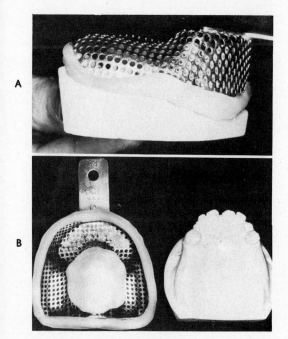

Fig. 26-5. A, Peripheral border utility wax is added to a stock tray. The wax can also be added to the center of the palatal area of the maxillary tray, **B.**

Fig. 26-6. Diagnostic casts made from impressions in stock trays. The extra width of the trays tends to distort the border tissues *(arrows)*.

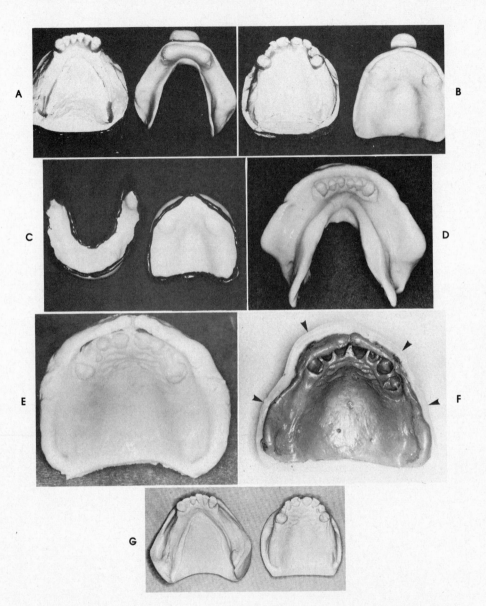

Fig. 26-7. A and **B,** Blocked-out undercuts and interproximal areas on casts, with custom autopoly-merizing resin trays. Notice that the wax spacers have been removed. **C,** Trays have been border molded with low-fusing modeling compound. **D** and **E,** Irreversible hydrocolloid impressions have been made. **F,** Thiokol rubber impression has been made of the maxillae, and the impression is prepared for boxing before the stone is poured in. **G,** Completed working casts.

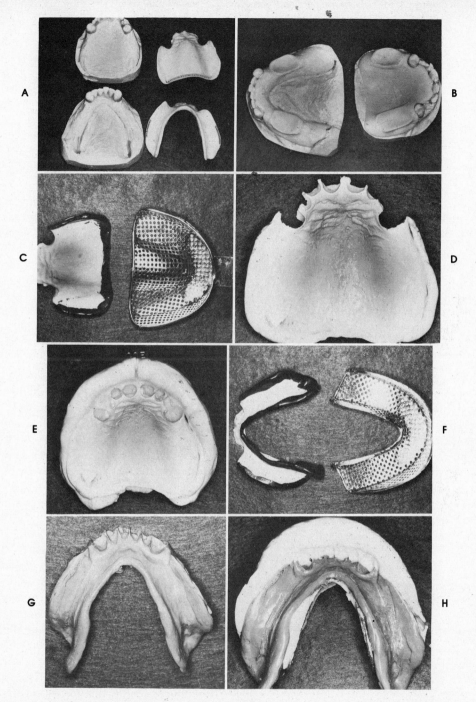

Fig. 26-8. Combination-method impression technique involves the use of custom trays, **A** and **B,** which conform to the edentulous segments of the jaws. The wax spacer has been removed from the tissue surface side of the custom trays, and the shadowed areas are those in which the resin contacts the mucosa. **C** to **H,** Border-molded resin trays and wash impressions made in zinc oxide–eugenol paste in the maxillae and in Thiokol rubber in the mandible. The secondary impression in the stock tray is made in irreversible hydrocolloid.

bodied Thiokol rubber impression material is to be used, space is provided in the tray over the ridge crest and over the center of the palate, and a rubber adhesive is applied. Either of these impression materials can be used to obtain excellent results.

The second technique involves a combination method (Fig. 26-8). Cold-curing resin trays are made to conform to the edentulous segments only. These trays have positive stops on the lingual surfaces of the remaining teeth and in the buccal shelf and posterior palatal seal areas. Roughened handles on the tongue side of the buccal areas will provide for retention of this section of the superimposed irreversible hydrocolloid in a stock tray. The clinical procedure for border molding the buccal, lingual, posterolingual, and posterior palatal seal areas is as described earlier. The tray is relieved by placement of several escape holes and is refined with a zinc oxide–eugenol impression. This sectional impression is checked in the usual manner (Chapters 8 and 10), all excess material is removed, and the impression is placed back in the mouth. A perforated stock tray that will accommodate the anterior teeth and their overlying mucolabial fold is selected, and the tray is filled with irreversible hydrocolloid impression material. Alginate is placed in the labial vestibule before insertion of the loaded tray into the mouth. When the irreversible hydrocolloid has set, the two sectional impressions are usually

removed together. Failure to do so simply necessitates that the resin tray be reoriented into the irreversible hydrocolloid impression. This technique can yield good final working casts (Fig. 26-9).

Jaw relation records

Jaw relation records are made by use of occlusion rims. Here again, both the laboratory and clinical procedures undertaken are practically identical to those of the usual complete denture construction. The objective of an accurate transfer of maxillomandibular relations is complicated slightly by the fact that it is not always possible to extend the anterior part of the trial denture base onto a stable area on the lingual surfaces of the anterior teeth. An extremely stable trial denture base is of paramount importance, and it is well worth the dentist's additional time to produce a trial base that fits the tissues very closely. Hard baseplate wax, reinforced wax, or cold-curing tray resin may be used for this purpose (Fig. 26-10). The indications for material selection are discussed in Chapter 11.

The presence of natural mandibular teeth can be a useful guide in establishment of the height of the occlusal plane, and the occlusion rims are constructed to that height (Fig. 26-11). Reference was made earlier to the importance of correcting any tooth-guided malposition of the mandible that patients may have acquired through the years in which they were becoming edentulous. If dentures are constructed with centric occlusion in an acquired eccentric position, deflective occlusal contacts can loosen the dentures and destroy underlying bone. *An occlusal adjustment of the remaining natural teeth may be necessary to ensure that centric occlusion and centric relation coincide.*

A study is made when the jaw relations are recorded to determine whether the occlusal vertical dimension is to be reproduced exactly (Fig. 26-12). An uneven loss of teeth, loosening of the remaining teeth, and tooth tissue wear have often led to reduced occlusal vertical dimension. If the occlusal vertical dimension is to be

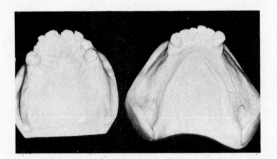

Fig. 26-9. Final working casts made with the combination-method impression technique.

increased, the amount of change should be determined at this time. The technique for registering centric relation is similar to that described in Chapter 18. The maxillary occlusion rim is contoured so that in centric relation it contacts the mandibular occlusion rim evenly and the clinically judged optimal interocclusal distance is achieved. Notches 5 mm deep are cut into the rims, and a centric relation registration is made with quick-setting plaster (thick, creamy consistency) (Fig. 26-13), beeswax, or zinc oxide–eugenol paste. A face-bow fork, especially prepared for removable partial and immediate dentures by grinding away the two anterior prongs, is attached to the occlusion rim (Fig. 26-14). The face-bow transfer is made in the usual

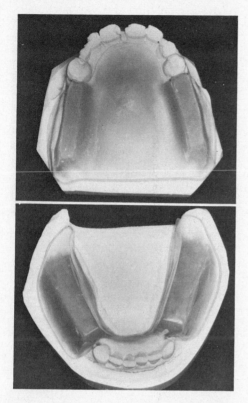

Fig. 26-10. Cold-curing tray resin is used as a recording base along with wax occlusion rims.

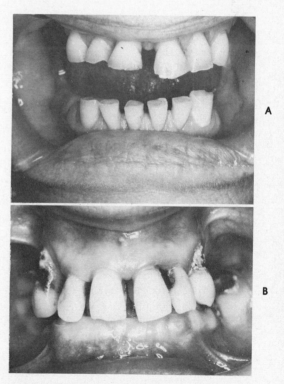

Fig. 26-12. A, Loss of posterior teeth has led to a dramatic loss of vertical dimension of occlusion. **B,** In this patient the dentist establishes the vertical dimension of occlusion in a manner similar to that employed when treating a completely edentulous patient.

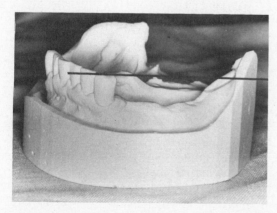

Fig. 26-11. Remaining mandibular teeth and retromolar pad are useful landmarks for the dentist in establishing height of occlusal plane.

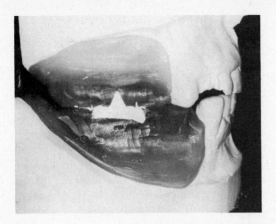

Fig. 26-13. When the occlusion rims have been trimmed so that they meet evenly when the jaws are in centric relation, the rims are grooved, and a quick-setting plaster record is made.

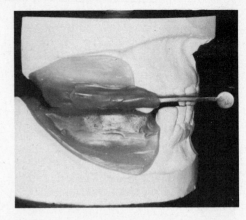

Fig. 26-14. Face-bow fork is sealed to buccal surfaces of maxillary occlusion rim. Notice that projections in concavity of the fork are removed to facilitate insertion of the fork's sides into the rim's buccal aspect.

manner, and the articulator mounting is completed (Fig. 26-15).

Protrusive relation records and articulator adjustment. The making of protrusive relation records and adjustment of the articulator are optional procedures and depend on whether cusp or cuspless teeth are to be used.

Cusp teeth. Whenever cusp teeth are employed, one of the two following procedures is carried out.

In the first procedure, approximately four layers of baseplate wax, cut in the shape of the arch, are placed over the maxillary anterior teeth and occlusion rims. The wax is softened, and the articulator is set 6 mm in protrusion, with an approximate condylar reading of 10 to 20 degrees. Then the articulator is closed into the soft wax. In the making of a protrusive record it is difficult to control the mandible in the amount of distance it goes forward when the record is made. For this reason, the record is first made on the articulator and is then chilled and placed in the mouth to rehearse the patient in what is desired. After the patient has an understanding of protruding the mandible into the wax indentations, this wax is again warmed in water of 135° F (57° C). Water is used instead of a flame

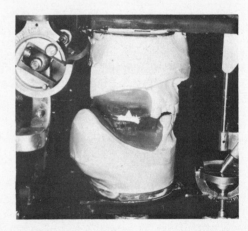

Fig. 26-15. Face-bow and centric relation–record transfers have been completed, and the casts are mounted on the articulator.

so that the indentations will preserved to guide the mandible. When the lower teeth are inserted lightly into the indentations, the patient is told to apply occlusal pressure. The wax is thick enough that the mandibular position can be recorded without penetration of the wax. The wax is chilled in the mouth, and the wax record and occlusion rims are placed on the casts in the articulator to test the adjustment. The locknuts for the condylar guidance adjustments are loosened so that the slot adjustments will move readily to adapt to the inclination that the patient has recorded in the warm wax. If the path on the articulator is too steep, the record will not touch the occlusion rim in back. If the path is too flat, the occlusion rims and teeth will not contact in front. These adjustments are placed at an inclination so that the entire surfaces of the mandibular and maxillary rims are in contact. When the dentist is satisfied, the condylar guidance slot adjustment locknuts are tightened, and the protrusive wax record is removed. The mandibular wax occlusion rim is removed from the metal framework, and the metal framework is placed again on the cast and is luted in place. The baseplates and occlusion rims of both casts are now disposed of because there are no further try-ins in this immediate denture procedure.

An equally effective alternate method of making a protrusive maxillomandibular relation record for immediate dentures involves the use of impression plaster. This method has the advantages of requiring the minimum of pressure at the time the record is made. One makes the protrusive record by instructing the patient to protrude the mandible and to close easily on the front teeth. However, this closure must be stopped just before the teeth touch. When the plaster has set, the occlusion rims are removed from the mouth, and this record is used to adjust condylar guidances on the articulator.

Cuspless teeth. The use of cuspless or nonanatomic teeth is described in Chapter 21. The same principles governing their selection for conventional complete dentures may be applied to immediate denture service.

Positioning the posterior teeth

The articulated casts can now be used for setting up the posterior teeth. The principles described earlier are adopted, and the teeth are set up in tight centric occlusion (Fig. 26-16). The trial denture bases are tried in the patient's mouth, and centric relation is confirmed. If the

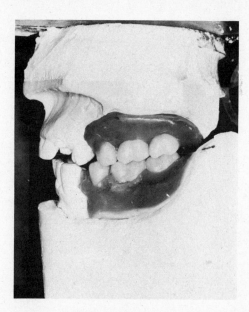

Fig. 26-16. Trial denture bases with the posterior teeth set up in tight, intercuspated fashion can now be returned to the mouth to confirm the accuracy of the original centric relation record.

previous maxillomandibular relation record was an incorrect one, centric relation and centric occlusion will not coincide. The mandibular posterior teeth are removed from the trial base, a new centric relation record is made, and the mandibular cast is remounted. The teeth are then reset to the new articulator mounting and retried in the mouth before the patient is dismissed.

Tooth selection

Tooth selection is easily carried out, since the patient's remaining natural teeth are an excellent starting point for form, size and shade selection.

Positioning of the anterior teeth

Positioning of the anterior teeth depends on whether the dentist wants to duplicate the patient's natural tooth arrangement. Whereas the latter is desirable for the majority of patients, some patients do present with rather

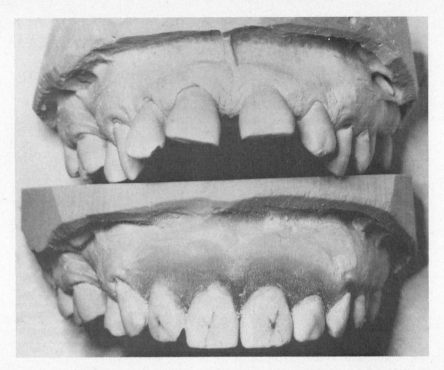

Fig. 26-17. The proposed immediate replacement of these anterior teeth is designed to provide the patient with an optimal cosmetic result. The stone teeth are waxed onto the diagnostic cast in their preferred position, and they will serve as a guide for final artificial tooth placement. (Courtesy Dr. A.H. Fenton, University of Toronto.)

unesthetic arrangements, which are usually the result of advanced periodontal disease and drifting of the teeth (Fig. 26-3, *A*, *B*, *E*, and *F*). Quite clearly these situations will demand a positioning of the prosthetic teeth that offers the maximum cosmetic result (Fig. 26-17). In these patients, the casts are rendered edentulous and the desired tooth arrangement is created irrespective of where the natural tooth or teeth were. When the dentist decides to position the anterior teeth in their original locale, he can proceed in one of two ways.

Fig. 26-18 demonstrates the first technique. Alternate teeth are cut away on the cast, and the labial root portion of the teeth is excavated to a minimal depth (approximately 1 mm) on the labial side and flush with the gingival margin on the lingual or palatal side. The slight depression carved in the labial region will accommodate the

ridge laps of the artificial teeth. Quite obviously, in mouths with periodontal disease accompanied by gingival recession and bone loss, little or no labial stone has to be removed. Minimal trimming to the cast will allow the construction of a denture that will provide an adequate matrix for a full, rounded ridge in the immediate area. The best results are obtained if no bone is removed at the time the dentures are inserted. The selected teeth are placed in their specific positions and modified as required.

The artificial right central incisor is usually the first tooth to be placed in position and is secured with wax. Then alternate teeth are removed and replaced until all are set. By removing only one tooth at a time, its replacement can duplicate any delicate irregularities that may exist. The muscles of facial expression depend on duplication of the dental arch; hence

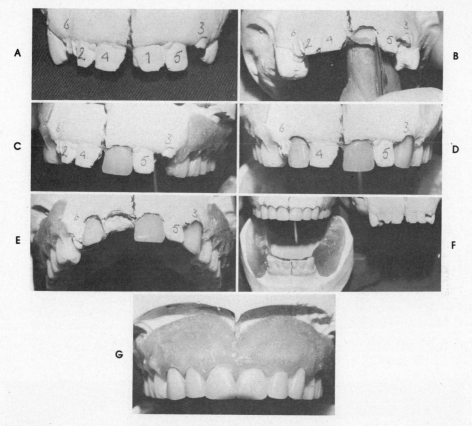

Fig. 26-18. A, Teeth to be "extracted" are numbered. Alternate teeth are cut away, **B,** and replaced with the selected artificial teeth, **C** to **F.** The minimal excavation at the cervical aspect of labial portion of the root allows for a ridge-lapping effect of the artificial teeth. **G,** Tooth setup is completed. Compare the appearance of the teeth to the cast of the natural dentition, **A.**

one tooth is placed at a time in order also to preserve this position. The lateral incisors are then cut away on the cast and replaced by artificial teeth. The remaining maxillary teeth (i.e., the left central incisor and right and left canines) are set in the place of those on the stone cast. A Boley gage is used to measure the distance between the labial surfaces of the canines on the stone cast so that their replacements will have an identical distance between their labial surfaces.

By the method just described, it is easier to attain accurate duplication of appearance, positions of individual teeth, and position of the dental arch.

In the second method (Fig. 26-19), the casts are trimmed to the single line drawn corresponding to the depth of the gingival sulcus. The teeth are broken off the cast at their cervical aspect, and the ridge is rounded to simulate a non–bone trimming procedure, except in interproximal areas. This procedure is carried out on one half of the remaining tooth segment and then on the other. The segments of artificial teeth can be set up alternately, or the entire cast may be rendered edentulous and the diagnostic cast used as a guide for tooth placement (Fig. 26-20).

The second method offers the advantage of ensuring that the cast preparation is completely

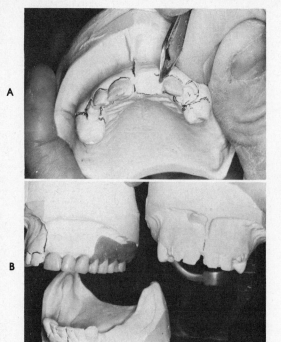

Fig. 26-19. A, Casts are trimmed to lines drawn on cast, corresponding to depth of gingival sulcus. **B,** One half of the trimming is done, and this segment of artificial teeth is set up, with the diagnostic cast being used as a guide. The other side is completed in a similar fashion.

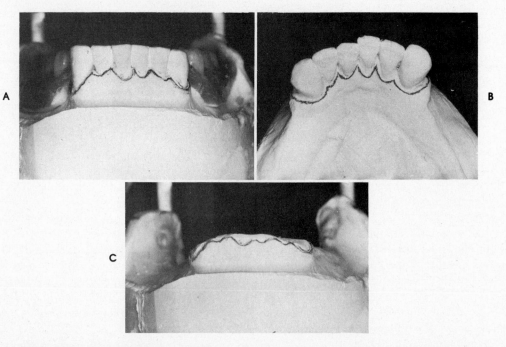

Fig. 26-20. A and **B,** Two views of an entire cast that is to be rendered "edentulous'" by the dentist. Line represents depth of gingival sulcus. **C,** Teeth have been broken at their cervical aspect, and the residual ridge area has been rounded off.

carried out by the dentist, rather than delegated to the technician. Final cast trimming in the first method has to be completed at the wax boil-out stage and, for reasons of convenience, is frequently done by the dental technician. The risk of unnecessary simulated bone trimming may then be created.

The patient whose pictures have been used to illustrate the previously described procedures desired a more even arrangement to her artificial teeth than had existed in her natural teeth. This desire was respected (Fig. 26-21), and her

incisal guidance, which was determined by the vertical and horizontal overlap, was advisedly modified. The condylar guidance was obtained with the interocclusal record as described. Her artificial occlusion was adjusted to harmonize with the two end factors governing the movement of the articulator (Chapter 21). Had cuspless (nonanatomic) teeth been selected for this patient, a more neutral incisal guidance would have been developed, with a minor alteration of the anterior cosmetic tooth arrangement.

If deep, sharp vertical overlap of the natural

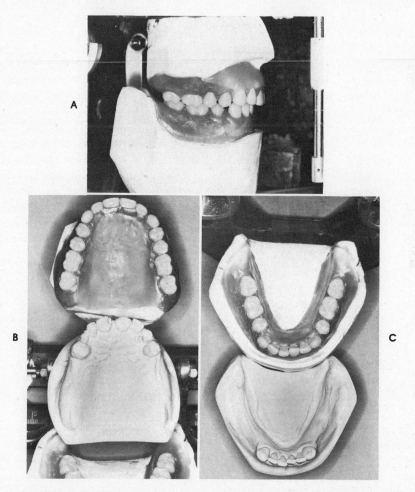

Fig. 26-21. A, Tooth setup has been completed. **B** and **C,** Both dental arches have been designed to conform to guides given by residual dentition. Incisal guidance has been modified to suit cosmetic dictates as determined by the dentist.

teeth exists, a reproduction of the same vertical overlap may be detrimental to complete denture stability. A deep vertical overlap results in a steep incisal guide angle, which in turn necessitates sharp inclines in all the anterior and posterior teeth. These steep inclines are a disturbing factor in the stability of dentures. However, esthetics can be maintained by introduction of some horizontal overlap. This may be done by reduction of the labiolingual thickness of the anterior teeth while the anteroposterior position of the labial face of the teeth and vertical occlusal relation are still maintained.

Waxing and flasking

The upper labial border of the denture is filled in with wax, according to the fullness of the border on the cast. An adequate thickness of the denture border is necessary to protect the patient's tissues from being cut by the denture flange if edema follows the removal of the teeth and insertion of the denture. The fullness of the border is reduced after the completion of the denture when all danger of swelling from the surgery is past. There can be no try-in of the trial denture other than to check the accuracy of the cast mounting before the anterior teeth are set. The rest of the waxing is done according to the principles described in Chapter 22.

Flasking is carried out in the usual way. After the wax boil-out and cleansing, a careful study of the radiographs is carried out to determine the amount of bone that has been destroyed by disease process. The need for this step at this stage can be avoided by the dentist's preparation of the casts as described in the second method of tooth positioning. The ridge area is trimmed to the desired form as specified by the dentist on his prescription, or the cast is trimmed by the dentist. Occasionally it is necessary to further estimate the necessary amount of bone to be removed during the surgical process should an alveolectomy be indicated. The cast is trimmed to reduce and smooth the anterior alveolar prominence for favorable reception of the denture. Any slight projections that are left in the

finished denture to conform to ridge irregularities can be removed from the inside of the finished denture before it is inserted in the patient's mouth. A well-rounded, full ridge that is convex and balloon-shaped will assure the denture's going into place and will afford an opportunity for the future ridge in the mouth to retain this desired from.

Preparation of surgical template

A transparent surgical template is made to be used as a guide for shaping of the ridge at the time the teeth are removed and the denture is inserted. The surgical template will reveal the location of places on the ridge where additional bone must be removed and will minimize the amount of surgery done at this time.

After the cast has been trimmed according to the plan just described, an impression is made of it in alginate (irreversible hydrocolloid). The cast in the flask is thoroughly soaked in water, and the impression material is placed in the same tray in which the original impression was made. (If the original impression was made in an individual acrylic resin tray, this impression tray will fit the cast perfectly.) The loaded tray is forced into position on the cast in such a way that no air is trapped in the impression material. When the material has set, the impression is removed, and plaster is poured into it to form a cast.

A wax pattern for the template is formed over the cast. This pattern should have a uniform thickness of 2 mm, except that it should fill the full contours produced by the borders of the impression.

The cast is half-flasked, and tinfoil is adapted over the wax pattern. Then the flasking is completed. The flask is heated in boiling water, and the wax is removed as for making a denture. When the flask is clean, tinfoil is adapted over the cast as described previously.

Tinfoil substitutes are not so good as tinfoil for protecting the resin during processing, because they do not seal the mold as tightly as tinfoil. As a result, templates made with a tinfoil substitute

Processing, occlusal corrections, and final preparation of the immediate denture(s)

Relief, if needed, is placed over any hard areas (e.g., median palatal raphe) by use of a sheet of 20- or 24-gage tin or lead that has been thinned on the edges and burnished to place. The dentures are processed, and resultant changes in occlusion are corrected before removal of the dentures from their casts for finishing. Articulating paper is used to locate deflective occlusal contacts in centric occlusion, and these are ground away with small mounted stones. Eccentric occlusions are not corrected at this time, since the final occlusal corrections are not made until the tissues have healed completely.

Before the time of surgery, the labial flange of the denture must be thinned to a minimum, except that the border must be well-rounded.

The prominences on the inner surface of the denture, representing the locations of fresh tooth sockets, must be trimmed. Identical changes must be made in the transparent surgical template. It is necessary that no early pressure be placed in the regions of immediate extractions. The anterior portion of the socket is particularly sensitive because the labial plate is very thin and sharp.

The inner surface of the denture should be reduced in the region where the socket prominences protrude. It must also be recessed in the area of the sharp labial plate. A stone capable of cutting both porcelain and resin, such as one of tungsten-carbide composition,* should be used to do this. Since the shape of this inner surface can be only an approximation of the postsurgical contour, it is necessary to remove an excess of denture material to spare the patient undue tissue pain and also to allow the ridge to fill to a better, broader bearing surface.

The inclination of the maxillary incisors causes an undercut in the labial region that need not be removed. The denture can be inserted on an

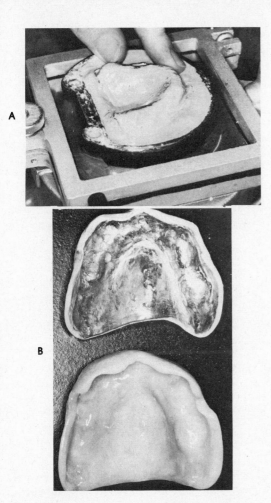

Fig. 26-22. A, Maxillary clear resin template is made with a vacuum-formed technique. **B,** Completed template compared to finished maxillary denture.

are somewhat cloudy instead of being transparent.

Colorless acrylic resin is packed in this mold and is processed in the same manner as a denture. Alternately, a clear resin template can be made by means of a vacuum-formed technique (Fig. 26-22).

The surgical template is a prescription for the surgical procedure and is an essential adjunct when any amount of bone trimming is necessary.

*Union Broach Co., Inc., Long Island City, N.Y.

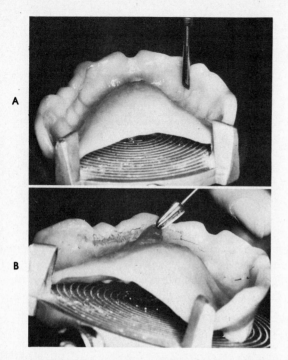

Fig. 26-23. A, Surveyor rod is used to demonstrate the entire undercut buccal segment of this denture and to explore variations in the path of denture insertion and withdrawal. Reduction of the resin undercut, **B,** is usually adequate to ensure comfort for the patient.

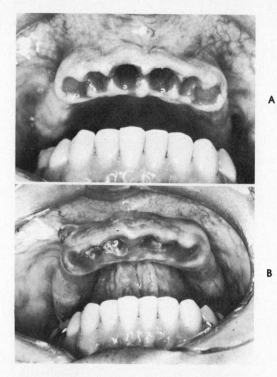

Fig. 26-24. A, Teeth are extracted. **B,** Template is tried in place before any surgical bone trimming is done.

upward and backward path, thus allowing the undercut to remain and give a better bearing surface.

Unilateral or bilateral undercuts of the posterior alveolar ridge are frequent. It is always tempting to eliminate these undercuts surgically, but the dentist is often able to cope with these undercuts by selecting an altered path of insertion and withdrawal of the denture combined with judicious trimming of the width of the resin flange in the undercut area (Fig. 26-23).

Surgery and insertion of the dentures

The surgical extraction procedure is well described in oral surgery textbooks.

The transparent surgical template is placed in the mouth *after* all the teeth have been removed but *before* any surgical trimming of bone or soft tissue is done (Fig. 26-24). When the template is securely seated against the palate or on the mandibular residual ridge, spots at the surgical site that are blanched from the pressure can be noticed. The template is removed, and soft tissue or bone is trimmed as indicated to relieve the spot of excessive pressure. In this procedure the surgical template must be seated perfectly, or it will not reveal the regions that must be trimmed. If the bone and soft tissues are not properly shaped to the contour of the template and the denture, the denture will not seat into its correct position. Failure to trim enough tissue so that the template will go to place or an excess amount of trimming will cause the denture to be in an incorrect position. These errors will cause occlusion to be incorrect and will cause unnecessary pain and discomfort to the patient. The dentures must seat in the mouth in exactly the position they were intended to occupy. The tissue flaps are approximated and sutured, and the denture, which had been previously sterilized in a cold sterilizing solution, is placed in the mouth. The patient is asked to close for the first check of occlusion. There should be no gross deflective occlusal contacts if the dentures have been seated correctly after surgery. Occlusal changes resulting from processing had been removed while the dentures were on the articulator. The patient is instructed to keep the dentures in position for 24 hours, at which time the dentist will remove them for the first time.

The versatility and usefulness of tissue conditioners can be taken advantage of at this stage. If the denture is loose (usually because of an ultra-conservative trim of the stone cast or an unanticipated need for extra surgical trimming of the socket sites), a temporary liner will compensate for the discrepancy in the fit and ensure patient comfort and denture stability. It must be emphasized that projections of the tissue conditioner material into socket sites should be trimmed, or they may interfere with normal socket healing.

Postoperative patient instructions (Fig. 26-25)

The dentures must be left in the mouth during the first 24 hours. The patient is cautioned that leaving the dentures out at first may result in swelling that will cause reseating to be either impossible or extremely painful. Any pain from the trauma of extraction will not be alleviated by removal of the dentures from the mouth. Within the first 24-hour period, ice packs may be held on the face to advantage, up to 15 minutes out of each hour. This is only a precautionary suggestion; as a general rule, the patient suffers no undue pain or discomfort. In case the patient cannot sleep because of nervousness or discomfort, a sedative is prescribed.

An immediate denture acts as a splint over the surgical field and helps to prevent a breakdown of the blood clot, which is often destroyed because of fluids in the mouth; therefore, troublesome hemorrhaging is rather rare.

The patient is advised to do no chewing during the first 24 hours, and a liquid diet is prescribed. Occlusion has not been finally adjusted; therefore mastication cannot be efficient in this time. Stability of the denture will improve when occlusion is perfected. Occlusion cannot be perfected until the swelling has disappeared, and occlusal perfection is usually done from 48 hours to 1 or 2 weeks after the dentures are inserted.

At the end of 24 hours the mouth is examined for border impingement and for excessive pressure spots at the site of recent extractions. It is not difficult to detect a spot that has not been trimmed sufficiently after removal of remaining teeth. This spot is manifest by a typical strawberry-red appearance. The spot is marked when one makes a ring around it with an indelible pencil, and the mark is transferred to the inner surface of the denture when the denture is pressed to place. The area thus marked on the denture is then relieved with a stone or scraper.

After 48 hours have elapsed, the denture is again examined for possible excessive border extension. In the postsurgical period, the template can be employed to confirm areas of pressure from the denture base (Fig. 26-26).

Perfection of occlusion

Occlusion may be perfected at the end of the 48-hour period because by that time most of the swelling has disappeared and the denture can be removed frequently without too much discomfort. However, it may be necessary to postpone occlusal correction for as long as 2 weeks. The comfort of the denture is enhanced greatly as soon as the imperfections in occlusion have been corrected.

The interocclusal record of centric relation is made in the same manner as for complete dentures. The impression plaster is placed on the

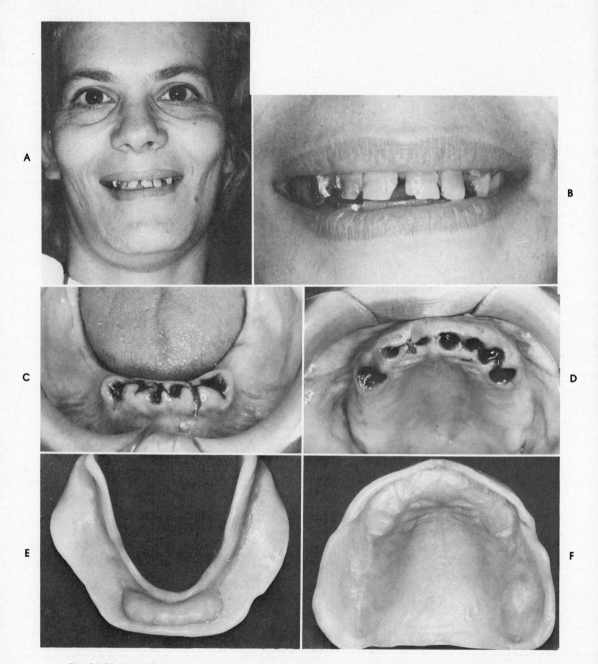

Fig. 26-25. A and **B,** Preoperative pictures. **C** and **D,** Operated sites 48 hours after surgery. **E** and **F,** Tissue surfaces of the completed dentures. **G** and **H,** Intraoral views 6 weeks after surgery. **I** and **J,** Posttreatment pictures.

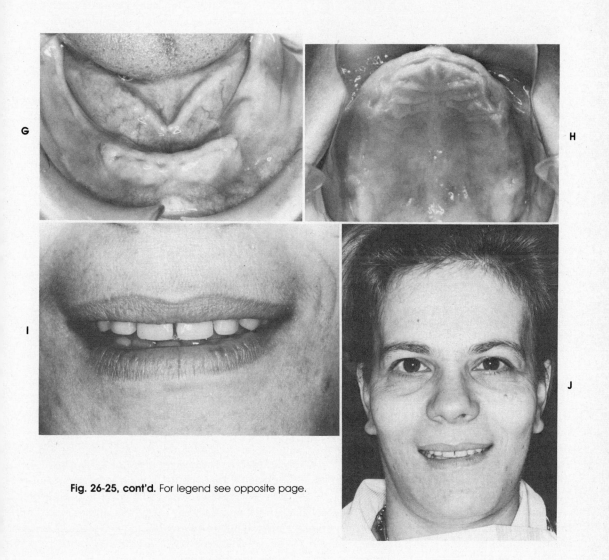

Fig. 26-25, cont'd. For legend see opposite page.

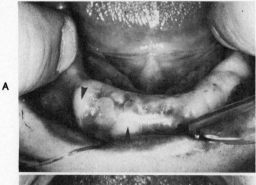

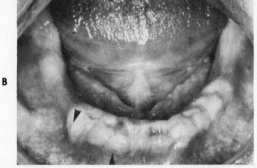

Fig. 26-26. Pressure areas *(arrows)*, which must be relieved on tissue surface side of denture. **A,** Surgical template is usefully employed in the postoperative period to identify such areas. **B,** Intraoral view of pressure areas.

lower premolars and molars, and the patient is instructed to pull the lower jaw back as far as it will go and to *close* on the back teeth. The word *bite* is avoided at this time because it implies protrusion to patients. Closure is stopped before any teeth touch. When the plaster is set, the interocclusal records are marked for identification and are laid aside.

If natural teeth or a partial lower denture opposes the immediate denture, an irreversible hydrocolloid impression of the entire arch is made in a stock metal tray with the partial denture (if any) in place. The partial denture is seated in the impression, and the undercuts are blocked out of it with wax or Moldine. Then a stone cast is made. This cast is mounted on the articulator by means of the interocclusal record

of centric relation, and the condylar guidances are adjusted by means of a protrusive interocclusal record.

The occlusion is corrected on the articulator when one follows the same principles and procedures as are described for complete dentures in Chapters 23 and 24.

SUBSEQUENT SERVICE FOR IMMEDIATE DENTURES

After the usual adjustments, the denture must be cared for in accordance with individual conditions, which vary greatly. The patient should be called for an appointment at least every 3 months to determine the amount of change that has taken place. If retention difficulties are encountered during this initial period, one of the tissue conditioners can be used on the tissue surface of the denture. The use of tissue conditioners is described in Section five. These materials have the property of flowing for a period of time, which allows for an equilization of tissue and occlusal pressure. When they harden, the tissues conditioners will frequently endure the stresses of usage for many weeks. This procedure can be repeated if required and enables the dentist to maintain the well-fitting status of the dentures during the time of rapid tissue changes. The danger of a changing occlusal relationship is largely controlled in this manner.

Wictorin (1969) indicates that socket calcification is complete 8 to 12 months after tooth extraction. His report indicates that a time lapse of almost 1 year is required before bone tissue completely regains its physical properties. He calculated that the bone volume of the alveolar ridge was reduced by 20% to 30% during the first 12 months after extraction of the teeth. An interval of 8 to 12 months should elapse before a hard acrylic resin refitting of the immediate dentures is carried out.

Wictorin (1964) also compared different types of dentitions in the mandible opposing immediate maxillary dentures. He found a tendency for increased vertical resorption in the operated maxillary ridge when remaining natural teeth

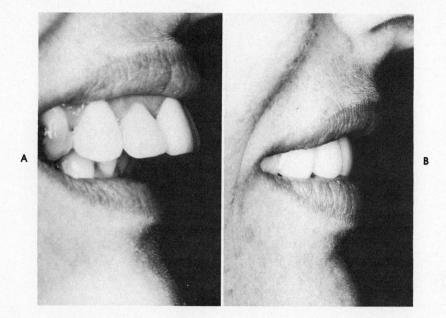

Fig. 26-27. Prominent premaxillary segment, **A,** has been dramatically modified by a maxillary alveolectomy and prosthodontic treatment, **B.**

were present in the lower jaw. Other studies (Hedegård and associates, 1967) demonstrated that in similar situations, mastication takes place mainly in the premolar and molar regions when these teeth have been artificially replaced. This explains why maxillary immediate denture construction combined with a simultaneous reconstruction of the lower jaw (should posterior mandibular teeth be missing) will result in less mobility of the maxillary denture and more normal mastication and thereby a lower rate of resorption in the anterior region of the upper jaw.

IMMEDIATE MAXILLARY DENTURES FOR PATIENTS REQUIRING AN EXTENSIVE ALVEOLECTOMY

Good evidence exists favoring a philosophy of no bone surgery in immediate denture mouth preparation. Despite this convincing evidence, a patient's jaw morphology can dictate a need for moderate to extensive bone trimming to achieve the desired cosmetic or functional results. The

following three specific situations deserve comment:

1. Patients with an Angle Class II, division 1, jaw appearance frequently desire a maxillary alveolectomy to improve their cosmetic appearance. The results obtained are frequently dramatic (Fig. 26-27). It must be pointed out, however, that the modification in lip support will unfortunately become quite evident as the patient gets older. The resultant effect is one of an inadequately supported labial vermilion border (Fig. 26-28). This procedure must be done with extreme caution because of the premature aging effect it can have on the lower third of the face as a result of improper support of the lips. It has been our frequent experience that these patients will require a more labial arrangement to their artificial teeth when their dentures are remade after several years.

2. Patients who have a short and thin upper lip and a prominent labial alveolar ridge will frequently require a modified alveolectomy to

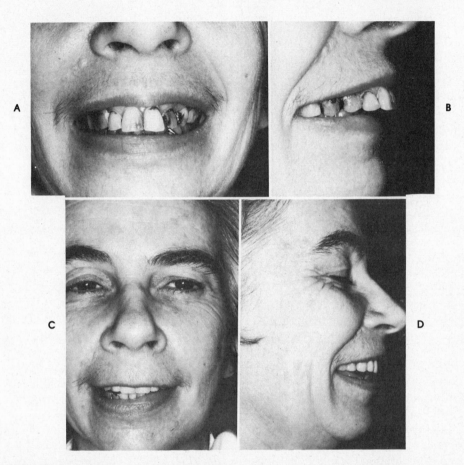

Fig. 26-28. A and **B,** Pretreatment appearance of a patient with a noticeable Angle Class II, division 1, appearance. **C** and **D,** Appearance 7 years after a maxillary alveolectomy and an immediate denture treatment. Notice the inadequately supported labial border. The best location for artificial teeth is in the same position as the natural teeth, unless the natural teeth are out of their normal position because of periodontal disease or problems in occlusion.

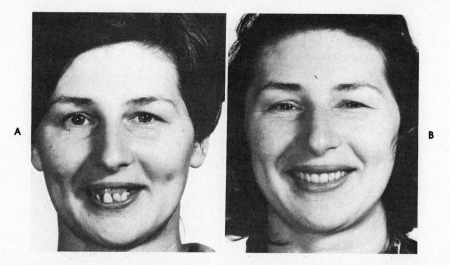

Fig. 26-29. Prominent labial alveolar ridge, **A,** has been reduced surgically, **B,** allowing for the artificial teeth to be positioned more superiorly but still in basically the same horizontal position. Notice the reduced prominence of the gingival tissues around the anterior maxillary teeth.

avoid a shortening or thickening of the upper lip after the insertion of an immediate denture (Fig. 26-29).

3. When diametrically opposed alveolar undercuts are present, the dentist may be tempted to correct one of them. If the undercuts are 1 mm or smaller, mucosal resiliency will usually compensate for the undercut. If the undercuts are more pronounced, a survey of the edentulous region of the master cast is essential. A path of denture insertion and withdrawal is selected with the purpose of covering the largest possible area of the labial or buccal slope of the residual ridge. Usually, a combination of cast surveying, mucosal resiliency, and careful relief of the acrylic resin engaging the undercut will suffice to overcome this problem.

REFERENCES

Carlsson, G.E., Bergman, B., and Hedegård, B.: Changes in contour of the maxillary alveolar process under immediate dentures; a longitudinal clinical and x-ray cephalometric study covering 5 years, Acta Odontol. Scand. **25:**1-31, 1967.

Carlsson, G.E., and Persson, G.: Morphologic changes of the mandible after extraction and wearing of dentures; a longitudinal clinical and x-ray cephalometric study covering 5 years, Odontol. Revy **18:**27-54, 1967.

Hedegård, B., Lundberg, M., and Wictorin, L.: Masticatory function—a cineradiographic investigation. I. Position of the bolus in full and partial lower denture cases, Acta Odontol. Scand. **25:**331-353, 1967.

Wictorin, L.: Bone resorption in cases with complete upper denture, Acta Radiol. [Diagn.], supp. 288, pp. 1-97, 1964.

Wictorin, L.: An evaluation of bone surgery in patients with immediate dentures, J. Prosthet. Dent. **21:**6-13, 1969.

27

Single complete dentures opposing natural teeth

MAXILLARY SINGLE DENTURES

When designing complete maxillary and mandibular dentures, the dentist has complete control over the tooth arrangement in the effort to ensure denture stability. This is rarely the case when a single complete denture is opposed by a residual natural dentition, e.g., maxillary denture opposing natural mandibular teeth or vice versa. In such situations, the objective of a balanced occlusion cannot always be met without significant correction of, or alteration to, the opposing natural teeth inclines and the occlusal plane. Patients needing maxillary single dentures are frequently encountered, and if careful attention is paid to the extra demands on the dentist's skills in occlusal design, good results are usually obtained. The reverse predicament is complicated by the reduced denture-bearing area of an ever-shrinking mandibular alveolar ridge. A useful analogy here is the use of a small hammer on a big anvil. Each heavy blow of the hammer tends to dislodge the hammer from the operator's hand.

The most common cause of difficulty with the occlusion of a maxillary denture and opposing natural teeth is the result of the inclination of some parts of the occlusal plane of the natural teeth. If the entire occlusal plane is not reasonably level, horizontal forces that reduce the stability of the denture are directed against it. For example, in an arch in which the mandibular

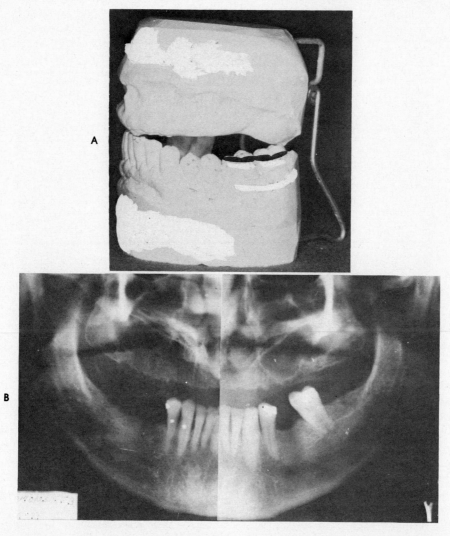

Fig. 27-1. A, Second and third molars have tipped forward into the first molar position. It is necessary to modify the occlusal morphology of these molars by extensive tooth grinding or the placement of cast restorations. If either is not possible, one or both teeth may have to be considered for extraction. **B,** A similar situation demonstrated in a panoramic radiograph. Here the patient's tooth No. 36 is extruded and must be reduced occlusally to avoid interference with the maxillary occlusal scheme.

first molars have been lost, the second and third molars will have tipped forward so that their occlusal surfaces face forward and up instead of facing upward (Fig. 27-1). If the teeth opposing these teeth have been lost, the second and third molars may have become elongated as well. The common error is to set the maxillary artificial teeth to meet the occlusal surfaces of the tipped teeth in the same way as they would if the natural teeth were in their correct alignment. This error causes a forward thrust to be exerted on that side whenever food is between these molar teeth. This forward thrust is the resolution of vertical functional and parafunctional forces and

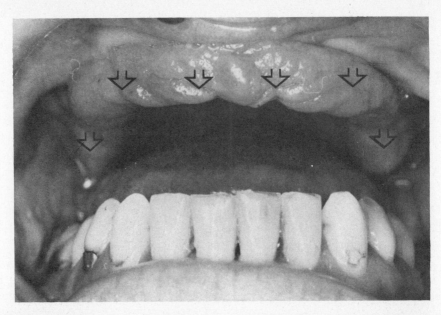

Fig. 27-2. This patient has worn a complete maxillary denture opposing a natural mandibular dentition for 12 years. The entire maxillary ridge has resorbed and been replaced by hyperplastic tissue.

is also exerted on the denture when the mandible is moved to the opposite side.

The forward thrust developed by the inclined occlusal surfaces causes the maxillary denture to tend to rotate. Obviously, rotation of a denture will break the intimate contact of the denture base with its basal seat, and retention of the denture will be lost. Eventually, the border seal will be broken, and bone under the denture will be destroyed. For these reasons, the occlusal plane of the natural teeth must be made reasonably level, or the artificial teeth must be set to contact only the highest parts of the natural teeth.

An excellent, well-fitting denture base is easily loosened when the mandible is moved into eccentric positions if there are steep inclines or deflective occlusal contacts in these positions. For that reason, it is necessary to prepare the teeth so that cross-arch balancing contacts are made possible.

For economic reasons it may be necessary to build a maxillary denture without restoration of some missing mandibular teeth. The question then arises as to how far it is permissible to go

and still have a favorable prognosis. It is essential to have some posterior teeth and some anterior teeth present on both sides of the arch. Building of a maxillary denture against six, eight, or even ten teeth in the anterior part of the mandibular arch may invite failure. Close contact is necessary in all the anterior teeth in such a setup. This necessitates steep inclines, which are likely to displace the denture. It is true some patients wear maxillary dentures against this combination of teeth in the mandibular arch, despite the tipping action that is constantly taking place. However, our clinical experience possibly indicates that when occlusal forces are localized to a small portion of the maxillary ridge, bone reduction is likely. This is frequently accompanied by the development of hyperplastic tissue (Fig. 27-2).

When a fixed or a removable partial denture is planned for the mandibular arch, it is important that the occlusal scheme be an integrated one, that is, *one developed when both arches are treated together* (Fig. 27-3). If the mandibular arch is not to be restored prosthetically, careful

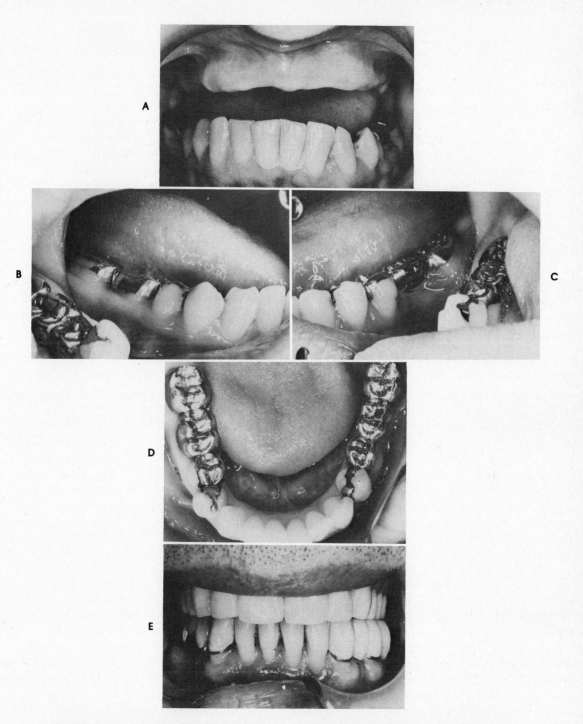

Fig. 27-3. The mandibular natural teeth in **A** to **D** were restored so that the fixed partial prostheses were designed and fabricated along with the maxillary complete denture to ensure an integrated occlusion. In **E,** a similar clinical and laboratory strategy enabled the dentist to ensure an optimal balanced occlusion and cosmetic result.

planning on articulated casts will ensure the dentist's control over an optimal occlusal plane.

Clinical and laboratory procedures

In the case of a single maxillary denture, an impression is made of both arches, and a maxillary occlusion rim is fabricated. If bilateral or a tripod of stable centric stops can be established on this rim, a centric relation record is made in wax or quick-setting plaster. If stable centric stops are not feasible because of a depleted mandibular dentition, a partial mandibular occlusion rim must be employed for the centric relation record. A face-bow registration is made, and the casts are mounted on a semiadjustable articulator. The condylar guidances on the articulator are either set to an average value or else by means of protrusive records.

The incisal guide is set at the angle that is considered necessary for occlusion of the denture. The more nearly horizontal it is possible to have the incisal guidance angle, the more the inclines will be reduced and the more stable will be the denture. Esthetics will influence the angle of the incisal guide because the vertical position of the anterior teeth varies with the amount of vertical overlap used.

The teeth are set up and arranged with the proper inclinations and vertical overlap without the exact contours of the manibular occlusal plane and intercuspation of the natural teeth being followed. The occlusal plane is oriented, and the teeth are inclined, with the anticipated necessary arrangement for occlusal balance. There are many dips in the occlusal plane of natural teeth because of tipping if any teeth of the arch have been lost. The mandibular first molar is the tooth most frequently missing, with resultant drifting of the second and third molars (Fig. 27-1). This causes extremely steep inclines so that the maxillary molars should not be set down into contact with these malpositioned teeth. The denture teeth are prepared with reduced inclines to diminish lateral stress and ensure stability from the standpoint of occlusion. The posterior teeth are set in occlusion in the hard baseplate-wax occlusion rim.

The articulator is moved into the various eccentric positions for study of the occlusal balancing contacts. The teeth are rearranged to obtain the best possible occlusal balancing contacts. However, it may be found that the natural teeth will prevent this balancing, and it will be necessary to grind the stone cast to remove interferences. After arrangement of the denture is complete, grinding of the interferences of the mandibular teeth on the stone cast is done by the movement of the maxillary teeth over the mandibular stone teeth.

If an opposing fixed or removable partial denture is part of the treatment, it is waxed-up at this stage. The objective is to insert all prostheses (fixed or removable partial dentures or the complete denture) at the same appointment to ensure optimal control and development of occlusal relations.

After the denture has been processed, it is placed in the mouth and is tested for retention, and the borders are checked for height.

A comparison of the natural teeth and the stone cast is made to note the areas to be ground. Preliminary grinding using diamond stones is preferably made on the teeth at the locations suggested by the stone cast.

Thin articulating paper is placed over the mandibular teeth, and an opening and closing movement is made to indicate the areas to be ground in centric relation. These areas are reduced by means of a fine soft Carborundum stone.

Next, simulated parafunctional or excursive movements are carried out, and gross discrepancies are reduced with diamond stones and refined with fine soft Carborundum stones.

Several dentists elect to place Carborundum grinding paste over the maxillary teeth and then instruct the patient to make all excursive movements. Care must be taken to prevent the grinding from producing an error in centric occlusion.

This grinding procedure is continued until it is felt that the minor interferences have been removed. This final grinding with a Carborundum paste, such as Kerr's abrasive paste, is done for removal of slight interferences. Under no circumstances should Carborundum powder or paste be employed for excessive grinding. Its use would establish improper inclines, since both the maxillary and mandibular teeth are being ground in the absence of one controlling end factor—the incisal guide control.

SUBSEQUENT PROBLEMS WITH SINGLE DENTURES AGAINST NATURAL TEETH

One of the major problems with dentures opposing natural teeth is that of abrasion.

The use of maxillary porcelain teeth, especially if they are ground during the occlusal correction, will lead to wear of the opposing natural tooth surfaces in a relatively short time. If this is allowed to continue, the pulps may even be exposed (Fig. 27-4, *E*).

Gold inlays on crowns and silver alloy restorations will wear away more rapidly than tooth enamel when they are opposed by porcelain complete denture teeth. This abrasion can destroy fine efforts at occlusal recontruction of the lower teeth, which might have been done to develop an ideal occlusal plane and curvature.

The use of acrylic resin teeth, in the single denture in this situation, is a clinically popular compromise, but the natural teeth or the gold or silver restorations can also wear away the occlusal surfaces of the resin teeth in a relatively short time in some patients.

Although modern resin teeth demonstrate excellent wear and hardness values, some dentists prefer to use gold occlusal surfaces on some of the denture teeth that oppose gold restorations or natural teeth (Fig. 27-5). When one or more gold occlusal surfaces are provided on each side of the single complete denture, it will stop the abrasion between unlike materials and protect the other teeth from abrasion. It is obviously not necessary to make all the posterior teeth

of gold. This is an accurate, albeit unnecessary, option and has limited application.

Formation of the gold surfaces

The procedure for making the gold occlusal surface involves the arrangement of plastic posterior teeth in the places where the gold surfaces are to be used. Porcelain or plastic teeth may be used in other places in the occlusal scheme. Once the occlusion has been balanced and perfected after the try-in, the plastic teeth to be converted are removed from the trial denture base.

The occlusal surfaces of the plastic teeth are cut off with a separating disk at right angles to the long axis of each tooth. A wax retention loop is attached to the cut surface, and the sprue for casting is attached to this surface also. The wax and resin patterns are invested, burned out, and cast, and the castings are polished. White inlay wax is used to restore the original buccal and lingual contours of the teeth. Then the gold occlusal surfaces with their wax buccal and lingual patterns are invested, and tooth-colored acrylic resin is processed to the gold occlusal surfaces. The teeth made of gold and acrylic resin are replaced in the positions they occupied when they were made only of acrylic resin. Since the occlusal surfaces had been corrected for occlusal contact before the castings were made, the gold occlusal surfaces assist in their being replaced in the original positions as guided by the opposing occlusion.

MANDIBULAR SINGLE DENTURES

The single mandibular denture opposing a restored complete or partial maxillary arch poses an even greater problem. This situation is frequently compounded by advanced residual ridge resorption of the edentulous mandible, and it is tempting to conclude that such patients are better off with all their remaining teeth extracted and complete upper and lower dentures constructed. Fig. 27-6 shows an example of the terrific destruction of bone from the lower

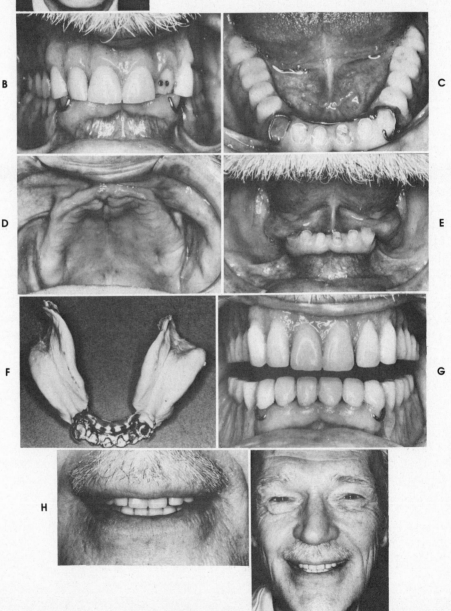

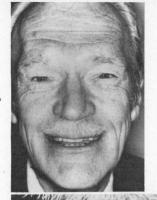

Fig. 27-4. A, A pictorial case history of the effects of a single maxillary denture with porcelain teeth opposing a few mandibular anterior teeth and an unserviced distal-extension removable partial denture. The long-term wear of this prosthesis resulted in, **B,** loss of vertical dimension of occlusion; **C** and **E,** excessive tooth abrasion and alveolar ridge resorption of the maxilla, **D. F** to **I,** Treatment restored occlusal vertical dimension and developed an incisal guidance that discouraged anterior tooth contacts except in excessive protrusive excursions. Note that a partial type of overdenture was used, **F** and **G.** (From Zarb, G.A., Bergman, B., Clayton, J.A., and MacKay, H.F., editors: Prosthodontic treatment for partially edentulous patients, St. Louis, 1978, The C.V. Mosby Co.)

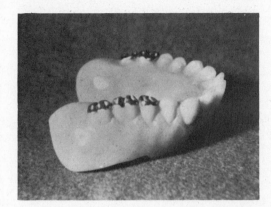

Fig. 27-5. Gold occlusal surfaces are made with acrylic resin teeth being used as patterns after the teeth have been set in occlusion. The resin part of the teeth with gold occlusal surfaces is processed from tooth-colored acrylic resin of the type used for fixed partial dentures.

A

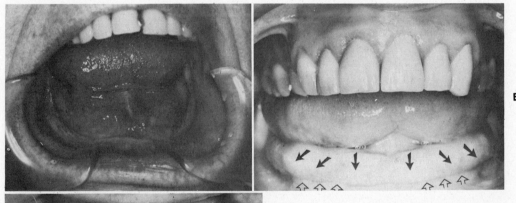

B

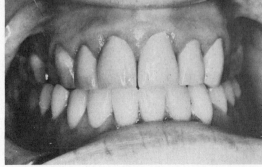

C

Fig. 27-6. A, Mandibular residual ridge has been destroyed by long-term, unserviced wear of a mandibular denture opposed by a natural dentition. In **B** and **C,** a similar situation exists—a pseudo–Class III occlusion is self-evident, and mandibular denture stability is further compromised by a high floor of the mouth attachment *(dark arrows)* and a resorbed ridge *(light arrows).*

jaw caused by such a complete mandibular denture. The mandibular ridge was destroyed in a relatively short time.

It is not always possible to convince the patient whose edentulous mandible opposes an intact or a restored maxillary dentition to have the remaining maxillary teeth extracted. Although the potential advanced residual ridge resorption in the mandible must be emphasized, along with the difficulties in denture stability that will be encountered, the dentist is frequently forced to compromise and attempt prosthodontic treatment for such a patient without further extractions.

The clinical and laboratory procedures are almost identical to the ones described earlier in this chapter. Clinical experience suggests, however, that the use of a resilient denture liner in the mandibular denture is a most useful adjunctive measure. At the conclusion of Chapter 1 (see Fig. 1-6) we speculated on the possible significance of employing permanent resilient (or for that matter, a series of temporary resilient) liners to reduce stresses to the residual alveolar ridges. The premise is that a stress-breaking or stress-reducing material may compensate for the gross imbalance in areas available to cope with functional and parafunctional pressures—somewhere in the region of 45 cm^2 of periodontal ligament for the maxillary dentition versus 12 cm^2 or less of mucosa-covered alveolar bone in an edentulous mandible. We and several of our colleagues have adopted this approach for most of our patients in this predicament, with consistently acceptable results.

SECTION FIVE

Supplemental prosthodontic procedures for edentulous patients

28

Relining and rebasing complete dentures

Materials used in complete denture prosthodontics are vulnerable to change, in that denture base materials or artificial teeth can fracture or abrade. However, the potential for irreversible change is greatest in the tissues supporting the prostheses. This point was emphasized in Section one, as an insidious and unavoidable sequel of the edentulous state. Meticulous attention and care in the construction of complete dentures (Sections two and three) will minimize adverse changes in the supporting tissues and in associated facial morphologic changes as well. However, these changes cannot be entirely avoided, and the need to "servicing" complete dentures to keep pace with the changing foundations becomes mandatory. The clinical efforts that aim at prolonging the useful life of complete dentures involve a reline or rebase procedure.

TREATMENT RATIONALE

As the denture foundations change, the impression surfaces of the dentures cease to fit the tissues properly. It is usually a simple matter to reestablish this denture-tissue relation more particularly when other relations are not (or else only slightly) disturbed by changes in the basal seals for the dentures. The procedure used is a *relining* one, and the dentist achieves this by adding new denture base material to the existing denture base, thereby refitting the denture.

Observed clinical changes include:
I   Loss of retention and stability
II Loss of vertical dimension of occlusion
III Loss of support for facial tissues
IV Horizontal shift of dentures: incorrect occlusal relationship
V   Reorientation of occlusal plane

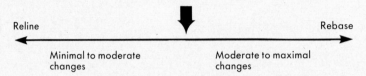

Reline   Rebase

Minimal to moderate   Moderate to maximal
changes   changes

Fig. 28-1. A, Loss of bone structure under both dentures permits the mandible to move upward to corresponding amount. As mandible rotates to closed position without translation of the condyles, body of mandible moves forward. The problem is to determine amount of change that has occurred in both basal seats. The occlusion may not appear to be correct when it is observed in the mouth, **B,** or else appears deceptively adequate. **C,** The extraoral close-mouthed appearance will be almost identical in both cases, however.

Rebasing of dentures is undertaken when the dentures need to be refitted and simultaneously reoriented as well. This is done so as to compensate for vertical and horizontal changes in both dentures' orientation, which have resulted from significant changes in the denture foundations and spatial reorientation of the mandible relative to the maxilla. In the rebasing procedure, a resurfacing of the fitting surface of the denture is also involved (as in the relining procedure). However, the bulk of new material that is added would be excessive unless an entirely new denture base were refitted. Both procedures involve making a new impression in the existing denture, but the indications for either procedure depend on the extent of adverse clinical changes observed (Fig. 28-1).

It is readily conceded that relining or rebasing a complete denture involves all the problems of making new dentures and the restriction that the dentist cannot move the teeth around as easily as with a new denture. *However, socioeconomic realities dictate that this service must be* *resorted to quite frequently, and clinical experience justifies its routine use.*

DIAGNOSIS

A thorough diagnosis of the changes that have occurred must be made before clinical procedures are started. It is necessary to determine the nature of the changes that have occurred, as well as the extent and location of the changes. It is therefore necessary to understand the changes that are possible and their symptoms.

Patients who have worn dentures successfully for a period of time may return for further service because of looseness, soreness, chewing inefficiency, or esthetic changes. These difficulties may be caused by (1) incorrect or unbalanced occlusion that existed at the time the dentures were inserted or (2) changes in one or both of the structures that support the dentures, which may or may not be associated with disharmonious occlusion. It is essential that the cause or causes of the difficulties be determined before any attempt is made to correct them.

Dentures with built-in errors in occlusion may not need relining. They may need only to have the occlusion corrected. Simple tests of the individual denture bases may show that stability and retention have not been lost even though the patient reports that the dentures are loose. In this situation the supporting tissues may show more irritation or inflammation on one side than on the other. The apparent looseness will have resulted from uneven occlusal contact that was not discernible at first.

The treatment involves keeping the dentures out of the mouth for 1 to 2 days or using a tissue conditioner, to allow the supporting tissues to become healthy. If occlusion was the cause of the gradual loss of retention, this rest, followed by a new centric relation record and remounting and regrinding procedures, will eliminate the cause and make the dentures comfortable and serviceable without relining.

Change in the basal seats of the denture may be obvious by comparison of the tissue contours with the contours of the tissue surfaces of the dentures, or it may be indicated by obvious looseness, general soreness and inflammation, loss of occlusal vertical dimension and esthetics, or disharmonious occlusal contacts. An examination of the oral mucosa under the dentures will reveal the state of its health. When this tissue is badly irritated, occlusal disharmony associated with loss of occlusal vertical dimension is to be suspected. Unsatisfactory changes in esthetics will indicate loss of occlusal vertical dimension even though the teeth may seem to occlude properly. If the supporting tissue is badly destroyed, surgical correction to eliminate excess hyperplastic tissue may be necessary before relining impressions are made.

The amount of change in the occlusal vertical dimension and esthetics that has resulted from the loss of supporting structure must be carefully noted. The problem is not simply one of change in the occlusal vertical dimension alone; the dentures may change in their horizontal relations to each other and to their basal seats. A loss of vertical dimension will automatically cause the mandible to have a more forward position in relation to the upper jaw than it would have at the original occlusal vertical dimension. This situation exists even though the jaws are maintained in centric relation with each other (Fig. 28-2).

Shrinkage of the bone of the maxillae usually permits the upper denture to move up and back in relation to its original position. However, the occlusion may force the maxillary denture forward. The lower denture usually moves down and forward, but it may move down and back in relation to the mandible as shrinkage occurs. Concurrently, the mandible moves to a higher position when the teeth are in occlusion than it occupied with the teeth in occlusion before the shrinkage occurred. This movement is rotary around a line approximately through the condyles. Since the occlusal plane and the body of the mandible are located below the level of this axis of rotation, the mandible moves forward as the space between the maxillae and the mandible is reduced from that existing when the dentures were constructed originally. This forward movement of the body of the mandible is not a change in centric relation, which may be retained despite the movement.

The effects of the rotary movement vary from patient to patient.

1. Mandibular rotation may cause loss of the proper centric occlusion of the dentures. The lower teeth may assume a protruded relation to the upper teeth so that if cusp teeth are used, the tooth contacts that occur at centric relation are between the mesial inclines of the cusps of the lower teeth and the distal inclines of the cusps of the upper teeth. This effect may progress so far as to allow the lower teeth to contact the upper teeth a full cusp width anterior to the relation in which they were originally arranged.

2. Mandibular rotation may cause changes in the structures that support the upper denture. The upper denture may be forced forward on the upper ridge instead of backward, as would be expected (Fig. 28-2). This would result from

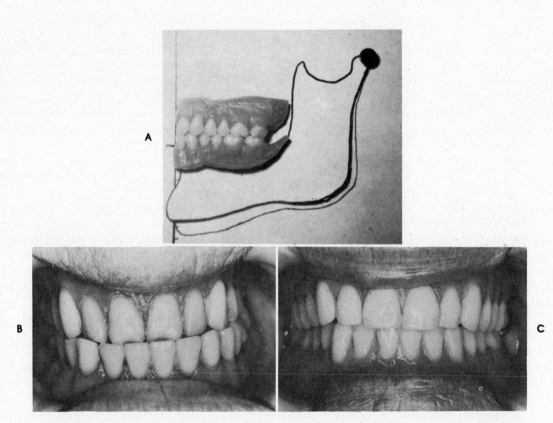

Fig. 28-2. A, Loss of bone structure under both dentures permits the mandible to move upward a corresponding amount. As mandible rotates to closed position without translation of the condyles, body of mandible moves forward. The problem is to determine amount of change that has occurred in both basal seats. The occlusion may not appear to be correct when it is observed in the mouth, **B,** or else appears deceptively adequate, **C.** The extraoral close-mouthed appearance will be almost identical in both cases, however.

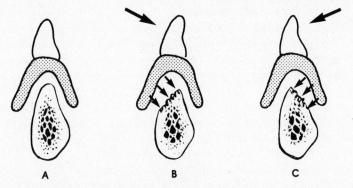

Fig. 28-3. Effect of reduction of occlusal vertical dimension on anterior part of mandibular residual ridge. **A,** Cross-section shape of ridge when denture was made. **B,** Inclined planes of cusps of teeth force mandibular denture posteriorly and cause destruction of labial side of ridge. **C,** Direction of force is changed when lower denture has moved forward far enough to develop contacts between distal side of lower cusps and mesial side of upper cusps. This force may cause destruction of lingual side of mandibular ridge.

the heavy, inclined plane contacts between the mesial inclines of the cusps of the lower teeth and the distal inclines of the cusps of the upper teeth. The direction of such occlusal forces could cause destruction of the anterior maxillary part of the denture foundation.

3. Mandibular rotation may cause the lower denture to be forced backward on the lower ridge by the changed relation of the incline planes of the cusps of the teeth. The occlusal forces of closures in centric position would force the denture distally and thus cause destruction of the labial side of the lower ridge (Fig. 28-3).

4. Mandibular rotation may cause the lower denture to be forced anteriorly by the incline planes of the teeth if the vertical dimension is reduced by shrinkage until the occlusion occurs one cusp forward of its intended relation. The tooth contacts are made, then, between the distal inclines of the cusps of the lower teeth and the mesial inclines of the cusps of the upper teeth. This causes the occlusal forces to be directed posteriorly on the upper denture and anteriorly on the lower denture (Fig. 28-3). These forces *tend* to destroy the bone on the lingual side of the lower ridge.

It appears, then, that mandibular rotation can

elicit severe damage from denture-supporting tissues over a long period of unsupervised denture wear. The stresses that cause such damage are probably augmented by the use of cusp posterior teeth and resultant incisal guidance, which now "locks" the mandibular denture into the maxillary one, or vice versa. Although proponents of the noncusp school of thought frequently indict cusp teeth as accelerating tissue damage in such situations, *no research evidence is available to support either school's claim that their tooth choice minimizes changes in the denture-supporting tissues.*

The horizontal position of each denture in relation to its own supporting ridge must be considered to determine whether the denture has moved forward or backward as a result of interocclusal forces applied on the dentures. Furthermore, one or both dentures may have rotated in relation to the supporting structures. Occlusion of the teeth in the mouth must not be the guide to horizontal repositioning of either denture. A new determination of the vertical dimension of the face by reestablishment of a normal interocclusal distance will be helpful in repositioning the dentures in a vertical direction.

Examination of the esthetics in profile, as far

as the support of the lips in an anteroposterior direction is concerned, will serve as a guide to the orientation of the dentures in relation to their respective foundations. The relation of the teeth to the ridges must be observed to determine the accuracy of the position. If shrinkage has been simply in the vertical direction, allowing the jaws to approach each other more closely than they should when occlusal contacts are made, the occlusion of the teeth cannot be correct even though there has been no forward or backward movement by the dentures.

It must be determined whether shrinkage of the jaws has been uniform under both dentures or one ridge has been destroyed more than the other one. Greater shrinkage in one arch than in the other will change the orientation of the occlusal plane. This will cause occlusal disharmony in eccentric occlusions even though the occlusal vertical dimension is reestablished by relining. A visual comparison of the size of the ridge with the size of the alveolar groove in the denture will serve as a guide.

PRELIMINARY TREATMENT

Most of the preceding points related to the need for a rebase procedure as suggested in Fig. 28-1. Their clinical handling demands some preliminary steps before the actual clinical procedure itself is undertaken. These clinical steps aim at the following objectives:

1. Reestablishment of the vertical dimension of occlusion
2. Resoration of esthetics by reorientation of the dentures anteroposteriorly
3. Reorientation of each denture to its foundation
4. Reorientation of the occlusal plane
5. Reestablishment of centric relation of the jaws
6. Correction of the impression surfaces

Most of these objectives are achieved more or less automatically by use of a tissue conditioner. This is particularly so if the adverse changes to be corrected are of the mild-to-moderate variety

(see Fig. 28-1). On the other hand, more severe changes and hence the clinical need for a rebase are usually rather easily carried out by use of combinations of compound stops, tissue conditioners, occlusal adjustment, and autopolymerizing augmentation of the occlusal surface or surfaces. This technique is used routinely to provide relief from mandibular dysfunction, which can result from vertical occlusal changes in complete denture wearers.

The obvious advantages of using tissue conditioners include those referred to in Chapter 6, such as restoration of a healthy condition of the basal seats and the ease with which they can be modified to prognosticate maximal function and cosmetic result.

After making certain that the tissues are healthy, the dentist looks for errors in the occlusion, occlusal vertical demension that should be corrected, and other changes that should be made before the final clinical procedure is undertaken.

The clinical relining or rebasing can be achieved by use of at least three ways, as follows: (1) the static impression technique, (2) the functional impression technique, and (3) the so-called chairside reline technique.

CLINICAL PROCEDURES
The static impression technique:
closed and open mouth relines

There are two major variations on the static-impression theme. In one variation the dentures are used as impression trays, and either the existing centric occlusion is used as a means to seat the dentures with the lining impression material, or else the centric relation is recorded (by use of the registration medium of choice) *before* the impressions are made.

The so-called *open mouth* technique was described by Boucher (1973) and implies the following:

1. It is a method for relining both maxillary and mandibular dentures at the same appointment.

2. The dentures are essentially being used as trays for making the new impressions.
3. The existing centric occlusion is not utilized, and a new centric relation record is accomplished *after* the impressions are made.

It is a demanding and laborious technique but quite a good one.

We prefer the closed-mouth reline technique when we choose the static impression method. Several techniques have been suggested (Bowman and Jaird, 1977), and they are all variations upon the same theme. Each denture is used as an impression tray, and the dentures' occlusion (corrected as part of the preliminary treatment or stabilized intraorally with wax or compound) is used to stabilize the trays while the impression material sets. Table 5 sums up some of the techniques frequently used. It must be emphasized that each technique has its merits and, if meticulously followed, will lead to repeatably good results. The dentures are sent to the laboratory with an accompanying work authorization form, which includes specific directions to the laboratory technician and information required by law. The directions include specifications for alterations, materials, finish, remount casts, and remounting of the upper denture.

For many years it was believed that the strains inherent in the processed denture base could be released on subsequent processing and cause some degree of warpage. However, the evidence presented by Smith and associates (1967) indicates that dentures can be adequately relined with the use of one of the autopolymerizing resins. This technique offers the advantages of a simplified and less costly laboratory procedure.

The processed dentures are usually ready to be inserted on the same day the impressions are made. The protocol described in Chapter 24 is followed, and occlusal refinement is carried out intraorally, or on an articulator. Follow-up instructions tend to be similar to those provided at the time of the insertion of new dentures.

Table 5

Different steps that can be considered as an integral part of a closed-mouth reline technique

Centric relation	Existing intercuspation is used to stabilize dentures
	Interocclusal record is made by use of wax or compound
	Corrected during the reestablishment of a new vertical dimension of occlusion by grinding or use of autopolymerizing resin
Denture preparations	Large undercuts relieved
	Hard resin surfaces relieved 1.5 to 2 mm
	Tissue conditioner removed or relieved
	"Escape" holes drilled particularly in a maxillary base; this will also assist in easy removal of the palatal portion during packing and processing
	Denture periphery shortened to create a flat border
Impression procedure	Border molding can be achieved with a low-fusing compound material
	A posterior palatal seal is achieved with low-fusing compound
	Border molding retained from the polymerized tissue-conditioning material
	Border molding achieved by choosing an impression material that is soft and yet viscous enough to support and register peripheral detail (one of the polyether impression materials)

The functional impression technique

The functional impression technique is both simple and practical and has gained considerable support during the past few years. It is the one we routinely use in our practice. It depends on a thorough understanding of the versatile properties of the tissue conditioners as functional impression materials. The relative ease with which these temporary soft liners can be

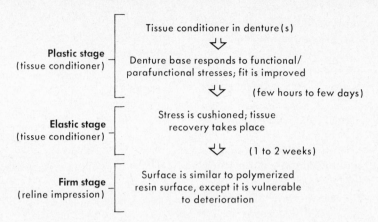

Plastic stage
(tissue conditioner)

Tissue conditioner in denture(s)
⇩
Denture base responds to functional/
parafunctional stresses; fit is improved

⇩　　(few hours to few days)

Elastic stage
(tissue conditioner)

Stress is cushioned; tissue
recovery takes place

⇩　　(1 to 2 weeks)

Firm stage
(reline impression)

Surface is similar to polymerized
resin surface, except it is vulnerable
to deterioration

Fig. 28-4. The different physical stages of tissue conditioner/treatment liners allow the dentist to use them for different objectives.

employed as functional impression materials has led to their abuse and to criticism by many dentists. It must be conceded, however, that they are an excellent adjunct in refitting complete dentures if used carefully and meticulously. Improvements in these materials include the economic advantage of retention of material compliance for many weeks, good dimensional stability, and excellent bonding to the resin denture base (Braden, 1970).

When a denture needs to be refitted, the patient's complaint or the dentist's oral prosthetic evaluation usually indicate undermined retention of the denture. Often one may see a variable hyperemia of the mucosa that may be accompanied by the presence of sore spots in the denture-bearing mucosa. The denture is checked intraorally to assess the need for peripheral reduction or extension, and a posterior palatal seal extension is developed with modeling compound on maxillary dentures. Occasionally three compound stops may be required on the impression surface of the denture to reestablish a proper occlusal relationship or improved occlusal plane orientation. A treatment liner is placed inside the denture. The lining material should flow evenly to cover the whole of the impression surface and the borders

of the denture with a thin layer of the material. If voids are evident, they should be filled with a fresh mix of the liner material. Unsupported areas of the liner may occur on the periphery of the denture, and this is indicative of the need for localized border molding with stick modeling compound before the placement of a fresh mix of liner. Occasionally borders are formed that are low and narrow, and this too is indicative of inadequate peripheral extension of the denture. Here again, the borders must be corrected by border molding with compound or one of the autopolymerizing resins before they are covered with the lining material. It must be emphasized that these materials have a tendency to slump during setting unless adequately supported. This slumping phenomenon probably accounts for the undermined peripheral integrity that can reduce denture retention. The patient's mandible is guided into a retruded position, which is hopefully one of maximum intercuspation, to help stabilize the denture while the lining material is setting. Excess material is trimmed away with a hot scalpel. Most of the materials used for this purpose progress through plastic and then elastic stages before hardening (Wilson and associates, 1966), and this procedure takes place over several days (Fig. 28-4). The plastic stage permits movement of the denture base or bases so that its position becomes compatible with the existing occlusion. This also allows the displaced tissues to recover and assume their original position. The patient is instructed regarding care of the prosthesis and its lining material.

Klinger and Lord (1973) have shown that a number of denture cleansers and other preparations, which may be of value in the control of plaque on dentures, can cause significant deterioration of tissue conditioners in a short time. Apparently simple rinsing of the temporarily lined denture combined with gentle brushing with a soft toothbrush are good interim measures to minimize damage to the lining. Clinical experience indicates that 10 to 14 days may elapse before the material is firm enough to proceed with the clinical reline sequence.

At the next appointment the dentist will usually find the temporarily relined denture to be well retained, with well-rounded peripheral borders and a healthy-appearing mucosa. Wilson and associates have pointed out that the physical properties of tissue-conditioning materials may create problems when used for impressions. The gradually increasing elasticity of the material in the mouth may result in a recovery of the compressed material when the load is removed, that is, when the impression is removed from the mouth. Hence the importance of pouring the cast when the material has reached the firm stage (Fig. 28-4).

Furthermore, these materials tend to deteriorate in some mouths, which precludes their use in this manner. If the dentist has any doubt about the quality of the surface appearance of the hardened liner, the reline procedure can be carried out as described earlier in the chapter, after the interim treatment liner has been removed. If the surface or peripheral deterioration is slight, these areas can be trimmed with a carbide bur, and the denture or dentures are prepared for a secondary, or wash, impression.

The stone cast must be poured immediately after removal of the relined denture base from the mouth. The material should not be plastic, or "self-flow," because the material's own weight may deform the impression (Erhardson and Johansson, 1970; Starcke and associates, 1972). It is also possible that the weight of the stone poured into the impression surface will cause distortion of the impression. Maxillary casts may have to be scored in the selected posterior palatal seal area, since the long period of plasticity of the material may not create sufficient displacement action in this area. Alternately, a thin bead of compound material may be used to augment the posterior palatal seal.

The laboratory phase of relining is well described in the literature (Sowter, 1968).

It must be emphasized that the making of a new centric relation record and the remount procedure are almost always necessary to ensure an optimal prosthodontic occlusion. The work of Tantanen and Siirilä (1972) showed that the functional status of dentures relined with treatment liners used as impression materials was as good as the status of dentures relined by border molding and then refined with a light-bodied impression material.

The chairside reline technique

Several attempts have been made to produce an acrylic or other plastic material that can be added to the denture and allowed to set in the mouth to produce an instant chairside reline. These have met with failure for several reasons: (1) the materials have often produced a chemical burn on the mucosa; (2) the resulting reline was often porous and subsequently developed a bad odor; (3) color stability was very low; and (4) if the denture was not positioned correctly, the material could not be removed easily in order to start again. Today, the chairside reline technique is of little use in clinical practice because of these attendant difficulties and has, for the most part, been discarded.

Both the static technique (or versions of it) and the functional impression technique are well accepted and experience-proved procedures. They can be used for both simple situations (denture settling is minimal) and complicated situations (excessive tissue changes have taken place). It appears that the choice between the two methods is based on the dentist's and the patient's convenience.

REFERENCES

Bergman, B., Carlsson, G.E., and Ericson, S.: Effect of differences in habitual use of complete dentures on underlying tissues, Scand. J. Dent. Res. **79**:449-460, 1971.

Bergman, B., and Carlsson, G.E., and Hedegård, B.: A longitudinal two-year study of a number of full denture cases, Acta Odontol. Scand. **22**:3-26, 1964.

Boucher, C.O.: The relining of complete dentures, J. Prosthet. Dent. **30**:521-526, 1973.

Bowman, J.F., and Javid, N.S.: Relining and rebasing techniques, Dent. Clin. North Am. **21**(2):369-378, 1977.

Braden, M.: Tissue conditioners. I. Composition and structure, J. Dent. Res. **49**:145-148, 1970.

Erhardson, S., and Johansson, E.G.: Jämförande laboratorieundersökning av COE-comfort, COE-soft och Ivoseal som avtrycksmaterial, Svensk Tandläk. Tidskr. **63**:633-645, 1970.

Klinger, S.M., and Lord, J.L.: Effect of common agents on intermediary temporary soft reline materials, J. Prosthet. Dent. **30**:749-755, 1973.

Rantanen, T., and Siirilä, H.S.: Fast and slow setting functional impression materials used in connection with complete denture relinings, Suom. Hammaslaak. Toim. **68**:175-180, 1972.

Smith, D.E., Lord, J.L., and Bolender, C.L.: Complete denture relines with autopolymerizing resin processed in water under air pressure, J. Prosthet. Dent. **18**:103-115, 1967.

Sowter, J.B.: Dental laboratory technology, Chapel Hill, 1968, University of North Carolina.

Starcke, E.N., et al.: Physical properties of tissue-conditioning materials as used in functional impressions, J. Prosthet. Dent. **27**:111-119, 1972.

Wilson, H.J., Tomlin, H.R., and Osborne, J.: Tissue conditioners and functional impression materials, Br. Dent. J. **121**:9-16, 1966.

29

Repair of complete dentures and duplication of casts

REPAIR OF DENTURES

The repair of dentures can be a puzzling and difficult part of prosthesis construction. This problem can be handled as a laboratory procedure, but a knowledge of the preparation and of the technical phase is essential whether it is handled in the office or sent outside the office. Often this service is required by patients on an emergency basis becuase tooth and denture fractures seem to occur at most inopportune times.

It is well for the dentist to be aware of the hazards in repairing a denture. Many repairs are difficult to assemble correctly so that they will cause the dentures to be ill-fitting. If a second process of curing by heat is necessary, changes will occur because the old resin resoftens during processing. These changes may cause a change in occlusion and in the fit of the denture over the basal seat. For this reason, it may be advisable to make a new centric relation record, mount the denture, and regrind it after the repair has been completed. It is well to mount and regrind dentures after a period of time, even though repair has not been made; therefore these two services might as well be combined.

The availability of autopolymerizing or cold-curing resins for repairs simplifies the repair procedure. The technique avoids the potential warpage of the dentures that results from reprocessing, and the entire operation can be carried out in much less time than by the heat-curing method. It is not necessary to flask the denture to cure the new resin.

Breakage of individual teeth, as well as breakage of the entire denture, is often caused by a change in occlusal relations, and remounting and regrinding would then be essential to prevent breakage from occurring again. It is impossible in laboratory procedures to return a perfectly adjusted occlusion. It is also well to advise the patient that the tissues will change during the elapsed time that the denture is not worn, but that they will readjust in a short time. The patient must not think that the denture is entirely to blame when the denture does not feel the same immediately on insertion.

Maxillary fracture repair

The broken edges are cleaned of debris and other interferences so that the two parts will fit together well (Fig. 29-1).

The two halves are held together by means of an old bur, which is luted to the teeth and resin surfaces by means of sticky wax (Fig. 29-2). No wax is placed over the fracture so that the tissue and palatal sides of the fracture can be examined to see that they are in correct apposition.

Plaster is vibrated gently onto the palatal side to prevent air bubbles and is then set on the balance of the mix to form the cast (Fig. 29-3).

The procedures used in repairing dentures with cold-curing resin are described in Figs. 29-1 to 29-8.

Repairs using cold-curing resin

When dentures are to be repaired by use of cold-curing resins (Figs. 29-4 to 29-8), the same care, as with other methods, is necessary to assemble the broken and replacement parts accurately. All debris must be removed, and the parts must be brought tightly together and held with sticky wax, or matchsticks (bur) and sticky wax. Then tinfoil is adapted to the basal surface of the denture before a plaster cast is poured inside the denture. The cast is removed from the denture, and the resin on both sides of the

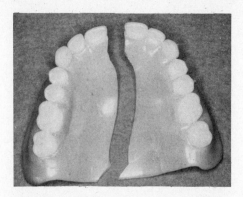

Fig. 29-1. Broken parts should be placed together to test for distortion or lost parts.

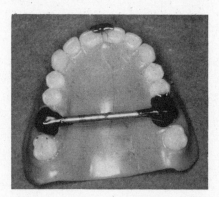

Fig. 29-2. Assembled parts held with sticky wax and an old bur.

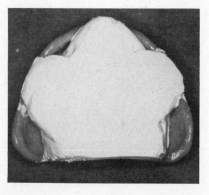

Fig. 29-3. Impression plaster is poured inside denture to retain position of parts.

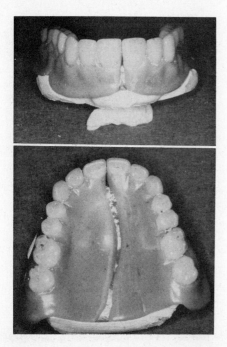

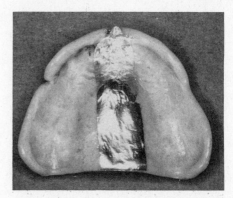

Fig. 29-5. Tinfoil over fracture line.

Fig. 29-4. Resin is cut away from fracture line, and the denture is reassembled on this plaster matrix after tinfoil has been placed over it.

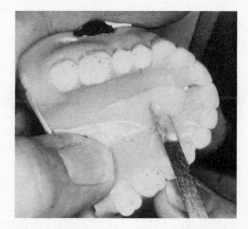

Fig. 29-6. Cold-curing acrylic resin is flowed into the open fracture over the tinfoil.

break is cut away and beveled. Then the cast is replaced, acrylic resin monomer is painted on the cut surfaces, and a cold-curing repair resin is placed in the break (Fig. 29-6). Alternate applications of monomer and polymer are made until the area to be repaired is filled. The area should be slightly overfilled to allow for finishing.

Curing under air pressure

Pressure can be maintained on the cold-curing resin while it cures if one places the denture in a pressure cooker after the resin has been forced into place. An air hose carrying 15 pounds (about 7 kg) or more of pressure is attached to the pressure cooker, and this pressure condenses the repair resin. This curing method can be used when the repair resin is added in small increments of powder (polymer) and liquid (monomer). Without this pressure,

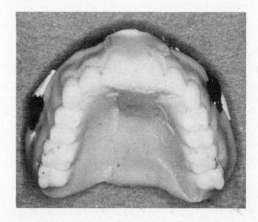

Fig. 29-7. Repair resin has polymerized.

the resin added in this manner is less dense than resin cured under pressure.

DUPLICATION OF CASTS

Duplication of casts has now become a comparatively simple and accurate process. These second casts are necessary in immediate denture construction for a second set of duplicate dentures and for casts poured in a refractory investment for partial and complete denture castings. Duplication can be carried out by use of one of these two techniques: (1) the reversible technique and (2) the irreversible hydrocolloid technique.

Reversible hydrocolloid technique

A mixture of one-half reversible hydrocolloid and one-half water by volume is placed in the upper part of a double-boiler. To facilitate rapid mixing of the water and hydrocolloid, one should break the hydrocolloid into small pieces when it is placed in the double boiler. New material may be used or scrap from hydrocolloid impressions may be used, inasmuch as it is not used in the mouth and is boiled during its preparation. This mixture is heated until it becomes smooth and homogeneous. While the mixture is cooling down, the cast is placed on the bottom plate of the special duplicating flask and is held in position by two pieces of Plasticine (Fig. 29-9). There are several types of duplicating flasks available, and the choice is based on laboratory convenience.

To ensure free flow of the material over the cast, the bottom plate of the flask and cast are immersed in warm water at 135° F (57° C). If the cast is not warm and well soaked, it will dry and cool the hydrocolloid material, thus preventing a smooth surface. During the cooling process, the hydrocolloid mixture in the double boiler is stirred to keep the mass at the same temperature throughout. It is cooled until a finger can be held in the mass without discomfort. This cooling is necessary to reduce shrinkage of the duplicating material and to prevent softening or melt-

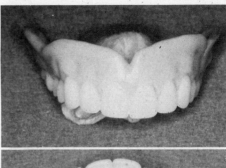
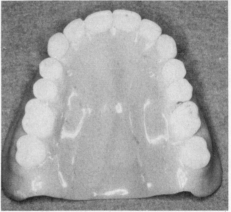

Fig. 29-8. Repair is complete.

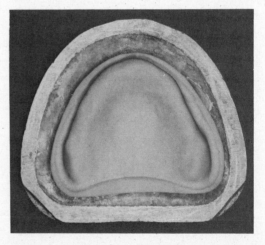

Fig. 29-9. Cast attached to base of duplicating flask with Plasticine.

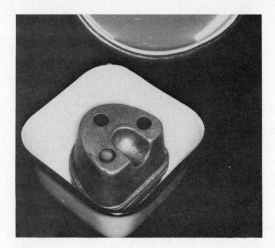

Fig. 29-10. Duplicating material ready to be poured into duplicating flask over the cast.

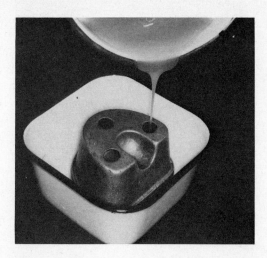

Fig. 29-11. Pouring of duplicating material into duplicating flask.

ing of any wax relief that may be in place on the cast to be duplicated.

A pan that is deeper than the height of the flask is used for cooling after pouring of the material. When the material is ready to pour, the flask is assembled with the cast inside on the bottom plate, and the assembly is placed in the pan (Fig. 29-10). The material is poured into the flask through one of the openings until the material flows out of the other opening. By pouring all the material into one opening instead of using both openings, one can prevent trapping air (Fig. 29-11). Ice and water are then placed in the pan to a level higher than the flask. The flask must not be opened until the mass is chilled thoroughly, a process that may take 20 minutes (Fig. 29-12). After chilling has been completed, the bottom plate is removed, and the hydrocolloid mass is trimmed with a knife around the bottom of the cast to facilitate its removal (Fig. 29-13). This cutting away of hydrocolloid material permits the cast to be grasped and gently withdrawn from the impression. The impression is now examined for incomplete flowing, spaces because of trapping of air, and excessive scarring because of improper removal (Fig. 29-14).

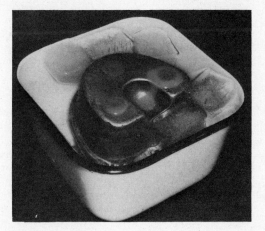

Fig. 29-12. Chilling of filled flask by means of ice and water.

If the impression is satisfactory, a mixture of stone or investment material, as may be required, is vibrated into the impression. The hydrocolloid material is of high water content and therefore becomes dehydrated and distorted rapidly. The fluid leaving the hydrocolloid mass is acid in reaction and will neutralize the alkaline of the stone and thereby soften and

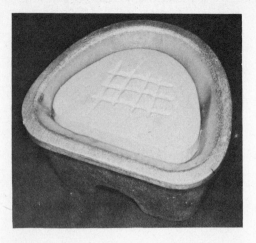

Fig. 29-13. Cutting away duplicating material to facilitate removal of the cast.

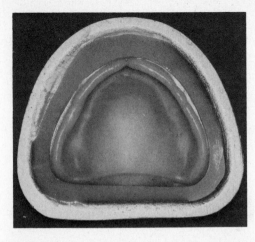

Fig. 29-14. Impression of cast in hydrocolloid material in the flask after removal of the cast.

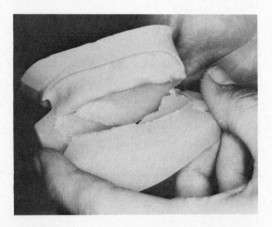

Fig. 29-15. Removal of hydrocolloid material and cast from the duplicating flask.

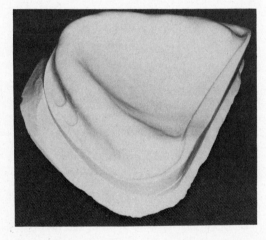

Fig. 29-16. Duplicated cast before trimming.

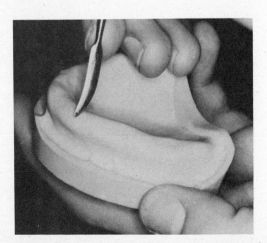

Fig. 29-17. The cast is carefully scrutinized for defects.

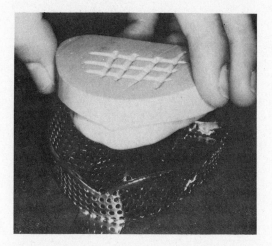

Fig. 29-18. An oversize stock tray is selected.

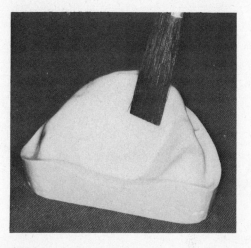

Fig. 29-19. Impression material is brushed onto the cast to ensure reproduction of detail.

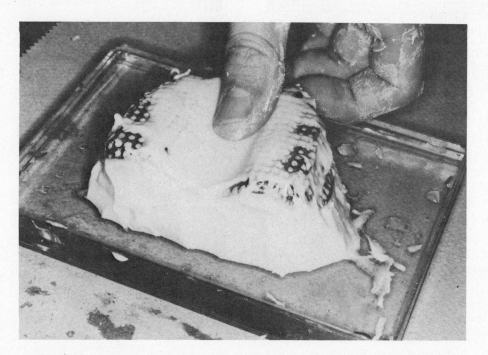

Fig. 29-20. Loaded impression tray is inverted onto the cast, which rests on a glass slab.

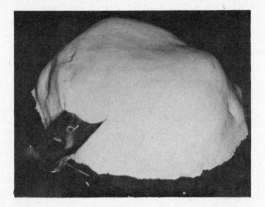

Fig. 29-21. Completed impression is covered with a thin plaster mix.

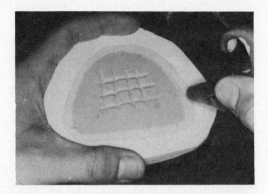

Fig. 29-22. A jet of air assists in separating master cast from "reinforced" impression.

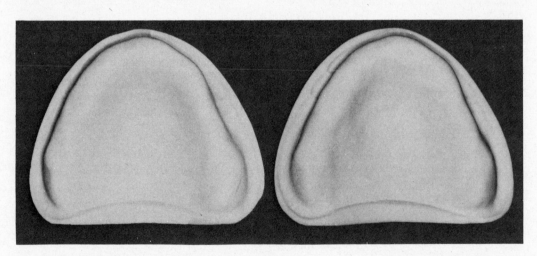

Fig. 29-23. Master and duplicate casts attest to accuracy of this technique.

roughen the surface of the cast. For that reason, the stone must be either poured immediately or kept in a canister. In the vibrating of the stone into the impression, a mass of stone about the size of a walnut is started in the area of the middle of the palate or between the ridges on a mandibular impression. This mass is spread when the impression is held at a sharp angle and is flowed to the other end of the impression. This mass is flowed back and forth several times to keep the layer very thin and thus prevent trapping and incorporation of air. In this manner, a smooth, pitless surface of the cast will be assured. Additional increasing amounts of stone are added until the impression is level full. After the stone has set, the hydrocolloid is slipped out of the flask, and the material is peeled away from the cast. The rough edges are trimmed off the cast, and it is ready to be used for the purpose intended (Figs. 29-15 and 29-16).

Irreversible hydrocolloid technique

The irreversible hydrocolloid technique is an even simpler method and one that is economical in terms of time, equipment, and materials. The cast is carefully examined for defects (Fig. 29-17). Nodules of stone are removed, and defects are filled with wax. An oversized rim-lock impression tray is selected, a thin mix of irreversible hydrocolloid is prepared, and an impression of the cast is made (Figs. 29-18 and 29-19). The loaded tray is inverted on the cast (Fig. 29-20), with care taken to place additional amounts of the hydrocolloid around the sides of the cast. When the impression material has set, the tray is entirely covered and surrounded with a thin mix of quick-setting plaster. This coating should be about ½ inch (12.5 mm) in thickness (Fig. 29-21). After the plaster has set, the glass slab is removed and the cast is separated from the impression. The use of an air syringe facilitates this separation (Fig. 29-22). If the impression is a correct one, a stone mix is poured into it and the duplicate cast is separated after 45 minutes. The result is usually indistinguishable from the original (Fig. 29-23).

30

Alternative treatment modalities for edentulous patients

It is tempting to conclude a text on the treatment of edentulous patients by suggesting that the applied content of the preceding chapters will ensure a happy complete denture experience for all our patients. However, clinical experience demands the admission that some edentulous patients simply cannot tolerate complete dentures. Such patient failure to do so is neither an indictment of our professional skills, nor necessarily an indictment of patient response to our clinical efforts. As clinicians we must accept the fact that many patients who wear complete dentures experience considerable difficulty adapting to their prostheses. In fact, some patients simply cannot wear their dentures at all, and their quality of life is profoundly affected by their predicament. Our treatment for these patients usually entails considerable efforts of both the clinical technical variety and the area of emotional support. Regrettably, we are even tempted at times to dismiss these patients as having difficult or impossible mouths, or worse as lacking motivation or learning skills. These clinical situations are very frustrating for both parties, and it is clear that conventional complete denture therapy is not the correct prescription for such patients. When all conventional methods including preprosthetic surgery have been attempted (Chapter 6), these patients have to be considered condidates for implant procedures.

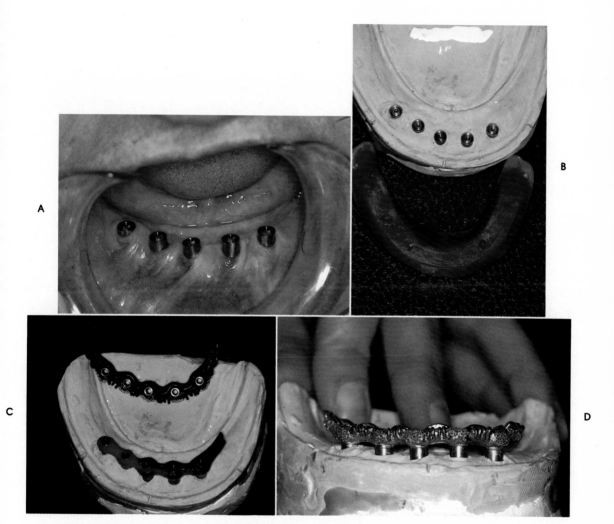

Plate 30–1. A, Clinical appearance of the transepithelial abutment component of the osseointe-grated fixture. **B,** Working cast produced from a custom tray and use of transfer copings. The brass fixture analogs can be "overdentured" by an occlusion rim, or else guide pins can be used to screw the trial base firmly into both brass analogs and titanium intraoral abutments. **C** and **D,** Wax-up reinforced with Duralay (Reliance Dental Mfg. Co., Alsip, Ill.), which is cast in a gold alloy or silver-palladium to act as a rigid framework for subsequent addition of stock teeth and resin replacement for lost gingival tissues. *Continued.*

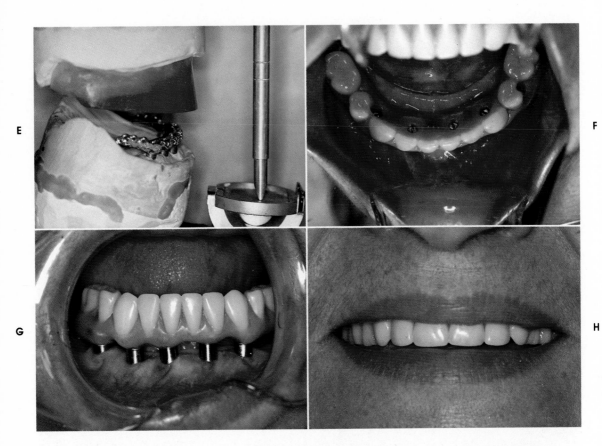

Plate 30–1, cont'd. E, Profile view of metal frame showing bulk of cantilevered portion to preclude metal fracture at this site. **F,** Openings in completed (resin-processed) prosthesis provide access for retaining screws. Screw holes are subsequently blocked out with an autopolymerizing resin. **G** and **H,** Prosthesis design allows for excellent scope for optimal home care procedures without undermining desired cosmetic result. (From Zarb, G.A., and Symington, J.M.: Osseointegrated dental Implants: preliminary report on a replication study, J. Prosth. Dent. **50**:271, Aug. 1983.)

The objective of this chapter is to review the current state of dental implants in clinical dentistry.

PATIENT CONSIDERATIONS

The psychological reactions to various forms of bodily organ loss have been investigated in patients who have undergone a hysterectomy or mastectomy. However remarkably little interest has been shown in the psychological reaction to tooth loss (Blomberg and Lindqvist, 1983). This apparent lack of interest is probably attributable to the prevalence of edentulism and the impressive success enjoyed by the dental profession in treating the condition. Furthermore edentulism is neither fatal, nor likely to elicit profound sympathy in a society that appears preoccupied with youthful appearances. The sense of shame and inferiority that many edentulous patients suffer is rendered even more poignant by the inability of some of them to tolerate a denture at all.

Patients who cannot wear dentures or else wear them with varying degrees of difficulty usually present with one or more of the following features:

1. Severe morphologic compromise of denture-supporting area or areas that significantly undermines denture retention.
2. Poor oral muscular coordination
3. Low tolerance of mucosal tissues
4. Parafunctional habit or habits leading to recurrent soreness and instability of prosthesis
5. Unrealistic prosthodontic expectations
6. Active or hyperactive gag reflex elicited by a removable prosthesis
7. Psychological inability to wear a denture, even if adequate denture retention or stability is present

The above patients are candidates for implant prescription. It should also be stated that even the most successful denture wearer frequently regrets his or her dependence on a removable prosthesis with all the risks of attendant sequelae. These patients, too, could be added to the list when longitudinal research in dental implants confirms the safe and easy availability of implant procedures. Such an advance could very well lead to therapeutic strategies in prosthodontics that will considerably reduce the conventional role of removable prostheses.

USE OF DENTAL IMPLANTS

The successful replacement of lost natural teeth by artificial tooth root analogs would advance dental treatment significantly. Both the dental literature and the presentations at dental meetings reflect the profession's ongoing concern with such a technique. It is clearly an exciting one and has fired the imagination of many dentists and researchers. However, the literature on oral implantology is dominated by anecdotal reports that have misled dentists into thinking that implantology is a clinical treatment method to be readily incorporated into their practices. Insufficient data are available to enable the clinician to predict the number of years of success of any alloplastic oral implant. Premature dissemination of alloplastic implant materials, methods, and techniques has preceded scientific animal and clinical research (Shulman, 1974; Boucher, 1976). There has been far too much testing of dental implants in humans and far too little evaluation of dental implant design and materials in laboratory animals (Hulbert, 1975).

At no time in the history of surgical implants has there been such an unrealistic reporting of results as in the dental implant field. Yet dentists all over the world persist in the endeavors to restore missing teeth with implants, frequently ignoring simpler, safer, and more predictable solutions for the prosthodontic problems confronting them. Implant placement on this basis is often tantamount to the creation of an instant, advanced periodontal disease–like situation insofar as a simulated attachment mechanism is achieved. Reported success is frequently a reflection of the stoicism of the individual patient, rather than significantly reliable evidence of the procedure's success.

It appears that most dental implants are

doomed to failure, with some types of implants failing more slowly than others. Hence the suggestion that subperiosteal implants, because of their large area, "fail slowly," thereby sustaining the illusion that some implants are more successful than others. The use of such clinical experimental techniques should be limited to those few situations in which the patient is aware of the experimental nature of the procedure and its short-lived potential. In 1959 Obwegeser concluded that implants should be advocated only as long as they are intended for use for a limited time. Johns (1976) observed that until the development of a pseudocementum that could evoke the formation of tissues analogous to Sharpey's fibers neither a satisfactory pseudojunctional epithelium nor a well-contoured bone support around an abutment may be possible.

It is regrettable that implant techniques as practiced in the past do not survive scientific scrutiny. It is therefore understandable that most North American university prosthodontic departments limit their teaching on dental implants to a mere presentation of scientific facts, coupled with a strong reluctance to prescribe the technique clinically.

In 1980, a conference sponsored by the National Institutes of Health (NIH) attempted to establish guidelines for the use of various types of implants already in clinical use. A group of dentists involved with dental implants looked at retrospective clinical data provided by several clinicians. These recommendations, while clearly limited by the retrospective nature of the study and the diversity of opinion offered by the conference participants, acknowledged the lack of well-controlled scientific documentation. A list of minimal clinical guidelines was, however, drawn up. Our observations reflect a dissatisfaction with the biomechanical implications of current implant techniques. However, this is not meant to indict the possible use of dental implants as a therapeutic concept. Several health disciplines are committed to a constant search for better tissue and organ replacements,

and clinical dentistry is no exception. However, a conscientious and tenacious commitment to research in the field of tooth and supporting alveolar bone replacement demands scientific methodology that has been lacking to a large extent. In this context, the following quotation from the Draft Statement re National Guidelines for Health Planning, U.S.A., 1978, is relevant: ". . . the effectiveness and safety of clinical procedures should be determined before they are incorporated into common practice, and monitored on a continuing basis; when found effective and safe, they should be introduced in ways that enhance economy, equity, and quality."

It is only the work of Brånemark and colleagues (1977, 1981) that indicates the possibility of a breakthrough in this field. Their clinical implant study is the only one that has survived longitudinal scientific scrutiny.

Brånemark and his colleagues (1977, 1981) have inserted over 4000 threaded, cylindrical, pure titanium implants into mandibular and maxillary sites, as well as tibial, temporal, and iliac bones. These implants were used for a large variety of dental and orthopedic restorative procedures. The titanium fixtures were implanted by use of a meticulous technique that aimed at a direct contact between living bone and implant material. This direct contact, or a development of interfacial osteogenesis, had alrady been hypothesized by several authors. The belief was that certain implant materials possess a dynamic surface chemistry that induces histologic changes at the implant interface that normally occur if the implant were not present. Branemark's laboratory and clinical results demonstrate a close spatial relationship between titanium and living bone. This interface zone was investigated by radiographs, histology, and scanning and transmission electron microscopy.

Furthermore, no wear products were seen in the bone or soft tissues despite implant loading of up to 90 months (Albrektsson et al., 1981).

Branemark refers to his results as ones in

which a predictable form of "osseointegration" is taking place. His definition of osseointegration indicates a highly differentiated bone response to the careful placement of pure titanium tooth root analogs. Moreover this response appears to become organized according to functional demands. Albrektsson and co-workers, (1981) have reported that osseointegration is also possible with various types of metals such as stainless steel, vitallium, and tantalum as well as titanium alloys. However none of these researchers has demonstated long-term clinical efficacy of their implants comparable to Brånemark's results. Brånemark's clinical application has now been replicated in several centers (Zarb and Symington, 1983) and indicates a very important advance in this field of tissue-integrated prostheses.

TISSUE INTEGRATION IN THE EDENTULOUS PATIENT
(Figs. 30-1 to 30-3 and Plate 30-1)

The entire objective in prescribing implants for patients is to provide them with an acceptable analog for their lost periodontal ligaments. For such an analog to be predictably safe and long lasting, it should rely upon a host bone response that is both highly differentiated and biomechanically adequate for functional and parafunctional stresses (Table 6). Such an achievement appears to depend on the following features:

1. Careful surgery that does not compromise the predictability of a favorable healing response as manifested by subsequent, great differentiation of the host tissue.

2. Use of an unalloyed titanium material, which means that the oxide layer that builds up over the metallic surface prevents an actual contact between bone and metal, suggestive of the possibility that the implant is similar to a ceramic surface. This layer is bound to affect the host tissue response albeit in an imperfectly understood way.

3. Design of a root analog that allows immediate stability of the implant and excellent scope for eventual stress distribution.

Table 6

Comparison of qualities of the periodontal ligament and the "attachment" mechanism induced with implants

MATERIAL	ATTACHMENT MECHANISM
1. Tooth	Periodontal ligament, which is also a sensory organ and a shock absorber, participates in remodeling and regulates osteogenesis
2. Implants in current use*	Poorly differentiated tissue Short- and long-term biomechanical behavior is unpredictable
3. Brånemark's tissue-integrated implants	Highly differentiated tissue Predictable long-term biomechanical behavior

*This method can be regarded as halfway technology, and such implants are a palliative at best.

4. Unloaded healing of the implant to ensure the predictability of an optimal healing response.

5. An impeccable fit of the prosthetic superstructure and correct occlusal relationships as well. These are standard objectives in prosthodontics, but the absence of resilient periodontal ligament support in tissue-integrated prostheses indicates a need for technical prosthodontic accuracy that may very well exceed what is required for tooth abutments.

Figs. 30-1 to 30-3 and Plate 30-1 outline the salient features involved in the clinical application of the osseointegration method.

It must be pointed out that the precise nature of the interfacial titanium-bone relationship is not completely clear, or is the information regarding the gingival response to the transepithelial part of the implant. Although clinical evidence of epithelial attachment to the implant post has been observed, its significance, or its relationship to the oral environment, is still under investigation. At this stage it is appropriate to suggest that the gingival cuff around an implant may not need to perform in an identical manner to the one around the natural tooth. At

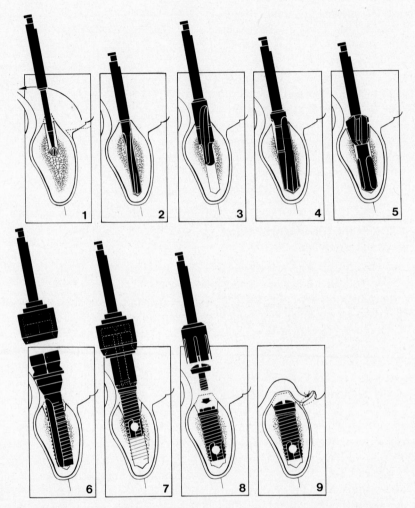

Fig. 30-1. First surgical stage. Scheme of the different steps undertaken at host bone site preparation to accommodate a titanium tooth root analog. *1-4,* Flap preparation, bone site preparation with gradual widening of bone fixture site; *5-9,* countersinking of access to fixture site, fixture installation, and placement of cover screw under mucoperiosteal flap. (Courtesy Dr. Ulf Lekholm, Institute of Applied Biotechnology, University of Göteborg, Göteborg, Sweden, 1983.)

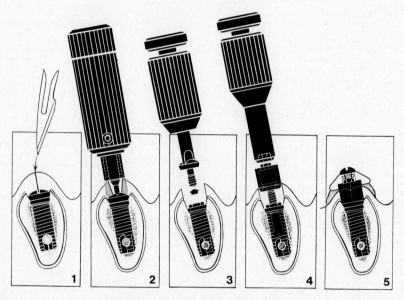

Fig. 30-2. Second surgical stage approximately 4 months later. Scheme of clinical steps required for abutment connection. *1,* Location of cover screw; *2,* circular excision of overlying mucosa; *3* and *4,* screw removal and abutment connection; *5,* abutment is in place, and a surgical pack is retained by means of a disposable healing cap. (Courtesy Dr. Ulf Lekholm, Institute of Applied Biotechnology, University of Göteborg, Göteborg, Sweden, 1983.)

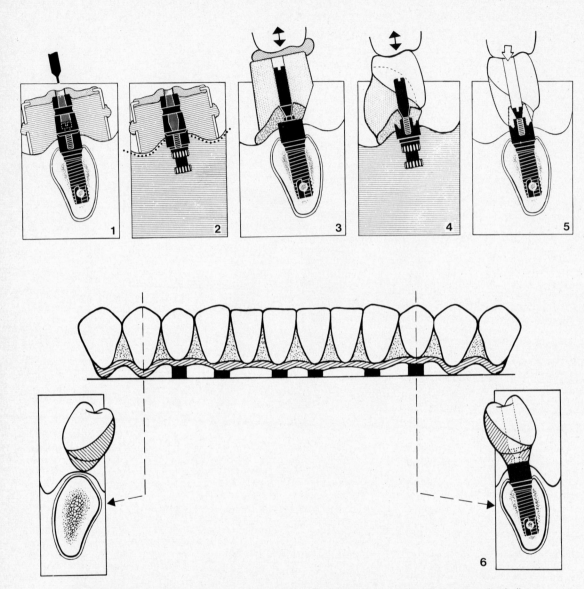

Fig. 30-3. Scheme of the prosthodontic procedure. *1,* Impression of transfer copings screwed onto the osseointegrated abutment. *2,* Brass abutment analogs are screwed to the copings, and a stone cast is poured. *3,* Guide pins are used to stabilize a trial denture base for jaw relation–recording purposes. *4,* Teeth are set up, tried in, indexed, and boiled out. *5,* A wax framework is designed to tie the teeth to the fixture analogs in a single cast unit, which allows for hygiene maintenance. *6,* The framework can be electively screwed into and unscrewed out of the osseointegrated tooth root analogs. (Courtesy Dr. Ulf Lekholm, Institute of Applied Biotechnology, University of Göteborg, Göteborg, Sweden, 1983.)

the Toronto Conference in 1982, Lindhe presented histologic and microbiologic evidence from 20 patients who had been treated with osseointegrated dental prostheses for several years. He found a relatively sparse inflammatory infiltrate in the connective tissue and a reduced pathogenicity of the microorganisms in the plaque on the fixtures. His results seemed to indicate that the epithelial interface with the pure titanium surface may be different from that with enamel or the root surface of the natural tooth. It is tempting to conclude that the soft tissue–titanium relationship cannot and perhaps should not be assessed by conventional dental indices and is not necessarily the "peri-implant" seal of consequence that implant literature suggests is necessary. In fact, Brånemark contends that osseointegration of the fixture into the host bone is adequate to ensure the ongoing viability of an abutment, even if an attachment apparatus coronal to the bone level does not occur. In this context Wennström's recent research (1982) suggests findings that may be extrapolated to the titanium-gingival unit. His experimental observations with dogs and humans showed two very important features: (1) mechanical plaque control can be maintained without signs of recession or attachment loss even in sites where attached or keratinized gingivae are lacking and (2) a free gingiva supported by loosely attached alveolar mucosa is not more susceptible to bacterial plaque infection than a free gingiva supported by a wide zone of attached gingiva.

We interpret Brånemark's work as not precluding the possibility that other materials or implant techniques will not produce the same results he reports. However at the time this text went to the printers, we were not aware of any other system or method that is supported by the same compelling evidence of a longitudinal nature as is Brånemark's.

It is tempting to suggest that Brånemark's work will lead to a rapid development of different methods, materials, and applications of the notion of tissue integration. Clinical prosthodontics appears to be entering a new era of therapy for edentulous patients. It should prove an exciting and gratifying one for patients and dentists.

REFERENCES

Adell, R., Lekholm, U., Rockler, B., and Brånemark, P.-I.: A 15-year study of osseointegrated implants in the treatment of the edentulous jaw, Int. J. Oral Surg. **6**:387, 1981.

Albrektsson, T., Brånemark, P.-I., Hansson, H.A., and Lindström, J.: Osseointegrated titanium implants, Acta Orthop. Scand. **52**:155, 1981.

Blomberg, S., and Lindqvist, L.W.: Psychological reactions to edentulousness and treatment with jawbone-anchored bridges, Acta Psychiatr. Scand. **68**:251, 1983.

Boucher, L.J.: Alloplastic tooth implants, J. Prosthet. Dent. **36**:567, 1976.

Brånemark, P.-I., Hansson, B.O., Adell, R., Breine, U., Lindström, J., Hallen, O., and Öhman, A.: Osseointegrated implants in the treatment of the edentulous jaw: experience from a ten-year period, monograph, Stockholm, 1977, Almqvist & Wiksell.

Dental Implants: Benefit and Risk, An NIH-Harvard Consensus Development Conference, U.S. Department of Health and Human Services, December 1980.

Hulbert, S.F.: Discussion on "biomaterials," J. Dent. Res. **54**(spec. issue B):174, 1975.

Johns, R.B.: Experimental studies on dental implants, Proc. R. Soc. Med. (Section of Odontology) **69**(1):1-7, 1976.

Lindhe, J.: Paper presented at the Toronto Conference on Osseointegration in Clinical Dentistry, May 1982.

Obwegeser, H.L.: Experiences with subperiosteal implants, Oral Surg. **12**:777, 1959.

Shulman, L.B.: Moderator summary, Section on implants, Symposium Proceedings, Dental biomaterials—research priorities, HEW Publ. Nos. 74-548, 134-137, 1974.

Wennström, J.L.: Keratinized and attached gingiva: regenerative potential and significance for periodontal health, doctoral thesis, University of Göteborg, Göteborg, Sweden, 1982.

Zarb, G.A., and Symington, J.M.: Osseointegrated dental implants: preliminary report on a replication study, J. Prosthet. Dent. **50**:271, 1983.

Bibliography

The bibliography is divided into two sections. The first is a list of books or general works on prosthodontic treatment of edentulous patients that are arranged alphabetically by author. The second section is made up of the periodical literature related to the prosthodontic treatment of edentulous patients. It is subdivided by subject headings with the references listed alphabetically by author.

The bibliography presents a general overview of the literature that has been taken mostly from dental journals that are well known to practicing dentists. As such, it provides a convenient source of reference as they seek to improve their ability to provide quality treatment for their patients.

GENERAL WORKS

Academy of Denture Prosthetics: Glossary of prosthodontic terms, edited by the Nomenclature Committee, ed. 4, St. Louis, 1977, The C.V. Mosby Co.

Adisman, I.K., and Laney, W.R.: Minimum acceptable laboratory procedures for maxillofacial prostheses, J. Prosthet. Dent. 27:91-93, 1972.

Alling, C.C., and Mahan, P.E.: Facial pain, ed. 2, Philadelphia, 1977, Lea & Febiger.

American Dental Association: Guide to dental materials and devices, ed. 6, Chicago, 1972-1973, American Dental Association.

Anderson, J.N.: Applied dental materials, ed. 5, Oxford, 1976, Blackwell Scientific Publications, Ltd.

Anderson, J.N., and Storer, R.: Immediate and replacement dentures, ed. 3, Oxford, 1981, Blackwell Scientific Publications.

Bell, W.H., Proffit, W.R., and White, R.P.: Surgical correction of dentofacial deformities, Philadelphia, 1980, W.B. Saunders, 2 vol.

Beresin, V.E., and Schiesser, F.J.: The neutral zone in complete and partial dentures, ed. 2, St. Louis, 1978, The C.V. Mosby Co.

Beumer, J., Curtis, T.A., and Firtell, D.N.: Maxillofacial rehabilitation: prosthodontic and surgical considerations, St. Louis, 1979, The C.V. Mosby Co.

Blakeslee, R.W., Renner, R.P., and Shiu, A.: Dental technology: theory and practice, St. Louis, 1980, The C.V. Mosby Co.

Blatterfein, L., Pearce, R.L., and Jackson, J.T.: Minimum acceptable procedures for satisfactory removable partial denture service, J. Prosthet. Dent. 27:84-87, 1972.

Brewer, A.A., and Morrow, R.M.: Overdentures, ed. 2, St. Louis, 1980, The C.V. Mosby Co.

Buchman, J.M., and Menekratis, A.: Complete and anchored dentures, Philadelphia, 1974, J.B. Lippincott Co.

Buckley, G., and Bruno, S.: Minimum aceptable laboratory procedures for satisfactory complete denture service, J. Prosthet. Dent. 27:81-83, 1972.

Caldarelli, D.D., guest editor: Symposium on Craniofacial Anomalies, Otolaryngol. Clin. North Am. 14(4):761-1031, 1981.

Craig, R.G., editor: Restorative dental materials, ed. 7, St. Louis, 1985, The C.V. Mosby Co.

Coelho, D.H.: Minimum acceptable laboratory procedures for satisfactory fixed partial dentures, J. Prosthet. Dent. 27:88-90, 1972.

Davis, W.H., and others: Mandibular vestibuloplasty with skin grafting: handbook for a technique of mandibular skin graft vestibuloplasty and lowering the floor of the mouth, ed. 3, Los Angeles, Calif., 1980, Southern California Oral Surgery Foundation.

DuBrul, E.L., editor: Sicher's oral anatomy, ed. 7, St. Louis, 1980, The C.V. Mosby Co.

Farrar, W.B., and McCarty, W.L.: Outline of temporomandibular joint diagnosis and treatment, Montgomery, Ala., 1979, The Normandie Study Group.

Federation of Prosthodontic Organizations: Guidelines for evaluation of completed prosthodontic treatment for complete dentures, J. Prosthet. Dent. 27:324-326, 1972.

Federation of Prosthodontic Organizations: Guidelines for evaluation of completed prosthodontic treatment for removable partial dentures. J. Prosthet. Dent. 27:326-328, 1972.

Federation of Prosthodontic Organization: Guidelines for determination of dentists who may be considered especially proficient in prosthodontics, J. Prosthet. Dent. 29:348-350, 1973.

Fish, E.W.: Principles of full denture prosthesis, ed. 4, London, 1948, Staples Press, Ltd.

Freedman, K.A.: Management of the geriatric dental patient, Chicago, 1979, Quintessence Publishing Co, Inc.

Fried, L.A.: Anatomy of the head, neck, face, and jaws, Philadelphia, 1976, Lea & Febiger.

Gehl, D.H., and Dresen, O.M.: Complete denture prosthesis, ed. 4, Philadelphia, 1958, W.B. Saunders Co.

Gelb, H.: Clinical management of head, neck and TMJ pain and dysfunction, Philadelphia, 1977, W.B. Saunders Co.

Glickman, I.: Glickman's clinical periodontology: prevention, diagnosis and treatment of periodontal disease in the practice of general dentistry, ed. 5, revised by Fermin A. Carranza, Philadelphia, 1979, W.B. Saunders Co.

Goldman, H.M., and Cohen, D.W.: Periodontal therapy, ed. 6, St. Louis, 1980, The C.V. Mosby Co.

Goldstein, R.E.: Esthetics in dentistry, Philadelphia, 1976, J.B. Lippincott Co.

Gray, H.: Anatomy of the human body, ed. 27, Philadelphia, 1959, Lea & Febiger.

Heartwell, C.M., and Rahn, A.O.: Syllabus of complete dentures, ed. 3, Philadelphia, 1980, Lea & Febiger.

Hiatt, J.L., and Gartner, L.P.: Textbook of head and neck anatomy, New York, 1981, Appleton-Century-Crofts.

Hudis, M.M.: Dental laboratory prosthodontics, Philadelphia, 1977, W.B. Saunders Co.

Jumber, J.E., Jumber, M.J., and Anderson, F.H.: An atlas of overdentures and attachments, Chicago, 1981, Quintessence Publishing Co., Inc.

Kawamura, Y., editor: Physiology of mastication: In Frontiers of oral physiology, vol. 1, Basel, Switz., 1974, S. Karger A.G.

Kratochvil, F.J., and Vig, R.G.: Principles of removable partial dentures, Los Angeles, 1979, University of California at Los Angeles.

Kruger, G.O., editor: Textbook of oral and maxillofacial surgery, ed. 5, St. Louis, 1979, The C.V. Mosby Co.

Laney, W.R., editor: Maxillofacial prosthetics, Postgraduate dental handbook series, vol. 4, Littleton, Mass., 1979, John Wright/PSG, Inc.

Laskin, M.: Oral and maxillofacial surgery, St. Louis, 1980, The C.V. Mosby Co.

Lefkowitz, W., editor: Proceedings of the Second International Prosthodontic Congress, St. Louis, 1979, The C.V. Mosby Co.

Leinfelder, K.F., and Taylor, D.F.: Laboratory and clinical dental materials. In Douglas Morr, D.V., editor: Dental laboratory technology, Chapel Hill, N.C., 1981, University of North Carolina Press.

Linkow, L.I.: Mandibular implants: a dynamic approach to oral implantology, North Haven, Conn., 1978, Glarus.

Lundeen, H.C., and Gibbs, C.H., editors: Advances in occlusion, Postgraduate dental handbook series, vol. 14, Littleton, Mass., C1981, John Wright/PSG, Inc.

Marquette University, Department of Removable Prosthodontics: Curriculum manual, 1976-1977, Milwaukee, 1977.

McCollum, B.B., and Stuart, C.E.: Research report on gnathology, South Pasadena, Calif., 1955, Scientific Press.

Morgan, D.H., et al., editors: Diseases of the temporomandibular apparatus: a multidisciplinary approach, ed. 2, St. Louis, 1982, The C.V. Mosby Co.

Morrow, R.M., and others: Dental laboratory procedures, St. Louis, 1980, The C.V. Mosby Co.

Morrow, R.M.: Handbook of immediate overdentures, St. Louis, 1978, The C.V. Mosby Co.

Nagle, R.J., and Sears, V.H.: Denture prosthetics, ed. 2, St. Louis, 1962, The C.V. Mosby Co.

National Association of Dental Laboratories, Education Committee: Trainer's manual for basic dental technology in complete and partial dentures and fixed crown and bridgework, Alexandria, Va., n.d., the Association.

Neill, D.M., and Nairn, R.I.: Complete denture prosthetics, Bristol, 1955, John Wright & Sons, Ltd.

Passamonti, G.: Atlas of complete dentures, Chicago, 1979, Quintessence Publishing Co. Inc.

Pokorny, D.K., and Blake, F.P.: Principles of occlusion, Anaheim, Calif. 1980, Dénar Co.

Preston, J.C., and Bergen, S.F.: Color science and dental art: a self-teaching program, St. Louis, 1980, The C.V. Mosby Co.

Ramfjord, S.P., and Ash, M., Jr.: Occlusion, ed. 2, Philadelphia, 1971, W.B. Saunders Co.

Reisbick, M.H., editor: Dental materials in clinical dentistry, Postgraduate dental handbook series, vol. II, Littleton, Mass., 1982, John Wright/PSG, Inc.

Renner, R.P.: Complete dentures: a guide for patient treatment, New York, 1981, Masson & Co.

Richardson, G.D.: Complete denture prosthodontics: the arrangement of artificial teeth, Los Angeles, 1977, Department of Removable Prosthodontics, School of Dentistry, University of Southern California.

Samson, E.: Art and the full prosthesis, London, 1974, William Heinemann Medical Books, Ltd.

Sarnat, B.G., and Laskin, D.M.: The temporomandibular joint: a biological basis for clinical practice, ed. 3, Springfield, Ill., 1980, Charles C Thomas, Publisher.

Sharry, J.J.: Complete denture prosthodontics, ed. 3, New York, 1974, McGraw-Hill Book Co.

Shillingburg, H.T., Hobo, S., and Whitsett, L.D.: Fundamentals of fixed prosthodontics, ed. 2, Chicago, 1981, Quintessence Publishing Co., Inc.

Silverman, M.M.: Occlusion in prosthodontics and in the natural dentition, Washington, D.C., 1962, Mutual Publishing Co.

Silverman, S.I.: Oral physiology, St. Louis, 1961, The C.V. Mosby Co.

Stanancought, D.: Laboratory procedures for full and partial dentures, edited by A.V. Newton, Oxford, 1978, Blackwell Scientific Publications.

Starshak, T.J., and Sanders, B.: Preprosthetic oral and maxillofacial surgery, St. Louis, 1980, The C.V. Mosby Co.

University of Michigan School of Dentistry: Clinic procedure manual, Ann Arbor, Mich., 1979, Overbeck.

Watt, D.M., and MacGregor, A.R.: Designing complete dentures, Philadelphia, 1976, W.B. Saunders Co.

Winkler, S., editor: Essentials of complete denture prosthodontics, Philadelphia, 1979, W.B. Saunders Co.

Wright, C.R., Swartz, W.H., and Godwin, W.C.: Facts you should know about your dentures, Toledo, 1963, Healthcare, Inc.

Zwemer, T.J., et al., editors: Boucher's clinical dental terminology: glossary of accepted terms in all disciplines of dentistry, ed. 3, St. Louis, 1982, The C.V. Mosby Co.

PERIODICAL LITERATURE
Anatomy of basal seat

Aguiar, A.E., Klein, I.A., and Beck, J.O., Jr.: Spongy bone architecture of edentulous mandibles: a television radiographic evaluation, J. Prosthet. Dent. 19:12-21, 1968.

Barrett, S.G., and Haines, R.W.: Structure of the mouth in the mandibular molar region and its relation to the denture, J. Prosthet. Dent. 12:835-847, 1962.

Boucher, C.O.: Complete denture impressions based upon the anatomy of the mouth, J. Am. Dent. Assoc. 31:1174-1181, 1944.

Graty, T.C., Tomlin, H.R., and Fox, E.D.: The mylohyoid ridge problem, Br. Dent. J. 116:203-208, 1964.

Harris, H.L.: The periphery of the full lower denture, Tex. Dent. J. 67:421-429, 1949.

Jani, R.M., and Bhargava, K.: A histologic comparison of palatal mucosa before and after wearing complete dentures, J. Prosthet. Dent. 36:254-260, 1976.

Józefowicz, W.: Pressure yielding of the maxillary mucoperiosteum, J. Prosthet. Dent. 27:600-606, 1972.

Kydd, W.L., and Mandley, J.: The stiffness of palatal mucoperiosteum, J. Prosthet. Dent. 18:116-121, 1967.

Luthra, S.P.: Measurement of the area of the maxillary basal seat for dentures, J. Prosthet. Dent. 30:25-27, 1973.

Lye, T.L.: The significance of the fovea palatini [sic] in complete denture prosthodontics, J. Prosthet. Dent. 33:504-510, 1975. [Properly fovea palatina.]

Maher, W.P., and Swindle, P.F.: Palatal vessels related to maxillary complete dentures, J. Prosthet. Dent. 22:143-155, 1969.

Markov, N.J.: Cytologic study of the effect of some biomechanical principles of complete denture construction on keratinization of the mucosa of the edentulous ridge, J. Prosthet. Dent. 21:132-135, 1969.

McMillan, D.R.: The cytological response of palatal mucosa to dentures, Dent. Pract. 22:302-304, 1972.

Mohl, N.D., and Drinnan, A.J.: Anatomy and physiology of the edentulous mouth, Dent. Clin. North Am. 21:199-217, 1977.

Nedelman, C., Gamer, S., and Bernick, S.: The alveolar ridge mucosa in denture and non-denture wearers, J. Prosthet. Dent. 23:265-273, 1970.

Pietrokovski, J.: The long residual ridge in man, J. Prosthet. Dent. 34:456-462, 1975.

Pietrokovski, J., and Massler, M.: Alveolar ridge resorption following tooth extraction, J. Prosthet. Dent. 17:21-27, 1967.

Pudwill, M.L., and Wentz, F.M.: Microscopic anatomy of edentulous residual ridges, J. Prosthet. Dent. 34:448-455, 1975.

Razek, M.K.A., and Shaaban, N.A.: Histochemical and histopathologic studies of alveolar mucosa under complete dentures, J. Prosthet. Dent. 39:29-36, 1978.

Schwarz, W.D.: The lingual crescent region of the complete lower denture, Br. Dent. J. 144:312-314, 1978.

Shannon, J.L.: The mentalis muscle in relation to edentulous mandibles, J. Prosthet. Dent. 27:477-484, 1972.

Silverman, S.I.: Denture prosthesis and the functional anatomy of the maxillofacial structures, J. Prosthet. Dent. 6:305-331, 1956.

Stephens, A.P., Cox, M., and Sharry, J.J.: Diurnal variation in palatal tissue thickness, J. Prosthet. Dent. 16:661-674, 1966.

Stram, J.R.: Topographical histology of the oral cavity, Otolaryngol. Clin. North Am. 5:201-206, 1972.

Turck, D.: A histologic comparison of the edentulous denture and non-denture bearing tissues, J. Prosthet. Dent. 15:419-434, 1965.

Uccellani, E.L.: Evaluating the mucous membranes of the edentulous mouth, J. Prosthet. Dent. 15:295-303, 1965.

Watson, I.B., and MacDonald, D.G.: Oral mucosa and complete dentures, J. Prosthet. Dent. **47**:133-140, 1982.

Watson, I.B., and McDonald, D.G.: Regional variations in the palatal mucosa of the edentulous mouth, J. Prosthet. Dent. **50**:853-859, 1983.

Articulators

Beck, H.O.: A clinical evaluation of the arcon concept of articulation, J. Prosthet. Dent. **9**:409-421, 1959.

Beck, H.O.: Choosing the articulator, J. Am. Dent. Assoc. **64**:468-475, 1962.

Beck, H.O.: Jaw registrations and articulators, J. Am. Dent. Assoc. **73**:863-869, 1966.

Bell, L.J., and Matich, J.A.: A study of the acceptability of lateral records by the Whip-Mix articulator, J. Prosthet. Dent. **38**:22-25, 1977.

Bellanti, N.D., and Martin, K.R.: The significance of articulator capability. Part II: The prevalence of immediate side shift, J. Prosthet. Dent. **42**:255-256, 1979.

Bellanti, N.D., and Martin K.R.: The significance of articulator capability. Part II: The prevalence of immediate side shift, J. Prosthet. Dent. **43**(3):255-256, 1979.

Celenza, F.V.: An analysis of articulators, Dent. Clin. North Am. **23**(2):305-326, 1979.

Coye, R.B.: A study of the variability of setting a fully adjustable gnathologic articulator to a pantographic tracing, J. Prosthet. Dent. **37**:460-465, 1977.

Davis, M.C.: Complete dentures and Transographics, J. Prosthet. Dent. **10**:61-77, 1960.

Finger, I.M., and Tanaka, H.: A new semiadjustable articulator. III. An investigation of the capability of the Hanau XP-51 articulator, J. Prosthet. Dent. **37**:310-319, 1977.

Gibbs, C.H., and Derda, H.J.: A new articulator emphasizing centric occlusion and the anterior determinants, J. Prosthet. Dent. **37**:382-393, 1977.

Guichet, N.F.: The Dénar system and its application in everyday dentistry, Dent. Clin. North Am. **23**(2):243-257, 1979.

Gysi, A.: An analysis of the development of the articulator (a reply to an article published under this title by R.E. Hall), J. Am. Dent. Assoc. **17**:1401-1424, 1930.

Gysi, A.: Some reasons for the necessity of using adaptable articulators, Dent. Dig. **37**:219-224, 1931.

Hall, R.E.: An analysis of the work and ideas of investigators and authors of relations and movements of the mandible, J. Am. Dent. Assoc. **16**:1642-1693, 1929.

Hall, R.E.: An analysis of the development of the articulator, J. Am. Dent. Assoc. **17**:3-51, 1930.

Hanau, R.L.: Dental engineering; the share of the condyle paths in the performance of mastication, and the importance of their correct reproduction in the articulator mechanism, Dent. Dig. **28**:2-7, 1922.

Hickey, J.C., Lundeen, H.C., and Bohannan, H.: A new articulator for use in teaching and general dentistry, J. Prosthet. Dent. **18**:425-437, 1967.

Irish, E.F.: The dupli-functional articulator, J. Prosthet. Dent. **15**:642-650, 1965.

Javid, N.S.: A comparative study of sagittal and lateral condylar paths in different articulators, J. Prosthet. Dent. **31**:130-136, 1974.

Kafandaris, N.M.: and Theodorou, P.T.: Modification of semiadjustable articulator to accept the patient's intercondylar width, J. Prosthet. Dent. **48**:385-387, 1982.

Lundeen, H.C.: Mandibular movement recordings and articulator adjustments simplified, Dent. Clin. North Am. **23**(2):231-241, 1979.

Mitchell, D.L., and Wilkie, N.D.: Articulators through the years. I. Up to 1940, J. Prosthet. Dent. **39**:330-338, 1978.

Mitchell, D.L., and Wilkie, N.D.: Articulators through the years, II. From 1940, J. Prosthet. Dent. **39**:451-458, 1978.

Mohamed, S.E., Schmidt, J.R., and Harrison, J.D.: Articulators in dental education and practice, J. Prosthet. Dent. **36**:319-325, 1976.

Myers, G.E.: Status report on articulators. Council on Dental Materials and Devices. J. Am. Dent. Assoc. **89**:1158-1161, 1974.

Needles, J.W.: Mandibular movements and articulator design, J. Am. Dent. Assoc. **10**:927-935, 1923.

Phillips, G.P.: Fundamentals in the reproduction of mandibular movements in edentulous mouths, J. Am. Dent. Assoc. **14**:409-415, 1927.

Phillips, G.P.: Graphic reproduction of mandibular movements in full denture construction, J. Am. Dent. Assoc. **17**:1489-1501, 1930.

Phillips, G.P.: Use of the occlusoscope, J. Am. Dent. Assoc. **26**:1332-1340, 1939.

Rihani, A.: Classification of articulators, J. Prosthet. Dent. **43**:344-347, 1980.

Sears, V.H.: Requirements of articulators in dentistry, Dent. Items Int. **48**:685-693, 1926.

Shanahan, T.E.J., and Leff, A.: Mandibular and articulator movements, J. Prosthet. Dent. **9**:941-945, 1959.

Shanahan, T.E.J., and Leff, A.: Mandibular and articulator movements. IV. Mandibular three dimensional movements, J. Prosthet. Dent. **12**:678-684, 1962.

Smith, B.J.: Adjustment of the lateral condylar guidance of Dentatus AR series of articulators, J. Prosthet. Dent. **34**:208-211, 1975.

Stansbery, C.J.: Functional position checkbite technic, J. Am. Dent. Assoc. **16**:421-440, 1929.

Stuart, C.E.: Use of the Stuart articulator in obtaining optimal occlusion, Dent. Clin. North Am. **23**(2):259-270, 1979.

Sweijd, F.: An articulator recording tridimensional condyle movements using impression materials, J. Prosthet. Dent. **44**:156-160, 1980.

Sweijd, F: An articulator recording tridimensional condyle movements using impression materials, J. Prosthet. Dent. **44**(2):156-160, 1980.

Tanaka, H.: The Teledyne Articulator System 154 as applied to complete denture construction, Dent. Clin. North Am. **23**(2):289-303, 1979.

Tanaka, H., and Beu, R.A.: A new semiadjustable articulator. I. Concept behind the new articulator, J. Prosthet. Dent. **33**:10-16, 1975.

Tanaka, H., Finger, I., and Porter, M.: A new semiadjustable articulator. II. Adjustment of a new concept articulator, J. Prosthet. Dent. **33**:158-168, 1975.

Tanaka, H., and Finger, I.M.: A new semiadjustable articulator. IV. An investigation of three semiadjustable articulators, J. Prosthet. Dent. **40**:288-293, 1978.

Thomas, C.J.: A classification of articulators, J. Prosthet. Dent. **30**:11-14, 1973.

Tradowsky, M.: Articulator adjustments using the transfer vise, J. Prosthet. Dent. **39**:47-55, 1978.

Weinberg, L.A.: An evaluation of basic articulators and their concepts. I. Basic concepts, J. Prosthet. Dent. **13**:622-644. II. Arbitrary, positional, semiadjustable articulators, **13**:645-663. IV. Fully adjustable articulators, **13**:1038-1054, 1963.

Winstanley, R.B.: Observations on the use of the Denar pantograph and articulator, J. Prosthet. Dent. **38**:660-672, 1977.

Basal seat, contours of mucosal surface impressions, casts, and dentures

Bolouri, A., Hilger, R.C., and Gowrylok, M.D.: Boxing impressions, J. Prosthet. Dent. **33**:692-695, 1975.

Davenport, J.C.: The denture surface, Br. Dent. J. **133**:101-105, 1972.

Dukes, B.S.: An evaluation of soft tissue responses following removal of ill-fitting dentures, J. Prosthet. Dent. **43**:251-253, 1980.

Gowman, D.J., Cornell, J., and Powers, C.M.: Effect of composition on dimensional stability of denture bases, J. Am. Dent. Assoc. **70**:1200-1203, 1965.

Grove, H.R., and Broering, L.F.: Impression boxing and cast pouring, J. Prosthet. Dent. **43**:112-115, 1980.

Hamrick, J.E.: A comparison of the retention of various denture-base materials, J. Prosthet. Dent. **12**:666-677, 1962.

Herlands, R.E.: The value of related diagnostic casts in complete denture planning, J. Conn. State Dent. Assoc. **55**(3):123-124, 1981.

Józefowicz, W.: Cushioning properties of the soft tissues forming the basal seat of dentures, J. Prosthet. Dent. **27**:471-476, 1972.

Kaiser, D.A., and Nicholls, J.I.: A study of distortion and surface hardness of improved artificial stone casts, J. Prosthet. Dent. **36**:373-381, 1976.

Kapur, K.K., Soman, S., and Stone, K.: The effect of denture factors on masticatory performance. I. Influence of denture base extension, J. Prosthet. Dent. **15**:54-64, 1965.

Kolb, H.R.: Variable denture-limiting structures of the edentulous mouth; maxillary border areas, J. Prosthet. Dent. **16**:194-201, 202-212, 1966.

Koran, A., 3d: Impression materials for recording the denture bearing mucosa, Dent. Clin. North Am. **24**(1):97-111, 1980.

Kydd, W.L., and Colin, H.D.: The biologic and mechanical effects of stress on oral mucosa, J. Prosthet. Dent. **47**:317-329, 1982.

Laney, W.R., and Gonzalez, J.B.: The maxillary denture: its palatal relief and posterior palatal seal, J. Am. Dent. Assoc. **75**:1182-1187, 1967.

McGivney, G.P.: Comparison of the adaptation of different mandibular denture bases, J. Prosthet. Dent. **30**:126-133, 1973.

Pietrokovski, J., and Chapman, R.J.: The form of the mandibular anterior lingual alveolar process in partially edentulous patients, J. Prosthet. Dent. **46**:371-375, 1981.

Powter, R.G., and Hope, M.: A method of boxing impressions, J. Prosthet. Dent. **45**:224-225, 1981.

Preiskel, H.W.: The posterior lingual extension of complete lower dentures, J. Prosthet. Dent. **19**:452-459, 1968.

Render, P.J.: Fabrication of custom trays from existing dentures, J. Prosthet. Dent. **43**:693-694, 1980.

Rudd, K.D., and Morrow, R.M.: A simplified method of mixing dental stone, J. Prosthet. Dent. **32**:675-678, 1974.

Rupp, N.W., Dickson, G., Lawson, M.E., Jr., and Sweeney, W.T.: Method for measuring the mucosal surface contours of impressions, casts and dentures, J. Am. Dent. Assoc. **54**:24-32, 1957.

Ryge, G., and Fairhurst, C.W.: The contour meter: an apparatus for comparison of mucosal surface contour of impressions, models, and dentures, J. Prosthet. Dent. **9**:676-682, 1959.

Ryge, G., and Fairhurst, C.W.: An evaluation of denture adaptation on the basis of contour meter recordings, J. Prosthet. Dent. **9**:755-760, 1959.

Shippee, R.W.: Accuracy of impressions made with elastic impression materials, J. Prosthet. Dent. **10**:381-386, 1960.

Swoope, C.C., Jr., and Kydd, W.L.: The effect of cusp form and occlusal surface area on denture base deformation, J. Prosthet. Dent. **16**:34-43, 1966.

Van Scotter, D.E., and Boucher, L.J.: The nature of supporting tissues for complete dentures, J. Prosthet. Dent. **15**:285-294, 1965.

Woelfel, J.B., Hickey, J.C., and Berg, T., Jr.: Contour variations, J. Am. Dent. Assoc. **67**:1-9, 1963.

Woelfel, J.B., Paffenbarger, G.C., and Sweeney, W.T.: Dimensional changes in complete dentures on drying, wetting and heating in water, J. Am. Dent. Assoc. **65**:495-505, 1962.

Young, J.M.: Surface characteristics of dental stone: impression orientation, J. Prosthet. Dent. **33**:336-341, 1975.

Baseplates, occlusion rims, and trial denture bases

Allred, H., Gear, V.D.A., Inglis, A.T., and Jenkins, M.A.: Thermoforming—a new aid in dentistry, Dent. Pract. **18**:419-422, 1968; **19**:2-7, 39-44, 1968.

Assadzadeh, A., and Yarmand, M.A.: A technique for making temporary bases for complete dentures, J. Prosthet. Dent. **33**:333-335, 1975.

Burnett, J.V.: Accurate trial denture bases, J. Prosthet. Dent. **19**:338-341, 1968.

de Gee, A.J., ten Harkel, E.C., and Davidson, C.L.: Measuring procedures for the determination of the three dimensional shape of dentures, J. Prosthet. Dent. **42**:149-153, 1979.

Desjardins, R.P.: Clinical evaluation of the wax trial denture, J. Am. Dent. Assoc. **104**(2):184-190, 1982.

Earnshaw, R., and Kleinberg, I.: Physical properties of synthetic resin baseplate materials. II. Cold-curing acrylic resins, Aust. Dent. J. **14**:255-263, 1969.

Garver, D.G.: Stabilization of record bases in the construction of complete dentures, J. Prosthet. Dent. **47**(3):342, 1982.

Gehl, D.H., and Payne, S.H.: A technique for making temporary bases for complete dentures, J. Prosthet. Dent. 33:333-335, 1975.

Graser, G.N.: Completed bases for removable dentures, J. Prosthet. Dent. 39:232-236, 1978.

Klein, M.B.: Occlusion rims with blocks of resin teeth, J. Prosthet. Dent. 33:17-21, 1975.

Kwong, W.K.: Fabricating acrylic resin baseplates for complete dentures, J. Prosthet. Dent. 50:127-128, 1983.

La Vere, A.M., and Freda, A.L.: Accurate-fitting record bases, J. Prosthet. Dent. 32:335-338, 1974.

McArthur, D.R.: Stalilized occlusion rims for small interarch spaces, J. Prosthet. Dent. 42(6):683-689, 1979.

Renner, R.P., and Blakeslee, R.W.: Basic wax contouring for complete dentures, J. Prosthet. Dent. 40:343-348, 1978.

Samant, A., and Martin, J.: Rigid, stable, maxillary denture bases, J. Prosthet. Dent. 49:731-732, 1983.

Schoen, P.E., and Stewart, J.L.: The effect of temporary bases on the accuracy of centric jaw relationship, J. Prosthet. Dent. 18:211-216, 1967.

Sears, V.H.: Essential factors in the trial base and the trial denture, J. Am. Dent. Assoc. 21:876-879, 1934.

Smith, D.C., Earnshaw, R., and McCrorie, J.W.: Some properties of modelling and baseplate waxes, Br. Dent. J. 118:437-442, 1965.

Terry, J.M., and Wahlberg, R.: Vacuum adaptation of baseplate materials, J. Prosthet. Dent. 16:26-33, 1966.

Travaglini, E.A.: Verification appointment in complete denture therapy, J. Prosthet. Dent. 44:478-483, 1980.

Bone

Baxter, J.C.: Relationship of osteoporosis to excessive residual ridge resorption, J. Prosthet. Dent. 46:123-125, 1981.

Chesnut, C.H., III, and Kribbs, P.J.: Osteoporosis: some aspects of pathophysiology and therapy, J. Prosthet. Dent. 48:4-7, 1982.

Dyer, M.R., and Ball, J.: Alveolar crest recession in the edentulous, Br. Dent. J. 149(10):290-292, 1980.

Hausman, E., and Ortman, L.: Present status of bone resorption in human periodontal disease, J. Periodontol. 50(4 Spec. No.):7-10, 1979.

Israel, H.: Evidence for continued apposition of adult mandibular bone from skeletalized materials, J. Prosthet. Dent. 41:101-104, 1979.

Kribbs, P.J., Smith, D.E., and Chesnut, C.H.: Oral findings in osteoporosis. Part I: Measurement of mandibular bone, J. Prosthet. Dent. 50:576-579, 1983.

Kribbs, P.J., Smith, D.E., and Chesnut, C.H.: Oral findings in osteoporosis. Part II: Relationship between residual ridge and alveolar bone resorption and generalized skeletal osteopenia, J. Prosthet. Dent. 50:719-724, 1983.

Landesman, H.M., Davis, W.H., Martinoff, J., and Kaminishi, R.: Resorption of the edentulous mandible after a vestibuloplasty with skin grafting, J. Prosthet. Dent. 49:619-622, 1983.

Mercier, P., and Inoue, S.: Bone density and serum minerals in cases of residual alveolar ridge atrophy, J. Prosthet. Dent. 46:250-256, 1981.

Parkinson, C.F.: Similarities in resorption patterns of maxillary and mandibular ridges, J. Prosthet. Dent. 39:598-602, 1978.

Penhall, B.: Preventive measures to control further bone loss and soft tissue damage in denture wearing, Aust. Dent. J. 25(6):319-324, 1980.

Rowe, D.J.: Bone loss in the elderly, J. Prosthet. Dent. 50:607-610, 1983.

Care of dentures (cleaning, etc.)

Abelson, D.C.: Denture plaque and denture cleansers, J. Prosthet. Dent. 45:376-379, 1981.

Altman, M.D., Yost, K.G., and Pitts, G.: A spectrofluorometric protein assay of plaque on dentures and of denture cleaning efficacy, J. Prosthet. Dent. 42(5):502-506, 1979.

Backenstose, W.M., and Wells, J.G.: Side effects of immersion-type cleansers on the metal components of dentures, J. Prosthet. Dent. 37:615-621, 1977.

Budtz-Jørgensen, E.: Materials and methods for cleaning dentures, J. Prosthet. Dent. 42:619-623, 1979.

Connor, J.N.E., Schoenfeld, C.M., and Taylor, R.L.: An evaluation of an enzyme denture cleanser, J. Prosthet. Dent. 37:147-157, 1977.

DePaola, L.G., and Minah, G.E.: Isolation of pathogenic microorganisms from dentures and denture-soaking containers of myelosuppressed cancer patients, J. Prosthet. Dent. 49:20-24, 1983.

Ghalichebaf, M., Graser, G.N., and Zander, H.A.: The efficacy of denture-cleansing agents, J. Prosthet. Dent. 48:515-520, 1982.

Gwinnett, A.J., and Caputo, L.: The effectiveness of ultrasonic denture cleaning: a scanning electron microscope study, J. Prosthet. Dent. 50:20-25, 1983.

Muenchinger, F.S.: Evaluation of an electrosonic denture cleaner, J. Prosthet. Dent. 33:610-614, 1975.

Mueller, H.J., and Greener, E.H.: Characterization of some denture cleansers, J. Prosthet. Dent. 43:491-496, 1980.

Myers, H.M., and Krol, A.J.: Effectiveness of a sonic-action denture cleaning program, J. Prosthet. Dent. 32:613-618, 1974.

Neill, D.J.: A study of materials and methods employed in cleaning dentures, Br. Dent. J. 124:107-115, 1968.

Nicholson, R.J., Stark, M.M., and Scott, H.E., Jr.: Calculus and stain removal from acrylic resin dentures, J. Prosthet. Dent. 20:326-329, 1968.

Pleasure, M.A., Duerr, E.L., and Goldman, M.: Eliminating a health hazard in prosthodontic treatment of patients with pulmonary tuberculosis, J. Prosthet. Dept. 9:818-824, 1959.

Rustogi, K.N., Melberg, J.R., Schlissel, H.J., et al.: The clinical efficacy of denture cleansers, Q. Natl. Dent. Assoc. 37(3):100-106, 1979.

Tarbet, W.J.: Denture plaque: quiet destroyer, J. Prosthet. Dent. 48:647-652, 1982.

Tucker, K.M., and King, W.H.: Found: a new soaking solution for dentures, J. Am. Dent. Assoc. 87:169-170, 1973.

Vieira, D.F., and Phillips, R.W.: Influence of certain variables on the abrasion of acrylic resin veneering materials, J. Prosthet. Dent. 12:720-731, 1962.

Casts

Carlyle, L.W.: Compatibility of irreversible hydrocolloid impression materials with dental stones, J. Prosthet. Dent. **49**:434-437, 1983.

Chong, J.A., Chong, M.P., and Docking, A.R.: The surface of gypsum cast in alginate impressions, Dent. Pract. **16**:107-109, 1965.

Henry, R.W., and Phillips, R.W.: Influence of particle size of stone on surface detail of cast, J. Prosthet. Dent. **11**:169-173, 1962.

Leung, R.L., and Schonfeld, S.E.: Gypsum casts as a potential source of microbial cross-contamination, J. Prosthet. Dent. **49**:210-211, 1983.

Mora, A.F., and Boone, M.E.: Rapid boxing of impressions, J. Prosthet. Dent. **49**:583-584, 1983.

Morris, J.C., Khan, Z., and Fields, H.: Effect on surface detail of casts when irreversible hydrocolloid was wetted before impression making, J. Prosthet. Dent. **49**:328-330, 1983.

Centric relation (see also Maxillomandibular relations and mandibular movements, Maxillomandibular relation records, and Vertical maxillomandibular relations)

Akerly, W.B.: A tripodal method of recording centric relation, J. Prosthet. Dent. **42**:461-465, 1979.

El-Aramany, M.A., George, W.A., and Scott, R.H.: Evaluation of the needle point tracing as a method for determining centric relation, J. Prosthet. Dent. **15**:1043-1054, 1965.

Avant, W.E.: Using the term "centric," J. Prosthet. Dent. **25**:12-15, 1971.

Azarbal, M.: Comparison of Myo-Monitor centric position to centric relation and centric occlusion, J. Prosthet. Dent. **38**:331-337, 1977.

Boos, R.H.: Centric relation and functional areas, J. Prosthet. Dent. **9**:191-196, 1959.

Dykins, W.R.: A consideration of centric relation, J. Prosthet. Dent. **20**:494-497, 1968.

Fletcher, A.M.: An investigation into the accuracy of three methods for recording centric jaw relation in the edentulous patient, Apex **5**:124-125, 1971.

Gottsegen, R.: Centric relation: the periodontist's viewpoint J. Prosthet. Dent. **16**:1034-1038, 1966.

Helkimo, M., Ingervall, B., and Carlsson, G.E.: Comparison of different methods in active and passive recording of the retruded position of the mandible, Scand. J. Dent. Res. **81**:265-271, 1973.

Hight, F.M.: Taking of registrations for securing centric jaw relation, J. Am. Dent. Assoc. **23**:1447-1450, 1936.

Hughes, G.A.: Discussion of "Factors influencing centric relation records in edentulous mouths," J. Prosthet. Dent. **14**:1066-1068, 1964.

Ismail, Y.H., George, W.A., Sassouni, V., and Scott, R.H.: Cephalometric study of the changes occurring in the face height following prosthetic treatment. I. Gradual reduction of both occlusal and rest face heights, J. Prosthet. Dent. **19**:321-337, 1968.

Jarvis, E.C.: A method of recording centric relation, J. Prosthet. Dent. **13**:617-621, 1963.

Lupkiewicz, S.M., Gibbs, C.H., Mahan, P.E., et al.: The instantaneous hinge axis—its reproducibility and use as an indicator for dysfunction, J. Dent. Res. **61**(1):2-7, 1982.

Kingery, R.H.: Maxillomandibular relationship of centric relation, J. Prosthet. Dent. **9**:922-926, 1959.

Koper, A.: Centric registration using a pneumographic procedure, J. Am. Dent. Assoc. **59**:674-682, 1959.

Lucia, V.O.: Centric relation—theory and practice, J. Prosthet. Dent. **10**:849-856, 1960.

Michman, J., and Langer, A.: Comparison of three methods of registering centric relation for edentulous patients, J. Prosthet. Dent. **13**:248-254, 1963.

Murphy, W.M.: Rest position of the mandible, J. Prosthet. Dent. **17**:329-332, 1967.

Nasr, M.F., and Griffiths, N.H.C.: Exercise therapy for accurate recording of centric relation, J. Prosthet. Dent. **29**:5-9, 1973.

Noble, W.H.: Anteroposterior position of "Myo-Monitor centric," J. Prosthet. Dent. **33**:398-402, 1975.

Owens, S.E., Lehr, R.P., Jr., and Biggs, N.L.: The functional significance of centric relation as demonstrated by electro-myography of the lateral pterygoid muscles, J. Prosthet. Dent. **33**:5-9, 1975.

Remien, J.C., and Ash, M.M., Jr.: "Myo-Monitor centric": an evaluation, J. Prosthet. Dent. **31**:137-145, 1974.

Saizar, P.: Centric relation and condylar movement: anatomic mechanism, J. Prosthet. Dent. **26**:581-591, 1971.

Shafagh, I., Yoder, J.L., and Thayer, K.E.: Diurnal variance of centric relation position, J. Prosthet. Dent. **34**:574-582, 1975.

Uccellani, E.L.: Use of a muscle relaxant as an aid in obtaining centric registration, J. Prosthet. Dent. **10**:92-94, 1960.

Williamson, E.H.: Laminagraphic study of mandibular condyle position when recording centric relation, J. Prosthet. Dent. **39**:561-564, 1978.

Yurkstas, A.A., and Kapur, K.K.: Factors influencing centric relation records in edentulous mouths, J. Prosthet. Dent. **14**:1054-1065, 1964.

Conditioning tissue of basal seat

Boos, R.H.: Preparation and conditioning of patients for prosthetic treatment, J. Prosthet. Dent. **9**:4-10, 1959.

Boos, R.H.: Preliminary treatment of prosthetic patients, J. Prosthet. Dent. **15**:1002-1009, 1965.

Chase, W.W.: Tissue conditioning utilizing dynamic adaptive stress, J. Prosthet. Dent. **11**:804-815, 1961.

Desjardins, R.P., and Tolman, D.E.: Etiology and management of hypermobile mucosa overlying the residual alveolar ridge, J. Prosthet. Dent. **32**:619-638, 1974.

Gazabatt, C., Nany, P.J., and Meissner, E.: A comparison of bone resorption following intraseptal alveolotomy and labial alveolectomy, J. Prosthet. Dent. **15**:435-443, 1965.

Hickey, J.C., and Stromberg, W.R.: Preparation of the mouth for complete dentures, J. Prosthet. Dent. **14**:611-622, 1964.

Kelly, E.: Tissue preparation for the complete denture patient—a simplified approach, Dent. Clin. North Am. **14**:441-452, 1970.

Klein, I.E.: Discussion of "Preliminary treatment of prosthetic patients," J. Prosthet. Dent. **15**:1010-1012, 1965.

Klein, I.E., and Miglino, J.C.: Uses and abuses of the tissue treatment materials, J. Prosthet. Dent. **16**:5-12, 1966.

Lytle, R.B.: management of abused oral tissues in complete denture construction, J. Prosthet. Dent. **7**:27-42, 1957.

Parry, L.G.: Tissue considerations in complete denture procedures, J. Prosthet. Dent. **6**:629-636, 1956.

Sharp, G.S.: Treatment for low tolerance to dentures: supplemental report, J. Prosthet. Dent. **17**:222-226, 1967.

Tautin, F.S.: The beneficial effects of tissue massage for the edentulous patient, J. Prosthet. Dent. **48**:653-656, 1982.

Wilson, H.J., Tomlin, H.R., and Osborne, J.: Tissue conditioners and functional impression materials, Br. Dent. J. **121**:9-16, 1966.

Denture adhesives

Karlsson, S., and Swartz, B.: Denture adhesives—their effect on the mobility of full upper dentures during chewing: a cineradiographic study, Swed. Dent. J. **5**(5-6):207-211, 1981.

Koudelka, B.M., Nelson, J.F., and Webb, J.G.: Denture self-repair: experimental soft tissue response to selected commercial adhesives, J. Prosthet. Dent. **43**:143-148, 1980.

Ow, R.K.K., and Bearn, E.M.: A method of studying the effect of adhesives on denture retention, J. Prosthet. Dent. **50**:332-337, 1983.

Segall, B.W., and Glassman, A.: Use of a medical-grade silicone adhesive as a denture liner in the treatment of idiopathic oral mucosal irritation, J. Prosthet. Dent. **47**:85-87, 1982.

Tarbet, W.J., Boone, M., and Schmidt, N.F.: Effect of a denture adhesive on complete denture dislodgement during mastication, J. Prosthet. Dent. **44**:374-378, 1980.

Tarbet, W.J., and Grossman, E.: Observations of denture-supporting tissue during six months of denture adhesive wearing, J. Am. Dent. Assoc. **101**(5):789-791, 1980.

Denture base materials

Academy of Denture Prosthetics: Final report of the workshop on clinical requirements of ideal denture base materials, J. Prosthet. Dent. **20**:101-105, 1968.

Anthony, D.H., and Peyton, F.A.: Dimensional accuracy of various denture-base materials, J. Prosthet. Dent. **12**:67-81, 1962.

Antonopoulos, A.N.: Dimensional and occlusal changes in fluid resin dentures, J. Prosthet. Dent. **39**:605-615, 1978.

Austin, A.T., and Basker, R.M.: The level of residual monomer in acrylic denture base materials with particular reference to a modified method of analysis, Br. Dent. J. **149**(10):281-286, 1980.

Axinn, S., Kopp, E.N., and Hanson, J.G.: Trouble shooting the pour resins, J. Prosthet. Dent. **33**:689-691, 1975.

Bates, J.F., and Stafford, G.D.: Polymeric denture base specifications, Biomed. Eng. **8**:288-291, 1973.

Barsby, M.J., and Braden, M.: A hydrophilic denture base resin, J. Dent. Res. **58**(6):1581-1584, 1979.

Barsby, M.J., and Braden, M.: Visco-elastic properties of pour (fluid) denture base resins, J. Dent. Res. **60**(2):146-148, 1981.

Bell, D.H., Finnegan, F.J., and Ward, J.E.: Pros and cons of hard and resilient denture base materials, J. Am. Dent. Assoc. **94**:511-518, 1977.

Bernhausen, E.R.: Resilient material used between the teeth and the denture base: a preliminary report, J. Prosthet. Dent. **25**:258-264, 1971.

Beyli, M.S., and von Fraunhofer, J.A.: An analysis of causes of fracture of acrylic resin dentures, J. Prosthet. Dent. **46**:238-241, 1981.

Boersma, H.: A method for making dental casts with cold-curing polyester resin, J. Am. Dent. Assoc. **74**:1265-1267, 1967.

Braden, M.: The absorption of water by acrylic resins and other materials, J. Prosthet. Dent. **14**:307-316, 1964.

Brauer, G.M.: Dental applications of polymers: a review, J. Am. Dent. Assoc. **72**:1151-1158, 1966.

Chevitarese, O., Craig, R.G., and Peyton, F.A.: Properties of various types of denture-base plastics, J. Prosthet. Dent. **12**:711-719, 1962.

Choudhary, S.C., Terry, J.M., Gehl, D.H., and Ryge, G.: Dimensional stability and fluid sorption in porcelain base dentures, J. Prosthet. Dent. **14**:442-455, 1964.

Dootz, E.R.: Fabricating non-precious metal bases, Dent. Clin. North Am. **24**(1):113-122, 1980.

Drew, R.E., and Kaldenburg, B.: The circumferential rib and its applications, Br. Dent. J. **136**:119-121, 1974.

Eick, J.D.: Biological properties of denture base resins, Dent. Clin. North Am. **21**:459-464, 1977.

Ellis, B., and Faraj, S.A.: The structure and surface topography of acrylic denture base materials, J. Dent. **8**(2):102-108, 1980.

Elzay, R.P., Pearson, G.O., and Irish, E.F.: Clinical and histologic evaluation of commercially prepared radiopaque denture material, J. Prosthet. Dent. **25**:251-257, 1971.

Fairchild, J.M., and Kelly, E.K.: Centrifugal casting process for resin-base dentures, J. Prosthet. Dent. **21**:607-612, 1969.

Faraj, S.A., and Ellis, B.: The effect of processing temperatures on the exotherm, porosity and properties of acrylic denture base, Br. Dent. J. **147**(8):209-212, 1979.

Firtell, D.N., Walsh, J.F., and Elahi, J.M.: The effect of gypsum products and separating materials on the typography of denture base materials, J. Prosthet. Dent. **44**:254-258, 1980.

Gay, W.D., and King, G.E.: An evaluation of the cure of acrylic resin by three methods, J. Prosthet. Dent. **42**(4):437-440, 1979.

Grant, A.A., and Atkinson, H.F.: Comparison between dimensional accuracy of dentures produced with pour-type resin and with heat-processed materials, J. Prosthet. Dent. **26**:296-301, 1971.

Grunewald, A.H., Paffenbarger, G.C., and Dickson, G.: Effect of molding processes on some properties of denture resins, J. Am. Dent. Assoc. **44**:269-284, 1952.

Halperin, A.R.: The cast aluminum denture base. Part I: Rationale, J. Prosthet. Dent. **43**(6):605-610, 1980.

Halperin, A.R., and Halperin, G.C.: The cast aluminum denture base. Part II: Technique, J. Prosthet. Dent. 44(1):94-100, 1980.

Hardy, F.: Comparison of fluid resin and compression molding methods in processing dimensional changes, J. Prosthet. Dent. 39:375-377, 1978.

Hargreaves, A.S.: Equilibrium water uptake and denture base resin behaviour, J. Dent. 6(4):342-352, 1978.

Harrison, A., Huggett, R., and Handley, R.W.: A correlation between abrasion resistance and other properties of some acrylic resins used in dentistry, J. Biomed. Mater. Res. 13(1):23-34, 1979.

Harrison, A., Huggett, R., and Jagger, R.C.: The effect of a cross-linking agent on the abrasion resistance and impact strength of an acrylic resin denture base material, J. Dent. 6(4):299-304, 1978.

Hensten-Pettersen, A., and Wictorin, L: The cytotoxic effect of denture base polymers, Acta Odontol. Scand. 39(2):101-106, 1981.

Ishimura, S.M.: A comparison between heat cured denture base resin and fluid base resin, J. Hawaii Dent. Assoc. 13(1):8-11, 1982.

Jagger, R.G.: Effect of the curing cycle on some properties of a polymethylmethacrylate denture base material, J. Oral Rehabil. 5(2):151-157, 1978.

Johnston, E.P., Nicholls, J.I., and Smith, D.E.: Flexure fatigue of 10 commonly used denture base resins, J. Prosthet. Dent. 46:478-483, 1981.

Kelly, E.: Fatigue failure in denture base polymers, J. Prosthet. Dent. 21:257-266, 1969.

Kelly, E.K.: Flexure fatigue resistance of heat-curing and cold-curing polymethyl methacrylate, J. Am. Dent. Assoc. 74:1273-1276, 1967.

Kimura, H.: A study on the dental injection molding system with cartridge (part 1) polycarbonate denture base, J. Osaka Univ. Dent. Sch. 20:51-61, 1980.

Knoblauch, K.R., and Reynik, R.J.: Analysis of a clinical evaluation of materials used intraorally, J. Prosthet. Dent. 29:244-249, 1973.

Kusy, R.P., Lytwyn, B.J., and Turner, D.T.: Characterization of cross-linked two-phase acrylic polymers, J. Dent. Res. 55:452-459, 1976.

Kydd, W.L., and Wykhuis, W.A.: Modified epoxy resin as a denture base material, J. Am. Dent. Assoc. 56:385-388, 1958.

Lang, B.R.: The use of gold in construction of mandibular denture bases, J. Prosthet. Dent. 32:399-404, 1974.

Little, J.D., and Abbott, J.J.: Tensile testing of denture base acrylic, J. Bioeng. 2(6):469-476, 1978.

Littler, J.D., and Abbott, J.J.: Tensile testing of denture base acrylic, J. Bioeng. 2(6):469-476, 1978.

Lorton, L., and Phillips, R.W.: Heat-released stress in acrylic dentures, J. Prosthet. Dent. 42:23-26, 1979.

Lyon, F.F.: Flow patterns of some denture base materials, Br. Dent. J. 126:266-268, 1969.

McCabe, J.F., and Wilson, H.J.: The use of differential scanning calorimetry for the evaluation of dental materials. Part II. Denture base materials, J. Oral Rehabil. 7(3):235-243, 1980.

McCabe, J.F., Wilson, S.J., and Wilson, H.J.: Cadmium in denture base materials, Br. Dent. J. 144:167-170, 1978.

Mainieri, E.T., Boone, M.E., and Potter, R.H.; Tooth movement and dimensional change of denture base materials using two investment methods, J. Prosthet. Dent. 44:368-373, 1980.

Manley, T.R., Bowman, A.J., and Cook, M.: Denture bases reinforced with carbon fibres, Br. Dent. J. 146(1):25, 1979.

Moore, F.D.: Organic metal bases for dentures, J. Prosthet. Dent. 17:227-231, 1967.

Morrow, R.M., Reiner, P.R., Feldmann, E.E., and Rudd, K.D.: Metal reinforced silicone-lined dentures, J. Prosthet. Dent. 19:219-229, 1968.

Murphy, W.M., Bates, J.F., Huggett, R., et al.: A comparative study of 3 denture base materials, Br. Dent. J. 152(8):273-276, 1982.

Obeid, A.A., Stafford, G.D., and Bates, J.F.: Clinical studies of strain behaviour of complete dentures, J. Biomed. Eng. 4(I):49-54, 1982.

O'Brien, W.J., and Ryge, G.: Wettability of polymethyl methacrylate treated with silicone tetrachloride, J. Prosthet. Dent. 15:304-308, 1965.

Ortman, H.R., Winkler, S., and Morris, H.F.: Clinical and laboratory investigation of a ceramic-filled acrylic resin compound, J. Prosthet. Dent. 24:253-267, 1970.

Paffenberger, G.D., Sweeney, W.T., and Bowen, R.L.: Bonding porcelain teeth to acrylic resin denture bases, J. Am. Dent. Assoc. 74:1018-1023, 1967.

Payne, S.H.: Denture base materials and the refitting of dentures, J. Am. Dent. Assoc. 49:562-566, 1954.

Powers, J.M., and Koran, A.: Color of denture resins, J. Dent. Res. 56:754-761, 1977.

Powers, J.M., and Lepeak, P.J.: Parameters that affect the color of denture resins, J. Dent. Res. 56:1331-1335, 1977.

Primack, J.E.: Radiopaque denture materials, J. Prosthet. Dent. 28:363-368, 1972.

Quinlivan, J.T.: Characterization of denture bases, Dent. Clin. North Am. 19:321-332, 1975.

Ristau, B.: Shrinkage and warpage of denture base materials using the Ristau Platform and the Ristau Post Dam, Quintessence Dent. Technol. 5(7):671-674, 1981.

Ruyter, I.E., and Espevik, S.: Compressive creep of denture base polymers, Acta Odontol. Scand. 38(3):169-177, 1980.

Ruyter, I.E., and Svendsen, S.A.: Flexural properties of denture base polymers, J. Prosthet. Dent. 43:95-104, 1980.

Ruyter, I.E.: Release of formaldehyde from denture base polymers, Acta Odontol. Scand. 38(1):17-27, 1980.

Samaranayake, L.P., and Macfarlane, T.W.: An in-vitro study of the adherence of Candida albicans to acrylic surfaces, Arch. Oral Biol. 25(8-9):603-609, 1980.

Schoonover, I.C., Fischer, T.E., Serio, A.D., and Sweeney, W.T.: Bonding of plastic teeth to heat-cured denture base resins, J. Am. Dent. Assoc. 44:285-287, 1952.

Schreiber, C.K.: Polymethylmethacrylate reinforced with carbon fibers, Br. Dent. J. 130:29-30, 1971.

Schreiber, C.K.: The clinical application of carbon fibre/polymer denture bases, Br. Dent. J. 137:21-22, 1974.

Soni, P.M., Powers, J.M., and Craig, R.G.: Comparison of the accuracy of denture bases by a non-parametric method, J. Oral Rehabil. 6(1):35-39, 1979.

Stafford, G.D., Bates, J.F., Huggett, R., et al.: A review of the properties of some denture base polymers, J. Dent. 8(4):292-306, 1980.

Stafford, G.D., and Huggett, R.: Creep and hardness testing of some denture base polymers, J. Prosthet. Dent. 39:682-687, 1978.

Stafford, G.D., Huggett, R., and Causton, B.E.: Fracture toughness of denture base acrylics, J. Biomed. Mater. Res. 14(4):359-371, 1980.

Stafford, G.D., Lewis, T.T., and Huggett, R.: Fatigue testing of denture base polymers, J. Oral Rehabil. 9(2):139-154, 1982.

Stafford, G.D., and MacCulloch, W.T.: Radiopaque denture base materials, Br. Dent. J. 131:22-24, 1971.

Stafford, G.D., and Smith, D.C.: Some studies of the properties of denture base polymers, Br. Dent. J. 125:337-342, 1968.

Strain, J.C.: Coloring materials for denture-base resins. I. Research necessary for their acceptance, J. Prosthet. Dent. 11:668-672, 1961. II. Suitability for use, J. Prosthet. Dent. 17:54-59, 1967.

Strain, J.C.: Reactions associated with acrylic denture base resins, J. Prosthet. Dent. 18:465-468, 1967.

Stuart, B.K.: Denture base coloring for patients with deep gingival pigmentation, J. Prosthet. Dent. 22:631-632, 1969.

Swaney, A.C., Paffenbarger, G.C., Caul, H.J., and Sweeney, W.T.: American Dental Association specification No. 12 for denture base resin, second revision, J. Am. Dent. Assoc. 46:54-66, 1953.

von Frannhofer, J.A., and Suchatlampong, C.: The surface characteristics of denture base polymers. J. Dent. 3:105-109, 1975.

Waters, N.E.: The fatigue fracture of acrylic, Dent. Pract. 18:389-392, 1968.

Weaver, R.E., and Goebel, W.M.: Reactions to acrylic resin dental prostheses, J. Prosthet. Dent. 43:138-142, 1980.

Welker, W.A., Kramer, D.C., and Mercer, R.W.: A technique for finishing and polishing denture bases, J. Prosthet. Dent. 39:240-241, 1978.

Whiting, R., and Jacobsen, P.H.: Dynamic mechanical properties of resin-based filling materials, J. Dent. Res. 59(1):55-60, 1980.

Wiebelt, F.J., Duncanson, M.G., Jr., and Strattor, R.J.: Comparison of bond strengths of polymethyl methacrylate and alpha cyanoacrylate, J. Prosthet. Dent. 47:603-605, 1982.

Wilson, H.J., and Tomlin, H.R.: Soft lining materials: some relevant properties and their determination, J. Prosthet. Dent. 21:244-250, 1969.

Winkler, S.: The current status of pour resins, J. Prosthet. Dent. 28:580-584, 1972.

Winkler, S.: Construction of denture bases from pour resins, Dent. Clin. North Am. 19:243-254, 1975.

Winkler, S., and Vernon, H.M.: Coloring acrylic denture base resins, J. Prosthet. Dent. 40:4-7, 1978.

Winkler, S., et al.: Characterization of denture base for people of color, J. Am. Dent. Assoc. 81:1349-1352, 1970.

Winkler, S., et al.: Investing mediums for pour resins, J. Am. Dent. Assoc. 83:848-851, 1971.

Woelfel, J.B.: Processing complete dentures, Dent. Clin. North Am. 21:329-338, 1977.

Woelfel, J.B., Paffenbarger, G.C., and Sweeney, W.T.: Some physical properties of organic denture base materials, J. Am. Dent. Assoc. 67:489-504, 1963.

Woelfel, J.B., Paffenbarger, G.C., and Sweeney, W.T.: Clinical evaluation of complete dentures made of 11 different types of denture base materials, J. Am. Dent. Assoc. 70:1170-1188, 1965.

Wolfaardt, J.F., and Austin, J.C.: The effect of heat and compression on the behavior of flask press springs, J. Dent. Assoc. South Afr. 36(6):403-404, 1981.

Wood, B.F., Sorensen, S.E., and Ortman, H.R.: Denture mold separators as a cause of staining around porcelain denture teeth, J. Prosthet. Dent. 17:149-154, 1967.

Wozniak, W.T., Muller, T.P., Silverman, R., et al.: Photographic assessment of colour changes in cold and heat cure resins, J. Oral Rehabil. 8(4):333-339, 1981.

Denture construction in general

Academy of Denture Prosthetics, 1959: Principles, concepts, and practices in prosthodontics, J. Prosthet. Dent. 9:528-538, 1959.

Academy of Denture Prosthetics, 1960: Principles, concepts, and practices in prosthodontics, progress report II, J. Prosthet. Dent. 10:804-806, 1960.

Academy of Denture Prosthetics, 1963: Principles, concepts and practices in prosthodontics, progress report III, J. Prosthet. Dent. 13:283-294, 1963.

Academy of Denture Prosthetics, 1968: Principles, concepts, and practices in prosthodontics, J. Prosthet. Dent. 19:180-198, 1968.

Barrett, S.G.: Essential features of complete denture construction, Apex 6:137-139, 1972.

Bascom, P.W.: Preservation in prosthodontics, J. Prosthet. Dent. 25:489-492, 1971.

Benson, D.: Experimental utilization of auxiliaries in removable prosthodontics, J. Dent. Educ. 37:27-30, 1973.

Bishop, E.: The prosthodontist, the patient, and the public, J. Prosthet. Dent. 45:205-208, 1981.

Boucher, C.O.: What knowledge, technical ability and experience are essential to the graduating dental student in complete denture prosthesis? J. Ontario Dent. Assoc. 31:12-17, 1954.

Brewer, A.A.: Treating complete denture patients, J. Prosthet. Dent. 14:1015-1030, 1964.

De Marco, T.J., and Paine, S.: Mandibular dimensional change, J. Prosthet. Dent. 31:482-485, 1974.

DeVan, M.M.: Biological demands of complete dentures, J. Am. Dent. Assoc. 45:524-527, 1952.

Donahue, T.J.: The case against the edentulous ridge—and an alternative, J. Am. Dent. Assoc. 101(5):781-784, 1980.

Dukes, B.S., Barnett, M.O., Kniejski, M.E.: A method for the duplication of complete dentures, J. Am. Dent. Assoc. 101(3):490-491, 1980.

Elsey, H.J.: A modified technique for edentulous flat ridge lower cases, Br. Dent. J. 126:134-135, 1969.

Fee, A.D.: The dental mechanics of Canada, J. Prosthet. Dent. 31:10-21, 1974.

Gehl, D.H.: Investment in the future, J. Prosthet. Dent. 18:190-201, 1967.

Gerber, A.: Complete dentures, Quintessence Int. 5:27-32, 1974.

Halperin, A.R., and King, R.E.: Fabrication of a maxillary complete denture utilizing the neuromuscular or centric occlusion position, J. Am. Dent. Assoc. **100**(1):67-70, 1980.

Harrison, A., and Huggett, R.: The construction of complete dentures—variations on several themes, part 1, Dent. Tech. **31**(7):10-12, 1978.

Heath, J.R., and Johnson, A.: The versatility of the copy denture technique, Br. Dent. J. **150**(7):189-193, 1981.

Henkin, R.I., and Christiansen, R.L.: Taste thresholds in patients with dentures, J. Am. Dent. Assoc. **75**:118-120, 1967.

Jamieson, C.H.: Modern concept of complete dentures, J. Prosthet. Dent. **6**:582-593, 1956.

Jones, P.: Realistic approach to complete denture construction, J. Prosthet. Dent. **8**:220-229, 1958.

King, W.H., Burton, M.C., and Tucker, K.M.: Clinical manifestations of dentaural hearing, J. Prosthet. Dent. **32**:130-140, 1974.

Kingery, R.H.: Full dentures, W. Va. Dent. J. **23**:69-76, 90, 1948.

Klein, I.E.: Complete dentures—status in the 1980's, N.Y. State Dent. J. **48**(6):368-369, 1982.

Klein, I.E., Blatterfein, L., and Kaufman, E.G.: Minimum clinical procedures for satisfactory complete denture, removable partial denture, and fixed partial denture services, J. Prosthet. Dent. **22**:4-10, 1969.

Koper, A.: The perils of dental practice, J. South. Calif. Dent. Assoc. **37**:46, 1969.

Krajicek, D.D.: The future of complete prosthodontics, J. Prosthet. Dent. **37**:126-132, 1977.

Kurth, L.E.: Fundamentals of full denture construction, Illinois Dent. J. **17**:7-11, 41, 1948; Penn. Dent. J. **15**:339-344, 1948.

LaDue, J.B.: Principal factors in full denture service, Bull. N.C. Dent. Soc. **34**:70-85 (disc. 245-256), 1950.

Lang, B.R.: An analysis of an experimental approach to teaching preclinical complete denture prosthodontics, J. Prosthet. Dent. **33**:521-528, 1975.

Lauciello, F.R., and Conti, S.P.: A combined clinical and laboratory techniques for the construction of complete dentures, Quintessence Dent. Technol. **3**(4)9-17, 1979.

Litvak, H., Silverman, S.I., and Garfinkel, L.: Oral stereognosis in dentulous and edentulous subjects, J. Prosthet. Dent. **25**:139-151, 1971.

Lombardi, R.E.: Work simplification in treatment with complete dentures, J. Prosthet. Dent. **31**:506-513, 1974.

Lukens, E.M., Saxton, R.N., and Bolender, C.L.: Development of a nursing home dental program, J. Prosthet. Dent. **33**:22-26, 1975.

Lytle, R.B., Atwood, D.A., and Beck, H.O.: Minimum standards of adequate prosthodontic service, J. Prosthet. Dent. **19**:108-110, 1968.

MacEntee, M.I., and Campbell, T.: Personal identification using dental prostheses, J. Prosthet. Dent. **41**:377-381, 1979.

Mack, A.: Complete dentures. I. General considerations, Br. Dent. J. **116**:372-375, 1964.

Mulrooney, R.: Dentures improperly constructed, Ont. Dent. **51**:12-14, 1974.

Nairn, R.I.: Interrelated factors in complete denture construction, J. Prosthet. Dent. **15**:19-24, 1965.

Pound, E.: Computerizing denture construction, J. South. Calif. Dent. Assoc. **41**:398-400, 1973.

Pound, E., and Murrell, G.A.: An introduction to denture simplification, J. Prosthet. Dent. **26**:570-580, 1971.

Ramstad, T., Norheim, P.W., and Eckersberg, T.: The reliability of clinical evaluation of some characteristics in complete prosthetics, J. Oral Rehabil. **7**(1):11-19, 1980.

Rayson, J.H.: Teaching complete denture prosthodontics, J. Dent. Educ. **35**:546-548, 1971.

Schabel, R., and Regli, C.P.: Prosthodontics for teen-age patients, J. Prosthet. Dent. **21**:251-256, 1969.

Schuyler, C.H.: Complete dentures, Penn. Dent. J. **21**:3-7, 1954.

Sears, V.H.: Questions and answers on full denture construction, N.Z. Dent. J. **48**:192-197, 1952.

Sears, V.H.: Some differing concepts of denture service, J. Prosthet. Dent. **4**:761-768, 1954; J. Calif. Dent. Assoc. & Nevada Dent. Soc. **30**:362-367, 1954.

Stephens, A.P.: Preventive complete denture prosthetics, J. Prosthet. Dent. **28**:469-477, 1972.

Sussman, B.A.: Routine treatment by complete dentures, J. Prosthet. Dent. **16**:451-457, 1966.

Swenson, M.G.: Key points of success in dentures, Northwest Dent. **33**:81-88, 1954; J. Tenn. Dent. Assoc. **36**:362-371, 1956.

Tanzer, G.: Space-saving lower total denture, Z.W.R. **82**:961-962, 1973.

Turner, C.E., and Shaffer, F.W.: Planning the treatment of complex prosthodontic case, J. Am. Dent. Assoc. **97**(6):992-993, 1978.

Tyson, J.A., and Dittfurth, P.R.: The dental assistant in complete denture prosthetics, Dent. Assist. **42**:15-18, 1973.

Vig, R.G.: Reducing laboratory aerosol contamination, J. Prosthet. Dent. **22**:156-157, 1969.

Vig, R.G.: Taking advantage of existing dentures, J. Prosthet. Dent. **26**:247-250, 1971.

Wormley, J.H.: How to maintain quality in economy dentures, J. Am. Dent. Assoc. **98**(2):215-218, 1979.

Yoshizumi, D.T.: An evaluation of factors pertinent to the success of complete denture service, J. Prosthet. Dent. **14**:866-878, 1964.

Young, J.M.: Prosthodontics in the general practice residency, J. Prosthet. Dent. **31**:615-627, 1974.

Denture retention and stability

Abdullah, M.A.: Surface tension in retention of complete dentures, J. Prosthet. Dent. **28**:141-144, 1972.

Ali, M.M.: A new approach to posterior palatal seal, Iraqi Dent. J. **2**:58-66, 1973.

Barbenel, J.C.: Physical retention of complete dentures, J. Prosthet. Dent. **26**:592-600, 1971.

Bláhová, Z., and Neuman, M.: Physical factors in retention of complete dentures, J. Prosthet. Dent. **25**:230-235, 1971.

Boucher, L.J., Ellinger, C., Lutes, M., and Hickey, J.C.: The effects of a microlayer of silica on the retention of mandibular complete dentures, J. Prosthet. Dent. **19**:581-586, 1968.

Brill, N., Tryde, G., and Schubeler, S.: The role of exteroceptors in denture retention, J. Prosthet. Dent. **9**:761-768, 1959.

Calomeni, A.A., Feldmann, E.E., and Kuebker, W.A.: Posterior palatal seal location and preparation on the maxillary complete denture cast, J. Prosthet. Dent. 49:628-630, 1983.

Carroll, E.A., and Shaffer, F.W.: Redefining the posterior palatal seal on a complete denture, J. Prosthet. Dent. 43:105-107, 1980.

Chen, M.: Reliability of the fovea palatini [sic] for determining the posterior border of the maxillary denture, J. Prosthet. Dent. 43:133-137, 1980. [Properly fovea palatina.]

Colón, A., Kotwal, K., and Mangelsdorff, A.D.: Analysis of the posterior palatal seal and the palatal form as related to the retention of complete dentures, J. Prosthet. Dent. 47:23-27, 1982.

Craig, R.G., Berry, G.C., and Peyton, F.A.: Physical factors related to denture retention, J. Prosthet. Dent. 10:459-467, 1960.

Csögör, A., and Michman, J.: Initial retention of complete mandibular dentures, J. Prosthet. Dent. 23:503-511, 1970.

Davis, D.J.: The vestibuloplasty—boon or bane? The aim is increased denture stability and retention, Oral Health 72(6):13-15, 1982.

Debba, G., and Razek, M.K.: Effects of the posterior palatal seal on denture retention, Egypt. Dent. J. 19:181-186, 1973.

Ettinger, R.L., and Scandrett, F.R.: The posterior palatal seal: a review, Aust. Dent. J. 25(4):197-200, 1980.

Faber, B.L.: Retention and stability of mandibular dentures, J. Prosthet. Dent. 17:210-218, 1967.

Frechette, A.R.: Complete denture stability related to tooth position, J. Prosthet. Dent. 11:1032-1037, 1961.

Gerber, A.: Complete dentures. II. The stability of maxillary dentures during mastication, Quintessence Int. 5:27-32, 1974.

Gesser, H.D., and Castaldi, C.R.: The preparation and evaluation of wetting dentures for adhesion and retention, J. Prosthet. Dent. 25:236-243, 1971.

Green, A.J., and Harman, L.: Influence of diuretics on complete denture retention: a preliminary report, J. Prosthet. Dent. 43:506-507, 1980.

Halperin, A.R., and Graser, G.N.: Adding a posterior palatal seal to a denture after a denture is completed, J. Mass. Dent. Soc. 30(2):104-107, 1981.

Hardy, I.R., and Kapur, K.K.: Posterior border seal—its rationale and importance, J. Prosthet. Dent. 8:386-397, 1958.

Jacobson, T.E., and Krol, A.J.: A contemporary review of the factors involved in complete denture retention, stability, and support. Part I: Retention, J. Prosthet. Dent. 49:5-15, 1983.

Jacobson, T.E., and Krol, A.J.: A contemporary review of the factors involved in complete dentures. Part II: Stability, J. Prosthet. Dent. 49:165-172, 1983.

Jacobson, R.E., and Krol, A.J.: A contemporary review of the factors involved in complete dentures. III. Support, J. Prosthet. Dent. 49:306-313, 1983.

Jones, H.S.: Improving the palatal seal in complete upper dentures, Dent. Surv. 51:54-55, 1975.

Kabcenell, J.L.: More retentive complete dentures, J. Am. Dent. Assoc. 80:116-120, 1970.

Kapur, K.K.: A clinical evaluation of denture adhesive, J. Prosthet. Dent. 18:550-558, 1967.

Kapur, K.K., and Soman, S.: The effect of denture factors on masticatory performance. II. Influence of the polished surface contour of denture base, J. Prosthet. Dent. 15:231-240, 1965.

Kawazoe, Y., and Hamada, T.: The role of saliva in retention of maxillary complete dentures, J. Prosthet. Dent. 40:131-136, 1978.

Kelly, E.K.: Retentive complete dentures for patients with perforated palates, J. Prosthet. Dent. 12:425-428, 1962.

Kudyba, P.J.: Establishing physiologic postpalatal seal with elastic material, J. Acad. Gen. Dent. 20:28-29, 1972.

Lauciello, F.R., and Conti, S.P.: A method of correcting the posterior palatal seal area of a maxillary complete denture, J. Prosthet. Dent. 42(6):690-692, 1979.

Levin, B.: Current concepts of obtaining stability and retention for complete dentures, Gen. Dent. 24:27-29, 1976.

Lindstrom, R.E., Pawelchak, J., Heyd, A., and Tarbet, W.J.: Physical-chemical aspects of denture retention and stability: a review of the literature, J. Prosthet. Dent. 42:371-375, 1979.

Lundquist, D.O.: An electromyographic analysis of the function of the buccinator muscle as an aid to denture retention and stabilization, J. Prosthet. Dent. 9:44-52, 1959.

Mack, A.: Complete dentures. VIII. Aids to retention, Br. Dent. J. 117:128-131, 1964.

Moore-Stevenson, P., Daly, C.H., and Smith, D.E.: Indicator pastes: their behavior and use, J. Prosthet. Dent. 41:258-265, 1979.

Morris, D.R., and Elliott, R.W., Jr.: Effect of ultrasonic cleaning upon stability of resin denture bases, J. Prosthet. Dent. 27:16-20, 1972.

Nikoukari, H.: A study of posterior palatal seals with varying palatal forms, J. Prosthet. Dent. 34:605-613, 1975.

O'Brien, W.J.: Base retention, Dent. Clin. North Am. 24(1):123-130, 1980.

Östlund, S.G.: Saliva and denture retention, J. Prosthet. Dent. 10:658-663, 1960.

Oursland, L.E.: Stabilizing mandibular dentures, J. Prosthet. Dent. 16:13-18, 1966.

Preiskel, H.: Prefabricated attachments for complete overlay dentures, Br. Dent. J. 123:161-167, 1967.

Sabet, E.M.: A new approach for determining the posterior limit of the upper denture for post damming, Egypt. Dent. J. 18:245-256, 1972.

Schiesser, F.J., Jr.: The neutral zone and polished surfaces in complete dentures, J. Prosthet. Dent. 14:854-865, 1964.

Schlissel, E.R., Newitter, D.A., Renner, R.R., and Gwinnett, A.J.: An evaluation of postadjustment polishing techniques for porcelain denture teeth, J. Prosthet. Dent. 43:258-265, 1980.

Sheppard, I.M.: Denture base dislodgment during mastication, J. Prosthet. Dent. 13:462-468, 1963.

Smith, D.E., Kydd, W.L., Wykhuis, W.A., and Phillips, L.A.: The mobility of artificial dentures during comminution, J. Prosthet. Dent. 13:839-856, 1963.

Steinhauser, E.W.: Free transplantation of oral mucosa for improvement of denture retention, J. Oral Surg. 27:955-961, 1969.

Strain, J.C.: Establishing stability for the mandibular complete denture, J. Prosthet. Dent. 21:359-363, 1969.

Swartz, M.L., Norman, R.D., and Phillips, R.W.: A method for measuring retention of denture adherents: an in vivo study, J. Prosthet. Dent. 17:456-463, 1967.

Swartz, W.H.: Retention forces with different denture base materials, J. prosthet. Dent. 16:458-463, 1966.

Tench, R.W.: Method for securing stability of lower dentures, Dent. Dig. 25:129-137, 1919.

Tench, R.W.: Retention of full upper and lower dentures, Dent. Dig. 25:385-393, 1919.

Terrell, W.H.: Retention and stability for full dentures, J. Am. Dent. Assoc. 23:1194-1204, 1936.

Tyson, K.W.: Physical factors in retention of complete upper dentures, J. Prosthet. Dent. 18:90-97, 1967.

Von Krammer, R.: Sublingual extension, J. Am. Dent. Assoc. 88:585-587, 1974.

Winkler, S., Ortman, H.R., and Ryczek, M.T.: Improving the retention of complete dentures, J. Prosthet. Dent. 34:11-15, 1975.

Wright, C.R.: Evaluation of the factors necessary to develop stability in mandibular dentures, J. Prosthet. Dent. 16:414-430, 1966.

Denture techniques

Becker, C.M., Swoope, C.C., and Schwalm, C.A.: Emergency dentures, J. Prosthet. Dent. 32:514-519, 1974.

Beresin, V.E., and Schiesser, F.J.: The neutral zone in complete dentures, J. Prosthet. Dent. 36:356-367, 1976.

Bocage, M., and Lehrhaupt, J.: Labial flange design in complete dentures, J. Prosthet. Dent. 37:499-506, 1977.

Boos, R.H.: Complete denture technique, including preparation and conditioning, Dent. Clin. North Am. 1:215-230, 1957.

Boucher, C.O.: Full dentures, J. Am. Dent. Assoc. 40:676-677, 1950.

Boucher, C.O.: The current status of prosthodontics, J. Prosthet. Dent. 10:411-425, 1960.

Boucher, C.O.: Essentials of complete denture service, J. Prosthet. Dent. 11:445-455, 1961.

Chalifoux, P.R.: Transitional denture technique, J. Prosthet. Dent. 40:682-683, 1978.

Curtis, T.A., Griffith, M.R., and Firtell, D.N.: Complete denture prosthodontics for the radiation patient, J. Prosthet. Dent. 36:66-76, 1976.

Geller, J.W.: Prosthetic dentistry, J. Prosthet. Dent. 10:33-36, 1960.

Gerber, A.: Complete dentures, III. Better dentures for the edentulous mandible, Quintessenz 24:59-64, 1973.

Hall, R.E.: Full denture construction, J. Am. Dent. Assoc. 16:1157-1198, 1929.

Hanau, R.L.: What are the physical requirements for and of prosthetic dentures? J. Am. Dent. Assoc. 10:1044-1049, 1923.

Harrison, A.: Prosthodontic techniques and the timing of complete denture procedures—a survey, J. Prosthet. Dent. 37:274-279, 1977.

Hickey, J.C., Boucher, C.O., and Woelfel, J.B.: Responsibility of the dentist in complete dentures, J. Prosthet. Dent. 12:637-653, 1962.

Hight, F.M., and Clapp, G.W.: Some essentials in full denture technic, Dent. Dig. 37:427-430, 515-519, 587-590, 669-673, 742-748, 810-814, 1931.

Holt, R.A., Jr.: A hollow complete lower denture, J. Prosthet. Dent. 45:452-454, 1981.

Hughes, G.A.: Discussion of "present-day concepts in complete denture service," J. Prosthet. Dent. 10:39-41, 1960.

Jaggers, J.H., and Maston, B.: Bilaterally hinged complete denture for a severely undercut maxillary arch: solution to a problem, J. Prosthet. Dent. 41:373-376, 1979.

Jankelson, B., and Radke, J.C.: The Myo-monitor: its use and abuse (II), Quintessence Int. 9(3):35-39, 1978.

Jones, P.M.: A realistic approach to complete denture construction, J. Prosthet. Dent. 8:220-229, 1958.

Jones, P.M.: Eleven aids for better complete dentures, J. Prosthet. Dent. 12:220-228, 1962.

Kafandaris, N.M., and Theodorou, T.P.: Complete denture technique using natural anterior teeth, J. Prosthet. Dent. 33:571-574, 1975.

Landesman, H.M.: A technique for the delivery of complete dentures, J. Prosthet. Dent. 43:348-351, 1980.

Levin, B.: Current concepts of lingual flange design, J. Prosthet. Dent. 45:242-252, 1981.

Lytle, R.B.: Complete denture construction based on a study of the deformation of the underlying soft tissues, J. Prosthet. Dent. 9:539-551, 1959.

Martone, A.L.: Clinical applications of concepts of functional anatomy and speech science to complete denture prosthodontics. VII. Recording phases, J. Prosthet. Dent. 13:4-33, 1963.

Martone, A.L.: Clinical applications of concepts of functional anatomy and speech science to complete denture prosthodontics. VIII. The final phases of denture construction, J. Prosthet. Dent. 13:204-228, 1963.

McGrane, H.F.: Full denture construction, Minneapolis Dist. Dent. J. 28:53-58, 1944.

McGrane, H.F.: Five basic principles of the McGrane full denture procedure, J. Fla. Dent. Soc. 20:5-8, 1949.

Meyer, F.S.: Construction of full dentures with balanced functional occlusion, J. Prosthet. Dent. 4:440-445, 1954.

Monson, G.S.: Monson technic for full denture construction, Transactions of the fifty-seventh annual meeting of the Illinois State Dental Society, pp. 89-95, 1921.

Moses, C.H.: Full denture procedure, J. Ontario Dent. Assoc. 20:494-509, 1945.

Murrell, G.A.: The management of difficult lower dentures, J. Prosthet. Dent. 32:243-250, 1974.

Phillips, G.: Full denture construction, J. Am. Dent. Assoc. 17:503-506, 1930.

Plainfield, S.: Myofunctional therapy for complete denture patients, J. Prosthet. Dent. 38:131-137, 1977.

Pound, E.: Conditioning of denture patients, J. Am. Dent. Assoc. 64:461-468, 1962.

Roberts, A.L.: Present-day concepts in complete denture service, J. Prosthet. Dent. 9:900-913, 1959.

Sears, V.H.: Escaping the commonplace in full denture construction, J. Am. Dent. Assoc. 23:212-215, 1936.

Sears, V.H.: Denture construction. Suitable sequence, Ill. Dent. J. **20**:523-530, 1951.

Sears, V.H.: Comprehensive denture service, J. Am. Dent. Assoc. **64**:531-552, 1962.

Sprigg, R.H.: Diagnostic procedures using the patient's existing dentures, J. Prosthet. Dent. **49**:153-161, 1983.

Stansbery, C.J.: Complete full denture technique, Dent. Dig. **39**:156-159, 178-182, 236-241, 258-260, 302-305, 339-343, 388-390, 1933; **40**:9-11, 1934.

Sussman, B.A.: Procedures in complete denture prosthesis, J. Prosthet. Dent. **10**:1011-1021, 1960.

Swanson, K.H.: Complete dentures using the TMJ articulator, J. Prosthet. Dent. **41**:497-506, 1979.

Swoope, C.C., Depew, T.E., Wisman, L.J., and Wands, D.H.: Interim dentures, J. Prosthet. Dent. **32**:604-612, 1974.

Tench, R.W.: Five essentials to successful full denture service, Dent. Dig. **30**:875-882, 1924; **31**:1-9, 77-84, 1925.

Terrell, W.H.: A simplified improved full denture technic, J. Am. Dent. Assoc. **22**:926-939, 1935.

Terrell, W.H.: Precision technique producing dentures that fit and function, J. Prosthet. Dent. **1**:353-377, 1951; Dent. J. Aust. **22**:484-508, 1950; Aust. J. Dent. **55**:100-118, 1951.

Terrell, W.H.: Fundamentals important to good complete denture construction, J. Prosthet. Dent. **8**:740-752, 1958.

Tupac, R.G.: A technique for fabricating mandibular treatment dentures, J. Prosthet. Dent. **39**:110-114, 1978.

Vaughan, H.C.: Some important factors in complete denture occlusion, J. Prosthet. Dent. **6**:642-651, 1956.

Walsh, J.F., and Walsh, T.: Muscle-formed complete mandibular dentures, J. Prosthet. Dent. **35**:254-258, 1976.

Wilson, L.G., and Anderson, G.A.: A denture tray technique for remake dentures, J. Prosthet. Dent. **34**:81-85, 1975.

Wormley, J.H., and Brunton, D.A.: Weighted mandibular dentures, J. Prosthet. Dent. **32**:101-102, 1974.

Diagnosis and treatment planning

Applegate, O.C.: Conditions which may influence the choice of partial or complete denture service, J. Prosthet. Dent. **7**:182-196, 1957.

Barone, J.V.: Diagnosis and prognosis in complete denture prosthesis, J. Prosthet. Dent. **14**:207-213, 1964.

Beeson, P.E.: The mouth examination for complete dentures: a review, J. Prosthet. Dent. **23**:482-488, 1970.

Bell, D.H., Jr.: Problems in complete denture treatment, J. Prosthet. Dent. **19**:550-560, 1968.

Bolender, C.L., Swoope, C.C., and Smith, D.E.: The Cornell Medical Index as a prognostic aid for complete denture patients, J. Prosthet. Dent. **22**:20-29, 1969.

Boucher, C.O.: Differential diagnosis for dentures, J. Mo. Dent. Assoc. **31**:425-437, 1951; J. Fla. Dent. Soc. **23**:9-12, 1953.

Bowman, A.J., and Green, R.M.: Preprosthetic conservation, Dent. Pract. **18**:249-251, 1968.

Braun, J.M., and Shotwell, J.L.: An evaluation of a polyvinyl occlusal splint for improving the health of inflamed maxillary supporting mucosa of complete denture patients, J. Prosthet. Dent. **42**:614-618, 1979.

Casey, D.M., and Lauciello, F.R.: A method for marking the functional depth of the floor of the mouth, J. Prosthet. Dent. **43**(1):108-111, 1980.

Conny, D.J., and Tedesco, L.A.: The gagging problem in prosthodontic treatment. I. Description and causes, J. Prosthet. Dent. **49**:601-606, 1983.

Conny, D.J.: The gagging problem in prosthodontic treatment. II. Patient management, J. Prosthet. Dent. **49**:757-761, 1983.

DeVan, M.M.: Physical, biological and psychological factors to be considered in the construction of dentures, J. Am. Dent. Assoc. **42**:290-293, 1951.

DeVan, M.M.: Procedures preceding the prosthodontic prescription, J. Prosthet. Dent. **13**:1006-1010, 1963.

Eglitis, I.I., Malone, W.F., Toto, P.D., and Gerhard, R.: The presence of immunoglobulin IgC and complement factor C3 in inflammatory papillary hyperplasia associated with maxillary dentures, J. Prosthet. Dent. **46**:201-214, 1981.

Emory, L.: The face in patient evaluation and diagnosis, J. Prosthet. Dent. **35**:247-253, 1976.

Ettinger, R.: Some observations on the diagnosis and treatment of complete denture problems, Aust. Dent. J. **23**(6):457-464, 1978.

Friedman, S.: Diagnosis and treatment planning, Dent. Clin. North Am. **21**:237-247, 1977.

Gordon, D.F.: Are new dentures necessary? J. Prosthet. Dent. **23**:512-521, 1970.

Harvey, W.L., Hoffman, W., Hochstetter, R., and Rouland, D.: Large edentulous ridges—are they better for dentures than small ridges? J. Prosthet. Dent. **47**:595-599, 1982.

Heartwell, C.M., Jr., and Peters, P.B.: Surgical and prosthodontic management of atrophied edentulous jaws. I. The evaluation of edentulous jaws, J. Prosthet. Dent. **16**:613-620, 1966.

Kabcenell, J.L.: Planning for individualized prosthetic treatment, J. Prosthet. Dent. **34**:389-392, 1975.

Kelly, K.: The prosthodontist, the oral surgeon, and the denture-supporting tissues, J. Prosthet. Dent. **16**:464-478, 1966.

Koper, A.: The initial interview with complete-denture patients: its structure and strategy, J. Prosthet. Dent. **23**:590-597, 1970.

Krajicek, D.D.: Periodontal considerations for prosthetic patients, J. Prosthet. Dent. **30**:15-18, 1973.

Landa, J.S.: Diagnosis of the edentulous mouth and the probable prognosis of its rehabilitation, Dent. Clin. North Am. **1**:187-201, 1975.

La Vere, A.M.: Denture education for edentulous patients, J. Prosthet. Dent. **16**:1013-1018, 1966.

Levin, B., and Landesman, H.M.: A practical questionnaire for predicting denture success or failure, J. Prosthet. Dent. **35**:124-130, 1976.

McCartney, J.E.: Prosthetic problems resulting from facial and intraoral changes in the edentulous patient, J. Dent. **9**(1):71-83, 1981.

Mack, A.: Complete dentures. II. The type of mouth, Br. Dent. J. **116**:426-429, 1964.

Marbach, J.J., et al.: Facial pains and anxiety levels: considerations for treatment, J. Prosthet. Dent. **40**:434-437, 1978.

Margolese, M.S.: The role of endocrines in prosthodontics, J. Prosthet. Dent. **23**:607-611, 1970.

Martone, A.L.: Clinical applications of concepts of functional anatomy and speech science to complete denture prosthodontics. VI. The diagnostic phase, J. Prosthet. Dent. **12**:817-834, 1962.

Meyer, R.A.: Management of denture patients with sharp residual ridges, J. Prosthet. Dent. **16**:431-437, 1966.

Mikhail, M.G., and Rosen, H.: The validity of temporomandibular joint radiographs using the head positioner, J. Prosthet. Dent. **42**:441-446, 1979.

Monaco, J.G., and Pickett, A.B.: The role of *Candida* in inflammatory papillary hyperplasia, J. Prosthet. Dent. **45**:470-471, 1981.

Murphy, W.M.: A clinical survey of gagging patients, J. Prosthet. Dent. **42**:145-148, 1979.

Nakamoto, R.Y.: Bony defects on the crest of the residual alveolar ridge, J. Prosthet. Dent. **19**:111-118, 1968.

Nassif, J.: Examination forms for edentulous patients—a survey, J. Prosthet. Dent. **35**:222-227, 1976.

Olson, J.W., Miller, R.L., Dukes, B.S., and Fields, H.: Hereditary hemorrhagic telangiectasia: prosthetic management and considerations, J. Prosthet. Dent. **50**:767-770, 1983.

Perrelet, L.A., Bernhard, M., and Spirgi, M.: Panoramic radiography in the examination of edentulous patients, J. Prosthet. Dent. **37**:494-498, 1977.

Perry, C.: Examination, diagnosis, and treatment planning, J. Prosthet. Dent. **10**:1004-1010, 1960.

Plainfield, S.: The transition from natural to artificial teeth, J. Prosthet. Dent. **33**:489-494, 1975.

Potgieter, P.J., and Carey, P.D.: The use of graphoanalysis for complete denture patient evaluation, J. Prosthet. Dent. **50**:623-626, 1983.

Regenbaum, G.: Prosthodontics and preventive diagnosis: a contradiction? Dent. Surv. **54**:47-49, 1978.

Rieder, C.E.: The interrelationships of various temporomandibular joint examination data in an initial survey population, J. Prosthet. Dent. **35**:299-306, 1976.

Rudd, K.D.: Making diagnostic casts is not a waste of time, J. Prosthet. Dent. **20**:89-100, 1968.

Schuyler, C.H.: Elements of diagnosis leading to full or partial dentures, J. Am. Dent. Assoc. **41**:302-305, 1950.

Setyaadmadja, A.T.S.H., Cheraskin, E., Ringsdorf, W.M., Jr., and Barrett, R.A.: Predictive prosthodontics. I. General health status and edentulousness, J. Prosthet. Dent. **21**:475-479, 1969.

Skinner, C.N.: Neuromuscular stimulator and conditioner of the hard and soft tissues, J. Prosthet. Dent. **23**:612-613, 1970.

Swenson, H.M., and Hudson, J.R.: Roentgenographic examination of edentulous patients, J. Prosthet. Dent. **18**:304-317, 1967.

Swoope, C.C.: Predicting denture success, J. Prosthet. Dent. **30**:860-865, 1973.

Tau, S., Mersel, A., Almagor, R., and Pietrokovski, J.: Spatial relationship between anatomic landmarks in edentulous patients: a radiographic study, J. Prosthet. Dent. **50**:314-318, 1983.

Thomson, J.C.: Diagnosis in full denture intolerance, Br. Dent. J. **124**:388-391, 1968.

Tucker, T.N.: Allergy to acrylic resin denture base, J. Prosthet. Dent. **46**:602, 1981.

Wright, S.M.: Medical history, social habits, and individual experiences of patients who gag with dentures, J. Prosthet. Dent. **45**:474-478, 1981.

Wright, S.M.: The radiologic anatomy of patients who gag with dentures, J. Prosthet. Dent. **45**:127-133, 1981.

Wright, S.M.: The radiographic examination of edentulous patients, J. Prosthet. Dent. **50**:164-166, 1983.

Esthetics

Antonoff, S.J.: Esthetics without prosthetics, J. Am. Dent. Assoc. **88**:833-837, 1974.

Beder, O.E.: Esthetics—an enigma, J. Prosthet. Dent. **25**:588-591, 1971.

Berg, T., Jr.: Cameo and profile: effective records of anterior esthetics and occlusion, J. Prosthet. Dent. **23**:598-606, 1970.

Blackburn, B.A.: Duplicating denture cosmetics, Dent. Surv. **46**:30-31, 1970.

Brigante, R.F.: Patient-assisted esthetics, J. Prosthet. Dent. **46**:14-20, 1981.

Cade, R.E.: The role of the mandibular anterior teeth in complete denture esthetics, J. Prosthet. Dent. **42**:368-370, 1979.

Calomeni, A.A.: Gold crown fabrication for complete dentures, J. Prosthet. Dent. **50**:439-440, 1983.

DeVan, M.M.: The appearance phase of denture construction, Dent. Clin. North Am. **1**:255-268, 1957.

Dirksen, L.C.: Natural esthetic buccal and labial anatomic form for complete dentures, J. Prosthet. Dent. **5**:368-374, 1955.

Ellinger, C.W.: Radiographic study of oral structures and their relation to anterior tooth position, J. Prosthet. Dent. **19**:36-45, 1968.

Esposito, S.J.: Esthetics for denture patients, J. Prosthet. Dent. **44**:608-615, 1980.

Fisher, D.: Orthodontic aid as a guide to esthetic appearance during immediate denture service, J. Am. Dent. Assoc. **103**(1):55-56, 1981.

Fisher, R.D.: Esthetics in denture construction, Dent. Clin. North Am. **1**:245-254, 1957.

Frush, J.P., and Fisher, R.D.: Introduction to dentogenic restorations, J. Prosthet. Dent. **5**:586-595, 1955.

Frush, J.P., and Fisher, R.D.: How dentogenic restorations interpret the sex factor, J. Prosthet. Dent. **6**:160-172, 1956.

Frush, J.P., and Fisher, R.D.: Age factor in dentogenics, J. Prosthet. Dent. **7**:5-13, 1957.

Frush, J.P., and Fisher, R.D.: The dynesthetic interpretation of the dentogenic concept, J. Prosthet. Dent. **8**:558-581, 1958.

Frush, J.P., and Fisher, R.D.: Dentogenics: its practical application, J. Prosthet. Dent. **9**:914-921, 1959.

Goldstein, R.E.: Esthetics in dentistry, J. Am. Dent. Assoc. **104**(3):301-302, 1982.

Goldstein, R.E.: Study of need for esthetics in dentistry, J. Prosthet. Dent. **21**:589-598, 1960.

Hartono, R.: The occlusal plane in relation to facial types, J. Prosthet. Dent. **17**:549-558, 1967.

Hooper, B.L.: Prosthodontia as a fine art, Dent. Dig. **33**:691-703, 774-788, 1927.

Hughes, G.A.: Facial types and tooth arrangement, J. Prosthet. Dent. **1**:82-95, 1951.

Jacobs, R.M.: Accommodation of perioral tonus after insertion of complete dentures, J. Am. Dent. Assoc. **74**:420-422, 1967.

Kern, B.E.: Anthropometric parameters of tooth selection, J. Prosthet. Dent. **17**:431-437, 1967.

Krajicek, D.D.: Achieving realism with complete dentures, J. Prosthet. Dent. **13**:229-235, 1963.

Krajicek, D.D.: Providing a natural appearance for edentulous patients of long standing, J. Can. Dent. Assoc. **33**:502-505, 1967.

Krajicek, D.D.: Duplicating nature: a realistic guide to aesthetic dentures, J. Can. Dent. Assoc. **34**:128-131, 1968.

Krajicek, D.D.: Dental art in prosthodontics, J. Prosthet. Dent. **21**:122-131, 1969.

Lammie, G.A.: The position of the anterior teeth in complete dentures, J. Prosthet. Dent. **9**:584-586, 1959.

Landa, L.S.: Practical guidelines for complete denture esthetics, Dent. Clin. North Am. **21**:285-298, 1977.

Levin, E.I.: Dental esthetics and the golden proportion, J. Prosthet. Dent. **40**:244-252, 1978.

Levnhardt, A.: Incisors and facial harmony in complete denture cases, Zahnaertzl. Prax. **22**:197-198, 1971.

Lieb, N.D., Silverman, S.I., and Garfinkel, L.: An analysis of soft tissue contours of the lips in relation to the maxillary cuspids, J. Prosthet. Dent. **18**:292-303, 1967.

Lombardi, R.E.: A method for the classification of errors in dental esthetics, J. Prosthet. Dent. **32**:501-513, 1974.

Lombardi, R.E.: Factors mediating against excellence in dental esthetics, J. Prosthet. Dent. **38**:243-248, 1977.

Lunderhausen, K.: A new method of esthetic denture design, Quintessence Int. **3**:41-42, 1972.

Mack, A.: Complete dentures. V. Try-in stage, Br. Dent. J. **117**:8-10, 1964.

Martone, A.L.: Effects of complete dentures on facial esthetics, J. Prosthet. Dent. **14**:231-255, 1964.

Martone, A.L.: Physiographic cinematography studies of a prosthodontic patient: an initial report, J. Prosthet. Dent. **14**:1069-1079, 1964.

Martone, A.L.: Complete denture esthetics and its relation to facial esthetics, Dent. Clin. North Am. **11**:89-100, 1967.

Martone, A.L., and Edwards, L.F.: Anatomy of the mouth and related structures. I. The face, J. Prosthet. Dent. **11**:1009-1018, 1961.

Matthews, T.G.: The anatomy of a smile, J. Prosthet. Dent. **39**:128-134, 1978.

Miller, E.L., and Bodden, W.R., and Jamison, H.C.: A study of the relationship of the dental midline to the facial median line, J. Prosthet. Dent. **41**:657-660, 1979.

Murray, C.G.: Anterior tooth positions in prosthodontics, Aust. Dent. J. **22**:113-119, 1977.

Murrell, G.: Audio-anesthetics, J. South. Calif. State Dent. Assoc. **41**:401-404, 1973.

Murrell, G.A.: Occlusal considerations in esthetic tooth positioning, J. Prosthet. Dent. **23**:499-502, 1970.

Nassif, N.J.: The relationship between the mandibular incisor teeth and the lower lip, J. Prosthet. Dent. **24**:483-491, 1970.

Ortman, H.R.: Relationship of the incisive papilla to the maxillary central incisor, J. Prosthet. Dent. **42**:492-496, 1979.

Payne, A.G.L.: Factors influencing the position of artificial upper anterior teeth, J. Prosthet. Dent. **26**:26-32, 1971.

Penhall, B.: Aesthetic considerations in full denture prosthodontics, Aust. Dent. J. **23**(4):314-318, 1978.

Plack, W.F., 3d, Todd, R.A., and Woody, R.D.: A technique for the simulation of melanin in denture bases, J. Am. Dent. Assoc. **103**(1):53-54, 1981.

Pound, E.: Esthetics and phonetics in full denture construction, J. Calif. Dent. Assoc. **26**:179-185, 1950.

Pound, E.: Lost—fine arts in the fallacy of the ridges, J. Prosthet. Dent. **4**:6-16, 1954.

Pound, E.: Recapturing esthetic tooth position in the edentulous patient, J. Am. Dent. Assoc. **55**:181-191, 1957.

Pound, E.: The basic four reviewed, J. South. Calif. State. Dent. Assoc. **41**:419-420, 1973.

Rayson, J.H., et al.: Placement of teeth in a complete denture: a cephalometric study, J. Am. Dent. Assoc. **81**:420-424, 1970.

Roraff, A.R.: Instant photographs for developing esthetics, J. Prosthet. Dent. **26**:21-25, 1971.

Rosenthal, R.L., and Kemper, J.T.: The "blow-wax" technique for stippling dentures, J. Prosthet. Dent. **32**:344-347, 1974.

Schiffman, P.: Relation of the maxillary canines to the incisive papilla, J. Prosthet. Dent. **14**:469-472, 1964.

Sears, V.H.: The art side of denture construction, Dent. Dig. **29**:764-770, 1923.

Sears, V.H.: An analysis of art factors in full denture construction, J. Am. Dent. Assoc. **25**:3-12, 1938.

Sendax, V.I.: An approach to the psychology of dentofacial esthetics, Dent. Clin. North Am. **11**:3-9, 1967.

Silverman, S.I.: Physiologic factors in complete denture esthetics, Dent. Clin. North Am. **11**:115-122, 1967.

Smith, B.J.: The value of the nose width as an esthetic guide in prosthodontics, J. Prosthet. Dent. **34**:562-573, 1975.

Stade, E.H., Hanson, J.G., and Baker, C.L.: Esthetic considerations in the use of face-bows, J. Prosthet. Dent. **48**:253-256, 1982.

Stephens, A.P.: Points prosthetic. VIII. The appearance of full dentures, J. Irish Dent. Assoc. **16**:17-20, 1970.

Tallgren, A.: The effect of denture wearing on facial morphology, Acta Odontol. Scand. **25**:563-592, 1967.

Tautin, F.S.: Denture esthetics is more than tooth selection, J. Prosthet. Dent. **40**:127-130, 1978.

Vig, R.G.: The denture look, J. Prosthet. Dent. **11**:9-15, 1961.

Vig, R.G., and Brundo, G.C.: The kinetics of anterior tooth display, J. Prosthet. Dent. **39**:502-504, 1978.

Geriatrics and geriatric changes

Boitel, R.H.: Problems of old age in dental prosthetics and restorative procedures, J. Prosthet. Dent. **26**:350-356, 1971.

Boucher, C.O.: The dentist's responsibility in denture service for the elderly, N.Y. J. Dent. **40**:319, 1970.

Breustedt, A.: Physiological and social factors of importance for the older edentulous patient, Int. Dent. J. **29**(4):276-284, 1979.

Eichner, K.: Conservative and prosthetic rehabilitation procedures in the dentition of old people, Int. Dent. J. **29**(4):285-297, 1979.

Fellman, S.: Treatment of complete denture patients in a geriatric facility, J. Prosthet. Dent. **35**:512-525, 1976.

Grasso, J.E., and Catalanatto, F.A.: The effects of age and full palatal coverage on oral stereognostic ability, J. Prosthet. Dent. **41**:215-219, 1979.

Heath, M.R.: Dental state and bone loss in the elderly, Proc. R. Soc. Med. **66**:590-594, 1973.

Jamieson, C.H.: Geriatrics and the denture patient, J. Prosthet. Dent. **8**:8-13, 1958.

Kelly, E.K.: Selection of posterior tooth forms and management of occlusion for the aging and debilitated patient, J. Calif. Dent. Assoc. **42**:212-215, 1966.

Kowitz, M.D., Ness, J.C., Campbell, J.G., et al.: Prosthetic maintenance research program for the geriatric patient. A cooperative study by the dental profession and the Dental Laboratory Conference, CDA J. **7**(11):37-44, 1979.

Kydd, W.L., Daly, C.H., and Nansen, D.: Variations in the response to mechanical stress of human soft tissues as related to age, J. Prosthet. Dent. **32**:493-500, 1974.

Langer, A.: Long term preventive aspects in oral rehabilitation of adults and elderly. II. Treatment of patients with terminal dentition, J. Oral Rehabil. **5**(3):229-239, 1978.

Langer, A., Michman, J., and Seifert, I.: Factors influencing satisfaction with complete dentures in geriatric patients, J. Prosthet. Dent. **11**:1019-1031, 1961.

Leathers, L.L.: Modification of prosthetic procedures for the ill and aged, J. Am. Dent. Assoc. **72**:369-372, 1966.

Lechner, S.K.: Prosthetic management in the geriatric patient, Aust. Dent. J. **19**:17-24, 1974.

Levin, B.: Special considerations for the geriatric complete denture patient, J. Acad. Gen. Dent. **19**:20-21, 1971.

Liddelow, K.P.: The prosthetic treatment of the elderly, Br. Dent. J. **117**:307-314, 1964.

Lotzkar, S.: Dental care for the aged, J. Public Health Dent. **37**:201-208, 1977.

Massler, M.: Geriatric dentistry: the problem, J. Prosthet. Dent. **40**:324-325, 1978.

Massler, M.: Geriatric dentistry: root caries in the elderly, J. Prosthet. Dent. **44**:147-149, 1980.

Massler, M.: Geriatric patient care, J. Am. Soc. Geriatr. Dent. **14**(1):10-19, 1978.

Massler, M.: Predicting denture failure in the elderly, Compend. Contin. Educ. Dent., **1**(2):131-134, 1980.

Nater, J.P., Groenman, N.H., Wakkers-Garritsen, B.G., and Timmer, L.H.: Etiologic factors in denture sore mouth syndrome, J. Prosthet. Dent. **40**:367-373, 1978.

Nedelman, C.I., and Bernick, S.: The significance of age changes in human alveolar mucosa and bone, J. Prosthet. Dent. **39**:495-501, 1978.

Nedelman, C. and Bernick, S.: Changes in nerve supply to aging human gingiva, J. Prosthet. Dent. **45**:364-370, 1981.

Perry, C.: Nutrition for senescent denture patients, J. Prosthet. Dent. **11**:73-78, 1961.

Pickett, H.G., Appleby, R.G., and Osborn, M.O.: Changes in the denture-supporting tissues associated with the aging process, J. Prosthet. Dent. **27**:257-262, 1972.

Scher, E.A., and Ritchie, G.M.: Prosthodontic treatment of the elderly by incremental modification to old dentures, Quintessence Int. **9**(8):47-53, 1978.

Silverman, S., Jr.: Geriatrics and tissue changes—problem of the aging denture patient, J. Prosthet. Dent. **8**:734-739, 1958.

St. Marie, G.L.: Dental care for the chronically ill and aged, J. Prosthet. Dent. **14**:52-57, 1964.

Storer, R.: The effect of the climacteric and of aging on prosthetic diagnosis and treatment planning, Br. Dent. J. **118**:349-354, 1965.

Winkler, S.: The geriatric complete denture patient, Dent. Clin. North Am. **21**:403-425, 1977.

Zafran, J.N., and Zayon, G.M.: Prosthodontics and the stroke patient, J. Am. Dent. Assoc. **74**:1250-1254, 1967.

History

Frahm, F.W.: Sixty years of progress in the field of prosthodontia, Dent. Items Int. **60**:964-972, 1938.

George Washington's dentures, J. Am. Dent. Assoc. **76**:961, 1968.

Gerber, A.: Progress in full denture prosthesis, Int. Dent. J. **7**:325-356, 1957.

Johnson, W.W.: The history of prosthetic dentistry, J. Prosthet. Dent. **9**:841-846, 1959.

Marguerite, R.: Evolution of full denture prosthesis, Int. Dent. J. **2**:388-418, 1952.

Myers, M.L.: Centric relation records: historical review, J. Prosthet. Dent. **47**:141-145, 1982.

Schwarz, W.D.: A review of the practice of prosthetic dentistry in Britain today, J. Prosthet. Dent. **22**:178-184, 1969.

Sears, V.H.: Developments in the denture field during the past half century, J. Prosthet. Dent. **8**:61-67, 1958.

Immediate dentures

Anderson, J.N., and Storer, R.: Immediate and replacement dentures, ed. 2, Oxford, 1973, Blackwell Scientific Publications, Ltd.

Appelbaum, M.B.: The practical dynamics of the interim denture concept: a comparison with the conventional immediate denture technique, J.A.D.A. **106**:826-830, 1983.

Bennett, C.G.: Transitional restorations for function and esthetics, J. Prosthet. Dent. **15**:867-872, 1965.

Bolouri, A.: Double-custom tray procedure for immediate dentures, J. Prosthet. Dent. **37**:344-348, 1977.

Bruce, R.W.: Immediate denture service designed to preserve oral structures, J. Prosthet. Dent. **16**:811-821, 1966.

Campagna, S.J.: An impression technique for immediate dentures, J. Prosthet. Dent. **20**:196-203, 1968.

Casey, D.M.: Interim complete immediate dentures for a patient wearing removable partial dentures, J. Prosthet. Dent. **39**:466-468, 1978.

Chaney, S.A.: Immediate denture impression technique using zinc oxide and eugenol and rubber base impression material, Dent. J. **43**:130-131, 1977.

Chaney, S.A., Moller, K.T., and Goodkind, R.J.: Effects of immediate dentures on certain structural and perceptual parameters of speech, J. Prosthet. Dent. **40:**8-12, 1978.

Chierici, G., Parker, M.L., and Hemphill, C.D.: Influence of immediate dentures on oral motor skill and speech, J. Prosthet. Dent. **39:**21-28, 1978.

Cohen, H.V.: Immediate full denture construction: advantages of the intermediate or transitional denture, J. N.J. Dent. Assoc. **42:**18-19, 1970.

Dahlberg, J.P.: Reconstructing the natural appearance by immediate dentures, J. Prosthet. Dent. **15:**205-212, 1965.

Demer, W.J.: Minimizing problems in placement of immediate dentures, J. Prosthet. Dent. **27:**275-284, 1972.

Flores, S.S., and Abelson, R.A.: Immediate dentures simplified, J. Acad. Gen. Dent. **18:**24-28, 1970.

Goldfarb, G.: A transitional denture technique using silicone rubber molds, J. Prosthet. Dent. **58:**25-26, 1965.

Heartwell, C.M., and Salisbury, F.W.: Immediate complete dentures: an evaluation, J. Prosthet. Dent. **15:**615-624, 1965.

Hopkins, R.: The immediate denture, Br. Dent. J. **147**(3):71-72, 1979.

Ismail, Y.H.: Effect of immediate complete dentures on tooth eruption and jaw development, J. Prosthet. Dent. **27:**485-493, 1972.

Javid, N., Tanaka, H., and Porter, M.R.: Split-tray impression technique for immediate upper dentures, J. Prosthet. Dent. **32:**348-351, 1974.

Jerbi, F.C.: Trimming the cast in the construction of immediate dentures, J. Prosthet. Dent. **16:**1047-1053, 1966.

Johnson, K.: A clinical evaluation of upper immediate denture procedures, J. Prosthet. Dent. **16:**799-810, 1966.

Johnson, K.: Immediate denture treatment for patients with class II malocclusions, Aust. Dent. J. **23**(5):383-388, 1978.

Jones, H.S.: Immediate replcement of lower anterior teeth, Dent. Surv. **46:**28-30, 1970.

Kelly, E.K.: Follow-up treatment for immediate denture patients, J. Prosthet. Dent. **17:**16-20, 1967.

Kessler, L.A., Gitzy, J.A., and Taylor, F.: Transitional dentures, J. Prosthet. Dent. **14:**465-468, 1964.

Laird, W.R.E.: Immediate dentures for children, J. Prosthet. Dent. **24:**358-361, 1970.

Lambrecht, J.R.: Immediate denture construction: the impression phase, J. Prosthet. Dent. **19:**237-245, 1968.

La Vere, A.M., and Krol, A.J.: Immediate denture service, J. Prosthet. Dent. **29:**10-15, 1973.

Loo, W.D.: Ridge-preservation with immediate treatment dentures, J. Prosthet. Dent. **19:**3-11, 1968.

Lutes, M.R., Ellinger, C.W., and Terry, J.M.: An impression procedure for construction of maxillary immediate dentures, J. Prosthet. Dent. **18:**202-210, 1967.

Mackay, D.R.: Intraseptal alveolectomy for immediate dentures, J. Am. Dent. Assoc. **68:**549-553, 1964.

Marash, L.M.: An investigation of full immediate denture treatment, Aust. Dent. J. **21:**237-241, 1976.

Oliver, L.T., Smith, R.A., Wolfe, H.E., and Koblitz, F.F.: Immediate denture processing with fluid resin, J. Prosthet. Dent. **34:**216-220, 1975.

Passamonti, G., Kotrajarus, P., Gheewalla, R.K., Clark, R.E., and Manness, W.L.: The effect of immediate dentures on maxillomandibular relations, J. Prosthet. Dent. **45:**122-126, 1981.

Payne, S.H.: A transitional denture, J. Prosthet. Dent. **14:**221-230, 1964.

Payne, S.H.: The trial denture, Dent. Clin. North Am. **21:**321-328, 1977.

Pound, E.: An all-inclusive immediate denture technic, J. Am. Dent. Assoc. **67:**16-22, 1963.

Pound, E.: Preparatory dentures: a protective philosophy, J. Prosthet. Dent. **15:**5-18, 1965.

Pound, E.: Controlled immediate dentures, J. Prosthet. Dent. **24:**243-252, 1970.

Radue, J.T., Unger, J.W., and Molinari, J.A.: Avoiding cross-contamination in immediate denture treatment, J. Prosthet. Dent. **49:**576, 1983.

Schlosser, R.O.: Advantages of conservative procedure in complete immediate denture prosthesis, J. Can. Dent. Assoc. **14:**611-616, 1948.

Sears, V.H.: Immediate denture restoration, J. Am. Dent. Assoc. **10:**644-647, 1923.

Swenson, M.G.: Improving immediate dentures in general practice, J. Am. Dent. Assoc. **47:**550-556, 1953.

Tallgren, A., Lang, B.R., Walker, G.F., et al.: Roentgen cephalometric analysis of ridge resorption and changes in jaw and occlusal relationships in immediate denture wearers, J. Oral Rehabil. **7**(1):77-94, 1980.

Terrell, W.H.: Immediate restorations by complete dentures, J. Prosthet. Dent. **1:**495-507, 1951; Aust. J. Dent. **55:**288-297, 1951.

Tilton, G.E.: Throwaway immediate denture, J. Prosthet. Dent. **4:**291, 1954.

Walsh, J.F., Walsh, T., and Griffiths, R.: An immediate denture technique to reproduce labial alveolar contour, J. Prosthet. Dent. **37:**222-230, 1977.

Waltz, E.: Considerate post-operative care for immediate denture patients, J. Prosthet. Dent. **16:**822-828, 1966.

Wictorin, L.: An evaluation of bone surgery in patients with immediate dentures, J. Prosthet. Dent. **21:**6-13, 1969.

Implants and magnets for retention of dentures

Adell, R.: Clinical results of osseointegrated implants supporting fixed prostheses in edentulous jaws, J. Prosthet. Dent. **50:**251-254, 1983.

Albrektsson, T.: Direct bone anchorage of dental implants, J. Prosthet. Dent. **50:**255-261, 1983.

Behrman, S.J.: Magnets implanted in the mandible: aid to denture retention, J. Am. Dent. Assoc. **68:**206-215, 1964.

Bergman, B.: Evaluation of the results of treatment with osseointegrated implants by the Swedish National Board of Health and Welfare, J. Prosthet. Dent. **50:**114-115, 1983.

Bodine, R.L., Jr.: Prosthodontic essentials and an evaluation of the mandibular subperiosteal implant denture, J. Am. Dent. Assoc. **51:**654-664, 1955.

Bodine, R.L., Jr., and Kotch, R.L.: Mandibular subperiosteal implant denture technique, J. Prosthet. Dent. **4:**396-412, 1954.

Bodine, R.L., and Vakay, L.R.: Rigidity of implant denture substructure with the mesostructure bar, J. Prosthet. Dent. **39:**88-94, 1978.

Bolouri, A., and Williams, C.E.: An interdisciplinary approach to complete dentures over the ramus frame implant, Compend. Contin. Educ. Dent. 3(4):305-310, 1982.

Boyne, P.J.: Restoration of deficient edentulous ridges by bone grafting and the use of subperiosteal metal implants, Int. J. Oral Surg. 3:278-281, 1974.

Brånemark, P.I.: Osseointegration and its experimental background, J. Prosthet. Dent. 50:399-410, 1983.

Cranin, A.N., and Cranin, S.L.: The intramucosal insert: a method of maxillary denture stabilization, J. Am. Dent. Assoc. 57:188-193, 1958.

Cranin, A.N., and Cranin, S.L.: Simplifying the subperiosteal implant denture technique, Oral Surg. 22:7-20, 1966.

Evasic, R.W.: Intramucosal implants: a review of concepts and techniques—single inserts and tandem denserts, J. Prosthet. Dent. 49:695-701, 1983.

Garefis, P.N.: Complete mandibular subperiosteal implants for edentulous mandibles, J. Prosthet. Dent. 39:670-677, 1978.

Gillings, B.R.D.: Magnetic retention for overdentures. Part II, J. Prosthet. Dent. 49:607-618, 1983.

Hansson, H.A., Albrektsson, T., and Brånemark, P.I.: Structural aspects of the interface between tissue and titanium implants, J. Prosthet. Dent. 50:108-113, 1983.

Kasemo, B.: Biocompatibility of titanium implants: surface science aspects, J. Prosthet. Dent. 49:832-837, 1983.

Lekholm, U.: Clinical procedures for treatment with osseointegrated dental implants, J. Prosthet. Dent. 50:116-120, 1983.

Liposky, R.B.: Use of the mandibular staple bone plate with augmentation in bone grafts, J. Oral Maxillofac. Surg. 40(8)527-531, 1982.

Lundqvist, S., and Carlsson, G.E.: Maxillary fixed prostheses on osseointegrated dental implants, J. Prosthet. Dent. 50:262-270, 1983.

Parsegian, V.A.: Molecular forces governing tight contact between cellular surfaces and substrates, J. Prosthet. Dent. 49:838-842, 1983.

Pedersen, K.N.: Tissue reaction to submerged ceramic tooth root implants: an experimental study in monkeys, Acta Odontol. Scand. 37(6):347-352, 1979.

Skalak, R.: Biomechanical considerations in osseointegrated prostheses, J. Prosthet. Dent. 49:843-848, 1983.

Young, L., Michel, J.D., and Moore, D.J.: A twenty-year evaluation of subperiosteal implants, J. Prosthet. Dent. 49:690-694, 1983.

Zarb, G.A.: The edentulous milieu, J. Prosthet. Dent. 49:825-831, 1983.

Zarb, G.A., Smith, D.C., Levant, H.C., Graham, B.S., and Staatsexamen, W.Z.: The effects of cemented and uncemented endosseous implants, J. Prosthet. Dent. 42:202-210, 1979.

Zarb, G.A.: Introduction to osseointegration in clinical dentistry, J. Prosthet. Dent. 49:824, 1983.

Zarb, G.A., and Symington, J.M.: Osseointegrated dental implants: preliminary report on a replication study, J. Prosthet. Dent. 50:271-276, 1983.

Impression materials

Ayers, H.D., Jr., Phillips, R.W., Dell, A., and Henry, R.W.: Detail duplication test used to evaluate elastic impression materials, J. Prosthet. Dent. 10:374-380, 1960.

Barolet, R.Y., and Desautels, P.C.: New elastomeric impression materials, J. Can. Dent. Assoc. 40:488-489, 1974.

Braden, M.: The composition, structure, and flow properties of functional impression materials (tissue conditioners), Dent. Pract. 16:301-304, 1966.

Davis, G.B., Moser, J.B., and Brinsden, G.I.: The bonding properties of elastomer tray adhesives, J. Prosthet. Dent. 36:278-285, 1976.

Dresen, O.M.: The rubber base impression materials, J. Prosthet. Dent. 8:14-18, 1958.

Eames, W.B., Wallace, S.W., Suway, N.B., et al.: Accuracy and dimensional stability of elastomeric impression materials, J. Prosthet. Dent. 42(2):159-162, 1979.

Fairchild, J.M.: Versatile uses for alginate impression material, J. Prosthet. Dent. 31:266-269, 1974.

Gunther, G., and Welsh, S.L.: Evaluation of a rubber-base impression material, J. Prosthet. Dent. 39:95-99, 1978.

Harcourt, J.K.: A review of modern impression materials, Aust. Dent. J. 23(2):178-186, 1978.

Herfort, T.W., Gerberich, W.W., Macosko, C.W., and Goodkind, R.J.: Tear strength of elastomeric impression materials, J. Prosthet. Dent. 39:59-62, 1978.

Kaloyannides, T.M., and Kapari, D.J.: Mixtures of elastomer impression materials. I. Setting time and consistency, J. Prosthet. Dent. 53:809-813, 1974.

Koran, A., Powers, J.M., and Craig, R.G.: Apparent viscosity of materials used for making edentulous impressions, J. Am. Dent. Assoc. 95:75-79, 1977.

Lacy, A.M., Bellman, T., Fukui, H., and Jendresen, M.D.: Time-dependent accuracy of elastomer impression materials. I. Condensation silicones, J. Prosthet. Dent. 45:209-215, 1981.

Lorton, L., Phillips, R.W., and Swartz, M.L.: The effect of ultrasonic cleaning methods on rubber base impression materials, J. Dent. Res. 57(9-10):939, 1978.

McCabe, J.F., and Bowman, A.J.: The rheological properties of dental impression materials, Br. Dent. J. 15:(16): 179-83, 1981.

McCarthy, J.A., and Moser, J.B.: Undercut reproducibility of functional impression materials (tissue conditioners), J. Oral Rehabil. 5(3):287-292, 1978.

Marcinak, C.F., Young, F.A., Draughn, R.A., et al.: Linear dimensional changes in elastic impression materials, J. Dent. Res. 59(7):1152-1155, 1980.

Marcroft, K.R., Tencate, R.L., and Skinner, E.W.: The effects of heat, aging, and mold separation on the dimensional stability of silicone rubber, J. Prosthet. Dent. 14:1091-1098, 1964.

Miller, M.W.: Synergesis of alginate impression materials, Br. Dent. J. 139:425-430, 1975.

Mincham, W., Thurgate, S.M., and Lewis, A.J.: Measurement of dimensional stability of elastomeric impression materials by holographic inferometry, Aust. Dent. J. 26(6):395-399, 1981.

Myers, G.E., and Peyton, F.A.: Clinical and physical studies of the silicone rubber impression materials, J. Prosthet. Dent. 9:315-324, 1959.

Myers, G.E., Wepfer, G.G., and Peyton, F.A.: The Thiokol rubber base impression materials, J. Prosthet. Dent. 8:330-339, 1958.

Phillips, R.W.: Physical properties and manipulation of rubber impression materials, J. Am. Dent. Assoc. 59:454-458, 1959.

Phillips, R.W., and Schnell, R.J.: Electroformed dies from Thiokol and silicone impressions, J. Prosthet. Dent. 8:992-1002, 1958.

Reisbick, M.H., Garrett, R., and Smith, D.D.: Some effects of device versus handmixing of irreversible hydrocolloids, J. Prosthet. Dent. 47:92-94, 1982.

Rogers, O.W.: Electrodeposited copper individual impression trays, J. Prosthet. Dent. 16:19-25, 1966.

Shigeto, N., Kawazoe, Y., Hamada, T., and Yamada, S.: Adhesion between copper-plated acrylic tray resin and a polysulfide rubber impression material, J. Prosthet. Dent. 42:228-230, 1979.

Sneed, W.D., Miller, R., and Olson, J.: Tear strength of ten elastomeric impression materials, J. Prosthet. Dent. 49:511-513, 1983.

Stackhouse, J.A., Jr.: Impression materials and electrodeposits. I. Impression materials, J. Prosthet. Dent. 45:44-48, 1981.

Stankewitz, C.G., Carpenter, W.M., and Kate, W., Jr.: Bacteremia associated with irreversible hydrocolloid dental impressions, J. Prosthet. Dent. 44:251-253, 1980.

Starcke, E.N., Jr.: A historical review of complete denture impression materials, J. Am. Dent. Assoc. 91:1037-1041, 1975.

Starcke, E.N., Jr., Marcroft, K.R., Fischer, T.E., and Sweeney, W.T.: Physical properties of tissue-conditioning materials as used in functional impressions, J. Prosthet. Dent. 27:111-119, 1972.

Tang, R.Y., Gonzalez, J.B., and Roberts, G.D.: Polyurethane elastomer as a possible resilient material for denture prostheses: a microbiological evaluation, J. Dent. Res. 54:1039-1045, 1975.

Tolley, L.G., and Craig, R.G.: Viscoelastic properties of elastomeric impression materials: polysulphide, silicone and polyether rubbers, J. Oral Rehabil. 5(2):121-128, 1978.

Impression procedures

Apfelbaum, D.: Functional impression of edentulous maxillas with alginates, Rev. Asoc. Odontol. Argent. 61:199-205, 1973.

Barone, J.V.: Physiologic complete denture impressions, J. Prosthet. Dent. 13:800-809, 1963.

Basker, R.M., and Spence, D.: Some properties and clinical uses of a border trimming material, Br. Dent. J. 140:138-142, 1976.

Bauman, R.: Impression trays for functional border molding of complete denture prostheses, Gen. Dent. 28(4):46-48, 1980.

Bolouri, A.: The use of wax and self-curing acrylic resin in border molding, J. Prosthet. Dent. 37:89-91, 1977.

Boone, M.E.: How to handle secondary impression trays, J. Conn. State Dent. Assoc. 47:168-169, 1973.

Borgman, C.A., and Bolender, C.L.: Four-handed impression procedure, Dent. Clin. North Am. 14:471-477, 1970.

Boucher, C.O.: Fundamental approach to the problems of impressions for complete dentures, Trans. Am. Dent. Soc. Europe 62:43-51, 1956; Dent. Pract. 8:162-171, 1958.

Casey, D.M., and Lauciello, F.R.: A method for marking the functional depth of the floor of the mouth, J. Prosthet. Dent. 43:108-111, 1980.

Collett, H.A.: Complete denture impressions, J. Prosthet. Dent. 15:603-614, 1965.

Collett, H.A.: Final impressions for complete dentures, J. Prosthet. Dent. 23:250-264, 1970.

Cupero, H.M.: Impression technique for complete maxillary immediate denture, J. Prosthet. Dent. 39:108-109, 1978.

DeVan, M.M.: Basic principles in impression making, J. Prosthet. Dent. 2:26-35, 1952.

Douglas, W.H., Wilson, H.J., and Bates, J.F.: Pressures involved in taking impressions, Dent. Pract. 15:248-250, 1965.

Filler, W.H.: Modified impression technique for hyperplastic alveolar ridges, J. Prosthet. Dent. 25:609-612, 1971.

Frank, R.P.: Analysis of pressures produced during maxillary edentulous impressions procedures, J. Prosthet. Dent. 22:400-413, 1969.

Frank, R.P.: Controlling pressures during complete denture impressions, Dent. Clin. North Am. 14:453-470, 1970.

Freeman, S.P.: Impressions for complete dentures, J. Am. Dent. Assoc. 79:1173-1178, 1969.

Goyal, B.K.: Management of hypermobile soft tissue by dual impression technique, Compend. Contin. Educ. Dent. 1(2):94-97, 1980.

Hall, R.E.: A simplified impression technic that produces the maximum degree of denture base adaption and retention, J. Am. Dent. Assoc. 20:1215-1218, 1913.

Harris, H.L.: Impressions, J. Am. Dent. Assoc. 57:170-173, 1958.

Hight, F.M.: A simple technic to obtain maximum retention and stability in lower impressions, J. Am. Dent. Assoc. 12:778-783, 1925.

Horn, H.R.: Elastomeric impression making: biologic, psychologic, and physical considerations, Dent. Clin. North Am. 25(3):481-492, 1981.

Jogelkar, A.P., and Sinkford, J.C.: Impression procedure for problem mandibular complete dentures, J. Am. Dent. Assoc. 77:1303-1307, 1968.

Karlsson, S., and Hedegård, B.: A study of the reproducibility of the functional denture space with a dynamic impression technique, J. Prosthet. Dent. 41:21-25, 1979.

Khan, Z., Jaggers, J.H., and Shay, J.S.: Impressions of unsupported movable tissues, J. Am. Dent. Assoc. 103(4):590-592, 1981.

Knap, F.J.: Border molding in mandibular denture impressions, J. Prosthet. Dent. 42(3):351-352, 1979.

Kubalek, M.V., and Buffington, B.C.: Impressions by the use of subatmospheric pressure, J. Prosthet. Dent. **16**:213-223, 1966.

Kudyba, P., and Cinotti, W.R.: Impression technique for denture reconstruction, Int. Dent. J. **28**(4):434-439, 1978.

La Vere, A.M., and Freda, A.L.: An individualized impression tray utilizing the patient's existing denture, J. Prosthet. Dent. **36**:334-336, 1976.

Lee, R.E.: Mucostatics, Dent. Clin. North Am. **24**(1):81-96, 1980.

Loiselle, R.J.: A maxillary impression technic, J. Am. Dent. Assoc. **81**:146-147, 1970.

Lott, F., and Levin, B.: Flange technique: an anatomic and physiologic approach to increased retention, function, comfort, and appearance of dentures, J. Prosthet. Dent. **16**:394-413, 1966.

Marmor, D., and Herbertson, J.E.: The use of swallowing in making complete lower impressions, J. Prosthet. Dent. **19**:208-218, 1968.

McCracken, W.L.: Externally stabilized mandibular impressions, J. Prosthet. Dent. **14**:5-11, 1964.

Miller, E.L., and Smith, H.F.: Impression procedure for a severely atrophic mandible. J. Am. Dent. Assoc. **83**:1093-1096, 1971.

Morange, R.M.: Fournet-Tuller technique for lower dentures, Dent. Dig. **54**:406-409, 1948.

Neill, D.J., and Glaysher, J.K.: Identifying the denture space, J. Oral Rehabil. **9**(3):259-277, 1982.

Osborne, J.: Two impression methods for mobile fibrous ridges, Br. Dent. J. **117**:392-394, 1964.

Preiskel, H.: An impression technique for complete overlay denture, Br. Dent. J. **124**:9-13, 1968.

Rapuano, J.A.: Technic for recording the lingual flange of a mandibular complete denture, J. Am. Dent. Assoc. **77**:605-607, 1968.

Rihani, A.: Pressures involved in making upper edentulous impressions, J. Prosthet. Dent. **46**:610-614, 1981.

Rodegerdts, C.R.: The relationship of pressure spots in complete denture impressions with mucosal irritations, J. Prosthet. Dent. **14**:1040-1049, 1964.

Rowe, A.H., and Forrest, J.O.: Dental impressions: the probability of contamination and a method of disinfection, Br. Dent. J. **145**(6):184-186, 1978.

Rudd, K.D.: An aid in obtaining accurate complete denture impressions, J. Prosthet. Dent. **18**:86-89, 1967.

Schlosser, R.O.: Advantages of closed mouth muscle action for certain steps of impression taking, J. Am. Dent. Assoc. **18**:100-104, 1931.

Schlosser, R.O.: The tested functional impressions as a positive means for determining maximum surface extension and correct peripheral outline form for full denture bases, J. Am. Dent. Assoc. **21**:1053-1062, 1934.

Shanahan, T.E.J.: Stabilizing lower dentures on unfavorable ridges, J. Prosthet. Dent. **12**:420-424, 1962.

Shannon, J.L.: Edentulous impression procedure for region of the mentalis muscles, J. Prosthet. Dent. **26**:130-133, 1971.

Simmonds, C.R., and Jones, P.M.: A variation in complete mandibular impression form related to an anomaly of the mylohyoid muscle, J. Prosthet. Dent. **34**:384-388, 1975.

Smith, D.E., Toolson, L.B., Bolender, C.L., and Lord, J.L.: One-step border molding of complete denture impressions using a polyether impression material, J. Prosthet. Dent. **41**:347-351, 1979.

Smutko, G.E.: Making edentulous impressions, Dent. Clin. North Am. **21**:261-269, 1977.

Solomon, E.G.: Functional impression technique for complete denture construction with silicon elastomer, J. Indian Dent. Assoc. **45**:29-35, 1973.

Stansbery, C.J.: The negative pressure method of impression taking, J. Am. Dent. Assoc. **12**:438-445, 1925.

Stephens, A.P.: Special trays for full denture impressions, J. Irish Dent. Assoc. **15**:31-33, 1969.

Storer, R., and McCabe, J.F.: An investigation of methods available for sterilising impressions, Br. Dent. J. **151**:(7):217-219, 1981.

Stromberg, W.R., and Hickey, J.C.: Comparison of physiologically and manually formed denture bases, J. Prosthet. Dent. **15**:213-230, 1965.

Svenson, S.O.: Impressions for difficult complete lower dentures, Quintessence Int. **10**(1):39-42, 1979.

Taicher, S., Rosen, A.G., Arbree, N.S., Bergen, S.F., Levy, M., and Lepley, J.B.: The use of polydimethylsiloxane as a custom impression tray, J. Prosthet. Dent. **48**:562-564, 1982.

Tench, R.W.: Afterthoughts concerning impressions for full dentures, J. Am. Dent. Assoc. **15**:37-45, 1928.

Tench, R.W.: Impressions for dentures, J. Am. Dent. Assoc. **21**:1005-1018, 1934.

Tilton, G.E.: Denture periphery, J. Prosthet. Dent. **2**:290-306, 1952.

Travaglini, E.A.: Preliminary impressions for complete dentures, Dent. Dig. **75**:400-503, 1969.

Travaglini, E.A.: Alternative procedures for impressioning the edentulous mouth (II), Quintessence Int. **9**(7):39-43, 1978.

Travaglini, E.A.: Alternative procedures for impressioning the edentulous mouth (I), Quintessence Int. **9**(6):35-38, 1978.

Tryde, G., et al.: Dynamic impression methods, J. Prosthet. Dent. **15**:1023-1034, 1965.

Tucker, K.M.: Personalized impression trays, Dent. Dig. **77**:154-158, 1971.

Vahidi, F.: Vertical displacement of distal-extension ridges by different impression techniques, J. Prosthet. Dent. **40**:374-377, 1978.

Vig, R.G.: A modified chew-in and functional impression technique, J. Prosthet. Dent. **14**:214-220, 1964.

Vig, R.G., and Smith, R.C.: Applied plaster impressions for maxillary complete dentures, J. Prosthet. Dent. **27**:586-590, 1972.

Walter, J.D.: Composite impression procedures, J. Prosthet. Dent. **30**:385-390, 1973.

Weintraub, G.S.: Establishing the posterior palatal seal during the final impression procedure: a functional approach, J. Am. Dent. Assoc. **94**:505-510, 1977.

Woelfel, J.B.: Contour variations in impressions of one edentulous patient, J. Prosthet. Dent. **12**:229-254, 1962.

Zinner, I.D., and Sherman, H.: An analysis of the development of complete denture impression techniques, J. Prosthet. Dent. **46**:242-249, 1981.

Incisal guidance

Christensen, F.T.: The effect of incisal guidance on cusp angulation in prosthetic occlusion, J. Prosthet. Dent. 11:48-54, 1961.

Frahm, F.W.: Incisal guidance—its influence in compensation and balance, J. Am. Dent. Assoc. 13:771-785, 1926.

Grant, A.A.: Elevation of the incisal guide pin following attachment of casts to articulators, J. Prosthet. Dent. 13:664-668, 1963.

Schuyler, C.H.: An evaluation of incisal guidance and its influence in restorative dentistry, J. Prosthet. Dent. 9:374-378, 1959.

Schuyler, C.H.: The function and importance of incisal guidance in oral rehabilitation, J. Prosthet. Dent. 13:1011-1029, 1963.

Siebert, G.: Recent results concerning physiological tooth movement and anterior guidance, J. Oral Rehabil. 8(6):479-493, 1981.

Masticatory forces applied against basal seat

Atkinson, H.F., and Ralph, W.J.: Tooth loss and biting force in man, J. Dent. Res. 52:225-228, 1973.

Bearn, E.M.: Some masticatory force patterns produced by full denture wearers, Dent. Pract. 22:342-346, 1972.

Bearn, E.M.: Effect of different occlusal profiles on the masticatory forces transmitted by complete dentures: an evaluation, Br. Dent. J. 134:7-10, 1973.

Berg, T., Jr., Chase, W.W., and Ray, K.: Denture base pressure tests, J. Prosthet. Dent. 17:540-548, 1967.

Boucher, C.O.: Studies of displacement of tissues under dentures, J. Am. Dent. Assoc. 27:1476-1478, 1940.

Cutright, D.E., Brudvik, J.S., Gay, W.D., and Selting, W.J.: Tissue pressure under complete maxillary dentures, J. Prosthet. Dent. 35:160-170, 1976.

Finnegan, F.J.: Determination of maxillomandibular force generated during deglutition, J. Prosthet. Dent. 17:134-143, 1967.

Gerber, A.: Complete dentures (VI). Mastication-centric for fit and tissue comfort, Quintessence Int. 5:33-38, 1974.

Gerber, A.: Complete dentures. IV. The teamwork of complete dentures in chewing function, Quintessence Int. 5:41-46, 1974.

Haraldson, T., Karlsson, U., and Carlsson, G.E.: Bite force and oral function in complete denture wearers, J. Oral Rehabil. 6(1):41-48, 1979.

Jacobs, R.M.: The effects of preprosthetic muscle exercise upon perioral tonus, J. Prosthet. Dent. 18:217-221, 1967.

Johnson, W.: A study of stress distribution in complete upper dentures, Dent. Pract. 15:374-379, 1965.

Kelsey, C.C., Reid, F.D., and Coplowitz, J.A.: A method of measuring pressures against tissues supporting functioning complete dentures, J. Prosthet. Dent. 35:376-383, 1976.

Lambrecht, J.R.: The influence of occlusal contact area on chewing performance, J. Prosthet. Dent. 15:444-450, 1965.

Lim, Kheng A.: Biting forces in edentulous patients, Malaysian Dent. J. 6:18-31, 1966.

Lopuck, S., Smith, J., and Caputo, A.: Photoelastic comparison of posterior denture occlusions, J. Prosthet. Dent. 40:18-22, 1978.

Ohashi, M., Woelfel, J.B., and Paffenbarger, G.C.: Pressures exerted on complete dentures during swallowing, J. Am. Dent. Assoc. 73:625-630, 1966.

Pacer, F.J., and Bowman, D.C.: Occlusal force discrimination by denture patients, J. Prosthet. Dent. 33:602-609, 1975.

Parker, H.M.: Impact reduction in complete and partial dentures, a pilot study, J. Prosthet. Dent. 16:227-245, 1966.

Roedema, W.H.: Relationship between the width of the occlusal table and pressures under dentures during function, J. Prosthet. Dent. 36:24-34, 1976.

Roedema, W.H.: A comparison of two methods of quantifying masticatory pressures developed under dentures with variable occlusal width, J. Oral Rehabil. 6(1):67-80, 1979.

Scott, I., and Ash, M.M., Jr.: A six-channel intraoral transmitter for measuring occlusal forces, J. Prosthet. Dent. 16:56-61, 1966.

Skinner, E.W., Campbell, R.L., and Chung, P.: Clinical study of the forces required to dislodge maxillary denture bases of various designs, J. Am. Dent. Assoc. 47:671-680, 1953.

Stromberg, W.R.: Method of measuring forces of denture bases against supporting tissues, J. Prosthet. Dent. 5:268-288, 1955.

Thomson, J.C.: The load factor in complete denture intolerance, J. Prosthet. Dent. 25:4-10, 1971.

Yurkstas, A.A., and Emerson, W.H.: Decreased masticatory function in denture patients, J. Prosthet. Dent. 14:931-934, 1964.

Maxillomandibular relations and mandibular movements

Arstad, T.: The influence of the lips on mandibular rest position in edentulous patients, J. Prosthet. Dent. 15:27-34, 1965.

Baikie, M.W.: The Gothic arch tracing and facial dimensions in the edentulous patient, J. S. Afr. Dent. Assoc. 27:144-151, 1972.

Beck, H.O., and Morrison, W.E.: A method for reproduction of movements of the mandible, J. Prosthet. Dent. 12:873-883, 1962.

Bell, D.H., Jr.: Sagittal balance of the mandible, J. Am. Dent. Assoc. 64:486-495, 1962.

Block, L.S.: Muscular tensions in denture construction, J. Prosthet. Dent. 2:198-203, 1952.

Block, L.S.: Common factors in complete denture prosthetics, Ill. Dent. J. 22:710-720, 1953.

Boucher, C.O.: Maxillomandibular relations, Dent. Pract. 13:427-433, 1963.

Boucher, L.J.: Limiting factors in posterior movements of mandibular condyles, J. Prosthet. Dent. 11:23-25, 1961.

Boucher, L.J.: Anatomy of the temporomandibular joint as it pertains to centric relation, J. Prosthet. Dent. 12:464-472, 1962.

Boucher, L.J., and Jacoby, J.: Posterior border movements of the human mandible, J. Prosthet. Dent. 11:836-841, 1961.

Boyanov, B.: Determining vertical dimension of occlusion and centric relation, J. Prosthet. Dent. **24**:18-24, 1970.

Buxbaum, J.D., Parente, F.J., Ramsey, W.O., et al.: A comparison of centric relation with maximum intercuspation based on quantitative electromyography, J. Oral Rehabil. **9**(1):45-51, 1982.

Dawson, P.E.: Centric relation: its effect on occluso-muscle harmony, Dent. Clin. North Am. **23**(2):169-180, 1979.

Dombrady, L.: Investigation into the transient instability of the rest position, J. Prosthet. Dent. **16**:479-490, 1966.

Douglas, J.R., and Maritato, F.R.: "Open rest," a new concept in the selection of the vertical dimension of occlusion, J. Prosthet. Dent. **15**:850-856, 1965.

Dutrie, N., and Yemm, R.: Muscles involved in voluntary mandibular retrusion in man, J. Oral Rehabil. **9**(2): 155-159, 1982.

Dyer, E.H.: Importance of a stable maxillomandibular relation, J. Prosthet. Dent. **30**:241-251, 1973.

Finger, I.M., and Tanaka, H.: A new semiadjustable articulator. III. An investigation of the capability of the Hanau XP-51 articulator, J. Prosthet. Dent. **37**:310-319, 1977.

Fox, S.S.: Lateral jaw movements in mammalian dentitions, J. Prosthet. Dent. **15**:810-825, 1965.

Garnick, J.J., and Ramfjord, S.P.: Rest position, J. Prosthet. Dent. **12**:895-911, 1962.

Gibbs, C.H., Lundeen, H.C., Mahan, P.E., and Fujimoto, J.: Chewing movements in relation to border movements at the first molar, J. Prosthet. Dent. **46**:308-322, 1981.

Goodkind, R.J.: Mandibular movement with changes in the vertical dimension, J. Prosthet. Dent. **18**:438-448, 1967.

Granger, E.R.: The temporomandibular joint in prosthodontics, J. Prosthet. Dent. **10**:239-242, 1960.

Guichet, N.F.: Biologic laws governing functions of muscles that move the mandible. I. Occlusal programming, J. Prosthet. Dent. **37**:648-656, 1977.

Guichet, N.F.: Biologic laws governing functions of muscles that move the mandible. II. Condylar position, J. Prosthet. Dent. **38**:35-41, 1977.

Guichet, N.F.: Biologic laws governing functions of muscles that move the mandible, J. Prosthet. Dent. **38**:174-179, 1977.

Guichet, N.F.: Biologic laws governing functions of muscles that move the mandible. IV. Degree of jaw separation and potential for maximum jaw separation, J. Prosthet. Dent. **38**:301-310, 1977.

Gysi, A.: Practical application of research results in denture construction (mandibular movements), J. Am. Dent. Assoc. **16**:199-223, 1929.

Hall, R.E.: Movements of the mandible and approximate mechanical imitation of these movements for the arrangement and grinding of artificial teeth for the efficient restoration of lost masticatory function in edentulous cases, J. Natl. Dent. Assoc. **7**:677-686, 1920.

Hickey, J.C., et al.: Mandibular movements in three dimensions, J. Prosthet. Dent. **13**:72-92, 1963.

Hickey, J.C., Williams, B.H., and Woelfel, J.B.: Stability of mandibular rest position, J. Prosthet. Dent. **11**:566-572, 1961.

Hight, F.M., and Clapp, G.W.: Some essentials in full denture technic (importance of correct jaw relations), Dent. Dig. **37**:742-748, 1931.

Hildebrand, Y.: Studies in mandibular kinematics, Dent. Cosmos **78**:449-458, 1936.

Hodge, L.C., and Mahan, P.E.: A study of mandibular movement from centric occlusion to maximum intercuspation, J. Prosthet. Dent. **18**:19-30, 1967.

Isaacson, D.: A clinical study of the condyle path, J. Prosthet. Dent. **9**:927-935, 1959.

Javid, N.S., and Porter, M.R.: The importance of the Hanau formula in construction of complete dentures, J. Prosthet. Dent. **34**:397-404, 1975.

Jemt, T., Karlsson, S., and Hedegård, B.: Mandibular movements of young adults recorded by intraorally placed light-emitting diodes, J. Prosthet. Dent. **42**:669-673, 1979.

Jerge, C.R.: The neurologic mechanism underlying cyclic jaw movements, J. Prosthet. Dent. **14**:667-681, 1964.

Kovats, J.J.: Overclosure of the jaws: a clinical syndrome, J. Prosthet. Dent. **18**:311-315, 1967.

Krajicek, D.D., et al.: Clinical and electromyographic study of mandibular rest position, J. Prosthet. Dent. **11**:826-830, 1961.

Kurth, L.E.: Physics of mandibular movement related to full denture construction, J. Prosthet. Dent. **4**:611-620, 1954.

Kydd, W.L.: Rapid serial roentgenographic cephalometry for observing mandibular movements, J. Prosthet. Dent. **8**:880-885, 1958.

Landa, J.S.: A critical analysis of the Bennett movement. I. J. Prosthet. Dent. **8**:709-726, 1958.

Landa, J.S.: A critical analysis of the Bennett movement. II. J. Prosthet. Dent. **8**:865-879, 1958.

Lee, R.L.: Jaw movements engraved in solid plastic for articulator controls. II. Transfer apparatus, J. Prosthet. Dent. **22**:513-527, 1969.

Le Pera, F.: Understanding graphic records of mandibular movements, J. Prosthet. Dent. **18**:417-424, 1967.

Lundeen, H.C., and Wirth, C.G.: Condylar movement patterns engraved in plastic blocks, J. Prosthet. Dent. **30**:866-875, 1973.

Lundeen, H.C., Shryock, E.F., and Gibbs, C.H.: An evaluation of mandibular border movements: their character and significance, J. Prosthet. Dent. **40**:442-452, 1978.

Luthra, S.P.: An instrument to measure the maxillomandibular relationship, J. Indian Dent. Assoc. **44**:149-151, 1972.

Mahan, P.E., Wilkinson, T.M., Gibbs, C.H., Mauderli, A., and Brannon, L.S.: Superior and inferior bellies of the lateral pterygoid muscle EMG activity at basic jaw positions, J. Prosthet. Dent. **50**:710-718, 1983.

McCoy, R.B., Shryock, E.F., and Lundeen, H.C.: A method of transferring mandibular-movement data to computer storage, J. Prosthet. Dent. **36**:510-516, 1976.

Mongini, F.: Relationship between the temporomandibular joint and pantographic tracings of mandibular movements, J. Prosthet. Dent. **43**:331-337, 1980.

Monson, G.S.: Applied mechanics to the theory of mandibular movements, Dent. Cosmos **74**:1039-1053, 1932.

Moses, C.H.: Mandibular movements and the arrangement of teeth, J. Can. Dent. Assoc. **12**:3-10, 1946.

Nagasawa, T., Sasaki, H., and Tsuru, H.: Masseteric silent period after tooth contact in full denture wearers, J. Dent. Res. **55**:314, 1976.

Nairn, R.I.: Maxillomandibular relations and aspects of occlusion, J. Prosthet. Dent. **31**:361-368, 1974.

Nairn, R.I., and Cutress, T.W.: Changes in mandibular position following removal of the remaining teeth and insertion of immediate complete dentures, Br. Dent. J. **122**:303-306, 1967.

Needles, J.W.: Mandibular movements and occlusion, J. Am. Dent. Assoc. **14**:786-791, 1927.

Olsson, A., and Posselt U.: Relationship of various skull reference lines, J. Prosthet. Dent. **11**:1045-1049, 1961.

Pound, E.: Jaw relations—logic or judgement, Quintessence Int. **7**:33-38, 1976.

Preiskel, H.W.: Some observations on the postural position of the mandible, J. Prosthet. Dent. **15**:625-633, 1965.

Rajstein, J., and Sorbin, S.: Establishments of correct vertical maxillomandibular relations in complete dentures, Isr. J. Dent. Med. **19**:28-31, 1970.

Regli, C.P., and Kelly, E.K.: The phenomenon of decreased mandibular arch width in opening movements, J. Prosthet. Dent. **17**:49-53, 1967.

Roedema, W.H., Knapp, J.G., Spencer, J., and Dever, M.K.: Computer-graphic representation of mandibular movements in three dimensions. I. The horizontal plane, J. Prosthet. Dent. **39**:378-383, 1978.

Roedema, W.H., Knapp, J.G., Spencer, J., and Dever, M.K.: Computer-graphic representation of mandibular movements in three dimensions. II. The sagittal and frontal planes, J. Prosthet. Dent. **40**:385-391, 1978.

Rudd, K.D., Morrow, R.M., and Jendresen, D.: Fluorescent photoanthropometry: a method for analyzing mandibular motion, J. Prosthet. Dent. **21**:495-505, 1969.

Salomon, J.A., Waysenson, B.D., and Warshaw, B.D.: Computer-monitored radionuclide tracking of three-dimensional mandibular movements. II. Experimental setup and preliminary results: Posselt diagram, J. Prosthet. Dent. **41**:463-469, 1979.

Schaerer, P., Stallard, R.E., and Zander, H.: Occlusal interferences and mastication: an electromyographic study, J. Prosthet. Dent. **17**:438-449, 1967.

Scott, W.R.: Occlusal registrations using alginate (irreversible hydrocolloid) impression material, J. Prosthet. Dent. **40**:517-519, 1978.

Sears, V.H.: Terminology of jaw relations, tooth occlusions, and their corresponding records, J. Prosthet. Dent. **10**:215-220, 1960.

Sears, V.H.: Mandibular equilibration, J. Am. Dent. Assoc. **65**:45-55, 1962.

Seitlin, D.J.: The mandibular lever, J. Prosthet. Dent. **19**:342-349, 1968.

Shanahan, T.E.J., and Leff, A.: Mandibular and articulator movements. V. Vertical and sagittal axes myths, J. Prosthet. Dent. **13**:866-872, 1963.

Shanahan, T.E.J., and Leff, A.: Mandibular and articulator movements. VI. Intraoral three dimensional study of terminal masticatory cycles, J. Prosthet. Dent. **14**:22-29, 279-289, 1964.

Sheppard, I.M.: Anteroposterior and posteroanterior movements of the mandible and condylar centricity during function, J. Prosthet. Dent. **12**:86-94, 1962.

Sheppard, I.M.: Incisive and related movements of the mandible, J. Prosthet. Dent. **14**:898-906, 1964.

Sheppard, I.M.: The effect of extreme vertical overlap on masticatory strokes, J. Prosthet. Dent. **15**:1035-1042, 1965.

Sheppard, I.M., and Sheppard, S.M.: Range of condylar movement during mandibular opening, J. Prosthet. Dent. **15**:263-271, 1965.

Shotwell, J.L., Kotowicz, W.E., and Clayton, J.A.: Ability of edentulous subjects to reproduce mandibular border tracings, J. Prosthet. Dent. **44**:379-383, 1980.

Silverman, M.M.: Character of mandibular movement during closure, J. Prosthet. Dent. **15**:634-641, 1965.

Silvestri, A.R., Cohen, S.N., and Connolly, R.J.: Muscle physiology during functional activities and parafunctional habits, J. Prosthet. Dent. **44**:64-67, 1980.

Swerdlow, H.: Vertical dimension literature review, J. Prosthet. Dent. **15**:241-247, 1965.

Tallgren, A.: Changes in adult face height due to aging, wear, and loss of teeth and prosthetic treatment, Acta Odontol. Scand. **15**(supp. 24):1-122, 1957.

Trapozzano, V.R., and Lazzari, J.B.: The physiology of the terminal rotational position of the condyles in the temporomandibular joint, J. Prosthet. Dent. **17**:122-133, 1967.

Waysenson, B., and Salomon, J.: Three-dimensional records of envelopes of motion related to mandibular movements, J. Prosthet. Dent. **38**:52-60, 1977.

Williamson, E.H., Caves, S.A., Edenfield, R.J., et al.: Cephalometric analysis: comparisons between maximum intercuspation and centric relation, Am. J. Orthod. **74**(6):672-677, 1978.

Woelfel, J.B., Hickey, J.C., Stacy, R.W., and Rinear, L.: Electromyographic analysis of jaw movements, J. Prosthet. Dent. **10**:688-697, 1960.

Wood, G.N.: Centric occlusion, centric relation, and the mandibular posture, J. Prosthet. Dent. **20**:292-306, 1968.

Zola, A., and Rothschild, E.A.: Condyle positions in unimpeded jaw movements, J. Prosthet. Dent. **11**:873-881, 1961.

Maxillomandibular relation records

Akerly, W.B.: A tripodal method of recording centric relation, J. Prosthet. Dent. **42**(4):461-465, 1979.

Bailey, L.R.: Recording edentulous jaw relationships, Dent. Clin. North Am. **21**:271-283, 1977.

Balthazar-Hart, Y., Sandrik, J.L., Malone, W.F.P., Mazar, B., and Hart, T.: Accuracy and dimensional stability of four interocclusal recording materials, J. Prosthet. Dent. **45**:586-591, 1981.

Boos, R.H.: Physiologic denture technique, J. Prosthet. Dent. **6**:726-740, 1956.

Boucher, C.O.: Discussion of "Accuracy in measuring functional dimensions and relations in oral prosthesis" by Charles E. Stuart, J. Prosthet. Dent. **9**:237-239, 1959.

Buffington, B.C.: Stabilizing record bases with controlled subatmospheric pressure, J. Prosthet. Dent. **21**:14-18, 1969.

Cohn, L.A.: Two techniques for interocclusal records, J. Prosthet. Dent. **13**:438-443, 1963.

Dawson, P.E.: Centric relation: its effect on occluso-muscle harmony, Dent. Clin. North Am. **23**(2):169-180, 1979.

Douglas, J.R., and Maritato, F.R.: A roentgenographic method to determine the vertical dimension of occlusion for complete dentures, J. Prosthet. Dent. **17**:450-455, 1967.

Graser, G.N.: An evaluation of terminal hinge position and neuromuscular position in edentulous patients. I. Maxillomandibular recordings, J. Prosthet. Dent. **36**:491-500, 1976.

Graser, G.N.: An evaluation of terminal hinge position and neuromuscular position in edentulous patients II. Duplicate mandibular dentures, J. Prosthet. Dent. **37**:12-18, 1977.

Grasso, J.E., and Sharry, J.: The duplicability of arrow-point tracings in dentulous subjects, J. Prosthet. Dent. **20**:106-115, 1968.

Hakim-Abdel, A.M.: The swallowing position as a centric relation record, J. Prosthet. Dent. **47**:12-15, 1982.

Halperin, A.R., Graser, G.N., and Abadi, B.J.: Accurate mounting casts for complete dentures, J. Prosthet. Dent. **43**:469-472, 1980.

Harcourt, J.K.: Accuracy in registration and transfer of prosthetic records, Aust. Dent. J. **19**:182-190, 1974.

Helft, M., Cardash, H., and Kaufman, C.: Combining final impressions with maxillomandibular relation records in stabilized record bases, J. Prosthet. Dent. **39**:135-138, 1978.

Hemphill, C.D., Parker M.L., and Regli, C.P.: Effects of uneven occlusal contact when registering maxillomandibular relations, J. Prosthet. Dent. **28**:357-359, 1972.

Hight, F.M.: Registration and recording of maxillomandibular relations, J. Am. Dent. Assoc. **21**:1660-1663, 1934.

Howell, R.A.: A clinical study of horizontal jaw relationships in edentulous patients, J. Dent. **9**(4):318-327, 1981.

Hughes, G.A.: Maxillo-mandibular relations in the teaching of denture prosthesis, J. Dent. Educ. **13**:133-144, 1949.

Hull, C.A., and Junghans, J.A.: A cephalometric approach to establishing the facial vertical dimension, J. Prosthet. Dent. **20**:37-42, 1968.

Hunt, G.C., and Yoxsimer, J.N.: Edentulous gnathologic recordings utilizing "vacustatics," J. Prosthet. Dent. **35**:588-594, 1976.

Ismail, Y.H., and George, W.A.: The consistency of the swallowing technique in determining occlusal vertical relation in edentulous patients, J. Prosthet. Dent. **19**:230-236, 1968.

Ishmail, Y.H., and Rokni, A.: Radiographic study of condylar position in centric relation and centric occlusion, J. Prosthet. Dent. **43**(3):327-330, 1980.

Klein, I.E., and Soni, A.: Stabilized record bases for complete dentures, J. Prosthet. Dent. **42**:584-587, 1979.

Kurth, L.E.: Methods of obtaining vertical dimension and centric relation: a practical evaluation of various methods, J. Am. Dent. Assoc. **59**:669-673, 1959.

Kurth, L.E.: From mouth to articulator: static jaw relations, J. Am. Dent. Assoc. **64**:517-520, 1962.

Langer, A.: The validity of maxillomandibular records made with trial and processed acrylic resin bases, J. Prosthet. Dent. **45**:253-258, 1981.

Langer, A., and Michman, J.: Intraoral technique for recording vertical horizontal maxillomandibular relations in complete dentures, J. Prosthet. Dent. **21**:599-606, 1969.

Langer, A., and Michman, J.: Evaluation of lateral tracings of edentulous subjects, J. Prosthet. Dent. **23**:381-386, 1970.

La Vere, A.M.: Lateral interocclusal positional records, J. Prosthet. Dent. **19**:350-358, 1968.

Leff, A.: Gnathodynamics of four mandibular positions, J. Prosthet. Dent. **16**:844-847, 1966.

Luebke, R.J.: Stabilized interocclusal centric relation records utilizing acrylic resin indexes, J. Prosthet. Dent. **46**:102-104, 1981.

Lundeen, H.C.: Centric relation records: the effect of muscle action, J. Prosthet. Dent. **31**:244-253, 1974.

Lundquist, D.O., and Fiebiger, G.E.: Registrations for relating the mandibular cast to the maxillary cast based on Kennedy's classification system, J. Prosthet. Dent. **35**:371-375, 1976.

Lytle, R.B.: Vertical relation of occlusion by the patient's neuromuscular perception, J. Prosthet. Dent. **14**:12-21, 1964.

McArthur, D.R.: Stabilized occlusion rims for small interarch spaces, J. Prosthet. Dent. **42**:683-689, 1979.

McCartney, J.W.: Recording centric-protrusive jaw relationship, J. Prosthet. Dent. **43**(2):231-232, 1980.

Meyer, F.S.: The generated path technique in reconstruction dentistry, J. Prosthet. Dent. **9**:354-366, 1959.

Millstein, P.L., and Clark, R.E.: Differential accuracy of silicone-body and self-curing resin interocclusal records and associated weight loss, J. Prosthet. Dent. **46**:380-384, 1981.

Millstein, P.L., Clark, R.E., and Kronman, J.H.: Determination of the accuracy of wax interocclusal registrations. II. J. Prosthet. Dent. **29**:40-45, 1973.

Morris, J.C.: Displacement of the soft tissues beneath temporary denture bases while making interocclusal records, J. Prosthet. Dent. **16**:1019-1033, 1966.

Parker, M.L., Hemphill, C.D., and Regli, C.P.: Anteroposterior position of the mandible as related to centric relation registrations, J. Prosthet. Dent. **31**:262-265, 1974.

Pasternak, M.P.: Establishing vertical maxillomandibular relations with posterior resin blocks, J. Prosthet. Dent. **19**:469-474, 1968.

Posselt, U., and Franzen, G.: Registration of the condyle path inclination by intraoral wax records: variations in three instruments, J. Prosthet. Dent. **10**:441-454, 1960.

Posselt, U., and Nevstedt, P.: Registration of the condyle path inclination by intraoral wax records—its practical value, J. Prosthet. Dent. **11**:43-47, 1961.

Posselt, U., and Skytting, B.: Registration of the condyle path inclination: variations using the Gysi technique, J. Prosthet. Dent. **10**:243-247, 1960.

Pound, E.: Accurate protrusive registrations for patients edentulous in one or both jaws, J. Prosthet. Dent. **50**:584-586, 1983.

Preiskel, H.W.: Considerations of the check record in complete denture construction, J. Prosthet. Dent. **18**:98-102, 1967.

Sanghvi, S.J., Bhatt, N.A., and Bhargava, K.: An evaluation of cross-bite ridge relations: a study of articulated jaw records of 150 edentulous patients, J. Prosthet. Dent. **46**:24-29, 1981.

Schuyler, C.H.: Intra-oral method of establishing maxillomandibular relation, J. Am. Dent. Assoc. **19**:1012-1019, 1932.

Scott, W.R.: Occlusal registrations using alginate (irreversible hydrocolloid) impression material, J. Prosthet. Dent. **40**:517-519, 1978.

Sears, V.H.: Jaw relations and a means of recording the most important articulator adjustment, Dent. Cosmos **68**:1047-1054, 1926.

Shanahan, T.E.J., and Leff, A.: Interocclusal records, J. Prosthet. Dent. **10**:842-848, 1960.

Shanahan, T.E.J., and Leff, A.: Mandibular and articulator movements. II. Illusion of mandibular tracings, J. Prosthet. Dent. **12**:82-85, 1962.

Shannon, J.L.: A technique for verifying centric relation at the established vertical relation, J. Prosthet. Dent. **28**:585-588, 1972.

Sindledecker, L.: Effect of different centric relation registrations on the pantographic representation of centric relation, J. Prosthet. Dent. **46**:271-279, 1981.

Stephens, A.P.: Full denture try-in, J. Irish Dent. Assoc. **15**:126-128, 1969.

Stuart, C.E.: Accuracy in measuring functional dimensions and relations in oral prosthesis, J. Prosthet. Dent. **9**:220-236, 1959.

Tench, R.W.: Interpretation and registration of mandibulomaxillary relations and their reproducton in an instrument, J. Am. Dent. Assoc. **13**:1675-1693, 1926.

Vierheller, P.G.: A functional method for establishing vertical and tentative centric maxillomandibular relations, J. Prosthet. Dent. **19**:587-593, 1968.

Watt, D.M.: Clinical applications of gnathosonics, J. Prosthet. Dent. **16**:83-95, 1966.

Watt, D.M.: Gnathosonics—a study of sounds produced by the masticatory mechanism, J. Prosthet. Dent. **16**:73-82, 1966.

Wilkie, N.D., Hurst, T.L., and Mitchell, D.L.: Radiographic comparisons of condylar-fossa relationships during maxillomandibular registrations made by different methods, J. Prosthet. Dent. **32**:529-533, 1974.

Williamson, E.H., Steinke, R.M., Morse, P.K., et al.: Centric relation: a comparison of muscle-determined position and operator guidance, Am. J. Orthod. **77**(2):133-145, 1980.

Williamson, E.H.: Laminagraphic study of mandibular condyle position when recording centric relation, J. Prosthet. Dent. **39**:561-564, 1978.

Wormley, J.H., and Brudvik, J.S.: A simplified procedure for remounting dentures, J. Prosthet. Dent. **16**:675-684, 1966.

Metal denture bases

Bahrani, A.S., Blair, G.A.S., and Crossland, B.: Slow rate hydraulic forming of stainless steel dentures, Br. Dent. J. **118**:425-431, 1965.

Gruenwald, A.H.: Gold base lower dentures, J. Prosthet. Dent. **14**:432-441, 1964.

Halperin, A.R.: The cast aluminum denture base. I. Rationale, J. Prosthet. Dent. **43**:605-610, 1980.

Halperin, A.R., and Halperin, G.C.: The cast aluminum denture base. II. Technique, J. Prosthet. Dent. **44**:94-100, 1980.

Lundquist, D.O.: An aluminum alloy as a denture-base material, J. Prosthet. Dent. **13**:102-110, 1963.

Pansch, J.L., Callagham, N.R., and Appleby, R.C.: Effects of cast-gold mandibular dentures on the vertical dimension of rest position, J. Prosthet. Dent. **28**:21-25, 1972.

Nutrition

Barone, J.V.: Nutrition of edentulous patients, J. Prosthet. Dent. **15**:804-809, 1965.

Barone, J.V.: Nutrition—phase one of the edentulous patient, J. Prosthet. Dent. **40**:122-126, 1978.

Detroit Dental Clinic Club, Complete Denture Section: Nutrition for the denture patient, J. Prosthet. Dent. **10**:53-60, 1960.

Hartsook, E.I.: Food selection, dietary adequacy, and related dental problems of patients with dental prostheses, J. Prosthet. Dent. **32**:32-40, 1974.

Mäkilä, E.: Milk and vegetables in the diet of institutionalized elderly people in Finland, J. Prosthet. Dent. **45**:134-137, 1981.

Massler, M.: Geriatric nutrition. I. Osteoporosis, J. Prosthet. Dent. **42**:252-254, 1979.

Massler, M.: Geriatric nutrition. II. Dehydration in the elderly, J. Prosthet. Dent. **42**:489-491, 1979.

Massler, M.: Geriatric nutrition: III. The role of taste and smell in appetite, J. Prosthet. Dent. **43**:247-250, 1980.

Massler, M.: Geriatric nutrition. IV. The role of the fiber in the diet, J. Prosthet. Dent. **50**:5-7, 1983.

Ramsey, W.O.: The role of nutrition in conditioning edentulous patients, J. Prosthet. Dent. **23**:130-135, 1970.

Ramsey, W.O.: Nutritional problems of the aged, J. Prosthet. Dent. **49**:16-19, 1983.

Smith, J.F.: Nutrition suggestions for the prosthetic patient, J. Prosthet. Dent. **16**:829-834, 1966.

Swoope, C.C., and Hartsook, E.: Nutrition analysis of prosthodontic patients, J. Prosthet. Dent. **38**:208-215, 1977.

Wical, K.E., and Brussee, P.: Effects of a calcium and vitamin D supplement on alveolar ridge resorption in immediate denture patients, J. Prosthet. Dent. **41**:4-11, 1979.

Wical, K.E., and Swoope, C.C.: Studies of residual ridge resorption. I. Use of panoramic radiographs for evaluation and classification of mandibular resorption, J. Prosthet. Dent. **32**:7-12, 1974.

Wical, K.E., and Swoope, C.C.: Studies of residual ridge resorption. II. The relationship of dietary calcium and phosphorus to residual ridge resorption, J. Prosthet. Dent. **32**:13-22, 1974.

Wical, K.: Commonsense dietary recommendations for geriatric dental patients, J. Prosthet. Dent. **49**:162-164, 1983.

Yurkstas, A.A., and Emerson, W.H.: Dietary selections of persons with natural and artificial teeth, J. Prosthet. Dent. **14**:695-697, 1964.

Occlusal corrections

Cerveris, A.R.: Vibracentric equilibration of centric occlusion, J. Am. Dent. Assoc. **63**:476-483, 1961.

Langer, A., and Michman, J.: Occlusal perception after placement of complete dentures, J. Prosthet. Dent. **19**:246-251, 1968.

Lauritzen, A.G., and Wolford, L.W.: Occlusal relationships: the split-cast method for articulator techniques, J. Prosthet. Dent. **14**:256-265, 1964.

Medwedeff, F.M.: An instrumented technique for occlusal adjustment, J. Am. Dent. Assoc. **98**(3):417-418, 1979.

Schlosser, R.O.: Checking completed dentures for adaptation and retention and establishing balanced articulation, J. Am. Dent. Assoc. **15**:1717-1723, 1928.

Schuyler, C.H.: Fundamental principles in the correction of occlusal disharmony, natural and artificial, J. Am. Dent. Assoc. **22**:1193-1202, 1935.

Sears, V.H.: Occlusal refinements on completed dentures, J. Am. Dent. Assoc. **59**:1250-1252, 1959.

Shannon, J.L.: A bilaterally balanced occlusal scheme for patients with arch width and curvature discrepancies, J. Prosthet. Dent. **44**(1):101-103, 1980.

Sowter, J.B., and Bass, R.E.: Increasing the efficiency of resin posterior teeth, J. Prosthet. Dent. **19**:465-468, 1968.

Stromberg, W.R.: Use of vibration in the occlusion refinement of complete dentures, J. Prosthet. Dent. **11**:621-624, 1961.

Tench, R.W.: A method for accurately remounting vulcanized dentures in the articulator for regrinding, Dent. Dig. **26**:286-298, 1920.

Ziebert, C.J., and Donegan, S.J.: Tooth contacts and stability before and after occlusal adjustment, J. Prosthet. Dent. **42**(3):276-281, 1979.

Occlusion

Abrahams, R., and Carey, P.D.: The use of the ala-tragus line for occlusal plane determination in complete dentures, J. Dent. **7**(4):339-341, 1979.

Aull, A.E.: Condylar determinants of occlusal patterns, J. Prosthet. Dent. **15**:826-846, 1965.

Barsoum, W.M., and El-Ebrashi, M.K.: The construction of individualized plastic teeth from beryllium-copper molds, J. Prosthet. Dent. **17**:251-260, 1967.

Beck, H.O.: Occlusion as related to complete removable prosthodontics, J. Prosthet. Dent. **27**:246-256, 1972.

Boucher, C.O.: Discussion of "laws of articulation," J. Prosthet. Dent. **13**:45-48, 1963.

Brewer, A.A., Reibel, P.R., and Nassif, N.J.: Comparison of zero degree teeth and anatomic teeth on complete dentures, J. Prosthet. Dent. **17**:28-35, 1967.

Brudvik, J.S., and Wormley, J.H.: A method of developing monoplane occlusions, J. Prosthet. Dent. **19**:573-580, 1968.

Carey, P.D.: Occlusal plane orientation and masticatory performance of complete dentures, J. Prosthet. Dent. **39**:368-371, 1978.

Christensen, F.T.: Cusp angulation for complete dentures, J. Prosthet. Dent. **8**:910-923, 1958.

Christensen, F.T.: The effect of Bonwill's triangle on complete dentures, J. Prosthet. Dent. **9**:791-796, 1959.

Christensen, F.T.: Balkwill's angle for complete dentures, J. Prosthet. Dent. **10**:95-98, 1960.

Christensen, F.T.: The compensating curve for complete dentures, J. Prosthet. Dent. **10**:637-642, 1960.

Coble, L.G.: A complete denture technique for selecting and setting up teeth, J. Prosthet. Dent. **10**:455-458, 1960.

DeVan, M.M.: Synopsis: Stability in full denture construction, Penn. Dent. J. **22**:8-9, 1955.

Dubois, B.L.: Condylar guidance inclination changes, J. Prosthet. Dent. **16**:44-55, 1966.

Dyer, E.H.: Dental articulation and occlusion, J. Prosthet. Dent. **17**:238-246, 1967.

Gillis, R.R.: Setting up the full denture producing a balanced articulation, J. Am. Dent. Assoc. **17**:228-239, 1930.

Gosen, A.J.: Mandibular leverage and occlusion, J. Prosthet. Dent. **31**:369-376, 1974.

Gronas, D.G., and Stout, C.J.: Lineal occlusion concepts for complete dentures, J. Prosthet. Dent. **32**:122-129, 1974.

Gysi, A.: Some essentials to masticating efficiency in artificial dentures, Dent. Dig. **26**:669-678, 718-725, 1920.

Gysi, A.: Selecting a form of denture service (occlusion), Dent. Dig. **35**:73-84, 1929.

Hanau, R.L.: Articulation defined, analyzed and formulated, J. Am. Dent. Assoc. **13**:1694-1707, 1926.

Hanau, R.L.: Occlusal changes in centric relation, J. Am. Dent. Assoc. **16**:1903-1915, 1929.

Hardy, I.R., and Passamonti, G.: A method of arranging artificial teeth for class II jaw relations, J. Prosthet. Dent. **13**:606-610, 1963.

Heartwell, C.M.J.: The effect of tissue resiliency on occlusion in complete denture prosthodontics, J. Prosthet. Dent. **34**:602-604, 1975.

Hooper, B.L.: Functional factors in the selection and arrangement of artificial teeth, J. Am. Dent. Assoc. **21**:603-615, 1934.

Ismail, Y.H., and Bowman, J.F.: Position of the occlusal plane in natural and artificial teeth, J. Prosthet. Dent. **20**:407-411, 1968.

Ismail, Y.H., and Rokni, A.: Radiographic study of condylar position in centric relation and centric occlusion, J. Prosthet. Dent. **43**:327-330, 1980.

Javid, N.S.: A technique for determination of the occlusal plane, J. Prosthet. Dent. **31**:270-272, 1974.

Jones, H.S.: A method of securing the curve of Spee for complete dentures, Dent. Dig. **77**:340-343, 1971.

Jordan, L.G.: Arrangement of anatomic-type artificial teeth into balanced occlusion, J. Prosthet. Dent. **39**:484-494, 1978.

Kapur, K.K., and Soman, S.D.: Masticatory performance and efficiency in denture wearers, J. Prosthet. Dent. **14**:687-694, 1964; **15**:451-463, 662-670, 857-866, 1965.

Kurth, L.E.: Discussion of "Condylar determinants of occlusal patterns. I. Statistical report on condylar path variations. II. Condylar movements may affect the occlusal patterns of teeth," J. Prosthet. Dent. 15:847-849, 1965.

Laird, W.R.E.: Swallowing and denture occlusion, J. Prosthet. Dent. 40:614-618, 1978.

Lang, B.R., and Kelsey, C.C.: International Prosthodontic Workshop on complete denture occlusion, University of Michigan, pp. 54-88, 1973.

Lang, B.R., and Razzoog, M.E.: A practical approach to restoring occlusion for edentulous patients. I. Guiding principles of tooth selection, J. Prosthet. Dent. 50:455-458, 1983.

Lang, B.R., and Razzoog, M.E.: A practical approach to restoring occlusion for edentulous patients. II. Arranging the functional and rational mold combination, J. Prosthet. Dent. 50:599-606, 1983.

Larkin, J.D.: Means for measuring the interocclusal distance, J. Prosthet. Dent. 17:247-250, 1967.

Lauciello, F.R.: Articulator-generated amalgam stops for complete dentures, J. Prosthet. Dent. 41:16-20, 1979.

L'Estrange, P.R., and Vig, P.S.: A comparitive study of the occlusal plane in dentulous and edentulous subjects, J. Prosthet. Dent. 33:495-503, 1975.

Levin, B.: A reevaluation of Hanau's laws of articulation and the Hanau Quint, J. Prosthet. Dent. 39:254-258, 1978.

Lucia, V.O.: Principles of articulation, Dent. Clin. North Am. 23(2):199-211, 1979.

Lundquist, D.O.: Prosthetic aspects of occlusion, J. Ala. Dent. Assoc. 62(3):56-57, 1978.

Lundquist, D.O., and Luther, W.W.: Occlusal plane determination, J. Prosthet. Dent. 23:489-498, 1970.

Margarida, R.A.: Establishing individual occlusions for edentulous patients, J. Prosthet. Dent. 21:485-494, 1969.

McDonald, G.T., and Purcell, J.P.: A rational approach to occlusion for complete dentures, Quintessence Int. 8:27-29, 1977.

Mehringer, E.J.: Physiologically generated occlusion, J. Prosthet. Dent. 30:373-379, 1973.

Mjor, P.S.: The effect of the end controlling guidances of the articulator on cusp inclination, J. Prosthet. Dent. 15:1055-1075, 1965.

Mongini, F.: Anatomic and clinical evaluation of the relationship between the temporomandibular joint and occlusion, J. Prosthet. Dent. 38:539-551, 1977.

Monson, G.S.: Some important factors which influence occlusion, J. Natl. Dent. Assoc. 9:498-502, 1922.

Moses, C.H.: Tooth forms and masticatory mechanisms of natural and artificial teeth, J. Prosthet. Dent. 19:22-35, 1968.

Murphy, T.R.: Dynamic occlusion and its relation to masticatory movements in a denture wearer, Br. Dent. J. 121:359-365, 1966.

Murrell, G.A.: The problems of functional conflicts between anterior teeth, J. Prosthet. Dent. 27:591-599, 1972.

Nasr, M.F., George, W.A., Travaglini, E.A., and Scott, R.H.: The relative efficiency of different types of posterior teeth, J. Prosthet. Dent. 18:3-11, 1967.

Needles, J.W.: The mechanics of spherical articulation, J. Am. Dent. Assoc. 9:866-881, 1922.

Needles, J.W.: Practical uses of the curve of Spee, J. Am. Dent. Assoc. 10:918-927, 1923.

Needles, J.W.: The problem of articulation, J. Am. Dent. Assoc. 11:1220-1224, 1924.

Neill, D.J.: Studies of tooth contact in complete dentures, Br. Dent. J. 123:369-378, 1967.

Okeson, J.P., Dickson, J.L., and Kemper, J.T.: The influence of assisted mandibular movement on the incidence of nonworking tooth contact, J. Prosthet. Dent. 48:174-177, 1982.

Ortman, H.R.: The role of occlusion in preservation and prevention in complete denture prosthodontics, J. Prosthet. Dent. 25:121-138, 1971.

Parr, G.R., and Loft, G.H.: The occlusal spectrum and complete dentures, Compend. Contin. Educ. Dent. 3(4)241-250, 1982.

Payne, S.H.: Diagnostic factors which influence the choice of posterior occlusion, Dent. Clin. North Am. 1:203-213, 1957.

Payne, S.H.: Posterior occlusion, J. Am. Dent. Assoc. 57:174-176, 1958.

Pleasure, M.A., and Friedman, S.W.: Practical full denture occlusion, J. Am. Dent. Assoc. and Dent. Cosmos 25:1606-1617, 1938.

Ramfjord, S.P.: The significance of recent research on occlusion for the teaching and practice of dentistry, J. Prosthet. Dent. 16:96-105, 1966.

Rieder, C.E.: Occlusal considerations in preventive care, J. Prosthet. Dent. 28:462-468, 1972.

Roraff, A.R., and Stansbury, B.E.: Errors caused by dimensional change in mounting material, J. Prosthet. Dent. 28:247-252, 1972.

Schlosser, R.O.: The relation of physics and physiology to balanced occlusion, J. Am. Dent. Assoc. 15:1108-1110, 1928.

Schlosser, R.O.: Arrangement of teeth in artificial dentures in accordance with accepted laws of articulation, J. Am. Dent. Assoc. 16:1258-1265, 1929.

Schlosser, R.O.: Treatment of malocclusion and the loss of retention in full denture prosthesis, J. Am. Dent. Assoc. 20:803-815, 1933.

Schuyler, C.H.: Principles employed in full denture prosthesis which may be applied in other fields of dentistry, J. Am. Dent. Assoc. 16:2045-2054, 1929.

Schuyler, C.H.: Full denture service as influenced by our understanding of tooth selection and articulation, J. Prosthet. Dent. 2:730-736, 1952.

Sears, V.H.: Balanced occlusion, J. Am. Dent. Assoc. 12:1448-1451, 1925.

Sears, V.H.: Scientific management of factors in bilateral prosthetic occlusion, J. Am. Dent. Assoc. 37:542-553, 1948.

Sears, V.H.: Centric and eccentric occlusions, J. Prosthet. Dent. 10:1029-1036, 1960.

Shanahan, T.E.J.: The individual occlusal curvature and occlusion, J. Prosthet. Dent. **8:**230-240, 1958.

Shanahan, T.E.J., and Leff, A.: Mandibular and articulator movements. VIII. Physiologic and mechanical concepts of occlusion, J. Prosthet. Dent. **16:**62-72, 1966.

Sheppard, I.M., and Sheppard, S.M.: Denture occlusion, J. Prosthet. Dent. **26:**468-476, 1971.

Shiba, A., Hayashi, T., Yoshida, J., and Tanaka, O.: Functionally generated amalgam paths for complete dentures, J. Prosthet. Dent. **46:**494-497, 1981.

Stansbery, C.J.: Balanced occlusion in relation to lost vertical dimension, J. Am. Dent. Assoc. **25:**228-233, 1938.

Stephens, A.P.: Full dentures which occlude with natural teeth, Dent. Pract. **21:**37-42, 1970.

Trapozzano, V.R.: Tests of balanced and nonbalanced occlusions, J. Prosthet. Dent. **10:**476-487, 1960.

Trapozzano, V.R.: Laws of articulation, J. Prosthet. Dent. **13:**34-44, 1963.

Watt, D.M.: Gnathosonics in occlusal evaluation, J. Prosthet. Dent. **19:**133-143, 1968.

Watt, D.M., and Hedegård, B.: The stereostethoscope—an instrument for clinical gnathosonics, J. Prosthet. Dent. **18:**458-464, 1967.

Wipf, H.H.: Pathways to occlusion: TMJ sterographic analog and mandibular movement indicator, Dent. Clin. North Am. **23**(2):271-287, 1979.

Woda, A., Vigneron, P., and Kay, D.: Nonfunctional and functional occlusal contacts: a review of the literature, J. Prosthet Dent. **42:**335-341, 1979.

Wright, W.H.: An analysis of the "spherical theory" and comparison with "condylar adjustment" as applied to occlusion, J. Am. Dent. Assoc. **13:**911-929, 1926.

Wright, W.H.: Anatomic influences on the establishment of balanced jaw relations and balanced occlusions, J. Am. Dent. Assoc. **15:**1102-1107, 1928.

Wright, W.H.: Selection and arrangement of artificial teeth for complete prosthetic dentures, J. Am. Dent. Assoc. **23:**2291-2307, 1936.

Orientation of casts, face-bow, hinge bow, and hinge axis

Aull, A.E.: A study of the transverse axis, J. Prosthet. Dent. **13:**469-479, 1963.

Beard, C.C., and Clayton, J.A.: Studies on the validity of the terminal hinge axis, J. Prosthet. Dent. **46:**185-191, 1981.

Beck, D.B., Kass, C.A., and Knap, F.J.: Procedural problems in using the Dénar pantograph as a transfer-bow, J. Prosthet. Dent. **39:**166-168, 1978.

Beck, H.O.: Selection of an articulator and jaw registrations, J. Prosthet. Dent. **10:**878-886, 1960.

Borgh, O., and Posselt, U.: Hinge axis registration: experiments on the articulator, J. Prosthet. Dent. **8:**35-40, 1958.

Christiansen, R.L.: Rationale of the face-bow in maxillary cast mounting, J. Prosthet. Dent. **9:**388-398, 1959.

Fox, S.S.: The significance of errors in hinge axis location, J. Am. Dent. Assoc. **74:**1268-1272, 1967.

Gonzalez, J.B., and Kingery, R.H.: Evaluation of planes of reference for orienting maxillary casts on articulators, J. Am. Dent. Assoc. **76:**329-336, 1968.

Hockel, J.L.: The face bow: a primary diagnostic aid to gaining an organic occlusion, the goal of orthopedic gnathology, Int. J. Orthod. **18**(2):13-16, 1980.

Kotwal, K.R.: The need to use an arbitrary face-bow when remounting complete dentures with interocclusal records, J. Prosthet. Dent. **42:**224-227, 1979.

Lauciello, F.R., and Appelbaum, M.: Anatomic comparison to arbitrary reference notch on Hanau articulators, J. Prosthet. Dent. **40:**676-681, 1978.

Lauritzen, A.G., and Bodner, G.H.: Variations in location of arbitrary and true hinge axis points, J. Prosthet. Dent. **11:**224-229, 1961.

Loos, L.G.: One face-bow adapts to three articulators, J. Prosthet. Dent. **39:**469-472, 1978.

Lauritzen, A.G., and Wolford, L.W.: Hinge axis location on an experimental basis, J. Prosthet. Dent. **11:**1059-1067, 1961.

Long, J.H., Jr.: Location of the terminal hinge axis by intraoral means, J. Prosthet. Dent. **23:**11-24, 1970.

Loos, L.G.: One face-bow adapts to three articulators, J. Prosthet. Dent. **39:**469-472, 1978.

McCollum, B.B.: The mandibular hinge axis and a method of locating it, J. Prosthet. Dent. **10:**428-435, 1960.

Mid-States Odonto-Occlusal Symposium: Hinge axes: intercondylar versus intrafossal, J. Am. Dent. Assoc. **63:**55-60, 1961.

Moberg, C.T., Yoder, J.L., and Thayer, K.E.: The pantograph as a face-bow transfer instrument, J. Prosthet. Dent. **29:**139-145, 1973.

Preston, J.D.: A reassessment of the mandibular transverse horizontal axis theory, J. Prosthet. Dent. **41:**605-613, 1979.

Razek, M.K.A.: Clinical evaluation of methods used in locating the mandibular hinge axis, J. Prosthet. Dent. **46:**369-373, 1981.

Renner, R.P., and Lau, V.M.S.: Hinge-axis location and face-bow transfer for edentulous patients, J. Prosthet. Dent. **35:**352-356, 1976.

Sabet, E.M., and Michael, C.G.: A study on the relationship between the horizontal condylar path angle and the face-bow record, Egypt Dent. J. **25**(1):51-62, 1979.

Schwarz, W.D., and Gear, V.D.A.: Accurate location and relocation of casts on articulators, J. Prosthet. Dent. **34:**694-697, 1975.

Shanahan, T.E.J., and Leff, A.: Mandibular and articulator movements. III. The mandibular axis dilemma, J. Prosthet. Dent. **12:**292-297, 1962.

Smith, H.F.: A comparison of empirical centric relation records with location of terminal hinge axis and apex of the Gothic arch tracing, J. Prosthet. Dent. **33:**511-520, 1975.

Teo, C.S., and Wise, M.D.: Comparison of retruded axis articular mountings with and without applied muscular force, J. Oral Rehabil. **8**(4):363-376, 1981.

Thorp, E.R., Smith, D.E., and Nicholls, J.I.: Evaluation of the use of a face-bow in complete denture occlusion, J. Prosthet. Dent. **39:**5-15, 1973.

Trapozzano, V.R., and Lazzari, J.B.: A study of hinge axis determination, J. Prosthet. Dent. **11:**858-863, 1961.

Walker, P.M.: Discrepancies between arbitrary and true hinge axes, J. Prosthet. Dent. **43:**279-285, 1980.

Weinberg, L.A.: An evaluation of the face-bow mounting, J.

Prosthet. Dent. **11**:32-42, 1961.

Wilkie, N.D.: The anterior point of reference, J. Prosthet. Dent. **41**:488-496, 1979.

Winstanley, R.B.: Hinge axis location on the articulator, J. Prosthet. Dent. **42**:135-144, 1979.

Yanus, M., Finger, I.M., and Weinberg, R.: Comparison of a universal mounting jig to a face bow, J. Prosthet. Dent. **49**:623-627, 1983.

Yohn, L.K.: Skin-surface reference point for locating the condyle with teeth in centric occlusion, J. Prosthet. Dent. **31**:514-517, 1974.

Pathosis and prosthodontics

Al-Ani, S., Shklar, G., and Yurkstas, A.A.: The effect of dentures on the exfoliative cytology of palatal and buccal oral mucosa, J. Prosthet. Dent. **16**:513-521, 1966.

Arendorf, T.M., and Walter, D.M.: Oral candidal populations in health and disease, Br. Dent. J. **147**(10):267-272, 1979.

Atwood, D.A.: Reduction of residual ridges: a major oral disease entity, J. Prosthet. Dent. **26**:266-279, 1971.

Beganović, M., and Malić, M.: Efikasnost terapje kandide albikans nistatin suspenzijim kod proteznih stomatopatija [Nystatin therapy of *Candida albicans* in cases of denture stomatitis], Acta Stomatol. Croat. **8**:64-70, 1974.

Bickley, R.W., Royston, P., and Hastings, G.: Tissue reaction to acrylic resin, J. Prosthet. Dent. **35**:156-159, 1976.

Bolender, C.L., Swenson, R.D., and Yamane, G.: Evaluation of treatment of inflammatory papillary hyperplasia of the palate, J. Prosthet. Dent. **15**:1013-1022, 1965.

Bottomley, W.K., and Terezhalmy, G.T.: Management of patients with myasthenia gravis who require maxillary dentures, J. Prosthet. Dent. **38**:609-614, 1977.

Bowman, A.J., and Latham, R.A.: The differential development and structure of keratinizing mucosa, Dent. Pract. **18**:349-352, 1968.

Buchner, A., and Helft, M.: Pathologic conditions of the oral mucosa associated with ill-fitting dentures. I. Denture stomatitis, Isr. J. Dent. Med. **27**(4):5-9, 1978.

Budtz-Jørgensen, E.: Denture stomatitis. III. Histopathology of trauma- and *Candida*-induced inflammatory lesions of the palatal mucosa, Acta Odontol. Scand. **28**:551-579, 1970.

Budtz-Jørgensen, E.: The significance of *Candida albicans* in denture stomatitis, Scand. J. Dent. Res. **82**:151-190, 1974.

Budtz-Jørgensen, E., Stenderup, A., and Grabowski, M.: An epidemiologic study of yeasts in elderly denture wearers, Community Dent. Oral Epidemiol. **3**:115-119, 1975.

Budtz-Jørgensen, E.: Oral mucosal lesions associated with the wearing of removable dentures, J. Oral Pathol. **10**(2):65-80, 1981.

Cheraskin, E., and Ringsdorf, W.M., Jr.: The edentulous patient. I. Xerostomia and the serum cholesterol level, J. Am. Geriatr. Soc. **17**:962-965, 1969.

Cheraskin, E., and Ringsdorf, W.M., Jr.: The edentulous patient. II. Xerostomia and the blood sugar level, J. Am. Geriatr. Soc. **17**:966-968, 1969.

Cutright, D.E.: Morphogenesis of inflammatory papillary hyperplasia, J. Prosthet. Dent. **33**:380-385, 1975.

DePaola, L.G., Peterson, D.E., Leupold, R.J., and Overholser, C.D.: Prosthodontic considerations for patients undergoing cancer chemotherapy, J. Am. Den. Assoc. **107**:48-51, 1983.

Domb, G.H., and Chole, R.A.: The burning mouth and tongue, Ear Nose Throat J. **60**(7):310-314, 1981.

Eid, M. el-S., Abdel-Razek, M.K., and Kamer, A.A.: A study of the different types of microorganisms present under removable and fixed prosthodontics, Egypt. Dent. J. **20**:13-26, 1974.

Ettinger, R.L.: The etiology of inflammatory papillary hyperplasia, J. Prosthet. Dent. **34**:254-261, 1975.

Fairchild, J.M.: Inflammatory papillary hyperplasia of the palate, J. Prosthet. Dent. **17**:232-237, 1967.

Fregert, S., Kollander, M., and Poulsen, J.: Allergic contact stomatitis from gold dentures, Contact Dermatitis **5**(1):63-64, 1979.

Gardner, A.F.: White sponge nevus in the oral regions, J. Prosthet. Dent. **18**:39-45, 1967.

Giunta, J., and Zablotsky, N.: Allergic stomatitis caused by self-polymerization resin, Oral Surg. **41**:631-637, 1976.

Goebel, W.M., and Duquette, P.: Mycotic infections associated with complete dentures: report of three cases, J. Am. Dent. Assoc. **88**:842-844, 1974.

Jenkins, W.M., Thomas, H.C., and Mason, D.K.: Oral infections with *Candida albicans*, Scott. Med. J. **18**:192-200, 1973.

Jones, P.M.: Complete dentures and the associated soft tissues, J. Prosthet. Dent. **36**:136-149, 1976.

Kaaber, S., Thulin, H., and Nielsen, E.: Skin sensitivity to denture base materials in the burning mouth syndrome, Contact Dermatitis **5**(2)90-96, 1979.

Katberg, J.W.: Cross-contamination via the prosthodontic laboratory, J. Prosthet. Dent. **32**:412-419, 1974.

Kelly, E., and Nakamoto, R.Y.: Cleidocranial dysostosis—a prosthodontic problem, J. Prosthet. Dent. **31**:518-526, 1974.

Kiehl, R.L.: Oral fibrolipoma beneath complete mandibular denture, J. Am. Dent. Assoc. **100**(4):561-562, 1980.

King, W.H., Reid, P., and Belting, C.M.: The influence of extraction and replacement of teeth on hearing, J. Prosthet. Dent. **23**:148-153, 1970.

Lambson, G.O., and Anderson, R.R.: Palatal papillary hyperplasia, J. Prosthet. Dent. **18**:528-533, 1967.

Langer, A.: Prosthodontic failures in patients with systemic disorders, J. Oral Rehabil. **6**(1):13-19, 1979.

Larato, D.C.: Disinfection of pumice, J. Prosthet. Dent. **18**:534-535, 1967.

Lewars, P.H.: Chronic periostitis in the mandible underneath artificial dentures, Br. J. Oral Surg. **8**:264-269, 1971.

Love, W.D., Goska, F.A., and Mixson, R.J.: The etiology of mucosal inflammation associated with dentures, J. Prosthet. Dent. **18**:515-527, 1967.

Mäkilä, E.: Prevalence of angular stomatitis; correlation with composition of food and metabolism of vitamins and iron, Acta Odontol. Scand, **27**:655-680, 1969.

Markov, N.J.: Cytologic study of the effect of toothbrush physiotherapy on the edentulous ridge, J. Prosthet. Dent. **18**:122-125, 1967.

Markov, N.J.: Cytologic study of keratinization under complete dentures, J. Prosthet. Dent. **20:**8-13, 1968.

Martin, M.V., and Lamb, D.J.: Frequency of *Candida albicans* serotypes in patients with denture-induced stomatitis and in normal denture wearers, J. Clin. Pathol. **35**(8):888-891, 1982.

Masella, R.P., Dolan, C.T., and Laney, W.R.: The prevention of the growth of *Candida* on Silastic 390 soft liner for dentures, J. Prosthet. Dent. **33:**250-257, 1975.

McCabe, J.F., and Basker, R.M.: Tissue sensitivity to acrylic resin: a method of measuring the residual monomer content and its clinical application, Br. Dent. J. **140:**347-350, 1976.

McKendrick, A.J.W.: Denture stomatitis and angular cheilitis in patients receiving long-term tetracycline therapy, Br. Dent. J. **124:**412-417, 1968.

Miller, E.L.: Clinical management of denture-induced inflammations, J. Prosthet. Dent. **38:**362-365, 1977.

Nakamoto, R.Y.: Use of a saliva substitute in postradiation xerostomia, J. Prosthet. Dent. **42:**539-542, 1979.

Nater, J.P., Groenman, N.H., Wakkers-Garritsen, B.G., and Timmer, L.H.: Biologic factors in denture sore mouth syndrome, J. Prosthet. Dent. **40:**367-373, 1978.

Nortje, C.J., Farman, A.G., Thomas, C.J., and Watermeyer, G.J.J.: X-linked hypohidrotic ectodermal dysplasia—an unusual prosthetic problem, J. Prosthet. Dent. **40:**137-142, 1978.

Nyquist, G.: Study of denture sore mouth; an investigation of traumatic, allergic and toxic lesions of the oral mucosa arising from the use of full dentures, Acta Odontol. Scand. **10**(supp. 9):11-154, 1952.

Nyquist, G.: Influence of denture hygiene and the bacterial flora on the condition of the oral mucosa in full denture casts, Acta Odontol. Scand. **11:**24-60, 1953.

Olsen, I.: Denture stomatitis. Relapse tendency and removal of acquired discolorations in long-term denture disinfection with chlorhexidine, Acta Odontol. Scand. **33:**111-114, 1975.

Olsen, I., and Birkeland, J.M.: Denture stomatitis—yeast occurrence and the pH of saliva and denture plaque, Scand. J. Dent. Res. **85:**130-134, 1977.

Perry, H.T., Jr.: The symptomology of temporomandibular joint disturbance, J. Prosthet. Dent. **19:**288-298, 1968.

Phillips, J.D., and Shawkat, A.H.: Prosthetic implications of Eagle's syndrome, J. Prosthet. Dent. **34:**614-619, 1975.

Robinson, H.B.G.: Diagnosis of lesions associated with dentures, J. Prosthet. Dent. **7:**338-340, 1957.

Russotto, S.B.: The role of *Candida albicans* in the pathogenesis of angular cheilosis, J. Prosthet. Dent. **44:**243-246, 1980.

Samaranayake, L.P., McCourtie, J., and MacFarlane, T.W.: Factors affecting the in-vitro adherence of *Candida albicans* to acrylic surfaces, Arch Oral Biol. **25**(8-9):611-615, 1980.

Schabel, R.W.: Diagnosis of sickle-cell anemia in the prosthetic patient, J. Prosthet. Dent. **20:**116-119, 1968.

Scher, E.A., Ritchie, G.M., and Flowers, D.J.: Antimycotic denture adhesive in treatment of denture stomatitis, J. Prosthet. Dent. **40:**622-627, 1978.

Schneider, S.S., and Roistacher, S.: Aspiration of denture base materials, J. Prosthet. Dent. **25:**493-496, 1971.

Sela, M., and Taicher, S.: Intraoral radiation carrier for edentulous patients, J. Prosthet. Dent. **50:**815-817, 1983.

Sharp, G.S., and Fister, W.: The etiology and treatment of the sore mouth, J. Prosthet. Dent. **16:**855-860, 1966.

Stern, M.A., and Whitacre, R.J.: Avoiding cross-contamination in prosthodontics, J. Prosthet. Dent. **46:**120-122, 1981.

Sutcher, H.D., Beatty, R.A., and Underwood, R.B.: Orofacial dyskinesia: effective prosthetic therapy, J. Prosthet. Dent. **30:**252-262, 1973.

Tolentino, A.T.: Prosthetic management of patients with pemphigus vulgaris, J. Prosthet. Dent. **38:**254-260, 1977.

Tucker, K.M., and Heget, H.S.: The incidence of inflammatory papillary hyperplasia, J. Am. Dent. Assoc. **93:**610-613, 1976.

Turrell, A.J.W.: Vertical dimension as it relates to the etiology of angular cheilosis, J. Prosthet. Dent. **19:**119-125, 1968.

Wakefield, C.W.: Laboratory contamination of dental prostheses, J. Prosthet. Dent. **44:**143-146, 1980.

Wakkers-Garritsen, B.G., Timmer, L.H., and Nater, J.P.: Etiological factors in the denture sore mouth syndrome: an investigation of 24 patients, Contact Dermatitis **1:**337, 1975.

Walker, D.M., Stafford, G.D., Huggett, R., et al.: The treatment of denture-induced stomatitis: evaluation of two agents, Br. Dent. J. **151**(12):416-419, 1981.

Welker, W.A.: Prosthodontic treatment of abused oral tissues, J. Prosthet. Dent. **37:**259-263, 1977.

Woodward, J.D., Smith, J.R., and Beck, H.O.: Osteopetrosis—prosthodontic treatment, J. Prosthet. Dent. **35:**608-614, 1976.

Wooten, J.W., Tarsitano, J.J., and LaVere, A.M.: Oral psoriasiform lesions: a possible prosthodontic complication, J. Prosthet. Dent. **24:**145-147, 1970.

Zakhari, K.N., and McMurry, W.S.: Denture stomatitis and methods influencing its cure, J. Prosthet. Dent. **37:**133-140, 1977.

Phonetics

Agnello, J.G., and Wictorin, L.: A study of phonetic changes in edentulous patients following complete denture treatment, J. Prosthet. Dent. **27:**133-139, 1972.

Chierici, G., and Lawson, L.: Clinical speech considerations in prosthodontics: perspectives of the prosthodontist and speech pathologist, J. Prosthet. Dent. **29:**29-39, 1973.

Ghi, H., and McGivney, G.P.: Influence of tooth proprioception on speech articulation, J. Prosthet. Dent. **42:**609-613, 1979.

Goyal, B.K., and Greenstein, P.: Functional contouring of the palatal vault for improving speech with complete dentures, J. Prosthet. Dent. **48:**640-646, 1982.

Hansen, C.A.: Phonetic considerations of chromium alloy palates for complete dentures, J. Prosthet. Dent. **34:**620-624, 1975.

Harley, W.T.: Dynamic palatography—a study of linguopalatal contacts during the production of selected consonant sounds, J. Prosthet. Dent. **27:**364-376, 1972.

Lauciello, F.R., Vergo, T., Schaaf, N.G., and Zimmerman, R.: Prosthodontic and speech rehabilitation after partial and complete glossectomy, J. Prosthet. Dent. **43**:204-211, 1980.

Levy, T.P.: Speech and complete dentures, Dalhousie Dent. J. **11**:13-18, 1971.

Martone, A.L., and Black, J.W.: An approach to prosthodontics through speech science. IV. Physiology of speech, J. Prosthet. Dent. **12**:409-419, 1962.

Martone, A.L., and Black, J.W.: An approach to prosthodontics through speech science, V. Speech science research of prosthodontic significance, J. Prosthet. Dent. **12**:629-636, 1962.

Matsuki, N.: Speech disorders in complete denture wearers. I. Subjective disorders, J. Jpn. Stomatol. Soc. **38**:252-265, 1971.

Murrell, G.A.: Phonetics, function, and anterior occlusion, J. Prosthet. Dent. **32**:23-31, 1974.

Palmer, J.M.: Analysis of speech in prosthodontic practice, J. Prosthet. Dent. **31**:605-614, 1974.

Palmer, J.M.: Structural changes for speech improvement in complete upper denture fabrication, J. Prosthet. Dent. **41**:507-510, 1979.

Pound, E.: Controlling anomalies of vertical dimension and speech, J. Prosthet. Dent. **36**:124-135, 1976.

Pound, E.: Let /S/ be your guide, J. Prosthet. Dent. **38**:482-489, 1977.

Pound, E.: The mandibular movements of speech and their seven related values, J. Prosthet. Dent. **16**:835-843, 1966.

Pound, E.: Utilizing speech to simplify a personalized denture service, J. Prosthet. Dent. **24**:586-600, 1970.

Pound, E.: Utilizing speech to simplify a personalized denture service, J. South. Calif. Dent. Assoc. **38**:1020-1029, 1970.

Reichenbach, E.: Interrelations between speech disorders and stomatology, Int. Dent. J. **16**:296-303, 1966.

Shaffer, F.W., and Kutz, R.A.: Phonetics and swallowing to determine palatal contours of dentures, J. Prosthet. Dent. **28**:360-362, 1972.

Sherman, H.: Phonetic capability as a function of vertical dimension in complete denture wearers—a preliminary report, J. Prosthet. Dent. **23**:621-632, 1970.

Silverman, M.M.: The whistle and swish sound in denture patients, J. Prosthet. Dent. **17**:144-148, 1967.

Tanaka, H.: Speech patterns of edentulous patients and morphology of the palate in relation to phonetics, J. Prosthet. Dent. **29**:16-28, 1973.

Tench, R.W.: The influence of speech habits on the design of full artificial dentures, J. Am. Dent. Assoc. **14**:644-647, 1927.

Tobey, E.A., and Finger, I.M.: Active versus passive adaptation: an acoustic study of vowels produced with and without dentures, J. Prosthet. Dent. **49**:314-320, 1983.

Physiology of mastication

Anderson, E.L.: Eating patterns before and after dentures, J. Am. Diet. Assoc. **58**:421-426, 1971.

Atkinson, H.F., and Faulkner, K.D.: A reexamination of mandibular movement using a closed circuit television detector, Aust. Dent. J. **26**(6):390-394, 1981.

Atkinson, H.F., and Shepherd, R.W.: Masticatory movement in the absence of teeth in man, Arch. Oral Biol. **18**:855-860, 1973.

Edlund, J., and Lamm, C.J.: Masticatory efficiency, J. Oral Rehabil. **7**(2):123-130, 1980.

Ettinger, R.L.: Diet, nutrition, and masticatory ability in a group of elderly edentulous patients, Aust. Dent. J. **18**:12-19, 1973.

Feldman, E.F.: Tooth contacts in denture occlusion—centric occlusion only, Dent. Clin. North Am. **15**:875-887, 1971.

Gillbe, G.V.: The function of the disc of the temporomandibular joint, J. Prosthet. Dent. **33**:196-204, 1975.

Henkin, R.I., and Christiansen, R.L.: Taste thresholds in patients with dentures, J. Am. Dent. Assoc. **75**:118-120, 1967.

Hickey, J.C., Woelfel, J.B., Allison, M.L., and Boucher, C.O.: Influence of occlusal schemes on the muscular activity of edentulous patients, J. Prosthet. Dent. **13**:444-451, 1963.

Ingervall, B., and Carlsson, G.E.: Masticatory muscle activity before and after elimination of balancing side occlusal interference, J. Oral Rehabil. **9**(3):183-192, 1982.

Jankelson, B.: Neuromuscular aspects of occlusion: effects of occlusal position on the physiology and dysfunction of the mandibular musculature, Dent. Clin. North Am. **23**(2):157-168, 1979.

Jemt, T.: Chewing patterns in dentate and complete denture wearers—recorded by light-emitting diodes, Swed. Dent. J. **5**(5-6):199-205, 1981.

Jemt, T.: Positions of the mandible during chewing and swallowing recorded by light-emitting diodes, J. Prosthet. Dent. **48**:206-209, 1982.

Jemt, T., and Hedegård, B.: The relative movements of the chin and the mandible during chewing, J. Oral Rehabil. **9**(3):253-258, 1982.

Jemt, T., and Karlsson, S.: Computer-analysed movements in three dimensions recorded by light-emitting diodes: a study of methodological errors and of evaluation of chewing behaviour in a group of young adults, J. Oral Rehabil. **9**(4):317-326, 1982.

Juniper, R.P.: The superior pterygoid muscle? Br. J. Oral Surg. **19**(2):121-128, 1981.

Kapur, K.K., Collister, T., and Fischer, E.E.: Masticatory and gustatory salivary reflex secretion rates and taste thresholds of denture wearers, J. Prosthet. Dent. **18**:406-416, 1967.

Kelly, E.K.: Factors affecting the masticatory performance of complete denture wearers, J. Prosthet. Dent. **33**:122-136, 1975.

Lehr, R.P., Jr., and Owens, S.E., Jr.: An electromyographic study of the human lateral pterygoid muscles, Anat. Rec. **196**(4):441-448, 1980.

Lewin, A., and Nickel, B.: The full description of jaw movement, J. Dent. Assoc. S. Afr. **33**(5):261-267, 1978.

Mehringer, E.J.: Function of steep cusps in mastication of complete dentures, J. Prosthet. Dent. **30**:367-372, 1973.

Moses, C.H.: Studies of wear, arrangement and occlusion of the dentitions of humans and animals and their relationship to orthodontia, periodontia, and prosthodontia, Dent. Items Int. **68**:953-999, 1946.

Moses, C.H.: Biologic emphasis in prosthodontics, J. Prosthet. Dent. **12**:695-710, 1962.

Mushimoto, E., and Mitani, H.: Bilateral coordination pattern of masticatory muscle activities during chewing in normal subjects, J. Prosthet. Dent. **48**:191-197, 1982.

Neill, D.J., and Phillips, H.I.: The masticatory performance and dietary intake of elderly edentulous patients, Dent. Pract. **22**:384-389, 1972.

Pameijer, J.H.N., Brion, M., Glickman, I., and Roeber, F.W.: Intraoral occlusal telemetry. V. Effect of occlusal adjustment upon tooth contacts during chewing and swallowing, J. Prosthet. Dent. **24**:492-497, 1970.

Posselt, U.: Discussion of "The human temporomandibular joint: kinematics and actions of the masticatory muscles" by Johan Ulrich, J. Prosthet. Dent. **9**:407-408, 1959.

Rissin, L., House, J.E., Manly, R.S., and Kapur, K.K.: Clinical comparison of masticatory performance and electromyographic activity of patients with complete dentures, overdentures, and natural teeth, J. Prosthet. Dent. **39**:508-511, 1978.

Schmid, F.R., and Ogata, R.I.: The composition and examination of synovial fluid, J. Prosthet. Dent. **18**:449-457, 1967.

Schweitzer, J.M.: Masticatory function in man; mandibular repositioning, J. Prosthet. Dent. **12**:262-291, 1962.

Sessle, B.J., and Hannam, A.G.: Mastication and swallowing, biological and clinical correlates, Toronto, 1976, University of Toronto Press.

Sheppard, I.M.: The closing masticatory strokes, J. Prosthet. Dent. **9**:946-951, 1959.

Sheppard, I.M., and Markus, N.: Total time of tooth contacts during mastication, J. Prosthet. Dent. **12**:460-463, 1962.

Sheppard, I.M, and Sheppard, S.M.: Bolus placement during mastication, J. Prosthet. Dent. **20**:506-510, 1968.

Van Scotter, D.E., and Boucher, L.J.: The effect of denture base materials on the stratum corneum, J. Prosthet. Dent. **15**:45-53, 1965.

Wayler, A.H., and Chauncey, H.H.: Impact of complete dentures and impaired natural dentition on masticatory performance and food choice in healthy aging men, J. Prosthet. Dent. **49**:427-433, 1983.

Wictorin, L., Hedegård, B., and Lundberg, M.: Cineradiographic studies of bolus position during chewing, J. Prosthet. Dent. **26**:236-246, 1971.

Wood, G.D.: Recording the opening and closing cycle of the mandible, Br. Dent. J. **146**(10): 305-309, 1979.

Yaeger, J.A.: Mandibular path in the grinding phase of mastication—a review, J. Prosthet. Dent. **39**:569-573, 1978.

Yurkstas, A.A.: The masticatory act; a review, J. Prosthet. Dent. **15**:248-262, 1965.

Zarb, G.A.: Oral motor patterns and their relation to oral prostheses, J. Prosthet. Dent. **47**:472-478, 1982.

Postinsertion instructions and care of dentures

Bauman, R.: Inflammatory papillary hyperplasia and home-care instructions to denture patients, J. Prosthet. Dent. **37**:608-609, 1977.

Brill, N., Tryde, G., and Schüber, S.: The role of learning in denture retention, J. Prosthet. Dent. **10**:468-475, 1960.

Council on Dental Health: Guidelines on after care for denture patients, J. Am. Dent. Assoc. **94**:1187, 1977.

Friedman, S.: Diagnosis, treatment planning, trouble shooting the edentulous patient, N.Y. J. Dent. **41**:238-250, 1971.

Goldstein, G.R., Soni, A., and Broner, A.: Insertion procedures for complete dentures, N.Y. State Dent. J. **48**(6):371-373, 1982.

Gronas, D.G.: Preparation of pressure-indicator paste, J. Prosthet. Dent. **37**:92-94, 1977.

Kovats, J.J.: Clinical evaluation of the gagging denture patient, J. Prosthet. Dent. **25**:613-619, 1971.

Landa, J.S.: Trouble shooting in complete denture prosthesis. I. Oral mucosa and border extension, J. Prosthet. Dent. **9**:978-987, 1959.

Landa, J.S.: Trouble shooting in complete denture prosthesis. II. Lesions of the oral mucosa and their correction, J. Prosthet. Dent. **10**:42-46, 1960.

Landa, J.S.: Trouble shooting in complete denture prosthesis. III. Traumatic injuries, J. Prosthet. Dent. **10**:263-269, 1960.

Landa, J.S.: Trouble shooting in complete denture prosthesis. IV. Proper adjustment procedures, J. Prosthet. Dent. **10**:490-495, 1960.

Landa, J.S.: Trouble shooting in complete denture prosthesis. V. Local and systemic involvement, J. Prosthet. Dent. **10**:682-687, 1960.

Landa, J.S.: Trouble shooting in complete denture prosthesis. VI. Factors of oral hygiene, chemicotoxicity, nutrition, allergy, and conductivity, J. Prosthet. Dent. **10**:887-890, 1960.

Landa, J.S.: Trouble shooting in complete denture prosthesis. VII. Mucosal irritations, J. Prosthet. Dent. **10**:1022-1028, 1960.

Landa, J.S.: Trouble shooting in complete denture prosthesis. VIII. Interferences with anatomic structures, J. Prosthet. Dent. **11**:79-83, 1961.

Landa, J.S.: Trouble shooting in complete denture prosthesis. IX. Salivation, stomatopyrosis, and glossopyrosis, J. Prosthet. Dent. **11**:244-246, 1961.

Landa, J.S.: Trouble shooting in complete denture prosthesis. X. Nerve impingement and the radiolucent lower anterior ridge, J. Prosthet. Dent. **11**:440-444, 1961.

Lees, G.H.: Pressure-indicating paste: 2 simple formulas, N.Z. Dent. J. **68**:238-239, 1972.

Lutes, M.R., et al.: Denture modification during adjustment phase of complete denture service, J. Prosthet. Dent. **28**:572-579, 1972.

Means, C.R., and Flenniken, I.E.: Gagging—a problem in prosthetic dentistry, J. Prosthet. Dent. **23**:614-620, 1970.

Michman, J., and Langer, A.: Postinsertion changes in complete dentures, J. Prosthet. Dent. **34**:125-134, 1975.

Morstad, A.T., and Petersen, A.D.: Postinsertion denture problems, J. Prosthet. Dent. **19**:126-132, 1968.

Naylor, J.G.: What the patient should know about complete dentures, J. Prosthet. Dent. **9**:832-840, 1959.

Ortman, L.F.: Patient education and complete denture maintenance, Dent. Clin. North Am. **21**:359-367, 1977.

Perry, C.: Printed literature for denture patients, J. Am. Dent. Assoc. **64**:552-554, 1962.

Sherman, H.: Denture insertion, Dent. Clin. North Am. **21**:339-357, 1977.

Singer, I.L.: The marble technique: a method for treating the "hopeless gagger" for complete dentures, J. Prosthet. Dent. **29**:146-150, 1973.

Stephens, A.P.: Points prosthetic, IX. Fitting full dentures, J. Irish Dent. Assoc. **16**:26-28, 1970.

Tautin, F.S.: Should dentures be worn continuously? J. Prosthet. Dent. **39**:372-374, 1978.

Woelfel, J.B., and Paffenbarger, G.D.: Pressure-indicator paste patterns in duplicate dentures made by different processing technics for the same patient, J. Am. Dent. Assoc. **70**:339-343, 1965.

Pre-extraction records

Aboul-Ela, L.M., and Razek, M.K.A.: Pre-extraction records of the occlusal place and vertical dimension, J. Prosthet. Dent. **38**:490-493, 1977.

Bennett, D.T., and Smales, F.C.: Oriented study models, Dent. Pract. **18**:353-355, 1968.

Bliss, C.H.: Three-dimensional photography in prosthodontics, J. Prosthet. Dent. **9**:708-716, 1959.

Heintz, W.D., and Peters, G.W.: Esthetic occlusion rims providing for jaw relations, J. Prosthet. Dent. **9**:587-593, 1959.

LaVere, A.M., and Freda, A.L.: A simplified procedure for survey and design of diagnostic casts, J. Prosthet. Dent. **37**:680-683, 1977.

Smith, D.E.: The reliability of pre-extraction records for complete dentures, J. Prosthet. Dent. **25**:592-608, 1971.

Turner, L.C.: The profile tracer: method for obtaining accurate pre-extraction records, J. Prosthet. Dent. **21**:364-370, 1969.

Processing techniques and denture-base finishing

Becker, C.M., Smith, D.E., and Nicholls, J.I.: The comparison of denture-base processing techniques. I. Materials characteristics, J. Prosthet. Dent. **37**:330-338, 1977.

Becker, C.M., Smith, D.E., and Nicholls, J.I.: The comparison of denture-base processing techniques. II. Dimensional changes due to processing. J. Prosthet. Dent. **37**:450-459, 1977.

Choudhary, S.C., Craig, J.F., and Suls, F.J.: Characterizing the denture base for noncaucasian patients, J. Prosthet. Dent. **33**:73-79, 1975.

Dukes, B.S., Fields, H., Morris, J.C., and Jewell, A.: A comparative study of changes in vertical dimension of occlusion using different investing mediums, J. Prosthet. Dent. **49**:568-571, 1983.

Firtell, D.N., Green, A.J., and Elahi, J.M.: Posterior peripheral seal distortion related to processing temperature, J. Prosthet. Dent. **45**:598-601, 1981.

Fairhurst, C.W., and Ryge, G.: Effect of tinfoil substitutes on the strength of denture base resins, J. Prosthet. Dent. **5**:508-513, 1955.

Garfunkel, E.: Evaluation of dimensional changes in complete dentures processed by injection-pressing and the pack-and-press technique, J. Prosthet. Dent. **50**:757-761, 1983.

Gay, W.D., and King, G.E.: An evaluation of the cure of acrylic resin by three methods, J. Prosthet. Dent. **42**:437-440, 1979.

Hardy, F.: Comparison of fluid resin and compression molding methods in processing dimensional changes, J. Prosthet. Dent. **39**:375-377, 1978.

Heath, J.R., and Basker, R.M.: The dimensional variability of duplicate dentures produced in an alginate investment, Br. Dent. J. **144**:111-114, 1978.

Le Pera, F.: Avoiding the increase of the vertical dimension of dentures in processing, J. Prosthet. Dent. **19**:364-369, 1968.

Lerner, H., and Pfeiffer, K.R.: Minimum vertical occlusal changes in cured acrylic resin dentures, J. Prosthet. Dent. **14**:294-297, 1964.

Marcroft, K.R., Tencate, R.L., and Hurst, W.W.: Use of a layered silicone rubber mold technique for denture processing, J. Prosthet. Dent. **11**:657-664, 1961.

Mercer, R.W., DuFort, C.R., Kramer, D.C., and Welker, W.A.: Cast ejector, J. Prosthet. Dent. **37**:95-97, 1977.

Oliva, R.A., and Lowe, J.A.: Denture flasking: a comparative study of three techniques, J. Prosthet. Dent. **48**:736-739, 1982.

Peyton, F.A., and Anthony, D.H.: Evaluation of dentures processed by different techniques, J. Prosthet. Dent. **13**:269-282, 1963.

Renner, R.P., and Blakeslee, R.W.: Basic wax contouring for complete dentures, J. Prosthet. Dent. **40**:343-348, 1978.

Shepard, W.L.: Denture bases processed from a fluid resin, J. Prosthet. Dent. **19**:561-572, 1968.

Starcke, E.N., Jr.: The contours of polished surfaces of complete dentures: a review of the literature, J. Am. Dent. Assoc. **81**:155-160, 1970.

Vig, R.G.: Method of reducing the shifting of teeth in denture processing, J. Prosthet. Dent. **33**:80-84, 1975.

Welker, W.A., Kramer, D.C., and Mercer, R.W.: A technique for finishing and polishing denture bases, J. Prosthet. Dent. **39**:240-241, 1978.

Wesley, R.C., et al.: Processing changes in complete dentures: posterior tooth contacts and pin opening, J. Prosthet. Dent. **29**:46-54, 1973.

Wictorin, L., and Agnello, J.: Speech pattern changes during edentulous and denture conditions. I. Palatographic study, Acta Odontol. Scand. **28**:729-737, 1970.

Winkler, S., et al.: Processing changes in complete dentures constructed from pour resins, J. Am. Dent. Assoc. **82**:349-353, 1971.

Zakhari, K.N.: Relationship of investing medium to occlusal changes and vertical opening during denture construction, J. Prosthet. Dent. **36**:501-509, 1976.

Zani, D., and Vieira, D.F.: A comparative study of silicone as a separating medium for denture processing, J. Prosthet. Dent. **42**(4):386-391, 1979.

Zani, D., and Vieira, D.F.: A comparative study of silicone as a separating medium for denture processing, J. Prosthet. Dent. **42**:386-391, 1979.

Psychologic aspects of denture service

Ament, P., and Ament, A.: Body image in dentistry, J. Prosthet. Dent. **24**:362-366, 1970.

Barone, J.V.: Nutrition—phase one of the edentulous patient, J. Prosthet. Dent. **40**:122-126, 1978.

Baseheart, J.R.: Nonverbal communication in the dentist-patient relationship, J. Prosthet. Dent. **34**:4-10, 1975.

Bliss, C.H.: Psychologic factors involved in presenting denture service, J. Prosthet. Dent. **1**:49-63, 1951.

Carlsson, G.E., Otterland, A., and Wennström, A.: Patient factors in appreciation of complete dentures, J. Prosthet. Dent. **17**:322-328, 1967.

Cheney, H.G.: Effect of patient behavior and personality on treatment planning, Dent. Clin. North Am. **21**:531-538, 1977.

Collett, H.A.: Motivation: a factor in denture treatment, J. Prosthet. Dent. **17**:5-15, 1967.

Collett, H.A., and Briggs, D.L.: Some psychosomatic considerations in prosthetic dentistry, J. Prosthet. Dent. **5**:361-367, 1955.

DeVan, M.M.: Physical, biological and psychological factors to be considered in the construction of dentures, J. Am. Dent. Assoc. **42**:290-293, 1951.

Giddon, D.B.: Psychologic aspects of prosthodontic treatment for geriatric patients, J. Prosthet. Dent. **43**:374-379, 1980.

Grieder, A.: Psychologic aspects of prosthodontics, J. Prosthet. Dent. **30**:736-744, 1973.

Guckes, A.D., Smith, D.E., and Swoope, C.C.: Counseling and related factors influencing satisfaction with dentures, J. Prosthet. Dent. **39**:259-267, 1978.

Heartwell, C.M., Jr.: Educating patients to accept dentures, J. Prosthet. Dent. **21**:574-579, 1969.

Heartwell, C.M., Jr.: Psychologic considerations in complete denture prosthodontics, J. Prosthet. Dent. **24**:5-10, 1970.

Hirsch, B., Levin, B., and Tiber, N.: Effects of patient involvement and esthetic preference on denture acceptance, J. Prosthet. Dent. **28**:127-132, 1972.

Hirsch, B., Levin, B., and Tiber, N.: Effects of dentist authoritarianism on patient evaluation of dentures, J. Prosthet. Dent. **30**:745-748, 1973.

Koper, A.: Difficult denture birds, J. Prosthet. Dent. **17**:532-539, 1967.

Krol, A.J.: A new approach to the gagging problem, J. Prosthet. Dent. **13**:611-616, 1963.

Lowental, U., and Tau, S.: Effects of ethnic origin, age, and bereavement on complete denture patients, J. Prosthet. Dent. **44**:133-136, 1980.

Michman, J., and Langer, A.: Clinical and electromyographic observations during adjustment to complete dentures, J. Prosthet. Dent. **19**:252-262, 1968.

Nassif, J.: A self-administered questionnaire—an aid in managing complete denture patients, J. Prosthet. Dent. **40**:363-366, 1978.

Newton, A.V.: The difficult denture patient: a review of psychological aspects, Br. Dent. J. **138**:93-97, 1975.

Oral Health Committee of the Federation of Prosthodontic Organizations: Add youth to your smile by prosthodontics, J. Prosthet. Dent. **21**:570-573, 1969.

Plainfield, S.: Communication distortion: the language of patients and practitioners of dentistry, J. Prosthet. Dent. **22**:11-19, 1969.

Pound, E.: Achieving patient acceptance to immediate denture service, J. Am. Dent. Assoc. **66**:795-802, 1963.

Psychological Aspects of Treating Denture Patients. Highlights of a symposium held at Northwestern University, April 24, 1974, Morris Plains, N.J., 1974, Professional Relations Department, Warner-Lambert Co.

Ramsey, W.O.: The relation of emotional factors to prosthodontic service, J. Prosthet. Dent. **23**:4-10, 1970.

Savage, R.D., and MacGregor, A.R.: Behavior therapy in prosthodontics, J. Prosthet. Dent. **24**:126-132, 1970.

Schabel, R.W.: Patient education with prosthetic acrylic resin models, J. Prosthet. Dent. **17**:104-108, 1965.

Schabel, R.W.: Dentist-patient communication—a major factor in treatment prognosis, J. Prosthet. Dent. **21**:3-5, 1969.

Schuyler, C.H.: Nausea complicating the full denture problem, J. Dent. Soc. N.Y. **10**:43-45, 1944.

Silverman, S., Silverman, S.I., Silverman, B., and Garfinkel, L.: Self-image and its relation to denture acceptance, J. Prosthet. Dent. **35**:131-141, 1976.

Smith, M.: Measurement of personality traits and their relation to patient satisfaction with complete dentures, J. Prosthet. Dent. **35**:492-503, 1976.

Straus, R., Sandifer, J.C., Hall, D.S., and Haley, J.V.: Behavioral factors and denture status, J. Prosthet. Dent. **37**:264-273, 1977.

Swenson, M.G.: Neglected factor in denture service, J. Prosthet. Dent. **1**:71-77, 1951.

Swoope, C.C.: The try-in-a-time for communication, Dent. Clin. North Am. **14**:479-491, 1970.

Tau, S., and Lowental, U.: Some personality determinants of denture preference, J. Prosthet. Dent. **44**:10-12, 1980.

Rebasing and relining

Barco, M.T., Jr., Moore, B.K., Swartz, M.L., et al.: The effect of relining on the accuracy and stability of maxillary complete dentures—an in vitro and in vivo study, J. Prosthet. Dent. **42**(1):17-22, 1979.

Bell, D.H., Jr.: Clinical evaluation of a resilient denture liner, J. Prosthet. Dent. **23**:394-406, 1970.

Body, L.H.: Relining immediate dentures utilizing cephalometrics, J. Prosthet. Dent. **11**:864-872, 1961.

Bowman, J.F., and Javid, N.S.: Relining and rebasing techniques, Dent. Clin. North Am. **21**:369-378, 1977.

Burton, J.F.: Rebasing mandibular full dentures using a visco-elastic impression material, N.Z. Dent. J. **76**(344):70-73, 1980.

Christensen, F.T.: Relining techniques for complete dentures, J. Prosthet. Dent. **26**:373-381, 1971.

Feldman, E.E., Morrow, R.M., and Jameson, W.S.: Relining complete dentures with an oral cure silicone elastomer and a duplicate denture, J. Prosthet. Dent. **23**:387-393, 1970.

Friedman, S.: Rebasing the complete maxillary denture, N.Y. State Dent. J. **40**:19-22, 1974.

George, J.P., and Boone, M.E.: A clinical study of rest position using the Kinesiograph and Myomonitor, J. Prosthet. Dent. **41**:456-462, 1979.

Hardy, I.R.: Rebasing the maxillary denture, Dent. Dig. **55**:23-27, 1949.

Hooper, B.L.: Rebasing or duplicating dentures: a method of restoring facial contour and correcting faulty retention, Dent. Dig. **38**:206-213, 1932.

Levin, B.: A reliable reline-rebase technique, J. Prosthet. Dent. 36:219-225, 1976.

McCartney, J.W.: The complete denture reline: a simplified technique, J. Prosthet. Dent. 45:564-567, 1981.

Ortman, H.R., and Ortman, L.F.: Denture refitting with today's concepts and materials, Dent. Clin. North Am. 19:269-290, 1975.

Ostrem, C.T.: Relining complete dentures, J. Prosthet. Dent. 11:204-213, 1961.

Payne, S.H.: Denture base materials and the refitting of dentures, J. Am. Dent. Assoc. 49:562-566, 1954.

Schlosser, R.O.: Consideration of some of the main factors contributing to the development of maximum efficiency and to the prolongation of the service life of complete immediate dentures, J. Prosthet. Dent. 5:452-464, 1955.

Sears, V.H.: Functional impressions for rebasing full dentures, J. Am. Dent. Assoc. 23:1031-1035, 1936.

Shaffer, F.W., and Filler, W.H.: Relining complete dentures with minimum occlusal error, J. Prosthet. Dent. 25:366-370, 1971.

Shannon, J.L.: Use of the remount jig as an aid in relining upper dentures, J. Prosthet. Dent. 34:393-396, 1975.

Smith, D.E., Lord, J.L., and Bolender, C.L.: Complete denture relines with autopolymerizing acrylic resin processed in water under air pressure, J. Prosthet. Dent. 18:103-115, 1967.

Tautin, F.S.: Home reliners—where we have failed, J. Prosthet. Dent. 25:19-20, 1971.

Terrell, W.H.: Relines, rebases, or transfers and repairs, J. Prosthet. Dent. 1:244-253, 1951; Aust. Dent. J. 55:359-368, 1951.

Terry, J.M., Lutes, M., and Ellinger, C.: Do-it-yourself denture reline materials: a Contourator study, J. Prosthet. Dent. 18:31-38, 1967.

Tucker, K.M.: Relining complete dentures with the use of a functional impression, J. Prosthet. Dent. 16:1054-1057, 1966.

Repairs and duplication

Beyli, M.S., and von Fraunhofer, J.A.: Repair of fractured acrylic resin, J. Prosthet. Dent. 44:497-503, 1980.

Bolouri, A., and Bell, J.D.: The use of intraoral cores to repair complete and partial removable prostheses, J. Prosthet. Dent. 36:472-475, 1976.

Chamberlain, J.B., and Basket, R.M.: A method of duplicating dentures, Br. Dent. J. 122:347-349, 1967.

Chan, K.C., and Boyer, D.B.: Repair of conventional and microfilled composite resins, J. Prosthet. Dent. 50:345-350, 1983.

Cooper, J.S., and Watkinson, A.C.: Duplication of full dentures, Br. Dent. J. 141:344-348, 1976.

Davies, N.R.: A practical spare denture, CDT Dig. 1:4-6, 1970.

Halperin, A.R., Abadi, B.J., and Halperin, G.C.: Repair of broken dentures in resin undercuts, J. Prosthet. Dent. 44:224-228, 1980.

Hoyle, D.E.: Immediate stabilization of a broken maxillary denture, J. Prosthet. Dent. 50:289-292, 1983.

Jochen, D.G., and Caputo, A.A.: Composite resin repair of procelain denture teeth, J. Prosthet. Dent. 38:673-679, 1977.

Koudelka, B.M., Nelson, J.F., and Webb, J.G., Jr.: Denture self-repair: experimental soft tissue response to selected commercial adhesives, J. Prosthet. Dent. 43(2):143-148, 1980.

Marcroft, K.R.: Fabrication of identical duplicate dentures, J. Am. Dent. Assoc. 64:476-481, 1962.

Singer, I.L.: The "zipper" technique for duplicating dentures: final impressions replica dentures and a complete denture splint, J. Prosthet. Dent. 33:582-590, 1975.

Thomson, H.: Duplication of complete dentures, Dent. Pract. 17:173-175, 1967.

Research

Antonopoulos, A.: Making complete dentures for research purposes, J. Prosthet. Dent. 37:349-355, 1977.

Appleby, R.C., and Ludwig, T.F.: Patient evaluation for complete denture therapy, J. Prosthet. Dent. 24:11-17, 1970.

Atwood, D.A.: A critique of research of the rest position of the mandible, J. Prosthet. Dent. 16:848-854, 1966.

Atwood, D.A.: A critique of research of the posterior limit of the mandibular position, J. Prosthet. Dent. 20:21-36, 1968.

Atwood, D.A., and Coy, W.A.: Clinical, cephalometric, and densitometric study of reduction of residual ridges, J. Prosthet. Dent. 26:280-295, 1971.

Bando, E., Fukushima, S., Kawabata, H., and Kohno, S.: Continuous observations of mandibular positions by telemetry, J. Prosthet. Dent. 28:485-490, 1972.

Bearn, E.M.: A preliminary report on a hydraulic measuring device for the study of forces transmitted by dentures, Dent. Pract. 22:17-20, 1973.

Bergman, B., and Carlsson, G.E.: Review of 54 complete denture patients' opinions 1 year after treatment, Acta Odontol. Scand. 30:399-414, 1972.

Bernstein, P.R., McCall, W.C., Mohl, N.D., Bishop, B., and Uthman, A.A.: The effect of voluntary activity on the masseteric silence period duration, J. Prosthet. Dent. 46:192-195, 1981.

Bessette, R.W., and Quinlivan, J.T.: Electromyographic evaluation of the Myo-monitor, J. Prosthet. Dent. 30:19-24, 1973.

Blanchet, L.J., Bowman, D.C., and McReynolds, H.D.: Effects of methyl methacrylate monomer vapors on respiration and circulation in unanesthetized rats, J. Prosthet. Dent. 48:344-348, 1982.

Brehm, T.W., and Abadi, B.J.: Patient response to variations in complete denture technique. IV. Residual ridge resorption-cast evaluation, J. Prosthet. Dent. 44:491-494, 1980.

Coccaro, P.J., and Lloyd, R.: Cephalometric analysis of morphologic face height, J. Prosthet. Dent. 15:35-44, 1965.

Craig, R.G., Farah, J.W., and El-Tahawi, H.M.: Three-dimensional photoelastic stress analysis of maxillary complete dentures, J. Prosthet. Dent. 31:122-129, 1974.

De Boever, J.A., McCall, W.D., Jr., Holden, S., and Ash, M.M., Jr.: Functional occlusal forces: an investigation by telemetry, J. Prosthet. Dent. 40:326-333, 1978.

Deeley, R.A.: The effect of protein versus placebo supplementation upon denture tolerance, J. Prosthet. Dent. **15:**65-72, 1965.

DeFurio, A., and Gehl, D.H.: Clinical study of the retention of maxillary complete dentures with different base materials, J. Prosthet. Dent. **23:**374-380, 1970.

Didbin, G.H., and Griffiths, M.J.: An intra-oral telemetry system for the continuous recording of vertical jaw movement, Phys. Med. Biol. **20:**355-365, 1975.

Ellinger, C.W., Somes, G.W., Nicol, B.R., Unger, J.W., and Wesley, R.C.: Patient response to variations in denture technique. III. Five-year subjective evaluation, J. Prosthet. Dent. **42:**127-130, 1979.

Feingold, R.M., Ward, N., and Murphy, A.: Ability to function with full dentures, natural dentition, and no dentition, J. Conn. State. Dent. Assoc. **48:**267-269, 1974.

Fernström, A.I., Oquist, G., and Söremark, R.: Location of the allergenic monomer in warm-polymerized acrylic dentures. III. Testing of the theory of an 'allergenic film' in the vestibular surface before polishing, Swed. Dent. J. **6**(2):87-91, 1982.

Fleisch, L., and Austin, J.C.: A histologic study of the response of masticatory and lining mucosa to mechanical loading in the vervet monkey, J. Prosthet. Dent. **39:**211-216, 1978.

Frazier, Q.Z., et al.: The relative repeatability of plaster interocclusal eccentric records for articulator adjustment in construction of complete dentures, J. Prosthet. Dent. **26:**456-467, 1971.

Furuya, R., and Hedegård, B.: The silent period in the masseter and the anterior temporal muscles at repeated registrations, J. Oral Rehabil. **8**(5):377-387, 1981.

Gabay, E.L.: Flow rate, sodium and potassium concentration in mixed saliva of complete denture-wearers, J. Oral Rehabil. **7**(6):435-443, 1980.

Gates, G.N., and Nicholls, J.I.: Evaluation of mandibular arch width change, J. Prosthet. Dent. **46:**385-392, 1981.

Gillings, B.R.D.: Photoelectric mandibulography: a technique for studying jaw movements, J. Prosthet. Dent. **17:**109-121, 1967.

Goodkind, R.J., and Heringlake, C.B.: Mandibular flexure in opening and closing movements, J. Prosthet. Dent. **30:**134-138, 1973.

Grasso, J.E., and Catalanatto, E.A.: The effects of age and full palatal coverage on oral stereognostic ability, J. Prosthet. Dent. **41:**215-219, 1979.

Hairston, L.E., and Blanton, P.L.: An electromyographic study of mandibular position in response to changes in body position, J. Prosthet. Dent. **49:**271-273, 1983.

Harrison, A.: Clinical results of the measurement of occlusal wear of complete dentures, J. Prosthet. Dent. **35:**504-511, 1976.

Hellsing, G., and Klineberg, I.: The masseter muscle: the silent period and its clinical implications, J. Prosthet. Dent. **49:**106-112, 1983.

Hickey, J.C., Henderson, D., and Straus, R.: Patient response to variations in denture technique. I. Design of a study, J. Prosthet. Dent. **22:**158-170, 1969.

Hiniker, J.J., and Ramfjord, S.P.: Anterior displacement of the mandible in adult rhesus monkeys, J. Prosthet. Dent. **16:**503-512, 1966.

Hobo, S., and Mochizuki, S.: A kinematic investigation of mandibular border movement by means of an electronic measuring system. I. Development of the measuring system, J. Prosthet. Dent. **50:**368-373, 1983.

Holt, J.E.: Research on remounting procedures, J. Prosthet. Dent. **38:**338-341, 1977.

Ingervall, B., and Hedegård, B.: An electromyographic study of masticatory and lip muscle function in patients with complete dentures, J. Prosthet. Dent. **43:**266-271, 1980.

Ismail, Y.H.: Changes in soft-tissue profile following extraction and complete denture treatment, J. Prosthet. Dent. **26:**11-20, 1971.

Jankelson, B., Sparks, S., Crane, P.F., and Radke, J.C.: Neural conduction of the Myo-monitor stimulus: a quantitative analysis, J. Prosthet. Dent. **34:**245-253, 1975.

Jemt, T., Hedegård, B., and Wickberg, K.: Chewing patterns before and after treatment with complete maxillary and bilateral distal-extension mandibular removable partial dentures, J. Prosthet. Dent. **50:**566-570, 1983.

Johns, L.D., Boone, M.E., and House, J.E.: Use of in vitro test method as applied to denture surface identification, J. Prosthet. Dent. **33:**454-457, 1975.

Józefowicz, W.: The influence of wearing dentures on residual ridges: a comparative study, J. Prosthet. Dent. **24:**137-144, 1970.

Kapur, K.K.: Studies of biologic parameters for denture design. I. Comparison of masseter muscle activity during chewing of crisp and soggy wafers in denture and dentition groups, J. Prosthet. Dent. **33:**242-249, 1975.

Kapur, K.K., and Fischer, E.E.: Effect of denture base thermal conductivity on gustatory response, J. Prosthet. Dent. **46:**603-609, 1981.

Kapur, K.K., Soman, S., and Yurkstas, A.: Test foods for measuring masticatory performance of denture wearers, J. Prosthet. Dent. **14:**483-491, 1964.

Kydd, W.L., Harrold, W., and Smith, D.E.: A technique for continuously monitoring the interocclusal distance, J. Prosthet. Dent. **18:**308-310, 1967.

Lestrel, P.E., Kapur, K.K., and Chauncey, H.H.: A cephalometric study of mandibular cortical bone thickness in dentulous persons and denture wearers, J. Prosthet. Dent. **43:**89-94, 1980.

Levin, B., Gamer, S., and Francis, E.D.: Patient preference for a mandibular complete denture with a broad or minimal base: a preliminary report, J. Prosthet. Dent. **23:**525-528, 1970.

Lindholm, K., Hakala, P.E., and Mäkilä, E.: Leukocyte count and keratinization of the palatal denture-bearing mucosa, J. Prosthet. Dent. **47:**440-444, 1982.

McCall, W.D., Jr., Tallgren, A., and Ash, M.M., Jr.: EMG silent periods in immediate denture patients: a longitudinal study, J. Dent. Res. **58**(12):2353-2359, 1979.

Maeda, R., Stoltz, K., User, A., et al.: Mucosal temperature rises following long-term use of full dentures, J. Oral Rehabil. **6**(3):273-278, 1979.

Mäkilä, E.: Primary oral status and adaptation to complete dentures. A clinical follow-up study of groups over and under 65 years, Ann. Acad. Sci. Fenn. **164:**1-29, 1974.

Martin, J.S., Digioia, W.J., Werley, M.S., et al.: Inhibitory effects of inhaled methyl methacrylate vapor on amphibian skeletal muscle, J. Dent. Res. 60(6):1028-1030, 1981.

McCall, W.D., Jr., De Boever, J.A., and Ash, M.M., Jr.: Telemetry system to study functional occlusal forces, J. Prosthet. Dent. 40:98-102, 1978.

Messerman, T.: A means for studying mandibular movements, J. Prosthet. Dent. 17:36-43, 1967.

Moini, M.R., McCall, W.D., Jr., and Mohl, N.D.: Jaw muscle silent periods: the effect of acrylic splints, J. Dent. Res. 59(4):683-688, 1980.

Mushimoto, E.: The role in masseter muscle activities of functionally elicited periodontal afferents from abutment teeth under overdentures, J. Oral Rehabil. 8(5):441-455, 1981.

Nedelman, C.I.: The effect of injected silicones upon the tissues of animals, J. Prosthet. Dent. 23:25-35, 1970.

Neill, D.J., and Roberts, B.J.: The effect of denture fixatives on masticatory performance in complete denture patients, J. Dent. 1:219-222, 1973.

Nicol, B.R., Somes, G.W., Ellinger, C.W., Unger, J.W., and Fuhrmann, J.: Patient response to variations in denture technique. II. Five-year cephalometric evaluation, J. Prosthet. Dent. 41:368-372, 1979.

Nilsson, B.: Taste acuity of the human palate. II. Studies with electrogustometry on subjects in different age groups, Acta Odontol. Scand. 37(4):217-234, 1979.

Nilsson, B.: Taste acuity of the human palate. III. Studies with taste solutions on subjects in different age groups, Acta Odontol. Scand. 37(4):235-252, 1979.

Okane, H., Yamashina, T., Nagasawa, T., and Tsuru, H.: The effect of anteroposterior inclination of the occlusal plane on biting force, J. Prosthet. Dent. 42:497-501, 1979.

Peavy, D.C., Jr., and Kendrick, G.S.: The effects of tooth movement on the palatine rugae, J. Prosthet. Dent. 18:536-542, 1967.

Perry, H.T.: Application of cephalometric radiographs for prosthodontics, J. Prosthet. Dent. 31:254-261, 1974.

Pietrokovski, J., and Massler, M.: Residual ridge remodeling after tooth extraction in monkeys, J. Prosthet. Dent. 26:119-129, 1971.

Ramfjord, S.P., and Hiniker, J.J.: Distal displacement of the mandible in adult rhesus monkeys, J. Prosthet. Dent. 16:491-502, 1966.

Rayson, J.H., et al.: The value of subjective evaluation in clinical research, J. Prosthet. Dent. 26:111-118, 1971.

Reitz, P.V., et al.: A cephalometric study of tooth position as related to facial structure in profiles of human beings: a comparison of Japanese (Oriental) and American (Caucasian) adults, J. Prosthet. Dent. 29:157-166, 1973.

Rissin, L., House, J.E., Manly, R.S., and Kapur, K.K.: Clinical comparison of masticatory performance and electromyographic activity of patients with complete dentures, overdentures, and natural teeth, J. Prosthet. Dent. 39:508-511, 1978.

Sabes, W.R., Ellinger, C.W., Tucker, S.R., Grant, S., Unger, J.W., and Fuhrman, J.: Patient response to variations in denture technique. IV. Microscopic response of the oral mucosa, J. Prosthet. Dent. 45:11-13, 1981.

Setcos, J.C., Vrijhoef, M.M.A., Blumershine, R., and Phillips, R.W.: Airborne particles from alginate powders, J. Am. Dent. Assoc. 106:355-358, 1983.

Shannon, I.L., Terry, J.M., and Nakamoto, R.Y.: Palatal coverage and parotid flow rate, J. Prosthet. Dent. 24:601-607, 1970.

Sheppard, I.M., Schwartz, L.R., and Sheppard, S.M.: Survey of the oral status of complete denture patients, J. Prosthet. Dent. 28:121-126, 1972.

Sheppard, S.M., and Sheppard, I.M.: Incidence of lateral excursions during function with complete dentures, J. Prosthet. Dent. 26:258-265, 1971.

Shiba, A., Yoshida, J., Nakao, M., Sano, K., Cho, H., and Hayashi, T.: Sodium dodecyl sulfate electrophoretic analysis of the protein in palatine saliva, J. Prosthet. Dent. 47:246-251, 1982.

Silverman, S.I.: Dimensions and displacement patterns of the posterior palatal seal, J. Prosthet. Dent. 25:470-488, 1971.

Stafford, G.D., and Griffiths, D.W.: Investigation of the strain produced in maxillary complete dentures in function, J. Oral Rehabil. 6(3):241-256, 1979.

Swerdlow, H.: Roentgencephalometric study of vertical dimension changes in immediate denture patients, J. Prosthet. Dent. 14:635-650, 1964.

Tallgren, A.: Positional changes of complete dentures; a 7 year longitudinal study, Acta Odontol. Scand. 27:539-561, 1969.

Tallgren, A.: Alveolar bone loss in denture wearers as related to facial morphology, Acta Odontol. Scand. 28:251-270, 1970.

Tallgren, A.: The continuing reduction of the residual alveolar ridges in complete denture wearers: a mixed-longitudinal study covering 25 years, J. Prosthet. Dent. 27:120-132, 1972.

Tallgren, A., Holden, S., Lang, B.R., et al.: Jaw muscle activity in complete denture wearers—a longitudinal electromyographic study, J. Prosthet. Dent. 44(2):123-132, 1980.

Tallgren, A., Lang, B.R., Walker, G.F., and Ash, M.M.: Changes in jaw relations, hyoid position, and head posture in complete denture wearers, J. Prosthet. Dent. 50:148-156, 1983.

Vitti, M., and Basmajian, J.V.: Integrated actions of masticatory muscles: simultaneous EMG from eight intramuscular electrodes, Anat. Rec. 187:173-189, 1977.

Wessberg, G.A., Epker, B.N., and Elliott, A.C.: Comparison of mandibular rest positions induced by phonetics, transcutaneous electrical stimulation, and masticatory electromyography, J. Prosthet. Dent. 49:100-105, 1983.

Wescott, W.B.: Current and future considerations for a geriatric population, J. Prosthet. Dent. 49:113-120, 1983.

Wipf, H.H.: Pathways to occlusion: TMJ stereographic analog and mandibular movement indicator, Dent. Clin. North Am. 23(2):271-287, 1979.

Woelfel, J.B., Winter, C.M., and Igarashi, T.: Five-year cephalometric study of mandibular ridge resorption with different posterior occlusal forms. I. Denture construction and initial comparison, J. Prosthet. Dent. 36:602-623, 1976.

Wood, G.D., and Williams, J.E.: Gnathodynamometers: measuring opening and closing forces, Dent. Update 8(4):239-241, 243, 246-247 passim, 1981.

Yarmand, M.A., and Gehl, D.H.: Laboratory and clinical study on a permanent type base for transferring interocclusal records, J. Prosthet. Dent. 25:497-505, 1971.

Young, J.M.: A study of the accuracy of the apposition of palatal tissues to complete dentures, J. Prosthet. Dent. 23:136-147, 1970.

Resilient liners in dentures

Allison, R.T., and Douglas, W.H.: Micro-colonization of the denture-fitting surface by *Candida albicans*, J. Dent. 1:198-201, 1973.

Battersby, B.J., Gehl, D.H., and O'Brien, W.J.: Effect of an elastic lining on the retention of dentures, J. Prosthet. Dent. 20:498-505, 1968.

Bauman, R.: Chairside modification of dentures for tissue conditioning materials, J. Prosthet. Dent. 40:225-226, 1978.

Bláhová, Z., and Neumann, M.: Retention of complete dentures lined with soft-curing resins, J. Prosthet. Dent. 25:371-374, 1971.

Duran, R.L., Powers, J.M., and Craig, R.G.: Viscoelastic and dynamic properties of soft liners and tissue conditioners, J. Dent. Res. 58(8):1801-1807, 1979.

Ellis, B., Lamb, D.J., and McDonald, M.P.: A study of the composition and diffusion characteristics of a soft liner, J. Dent. 7(2):133-140, 1979.

Ellis, B., Lamb, D.J., and Al-Nakash, S.: Variations in the elastic modulus of a soft lining material, Br. Dent. J. 149(3):79-82, 1980.

Goll, G., Smith, D.E., and Plein, J.B.: The effect of denture cleansers on temporary soft liners, J. Prosthet. Dent. 50:466-472, 1983.

Harris, W.T., and Mack, J.F.: Conditioning dentures for problem patients, J. Prosthet. Dent. 34:141-144, 1975.

Harrison, A.: Temporary soft lining materials: a review of their uses, Br. Dent. J. 151(12):419-422, 1981.

Klinger, S.M., and Lord, J.L.: Effect of common agents on intermediary temporary soft reline materials, J. Prosthet. Dent. 30:749-755, 1973.

Lewis, A.J.: The nature and mode of action of tissue conditioners, Northwest Dent. 57(1):20-22, 1978.

McCarthy, J.A., and Moser, J.B.: Mechanical properties of tissue conditioners. I. Theoretical considerations, behavioral characteristics, and tensile properties, J. Prosthet. Dent. 40:89-97, 1978.

McCarthy, J.A., and Moser, J.B.: Mechanical properties of tissue conditioners. II. Creep characteristics, J. Prosthet. Dent. 40:334-342, 1978.

McCarthy, J.A., and Moser, J.B.: Tissue conditioners as functional impression materials, J. Oral Rehabil. 5(4):357-364, 1978.

Mäkilä, E., and Honka, O.: Clinical study of heat-cured silicone soft lining material, J. Oral Rehabil. 6(2):199-204, 1979.

Parker, S., and Braden, M.: New soft lining materials, J. Dent. 10(2):149-153, 1982.

Rantanen, T., and Lindholm, K.: Two new tissue conditioners and their ability to reproduce undercuts, Proc. Finn. Dent. Soc. 69:105-109, 1973.

Razek, M.K.A., and Mohamed, Z.M.: Influence of tissue-conditioning materials on the oral bacteriologic status of complete denture wearers, J. Prosthet. Dent. 44:137-142, 1980.

Razek, M.K.A.: Assessment of tissue conditioning materials for functional impressions, J. Prosthet. Dent. 42:376-380, 1979.

Reisbick, M.H.: Silicone as a denture mold liner, J. Prosthet. Dent. 26:382-386, 1971.

Schmidt, W.F., and Smith, D.E.: A six-year retrospective study of Molloplast-B-lined dentures. I. Patient response, J. Prosthet. Dent. 50:308-313, 1983.

Schmidt, W.F., and Smith, D.E.: A six-year study of Molloplast-B-lined dentures. II. Liner serviceability, J. Prosthet. Dent. 50:459-465, 1983.

Tassarotti, B.: A clinical and histologic evaluation of a conditioning material, J. Prosthet. Dent. 28:13-18, 1972.

Von Krammer, K.R.: Tissue conditions, J. Prosthet. Dent. 25:244-250, 1971.

Ward, J.E.: Effect of time lapse between mixing and loading on the flow of tissue conditioning materials, J. Prosthet. Dent. 40:499-508, 1978.

Williamson, J.J.: The effect of denture lining materials on the growth of *Candida albicans*, Br. Dent. J. 125:106-110, 1968.

Woelfel, J.B., and Paffenbarger, G.D.: Evaluation of complete dentures lined with resilient silicone rubber, J. Am. Dent. Assoc. 76:582-590, 1968.

Wright, P.S.: Characterization of the rupture properties of denture soft lining materials, J. Dent. Res. 59(3):614-619, 1980.

Wright, P.S.: Characterization of the adhesion of soft lining materials to poly(methyl methacrylate), J. Dent. Res. 61(8):1002-1005, 1982.

Single dentures

Bruce, R.W.: Complete dentures opposing natural teeth, J. Prosthet. Dent. 26:448-455, 1971.

Ellinger, C.W., Rayson, J.H., and Henderson, D.: Single complete dentures, J. Prosthet. Dent. 26:4-10, 1971.

Rudd, K.D., and Morrow, R.M.: Occlusion and the single denture, J. Prosthet. Dent. 30:4-10, 1973.

Stansbury, C.B.: Single denture construction against a nonmodified natural dentition, Aust. J. Dent. 57:79-83, 1953.

Surgical preparation of mouth for dentures

Amphlett, J., and Colwell, W.C.: Edentulous vestibuloplasty using the palatal graft technique, J. Prosthet. Dent. 48:8-14, 1982.

Axinn, S., and Brasher, W.J.: Frenectomy plus free graft, J. Prosthet. Dent. 50:16-19, 1983.

Bell, R.A., and Richardson, A.: Prosthodontic treatment of pendulous maxillary tuberosities, J. Am. Dent. Assoc. 103(6):894-895, 1981.

Bergendal, T., Heimdahl, A., and Isacsson, G.: Surgery in the treatment of denture-related inflammatory papillary hyperplasia of the palate, Int. J. Oral Surg. 9(4):312-319, 1980.

Bolender, C.L., and Swenson, R.D.: Cephalometric evaluation of a labial vestibular extension procedure, J. Prosthet. Dent. 13:416-431, 1963.

Curtis, T.A., and Ware, W.H.: Autogenous bone graft procedures for atrophic edentulous mandibles, J. Prosthet. Dent. 38:366-379, 1977.

Firtell, D.N., Oatis, G.W., Curtis, T.A., and Sugg, W.E., Jr.: A stent for a split-thickness graft vestibuloplasty, J. Prosthet. Dent. 36:204-210, 1976.

Fisher, S.J.: Preprosthetic surgery, J. Can. Dent. Assoc. 41:297-299, 1975.

Friedlander, A.H., and Renner, R.P.: Selective resection of the circumoral musculature for enhancement of mandibular denture stability, J. Prosthet. Dent. 37:602-607, 1977.

Glogoff, M., and Baum, S.M.: Vestibular preparation for dentures, J. Mercer Dent. Soc. 27:14-16, 1973.

Groetsema, W.R.: Interpositional bone grafts to augment the atrophic mandible, J. Prosthet. Dent. 50:618-622, 1983.

Gross, B.D., James, R.B., and Fister, J.: Use of pocket inlay grafts and tuberoplasty in maxillary prosthetic construction, J. Prosthet. Dent. 43(6):649-653, 1980.

Hamacher, E.N., and Fredrickson, E.J.: A dynamic flap and grooved denture technique for mandibular dentures, J. Prosthet. Dent. 19:460-464, 1968.

Heartwell, C.M., Jr., and Peters, P.B.: Surgical and prosthodontic management of atrophied edentulous jaws. II. The surgical and prosthodontic treatment, J. Prosthet. Dent. 16:621-635, 1966.

Held, A.J.: Oral vestibular surgery in periodontal or prosthetic treatment, Dent. Pract. 16:195-202, 1966.

Hopkins, R., and Stafford, G.D.: Experience of preprosthetic surgery on the atrophic edentulous mandible, Br. Dent. J. 137:341-346, 1974.

Jones, P.M., and Nakayama, L.K.: Surgical experiences of complete denture patients, J. Prosthet. Dent. 18:12-18, 1967.

Landesman, H.M., and Levin, B.: A patient survey of denture tolerance before and after a mandibular vestibuloplasty with skin grafting, J. Am. Dent. Assoc. 90:806-810, 1975.

Langer, B., and Calagna, L.: The alteration of lingual mucosa with free gingival grafts: protection of a denture bearing surface, J. Periodontol. 49(12):646-648, 1978.

Laskin, D.M.: A sclerosing procedure for hypermobile edentulous ridges, J. Prosthet. Dent. 23:274-278, 1970.

Linenberg, W.B.: Surgical preparation of the mouth for immediate dentures, J. Prosthet. Dent. 13:95-101, 1963.

MacEntee, M.I., Goldstein, B.M., and Price, C.: Submucosal root retention: a two-year clinical observation, J. Prosthet. Dent. 47:483-487, 1982.

Masella, R., and Mercier, P.: Surgical and prosthodontic reconstruction of the severely handicapped edentulous patient, J. Prosthet. Dent. 50:377-383, 1983.

Meister, M., Jr., Van Swol, R.L., Rank, D.F., et al.: Utilizing the free gingival graft for edentulous ridge augmentation, Greater Milw. Dent. Bull. 48(3):64-68, 1981.

Miller, E.L.: Sometimes overlooked: pre-prosthetic surgery, J. Prosthet. Dent. 36:484-490, 1976.

Mitchener, R.W.: Vertical space for denture bases—without surgery, J. Prosthet. Dent. 47:354-355, 1982.

Murray, C.G., and Adkins, K.F.: The elective retention of vital roots for alveolar bone preservation: a pilot study, J. Oral Surg. 37(9):650-656, 1979.

Nery, E.B., Lynch, K.L., and Rooney, G.E.: Alveolar ridge augmentation with tricalcium phosphate ceramic, J. Prosthet. Dent. 40:668-674, 1978.

Ogle, R.E.: Preprosthetic surgery, Dent. Clin. North Am. 21:219-236, 1977.

Phillips, H., Brown, A., and Prusin, W.S.: Maxillary and mandibular vestibuloplasty for improved denture retention, J. Can. Dent. Assoc. 41:569-571, 1975.

Prowler, J.R.: Ridge extension technique combined with skin graft, J. Prosthet. Dent. 17:343-349, 1967.

Roberts, B.J.: The efficiency of the mylohyoid ridge resection in improving success with the complete lower denture: a clinical assessment, Br. Dent. J. 142:151-155, 1977.

Roberts, B.J.: Mylohyoid ridge reductions as an aid to success in complete lower dentures, J. Prosthet. Dent. 37:486-493, 1977.

Sanders, B., and Beumer, J.: Augmentation rib grafting to the inferior border of the atrophic edentulous mandible: a 5-year experience, J. Prosthet. Dent. 47:16-22, 1982.

Schwartz, W.D.: Prosthetic treatment of patients after bone grafting procedures, Br. J. Oral Surg. 20(1):45-52, 1982.

Strain, F.E.: Bone obstacles to successful lower dentures and their surgical elimination, J. Prosthet. Dent. 17:333-342, 1967.

Stratigos, G.T., Cassara, A., and Birnbaum, M.: Reverse visor osteotomy for augmentation of the atrophic edentulous mandible, J. Oral Maxillofac. Surg. 40(4):231-233, 1982.

Stuller, C.B., and Schaberg, S.J.: Use of the segmented LeFort I osteotomy to correct severe extrusion of maxillary posterior teeth or tuberosities, J. Prosthet. Dent. 50:157-163, 1983.

Tortorelli, A.F.: A technique for vestibular sulcus extension, J. Prosthet. Dent. 20:14-20, 1968.

Walsh, J.P.: Surgical preparation of the mouth for dentures, N.Z. Dent. J. 42:172-177, 1946.

Wilkie, N.D.: The role of the prosthodontist in preposthetic surgery, J. Prosthet. Dent. 33:386-397, 1975.

Taste perception and oral tactility

Hammond, R., Beder, O.E., and Ratener, P.E.: Palatal receptor contribution to and effects of palatal alteration on taste acuity thresholds, J. Prosthet. Dent. 49:121-125, 1983.

Murphy, W.M.: The effect of complete dentures on taste perception, Br. Dent. J. 130:201-205, 1971.

Murphy, W.M., Morris, R.A., and O'Sullivan, D.C.: Effect of oral prosthesis upon texture perception of food, Br. Dent. J. 137:245-249, 1974.

Owall, B.: Oral tactility during chewing. III. Denture wearers, Odontol. Revy 25:255-271, 1974.

Temporomandibular joint disturbances

Bessette, R.W., Mohl, N.D., and DiCosimo, C.J., 2d.: Comparison of results of electromyographic and radiographic examinations in patients with myofascial pain-dysfunction syndrome, J. Am. Dent. Assoc. **89**:1358-1364, 1974.

Bohl, C.F., and Knap, F.J.: Evaluating occlusal relationships, mandibular dysfunction, and temporomandibular joint pain by palpation, J. Prosthet. Dent. **32**:80-86, 1974.

Bottger, H.: Prosthetic measures with reference to temporomandibular joint and the masticatory pathway, Dtsch. Zahnaerztl. Z. **102**:84-86, 1977.

Carlsson, G.E.: Symptoms of mandibular dysfunction in complete denture wearers, J. Dent. **4**:265-270, 1976.

Caryle, L.W., 3rd., and Richardson, J.T.: Temporomandibular joint syndrome in edentulous subjects, Tex. Dent. J. **99**(2):15-16, 1982.

Choy, E., and Smith, D.E.: The prevalence of temporomandibular joint disturbances in complete denture patients, J. Oral Rehabil. **7**(4):331-352, 1980.

Costen, J.B.: Correlation of x-ray findings in the mandibular joint with clinical signs, especially trismus, J. Am. Dent. Assoc. **26**:405-407, 1939.

Farrar, W.B.: Characteristics of the condylar path in internal derangements of the TMJ, J. Prosthet. Dent. **39**:319-323, 1978.

Farrar, W.B., and McCarty, W.L., Jr.: The TMJ dilemma, J. Ala. Dent. Assoc. **63**(1):19-26, 1979.

Freese, A.S.: Temporomandibular joint pain: etiology, symptomatology, and diagnosis, J. Prosthet. Dent. **10**:1078-1085, 1960.

Gelb, H.: Evaluation of static centric relation in the temporomandibular joint dysfunction syndrome, Dent. Clin. North Am. **19**:519-530, 1975.

Gelb, H., and Bernstein, I.: Clinical evaluation of two hundred patients with temporomandibular joint syndrome, J. Prosthet. Dent. **49**:234-243, 1983.

Goharian, R.K., and Neff, P.A.: Effect of occlusal retainers on temporomandibular joint and facial pain, J. Prosthet. Dent. **44**(2): 206-208, 1980.

Goodfriend, D.J.: The role of dental factors in the cause and treatment of ear symptoms and disease, Dent. Cosmos **78**:1292-1310, 1936.

Grandos, J.I.: The influence of the loss of teeth and attrition on the articular eminence, J. Prosthet. Dent. **42**:78-85, 1979.

Greene, C.S., and Laskin, D.M.: Long-term evaluation of conservative treatment for myofascial pain-dysfunction syndrome, J. Am. Dent. Assoc. **89**:1365-1368, 1974.

Helöe, B., Heiberg, A.N., and Krogstad, B.S.: A multiprofessional study of patients with myofascial pain-dysfunction syndrome. I. Acta Odontol. Scand. **38**(2):109-117, 1980.

Hilloowala, R.A.: The temporomandibular joint—a diginglymus joint, J. Prosthet. Dent. **33**:328-332, 1975.

Iroshnikova, E.S.: Prosthodontic treatment of patients with limited opening ability of the mouth, Stomatologiia (Mosk.) **53**:55-57, 1974.

Kelly, H.T., and Goodfriend, D.J.: Medical significance of equilibration of the masticating mechanism, J. Prosthet. Dent. **10**:496-515, 1960.

Kopp, S., and Rockler, B.: Relationship between clinical and radiographic findings in patients with mandibular pain or dysfunction, Acta Radiol. (Diagn.) (Stockh.) **20**(3):465-477, 1979.

Kopp, S.: Short term evaluation of counselling and occlusal adjustment in patients with mandibular dysfunction involving the temporomandibular joint, J. Oral Rehabil. **6**(2):101-109, 1979.

Kotani, H., Kawazoe, Y., Hamada, T., and Yamada, S.: Quantitative electromyographic diagnosis of myofascial pain-dysfunction syndrome, J. Prosthet. Dent. **43**:450-456, 1980.

Kovaleski, W.C., III, and DeBoever, J.: Influence of occlusal splints on jaw position and musculature in patients with temporomandibular joint dysfunction, J. Prosthet. Dent. **33**:321-327, 1975.

Lerman, M.D.: A complete hydrostatically derived treatment procedure for the TMJ pain-dysfunction syndrome, J. Am. Dent. Assoc. **89**:1351-1357, 1974.

Lerman, M.D.: The hydrostatic appliance: a new approach to treatment of the TMJ pain-dysfunction, J. Am. Dent. Assoc. **89**:1343-1350, 1974.

Lous, I.: Treatment of TMJ syndrome by pivots, J. Prosthet. Dent. **40**:179-182, 1978.

McCall, W.D., Uthman, A.A., and Mohl, N.D.: TMJ symptom severity and EMG silent periods, J. Dent. Res. **57**(5-6):709-714, 1978.

Magnusson, T.: Prevalence of recurrent headache and mandibular dysfunction in patients with unsatisfactory complete dentures, Community Dental Oral Epidemiol. **8**(3):159-164, 1980.

Magnusson, T.J.: Change in recurrent headache and mandibular dysfunction after treatment with new complete dentures, J. Oral Rehabil. **9**(2):95-105, 1982.

Manns, A., Miralles, R., Santander, H., and Valdivia, J.: Influence of the vertical dimension in the treatment of myofascial pain-dysfunction syndrome, J. Prosthet. Dent. **50**:700-709, 1983.

Ouellette, P.L.: TMJ sound prints: electronic auscultation and sonagraphic audiospectral analysis of the temporomandibular joint, J. Am. Dent. Assoc. **89**:623-628, 1974.

Pinto, O.F.: A new structure related to the temporomandibular joint and middle ear, J. Prosthet. Dent. **12**:95-103, 1962.

Rieder, C.E.: Comparison of the efficacy of a questionnaire, oral history, and clinical examination in detecting signs and symptoms of occlusal and temporomandibular joint dysfunction, J. Prosthet. Dent. **38**:433-440, 1977.

Rieder, C.E.: The prevalence and magnitude of mandibular displacement in a survey population, J. Prosthet. Dent. **39**:324-329, 1978.

Rieder, C.E.: Maximum mandibular opening in patients with and without a history of TMJ dysfunction, J. Prosthet. Dent. **39**:441-446, 1978.

Rieder, C.E.: The frequency of parafunctional occlusal habits compared with the incidence of mandibular displacement, J. Prosthet. Dent. **40**:75-82, 1978.

Rieder, C.E., Martinoff, J.T., and Wilcox, S.A.: The prevalence of mandibular dysfunction. I. Sex and age distribution of related signs and symptoms, J. Prosthet. Dent.
50:81-88, 1983.

Rieder, C.E., and Martinoff, J.T.: The prevalence of mandibular dysfunction. II. A multiphasic dysfunction profile,
J. Prosthet. Dent. **50:**237-244, 1983.

Roura, N., and Clayton, J.A.: Pantographic records on TMJ
dysfunction subjects treated with occlusal splints: a
progress report, J. Prosthet. Dent. **33:**442-453, 1975.

Rozencweig, D., and Martin, G.: Selective tomography of
the TMJ and the myofacial pain-dysfunction syndrome, J.
Prosthet. Dent. **40:**67-74, 1978.

Sheppard, I.M., and Sheppard, S.M.: Characteristics of
temporomandibular joint problems, J. Prosthet. Dent.
38:180-191, 1977.

Shields, J.M., Clayton, J.A., and Sindledecker, L.D.: Using
pantographic tracings to detect TMJ and muscle dysfunc-
tions, J. Prosthet. Dent. **39:**80-87, 1978.

Shore, N.A.: Recognition and recording of symptoms of
temporomandibular joint dysfunction, J. Am. Dent.
Assoc. **66:**19-23, 1963.

Simonet, P.F.: Influence of TMJ dysfunction on Bennett
movement as recorded by a modified pantograph. I. Literature review, J. Prosthet. Dent. **46:**437-442, 1981.

Standlee, J.P., Caputo, A.A., and Ralph, J.P.: The condyle
as a stress-distributing component of the temporomandibular joint, J. Oral Rehabil. **8**(5):391-400, 1981.

Travell, J.: Temporomandibular joint pain referred from
muscles of the head and neck, J. Prosthet. Dent. **10:**745-
763, 1960.

Vaughan, H.C.: External facial symptoms resulting from
indirect trauma in and about the infratemporal fossa, J.
Prosthet. Dent. **12:**486-492, 1962.

Weinberg, L.A.: Temporomandibular joint function and its
effect on concepts of occlusion, J. Prosthet. Dent. **35:**553-
566, 1976.

Weinberg, L.A.: An evaluation of stress in temporomandibular joint dysfunction-pain syndrome, J. Prosthet. Dent.
38:192-207, 1977.

Weinberg, L.A.: Treatment prostheses in TMJ dysfunction-
pain syndrome, J. Prosthet. Dent. **39:**654-669, 1978.

Weinberg, L.A.: An evaluation of occlusal factors in TMJ
dysfunction-pain syndrome, J. Prosthet. Dent. **41:**198-
208, 1979.

Weinberg, L.A.: Role of condylar position in TMJ dysfunction-pain syndrome, J. Prosthet. Dent. **41:**636-641,
1979.

Weinberg, L.A.: The etiology, diagnosis, and treatment of
TMJ dysfunction-pain syndrome. II. Differential diagnosis, J. Prosthet. Dent. **43:**58-70, 1980.

Weinberg, L.A.: The etiology, diagnosis, and treatment of
TMJ dysfunction-pain syndrome. III. Treatment, J. Prosthet. Dent. **43:**186-196, 1980.

Weinberg, L.A.: The role of stress, occlusion, and condyle
position in TMJ dysfunction-pain, J. Prosthet. Dent.
49:532-545, 1983.

Zarb, G.A., and Speck, J.E.: The treatment of temporomandibular joint dysfunction: a retrospective study, J. Prosthet. Dent. **38:**420-432, 1977.

Zarb, G.A., and Thompson, G.W.: Assessment of clinical
treatment of patients with temporomandibular joint dysfunction, J. Prosthet. Dent. **24:**542-554, 1970.

Tissue changes under dentures

Atwood, D.A.: Some clinical factors related to rate of resorption of residual ridges, J. Prosthet. Dent. **12:**441-450,
1962.

Atwood, D.A.: Postextraction changes in the adult mandible
as illustrated by microradiographs of midsagittal sections
and serial cephalometric roentgenograms, J. Prosthet.
Dent. **13:**810-824, 1963.

Atwood, D.A.: Bone loss of edentulous alveolar ridges, J.
Periodontol. **50**(4 Spec. No.):11-21, 1979.

Baylink, D.J., Wergedal, J.E., Yamamoto, K., and Manzke,
E.: Systemic factors in alveolar bone loss, J. Prosthet.
Dent. **31:**486-505, 1974.

Benson, D., Rothman, R.S., and Sims, T.N.: The effect of a
denture adhesive on the oral mucosa and vertical dimension of complete denture patients, J. South. Calif. Dent.
Assoc. **40:**533-535, 1972.

Berg, H., Carlsson, G.E., and Helkimo, H.: Changes in
shape of anterior parts of upper jaws after extraction of
teeth and prosthetic treatment, J. Prosthet. Dent. **34:**262-
268, 1975.

Bergman, B., Carlsson, G.E., and Ericson, S.: Effect of differences in habitual use of complete dentures on underlying tissues, Scand. J. Dent. Res. **79:**449-460, 1971.

Bodine, R.L.: Oral lesions caused by ill-fitting dentures, J.
Prosthet. Dent. **21:**580-588, 1969.

Danilewicz-Stysiak, Z.: Allergy as a cause of denture sore
mouth, J. Prosthet. Dent. **25:**16-18, 1971.

Enlow, D.H., Bianco, H.J., and Eklund, S.: The remodeling of the edentulous mandible, J. Prosthet. Dent.
36:685-693, 1976.

Kapur, K., and Shklar, G.: The effect of complete dentures
on alveolar mucosa, J. Prosthet. Dent. **13:**1030-1037,
1963.

Kelly, E.: Changes caused by a mandibular removable partial denture opposing a maxillary complete denture, J.
Prosthet. Dent. **27:**140-150, 1972.

Kelsey, C.C.: Alveolar bone resorption under complete
dentures, J. Prosthet. Dent. **25:**152-161, 1971.

Klein, I.: The effect of thyrocalcitonin and growth hormones
on bone metabolism, J. Prosthet. Dent. **33:**365-379,
1975.

Koran, A., Craig, R.G., and Tillitson, E.W.: Coefficient of
friction of prosthetic tooth materials, J. Prosthet. Dent.
27:269-274, 1972.

Lange, K.W., and Lange, K.O.: A new method of measuring
facial geometry, J. Prosthet. Dent. **29:**132-138, 1973.

Likeman, P.R., and Watt, D.M.: Morphological changes in
the maxillary denture bearing area: a follow up 14 to 17
years after tooth extraction, Br. Dent. J. **136:**500-503,
1974.

Michael, C.G., and Barsoum, W.M.: Comparing ridge
resorption with various surgical techniques in immediate
dentures, J. Prosthet. Dent. **35:**142-155, 1976.

Miller, E.L.: Types of inflammation caused by oral prostheses, J. Prosthet. Dent. **30:**380-384, 1973.

Miner, J.F.: The nature of a denture base: a key factor in denture sore mouth, J. Prosthet. Dent. **29**:250-255, 1973.

Ortman, H.R.: Factors of bone resorption of the residual ridge, J. Prosthet. Dent. **12**:429-440, 1962.

Page, M.E.: Systemic and prosthodontic treatment to prevent bone resorption in edentulous patients, J. Prosthet. Dent. **33**:483-488, 1975.

Parkinson, C.F.: Similarities in resorption patterns of maxillary and mandibular ridges, J. Prosthet. Dent. **39**:598-602, 1978.

Pietrokovski, J., and Sorin, S.: Size and shape of the residual ridge in man, Isr. J. Dent. Med. **22**:73-79, 1973.

Ritchie, G.M., Fletcher, A.M., Main, D.M.G., and Prophet, A.S.: The etiology, exfoliative cytology, and treatment of denture stomatitis, J. Prosthet. Dent. **22**:185-200, 1969.

Stungis, T.E., and Fink, J.N.: Hypersensitivity to acrylic resin, J. Prosthet. Dent. **22**:425-428, 1969.

Tautin, F.S.: Should dentures be worn continuously? J. Prosthet. Dent. **39**:372-374, 1978.

Vierheller, P.G., Speiser, W.H., and Al-Rahmani, A.F.: Measuring mandibular vertical bone resorption by radiographic cephalometry, J. Prosthet. Dent. **26**:33-40, 1971.

Watson, I.B.: The effect of complete dentures on oral mucosa, J. Dent. **6**(2):171-178, 1978.

Watt, D.M., and Likeman, P.R.: Morphological changes in the denture bearing area following the extraction of maxillary teeth, Br. Dent. J. **136**:225-235, 1974.

Wendt, D.C.: The degenerative denture ridge—care and treatment, J. Prosthet. Dent. **32**:477-492, 1974.

Wical, K.E., and Swoope, C.C.: Studies of residual ridge resorption. I. Use of panoramic radiographs for evaluation and classification of mandibular resorption, J. Prosthet. dent. **32**:7-12, 1974.

Wical, K.E., and Swoope, C.C.: Studies of ridge resorption. II. The relationship of dietary calcium and phosphorus to residual ridge resorption, J. Prosthet. Dent. **32**:13-22, 1974.

Winter, C.M., Woelfel, J.B., and Igarashi, T.: Five-year changes in the edentulous mandible as determined on oblique cephalometric radiographs, J. Dent. Res. **53**:1455-1467, 1974.

Woelfel, J.B., and Paffenbarger, G.C.: Change in occlusion of complete dentures caused by a pipe habit, J. Am. Dent. Assoc. **66**:478-485, 1963.

Yemm, R.: Stress-induced muscle activity: a possible etiologic factor in denture soreness, J. Prosthet. Dent. **28**:133-140, 1972.

Tongue

Desjardins, R.P.: The tongue as it relates to complete dentures, J. Am. Dent. Assoc. **88**:814-822, 1974.

Farman, A.G., et al.: Central papillary atrophy of the tongue and denture stomatitis, J. Prosthet. Dent. **40**:253-256, 1978.

Farman, A.G., van Wyk, C.W., Dreyer, W.P., Staz, J., Thomas, C.J., Louw, J.H., and Bester, D.: Central papillary atrophy of the tongue and denture stomatitis, J. Prosthet. Dent. **40**:253-256, 1978.

Fish, E.W.: Tongue space in full denture construction, Br. Dent. J. **83**:137-142, 1947.

Herring, H.W., Jr., and Akerly, W.B.: Aid to correct tongue position in the mandibular complete denture, J. Prosthet. Dent. **46**:676-677, 1981.

Kydd, W.L., and Toda, J.M.: Tongue pressures exerted on the hard palate during swallowing, J. Am. Dent. Assoc. **65**:319-330, 1962.

Rinaldi, P., and Sharry, J.: Tongue force and fatigue in adults, J. Prosthet. Dent. **13**:857-865, 1963.

Willigen, J.D. van: Movement of mandibular sulci during normal tongue and mouth movements, J. Prosthet. Dent. **27**:4-15, 1972.

Wright, C.R., et al.: Study of the tongue and its relation to denture stability, J. Am. Dent. Assoc. **39**:269-275, 1949.

Tooth forms and occlusal patterns

Brill, N., Schübeler, S., and Tryde, G.: Influence of occlusal patterns on movements of the mandible, J. Prosthet. Dent. **12**:255-261, 1962.

Buckner, H., and LaVelle, W.E.: Metal backings for denture teeth, J. Prosthet. Dent. **32**:579-581, 1974.

Clough, H.E., Knodle, J.M., Leeper, S.H., Pudwill, M.L., and Taylor, D.T.: A comparison of lingualized occlusion and monoplane occlusion in complete dentures, J. Prosthet. Dent. **50**:176-179, 1983.

Crispin, B.J.: Tissue response to posterior denture base-type pontics, J. Prosthet. Dent. **42**(3):257-261, 1979.

Dickson, R.L.: Mechanical analysis of posterior teeth in centric closure, J. Prosthet. Dent. **27**:358-363, 1972.

Engelmeier, R.L.: Fabricating denture teeth with custom anatomic and nonanatomic metal occlusal surfaces, J. Prosthet. Dent. **43**(3):352-356, 1980.

French, F.A.: Problem of building satisfactory dentures, J. Prosthet. Dent. **4**:769-781, 1954.

Gronas, D.G., and Stout, C.J.: Lineal occlusion concepts for complete dentures, J. Prosthet. Dent. **32**:122-129, 1974.

Gysi, A.: Resiliency and the like in its effect on the facet angulations of artificial teeth, Dent. Dig. **36**:623-628, 1930.

Hall, R.E.: The inverted cusp tooth, J. Am. Dent. Assoc. **18**:2366-2368, 1931.

Hardy, I.R.: Developing a correct occlusal pattern for a maxillary denture, Dent. Dig. **56**:526-530, 1950.

Harrison, A., and Huggett, R.: Measuring the rate of wear of artificial teeth in complete dentures, J. Prosthet. Dent. **33**:615-619, 1975.

Hickey, J.C., Kreider, J.A., Boucher, C.O., and Storz, O.: A method of studying the influence of occlusal schemes on muscular activity, J. Prosthet. Dent. **9**:498-505, 1959.

Kelly, E.: Centric relation, centric occlusion, and posterior tooth forms and arrangement, J. Prosthet. Dent. **37**:5-11, 1977.

Koyama, M., Inaba, S., and Yokoyama, K.: Quest for ideal occlusal patterns for complete dentures, J. Prosthet. Dent. **35**:620-623, 1976.

Lang, B.R., and Thompson, P.M.: The cusp angles of artificial mandibular first molars, J. Prosthet. Dent. **28**:26-35, 1972.

Levin, B.: A review of artificial posterior tooth forms including a preliminary report on a new posterior tooth, J. Prosthet. Dent. **38**:3-15, 1977.

Levy, P.H.: A form and functional concept of occlusion and the maxillomandibular relationship, J. Prosthet. Dent. **33**:149-157, 1975.

Lopuck, S., Smith, J., and Caputo, A.: Photoelastic comparison of posterior denture occlusions, J. Prosthet. Dent. **40**:18-22, 1978.

Miller, C.D., and Feldmann, E.: A device to aid in arrangement of nonanatomic tooth forms, J. Prosthet. Dent. **22**:37-45, 1969.

Moffa, J.P., Jenkins, W.A., and Weaver, R.G.: Silane bonding of porcelain denture teeth to acrylic resin denture bases, J. Prosthet. Dent. **33**:620-627, 1975.

Morrow, R.M., Matvias, F.M., Windeler, A.S., and Fuchs, R.J.: Bonding of plastic teeth to two heat-curing denture base resins, J. Prosthet. Dent. **39**:565-568, 1978.

Moses, C.H.: Human tooth form and arrangement from the anthropologic approach, J. Prosthet. Dent. **9**:197-212, 1959.

Myerson, R.L.: Use of porcelain and plastic teeth in opposing complete dentures, J. Prosthet. Dent. **7**:625-633, 1957.

Raptis, C.N., Powers, J.M., and Fan, P.L.: Frictional behavior and surface failure of acrylic denture teeth, J. Dent. Res. **60**(5):908-913, 1981.

Roraff, A.R.: Arranging artificial teeth according to anatomic landmarks, J. Prosthet. Dent. **38**:120-130, 1977.

Roydhouse, R.H.: Composite teeth—clinical observations, Quintessence Int. **13**(1):33-35, 1982.

Schneider, R.L.: Custom metal occlusal surfaces for acrylic resin denture teeth, J. Prosthet. Dent. **46**(1):98-101, 1981.

Schuyler, C.H.: Full denture service as influenced by tooth forms and materials, J. Prosthet. Dent. **1**:33-37, 1951.

Schuyler, C.H.: Discussion of "Human tooth form and arrangement from the anthropologic approach," J. Prosthet. Dent. **9**:213-214, 1959.

Sears, V.H.: Selection and management of posterior teeth, J. Prosthet. Dent. **7**:723-737, 1957.

Shannon, J.L.: A bilaterally balanced occlusal scheme for patients with arch width and curvature discrepancies, J. Prosthet. Dent. **44**:101-103, 1980.

Smith, D.E.: The simplification of occlusion in complete denture practice: posterior tooth form and clinical procedures, Dent. Clin. North Am. **14**:493-517, 1970.

Thomas, C.J.: The change from plastic to porcelain posterior teeth in full dentures, Diastema **3**:17-28, 1971.

Trapozzano, V.R.: Testing of occlusal patterns on the same denture base, J. Prosthet. Dent. **9**:53-69, 1959.

von Krammer, K.R.: Artificial occlusal surfaces, J. Prosthet. Dent. **30**:391-393, 1973.

von Krammer, K.R.: Modified artificial occlusal surfaces, J. Prosthet. Dent. **30**:394-402, 1973.

Woelfel, J.B., Hickey, J.C., and Allison, M.L.: Effect of posterior tooth form on jaw and denture movement, J. Prosthet. Dent. **12**:922-939, 1962.

Yurkstas, A.A.: The influence of geometric occlusal carvings on the masticatory effectiveness of complete dentures, J. Prosthet. Dent. **13**:452-461, 1963.

Tooth position in relation to basal seat

Davis, D.J.: Simplification of tooth arrangement in complete dentures, Quintessence Dent. Technol. **6**(2):119-122, 1982.

Fredrickson, E.J.: Comparison of posterior teeth, J. Am. Dent. Assoc. **92**:561-564, 1976.

Goyal, B.K., and Bhargava, K.: Arrangement of artificial teeth in abnormal jaw relations: maxillary protrusion and wider upper arch, J. Prosthet. Dent. **32**:107-111, 1974.

McGee, G.F.: Tooth placement and base contour in denture construction, J. Prosthet. Dent. **10**:651-657, 1960.

Murray, C.G.: Re-establishing natural tooth position in the edentulous environment, Aust. Dent. J. **23**(5):415-421, 1978.

Watt, D.M.: Tooth positions on complete dentures, J. Dent. **6**(2):147-160, 1978.

Weinberg, L.A.: Tooth position in relation to the denture base foundation, J. Prosthet. Dent. **8**:398-405, 1958.

Tooth selection (anterior)

Askinas, S.W., and Kaiser, D.A.: Technique for making a customized shade guide, J. Prosthet. Dent. **42**:234-235, 1979.

Barna, G.J., Taylor, J.W., King, G.E., and Pelleu, G.B.: The influence of selected light intensities on color perception within the color range of natural teeth, J. Prosthet. Dent. **46**:450-453, 1981.

Bell, R.A.: The geometric theory of selection of artificial teeth: is it valid? J. Am. Dent. Assoc. **97**(4):637-640, 1978.

Brewer, A.: Selection of denture teeth for esthetics and function, J. Prosthet. Dent. **23**:368-373, 1970.

Clapp, G.W.: How the science of esthetic tooth-form selection was made easy, J. Prosthet. Dent. **5**:596-608, 1955.

Cozza, V.J.: Comparison of the angle of taper of maxillary central incisors, maxillary dental arch, and skull, J. Prosthet. Dent. **24**:133-136, 1970.

Dummett, C.O., Sakumura, J.S., and Barens, G.: The relationship of facial skin complexion to oral mucosa pigmentation and tooth color, J. Prosthet. Dent. **43**:392-396, 1980.

Ela, L.M., and Razek, M.K.: A positive guide to the selection of anterior teeth, Egypt. Dent. J. **18**:281-290, 1972.

Kern, B.K.: Anthropometric parameters of tooth selection, J. Prosthet. Dent. **17**:431-437, 1967.

Mavroskoufis, F., and Ritchie, G.M.: Nasal width and incisive papilla as guides for the selection and arrangement of maxillary anterior teeth, J. Prosthet. Dent. **45**:592-597, 1981.

Mavroskoufis, F., and Ritchie, G.M.: The face-form as a guide for the selection of maxillary central incisors, J. Prosthet. Dent. **43**:501-505, 1980.

Mavroskoufis, F., and Ritchie, G.M.: Variations in size and form between left and right maxillary central incisor teeth, J. Prosthet. Dent. **43**:254-257, 1980.

Payne, S.H.: Construction of custom denture teeth, Dent. Clin. North Am. 19:333-346, 1975.

Saleski, C.G.: Color, light, and shade matching, J. Prosthet. Dent. 27:263-268, 1972.

Scandrett, F.R., Kerber, P.E., and Umrigar, Z.R.: A clinical evaluation of techniques to determine the combined width of the maxillary anterior teeth and the maxillary central incisor, J. Prosthet. Dent. 48:15-22, 1982.

Stephens, A.P.: The selection and setting-up of anterior teeth, J. Irish Dent. Assoc. 15:78-80, 1969.

Van Victor, A.: The mold guide cast—its significance in denture esthetics, J. Prosthet. Dent. 13:406, 415, 1963.

Wehner, P.J., Hickey, J.C., and Boucher, C.O.: Selection of artificial teeth, J. Prosthet. Dent. 18:222-232, 1967.

Tooth-supported complete dentures

Benington, I.C.: A method of using resilient anchorages in complete denture construction, J. Dent. 1:171-172, 1973.

Cozza, V.J.: A simple technique for tooth supported complete dentures, J. Colo. Dent. Assoc. 48:28-32, 1970.

Crum, R.J., and Rooney, G.E.: Alveolar bone loss in overdentures: a 5-year study, J. Prosthet. Dent. 40:610-613, 1978.

Davis, R.K., Renner, R.P., Antos, E.W., Schlissel, E.R., and Baer, P.N.: A two-year longitudinal study of the periodontal health status of overdenture patients, J. Prosthet. Dent. 45:358-363, 1981.

Dodge, C.A.: Prevention of complete denture problems by use of "overdentures," J. Prosthet. Dent. 30:403-411, 1973.

Duckmanton, N.A.: The role of the overlay denture in the prevention of mandibular ridge atrophy, Aust. Dent. J. 23(4):332-343, 1978.

Essenfeld, G.: The immediate overdenture, Dent. Surv. 54(8):18-22, 1978.

Feldstein, S., and Teitel, M.: The immediate overdenture, J. Am. Dent. Assoc. 93:775-778, 1976.

Fenton, A.H.: Interim overdentures, J. Prosthet. Dent. 36:4-12, 1976.

Fenton, A.H., Zarb, G.A., and MacKay, H.F.: Overdenture oversights, Dent. Clin. North Am. 23(1):117-130, 1979.

Foerth, D., and Renner, R.: An alternative to conventional mandibular overdenture service, Dent. Surv. 53(3):51-55, 1977.

Frantz, W.R.: The use of natural teeth in overlay dentures, J. Prosthet. Dent. 34:135-140, 1975.

Garver, D.G., Fenster, R.K., and Connole, P.W.: Vital root retention in humans: an interim report, J. Prosthet. Dent. 41:255-257, 1979.

Garver, D.G., and Muir, T.E.: The retention of vital submucosal roots under immediate dentures: a surgical procedure, J. Prosthet. Dent. 50:753-756, 1983.

Ghalichebaf, M., and Graser, G.N.: The cosmetic overdenture, J. Prosthet. Dent. 42:348-350, 1979.

Goerig, A.C.: Immediate overdenture, J. Am. Dent. Assoc. 88:356-359, 1974.

Graser, G.N., and Caton, J.G.: Influence of overdenture abutment tooth contour on the periodontium: a preliminary report, J. Prosthet. Dent. 49:173-177, 1983.

Guyer, S.E.: Selectively retained vital roots for partial support of overdentures: a patient report, J. Prosthet. Dent. 33:258-263, 1975.

Helft, M., Kaufman, C., and Cardash, H.S.: The overdenture: a concept, Isr. J. Dent. Med. 27(2):5-7, 5-6, 1978.

Johansson, J.: Overlay removable prostheses, J. Irish Dent. Assoc. 20:99-104, 1974.

Kabcenell, J.L.: Tooth-supported complete dentures, J. Prosthet. Dent. 26:251-257, 1971.

Kay, W.D., and Abes, M.S.: Sensory perception in overdenture patients, J. Prosthet. Dent. 35:615-619, 1976.

Kotwal, K.R.: Outline of standards for evaluating patients for overdentures, J. Prosthet. Dent. 37:141-146, 1977.

Lambert, P.M., Skerl, R.F., and Campana, H.A.: Free autogenous graft coverage of vital retained roots, J. Prosthet. Dent. 50:611-617, 1983.

Larkin, J.D.: Tooth supported complete dentures: twenty-seventh year of observation, Tex. Dent. J. 91:26-30, 1973.

Levin, A.C., Shifman, A., and Lepley, J.B.: Preservation of occlusal vertical dimension in overdentures, J. Am. Dent. Assoc. 97(5):838-839, 1978.

Loiselle, R.J., Crum, R.J., Rooney, G.E., Jr., and Stuever, C.H., Jr.: The physiologic basis for the overlay denture, J. Prosthet. Dent. 28:4-12, 1972.

Lord, J.L., and Teel, S.: The overdenture: patient selection, use of copings, and follow-up evaluation, J. Prosthet. Dent. 32:41-51, 1974.

Marquardt, G.L.: Dolder bar joint mandibular overdenture: a technique for nonparallel abutment teeth, J. Prosthet. Dent. 36:101-111, 1976.

Mascola, R.F.: The root-retained complete denture, J. Am. Dent. Assoc. 92:586-587, 1976.

Maurer, C.R.: Complete denture construction on an alveolar process containing endodontically treated roots, J. Prosthet. Dent. 30:756-758, 1973.

Mensor, M.C., Jr.: Attachment fixation of the overdenture, II. J. Prosthet. Dent. 39:16-20, 1978.

Morrow, R.M., et al.: Tooth-supported complete dentures: description and clinical evaluation of a simplified technique, J. Prosthet. Dent. 22:414-424, 1969.

Osburn, R.C.: Preservation of the alveolar ridge: a simplified technique for retaining teeth beneath removable appliances, J. Indiana State Dent. Assoc. 53:8-11, 1974.

Pardo, G.I., and Renner, R.P.: The telescoped overdenture: advantages and limitations, J. Am. Dent. Assoc. 101(6):932-934, 1980.

Perel, M.L.: Telescope dentures, J. Prosthet. Dent. 29:151-156, 1973.

Quinlivan, J.T.: An attachment for overlay dentures, J. Prosthet. Dent. 32:256-261, 1974.

Reitz, P.V., Weiner, M.G., and Levin, B.: An overdenture survey: preliminary report, J. Prosthet. Dent. 37:246-258, 1977.

Reitz, P.V., Weiner, M.G., and Levin, B.: An overdenture survey: second report, J. Prosthet. Dent. 43:457-462, 1980.

Robbins, J.W.: Success of overdentures and prevention of failure, J. Am. Dent. Assoc. 100(6):858-862, 1980.

Schweitzer, J.M., Schweitzer, R.D., and Schweitzer, J.: The telescoped complete denture; a research report at the clinical level, J. Prosthet. Dent. 26:357-372, 1971.

Thayer, H.H., and Caputo, A.A.: Effects of overdentures upon remaining oral structures, J. Prosthet. Dent. 37:374-381, 1977.

Thayer, H.H., and Caputo, A.A.: Photoelastic stress analysis of overdenture attachments, J. Prosthet. Dent. 43:611-617, 1980.

Thomas, C.J., and Nutt, G.M.: The in vitro fungicidal properties of Visco-Gel, alone and combined with nystatin and amphotericin B, J. Oral Rehabil. 5(2):167-172, 1978.

Toolson, L.B., and Smith, D.E.: A five-year longitudinal study of patients treated with overdentures, J. Prosthet. Dent. 49:749-756, 1983.

Warren, A.B., and Caputo, A.A.: Load transfer to alveolar bone as influenced by abutment designs for tooth-supported dentures, J. Prosthet. Dent. 33:137-148, 1975.

Welker, W.A., and Kramer, D.C.: Waxing tooth copings for overdentures, J. Prosthet. Dent. 32:668-671, 1974.

Welker, W.A., Jividen, G.J., and Kramer, D.C.: Preventive prosthodontics—mucosal coverage of roots, J. Prosthet. Dent. 40:619-621, 1978.

White, J.T.: Abutment stress in overdentures, J. Prosthet. Dent. 40:13-17, 1978.

Vertical maxillomandibular relations

Boos, R.H.: Vertical, centric and functional dimensions recorded by gnathodynamics, J. Am. Dent. Assoc. 59:682-689, 1959.

Boucher, L.J., Zwemer, T.J., and Pflughoeft, F.: Can biting force be used as a criterion for registering vertical dimension? J. Prosthet. Dent. 9:594-599, 1959.

Brill, N., Fujii, H., Stoltze, K., et al.: Dynamic and static recordings of the comfortable zone, J. Oral Rehabil. 5(2):145-150, 1978.

Broekhuijsen, M.L., and van Willigen, J.D.: The precision of measurement and the stability of the preferred vertical dimension of occlusion in man, Arch. Oral Biol. 27(6):487-491, 1982.

Cohen, B., and Kamen, A.: Regression equation for lower dentures, J. Dent. Res. 53:147, 1974.

Dikshit, J.V., and Mirza, F.D.: Muscle relaxant and rest position—a cephalometric study, J. Prosthet. Dent. 42:579-587, 1979.

Dukes, B.S., Fields, H., and Olson, J.W.: A laboratory study of changes in vertical dimension using acrylic resin and porcelain teeth, J. Am. Dent. Assoc. 106:842-843, 1983.

Feldman, S., Leupold, R.J., and Staling, L.M.: Rest vertical dimension determined by electromyography with biofeedback as compared to conventional methods, J. Prosthet. Dent. 40:216-219, 1978.

Gamon, J.A., and Wright, S.M.: Perception of vertical dimension, J. Oral Rehabil. 9(4):307-316, 1982.

Gattozzi, J.G., Nicol, B.R., Somes, G.W., and Ellinger, C.W.: Variations in mandibular rest positions with and without dentures in place, J. Prosthet. Dent. 36:159-163, 1976.

Harris, H.L.: Effect of loss of vertical dimension of anatomic structures of the head and neck, J. Am. Dent. Assoc. & Dent. Cosmos 25:175-193, 1938.

Heath, M.R.: The contact-relax method. To establish the 'rest position' and assess the inter-occlusal distance, Br. Dent. J. 149(6):181-182, 1980.

Joniot, B.: Physiologic mandibular resting posture, J. Prosthet. Dent. 31:4-9, 1974.

Kleinman, A.M., and Sheppard, I.M.: A direct procedure for indicating mandibular rest position, J. Prosthet. Dent. 28:19-20, 1972.

Kleinman, A.M., and Sheppard, I.M.: Mandibular rest levels with and without dentures in place in edentulous and complete denture–wearing subjects, J. Prosthet. Dent. 28:478-484, 1972.

Mackenna, B.R., and Turker, K.S.: Jaw separation and maximum incising force, J. Prosthet. Dent. 49:726-730, 1983.

McLean, L.F., Brenman, H.S., and Friedman, M.G.: Effects of changing body position on dental occlusion, J. Dent. Res. 52:1041-1045, 1973.

McNamara, J.A., Jr.: Electromyography of the mandibular postural position in the rhesus monkey (*Macaca mulatta*), J. Dent. Res. 53:945, 1974.

Owen, W.D., and Douglas, J.R.: Near or full occlusal vertical dimension increase of severely reduced interarch distance in complete dentures, J. Prosthet. Dent. 26:134-138, 1971.

Pound, E.: The vertical dimension of speech: the pilot of occlusion, J. Calif. Dent. Assoc. 6(2):42-47, 1978.

Provost, W.A., and Towle, H.J.: Determination of physiologic rest position by electronic measurement, J. Prosthet. Dent. 27:377-380, 1972.

Razek, M.K.A., and Abdalla, F.: Two-dimensional study of the neutral zone at different occlusal vertical heights, J. Prosthet. Dent. 46:484-489, 1981.

Rugh, J.D., and Drago, C.J.: Vertical dimension: a study of clinical rest position and jaw muscle activity, J. Prosthet. Dent. 45:670-675, 1981.

Sabet, E.: Critical analysis of vertical dimension in complete denture prosthodontics, Egypt. Dent. J. 16:135-144, 1970.

Sabet, E.M., and Abdalla, F.: A study on the effect of different impression techniques on constancy of occlusal vertical dimension, Egypt. Dent. J. 24(1):79-88, 1978.

Schweitzer, J.M.: Open bite from the prosthetic point of view, Dent. Clin. North Am. 1:269-283, 1957.

Sheppard, I.M., and Sheppard, S.M.: Vertical dimension measurements, J. Prosthet. Dent. 34:269-277, 1975.

Sheppard, I.M., and Sheppard, S.M.: The relationship of vertical dimension to atypical swallowing with complete dentures, J. Prosthet. Dent. 38:249-253, 1977.

Shirinian, G.H., and Strem, B.E.: Interocclusal distance: a comparison between American Caucasians and Negroes, J. Prosthet. Dent. 37:394-396, 1977.

Silverman, M.M.: The comparative accuracy of the closest-speaking-space and the freeway space in measuring vertical dimension, J. Acad. Gen. Dent. 22:34-36, 1974.

Singh, B.J.: A new method of recording vertical dimension of occlusion in complete denture prosthodontics, J. Indian Dent. Assoc. **42**:304-306, 1970.

Storey, A.T.: Physiology of a changing vertical dimension, J. Prosthet. Dent. **12**:912-921, 1962.

Timmer, L.H.: A reproducible method for determining the vertical dimension of occlusion, J. Prosthet. Dent. **22**:621-630, 1969.

Toolson, L.B., and Smith, D.E.: Clinical measurement and evaluation of vertical dimension, J. Prosthet. Dent. **47**:236-241, 1982.

Tryde, G., et al.: The fallacy of facial measurements of occlusal height in edentulous subjects, J. Oral Rehabil. **3**:353-358, 1976.

Tueller, V.M.: The relationship between the vertical dimension of occlusion and forces generated by closing muscles of mastication, J. Prosthet. Dent. **22**:284-288, 1969.

Turrell, A.J.W.: Clinical assessment of vertical dimension, J. Prosthet. Dent. **28**:238-246, 1972.

van Willigen, J.D., de Vos, A.L., and Broekhuijsen, M.L.: Psychophysical investigations of the preferred vertical dimension of occlusion in edentulous patients, J. Prosthet. Dent. **35**:259-266, 1976.

Wagner, A.G.: Comparison of four methods to determine rest position of the mandible, J. Prosthet. Dent. **25**:506-514, 1971.

Weinberg, L.A.: Vertical dimension: a research and clinical analysis, J. Prosthet. Dent. **47**:290-302, 1982.

Willigen, J.D., van de Vos, A.D., and Broekhuijsen, M.L.: Some psychophysical experiments into the vertical dimension of occlusion of edentulous subjects, Arch. Int. Physiol. Biochem. **82**:395-399, 1974.

Yemm, R., and Berry, D.C.: Passive control in mandibular rest position, J. Prosthet. Dent. **22**:30-36, 1969.

Yemm, R., El-Sharkawy, M., and Stephens, C.D.: Measurement of lip posture and interaction between lip posture and resting face height, J. Oral Rehabil. **5**(4):391-402, 1978.

Index